Diagnostic Techniques in Hematological Malignancies

Diagnostic Techniques in Hematological Malignancies

Editor

Wendy N. Erber
Addenbrooke's Hospital and University of Cambridge, Cambridge, UK

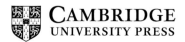

CAMBRIDGE UNIVERSITY PRESS
Cambridge, New York, Melbourne, Madrid, Cape Town, Singapore,
São Paulo, Delhi, Dubai, Tokyo, Mexico City

Cambridge University Press
The Edinburgh Building, Cambridge CB2 8RU, UK

Published in the the United States of America by Cambridge University Press,
New York

www.cambridge.org
Information on this title: www.cambridge.org/9780521111218

First published 2010

Printed in the United Kingdom at the University Press, Cambridge

A catalog record for this publication is available from the British Library

Library of Congress Cataloging in Publication data
Diagnostic techniques in hematological malignancies / editor, Wendy N. Erber.
    p. ; cm.
Includes bibliographical references and index.
ISBN 978-0-521-11121-8 (hardback)
1. Myeloproliferative disorders – Diagnosis.   2. Leukemia – Diagnosis.   3. Blood – Diseases – Diagnosis.
4. Blood – Analysis.   I. Erber, Wendy N., 1957–
[DNLM: 1. Hematologic Neoplasms – diagnosis. WH 525]
RC645.75.D53   2010
616.99′419–dc22

2010027648

ISBN 978-0-521-11121-8 Hardback

To Gary

For his enduring patience, encouragement, inspiration, support and advice.

Contents

Contributors

Philip A. Beer
Department of Haematology, University of Cambridge and Addenbrooke's Hospital, Cambridge, UK

Dario Campana
Departments of Oncology and Pathology, St. Jude Children's Research Hospital, and Department of Pediatrics, University of Tennessee Health Science Center, College of Medicine, Memphis, TN, USA

Elaine Coustan-Smith
Department of Oncology, St. Jude Children's Research Hospital, Memphis, TN, USA

Ahmet Dogan
Department of Laboratory Medicine and Pathology, Mayo Clinic, Rochester, MN, USA

Wendy N. Erber
Haematology Department, Addenbrooke's Hospital and University of Cambridge, Cambridge, UK

Pierre Fenaux
Service d'hématologie, Hôpital Avicenne (Assistance Publique – Hôpitaux de Paris), Paris 13 Université, Bobigny France and INSERM Unit 848, Institut Gustave Roussy, Villejuif France

Rafael Fonseca
Cancer Center, Mayo Clinic Arizona, Scottsdale, AZ, USA

Kathryn Foucar
Department of Pathology, University of New Mexico Health Sciences Center, and TriCore Reference Laboratories, Albuquerque, NM, USA

Anthony R. Green
Department of Haematology, University of Cambridge and Addenbrooke's Hospital, Cambridge, UK

David Grimwade
Department of Medical and Molecular Genetics, King's College, London, UK

Emma J. Gudgin
Department of Haematology, University of Cambridge, Cambridge, UK

Christine J. Harrison
Leukaemia Research Cytogenetics Group, Northern Institute for Cancer Research, Newcastle University, Newcastle upon Tyne, UK

Jennifer Herrick
Department of Laboratory Medicine and Pathology, Mayo Clinic, Rochester, MN, USA

Brian Huntly
Department of Haematology, University of Cambridge, Cambridge, UK

Raphael Itzykson
Service d'hématologie, Hôpital Avicenne (Assistance Publique – Hôpitaux de Paris), Paris 13 Université, Bobigny France and INSERM Unit 1009, Institut Gustave Roussy, Villejuif France

Michael J. Keating
Leukemia Department, University of Texas MD Anderson Cancer Center, Houston, TX, USA

Ken Mills
Centre for Cancer Research and Cell Biology (CCRCB), School of Medicine, Queen's University Belfast, Belfast, UK

Kaaren K. Reichard
Department of Pathology, University of New
Mexico Health Sciences Center, and TriCore
Reference Laboratories, Albuquerque, NM, USA

Hervé Roudot
Laboratoire d'hématologie, Hôpital Avicenne
(Assistance Publique – Hôpitaux de Paris),
Paris 13 Université, France

Claire Schwab
Leukaemia Research Cytogenetics Group, Northern
Institute for Cancer Research, Newcastle University,
Newcastle upon Tyne, UK

Mike A. Scott
Haematology Department, Addenbrooke's Hospital,
Cambridge, UK

Maryalice Stetler-Stevenson
Laboratory of Pathology, Center for Cancer Research,
National Cancer Institute, National Institutes of
Health, Bethesda, MD, USA

Constantine S. Tam
Hematology Department, St Vincent's Hospital,
Melbourne, Victoria, Australia

Riccardo Valdez
Department of Laboratory Medicine
and Pathology, Mayo Clinic Arizona, Scottsdale,
AZ, USA

Constance M. Yuan
Laboratory of Pathology, Center for Cancer Research,
National Cancer Institute, National Institutes of
Health, Bethesda, MD, USA

Preface

The diagnosis of hematological malignancies is complex, expensive and evolving rapidly. There is a myriad of tests available and these are of increasing importance in the diagnosis and ongoing assessment of hematological malignancies. Optimal test utilization requires knowledge of the many individual diseases and the range of tests available to investigate them. Morphology, cell phenotyping, cytogenetics and molecular genetics are all essential and these must be used in a structured approach with the results integrated to give an overall diagnosis. To use these tests appropriately requires an understanding of the principles and roles of each of these test types and how they supplement traditional morphological assessment. As director of a large hemato-oncology diagnostic service and supervisor of hematologists-in-training, I have seen the difficulties trainees have experienced, and the time, effort and resources wasted on poorly focused testing due to lack of knowledge in these areas. As a consequence, and in the absence of texts on this subject, I was motivated to write a book to explain the diagnostic techniques and how they should optimally be applied to hematological malignancies.

This multi-authored book by an international panel of experts gives a state-of-the-art account of the principles and applications of the laboratory investigations available in the analysis of hematological malignancies in blood and bone marrow. The first five chapters provide a succinct review of the diagnostic techniques covering morphology, immunocytochemistry, flow cytometry, cytogenetics and molecular genetics. For each the methodological principles, data interpretation and limitations are provided, and the role of the techniques illustrated by clinical examples. These are followed by a chapter describing how the results of these should be integrated to give an overall interpretation of the disorder and thereby add value to the individual results for the clinician. The second part of the book is devoted to the malignancies. Recognized clinical leaders have written comprehensive chapters on appropriate test utilization in each of the diseases or group of

disorders. For each, after a brief introduction, there is a structured account of how to best apply the range of laboratory investigations throughout the course of the disease. Although emphasis is on testing at diagnosis and for staging, additional evolving roles are highlighted. These include the use of the diagnostic techniques to identify prognostic markers, detect potential therapeutic targets, assess persistent low-level disease following therapy and disease monitoring for pending relapse. It is these additional roles that are becoming increasingly important as we move to greater use of targeted therapies and personalized medicine with curative intent.

This book is intended for hematologists- and pathologists-in-training, qualified hematologists and clinical scientists who wish to acquire a background to diagnostic testing in the hematological malignancies. It provides a useful guide to a rational structured (and hence economical) approach to the laboratory assessment of hematological malignancies. The book includes many high quality color illustrations and diagrams to demonstrate the key features and these should be useful resources for even experienced hematologists.

Due to the pace of change and the vast amount of information concerning these complex diseases, this book required a panel of experts to provide the most complete and up-to-date account of the techniques and diseases. I was delighted that each of the authors accepted the invitation to contribute with enthusiasm for the project. I am indebted to them and thank them most sincerely for the enormous amount of time, effort and expertise they have given in writing their excellent contributions, each with their own individual style. Without the authors' devotion this book would not have eventuated.

I also thank my colleagues in the Haemato-Oncology Diagnostic Service in the Haematology Department at Addenbrooke's Hospital, Cambridge for their assistance in preparing the book. Specific mention and thanks to Drs Lisa Cooke and Carolyn Grove for their constructive comments from the perspective of a hematology trainee, to Dr Anthony Bench, Bridget Manasse and Lisa Happerfield for their scientific contributions and Hannah Roberts for her secretarial support. I am most grateful to Cambridge University Press for instigating this project. Special and sincere thanks to Nicholas Dunton for his guidance and expertise in coordinating the project and keeping me and the book on track. Thanks also to Mark Boyd, Abigail Jones, and Joanna Souter for their help with various phases of this production.

This book should be a useful guide to a structured systematic approach to the analysis of hematological malignancies. I intend to use it myself and hope it also meets the needs of others.

Morphology

Wendy N. Erber

The diagnosis of hematological malignancies has benefited enormously from recent scientific advances. In spite of this, morphology remains critically important and is the key front-line diagnostic technique which must not be overlooked. The light microscopy appearances may be diagnostic but, in addition, they are the foundation upon which decisions about further scientific assessment are based. In the modern era that utilizes a multi-parameter approach to disease classification, morphology is the screening test that determines the further investigations necessary [1]. This opening chapter describes the principles of morphological assessment of the blood and bone marrow in the diagnosis, staging and monitoring of hematological malignancies. It will guide the reader through the process of blood and bone marrow microscopy and demonstrate how morphology alone can often give an indication of the underlying diagnosis. The chapter is not intended as a textbook or atlas of hematological neoplasms; for this, the reader is referred to one of numerous excellent monographs and atlases [2–5].

Peripheral blood

Abnormalities on a blood count, be they quantitative or qualitative, may be the first indication of a hematological malignancy and will generally lead to a blood film being examined [6]. Whereas currently this is most commonly performed by light microscopy, automated image capture methods are increasingly being used [7–8]. It is recommended for the assessment of neoplastic cells that morphological review be performed manually as a well-trained pair of eyes is more discriminating than a programmed computer. The abnormalities on the blood film may be diagnostic, or lead to a provisional diagnosis.

Blood film examination requires a well-prepared smear made from a fresh blood sample (i.e. < 2 hours in anticoagulant). The smear must be air-dried, fixed and stained with a Romanowsky stain (e.g. May–Grünwald Giemsa). A cover-slip, rather than oil, should be placed over the entire smear using mounting medium to provide permanent protection without interfering with the optics. Misidentification of significant and potentially diagnostic features can occur as a result of prolonged blood storage which causes EDTA-artefact, storage at the wrong temperature, poorly spread smears and poor quality stain.

The smear should be viewed macroscopically for its quality and staining appearances. Even without magnification abnormal color, which may indicate the presence of proteinemia, or pattern, due to red cell agglutination, may be evident. Microscopy should then commence with systematic scanning of the entire smear using a low-power (×10) objective, followed by ×20 or ×25 objectives to assess:

1. Background appearance of the blood, e.g. protein stain, abnormal agglutinates.
2. Erythrocyte distribution pattern, especially rouleaux or agglutination.
3. For a manual assessment of the leukocyte count to detect discrepancies with the automated blood count.
4. Leukocyte distribution and presence of abnormal cells.

Scanning at this low magnification can guide the microscopist to specific cells which appear abnormal, or areas of the film with an abnormal cellular distribution and which require more detailed review at higher magnification. This is crucial to avoid missing significant abnormal cells which may be "hidden" at

---

Diagnostic Techniques in Hematological Malignancies, ed. Wendy N. Erber. Published by Cambridge University Press.
© Cambridge University Press 2010.

the edge or in the tail of the film and otherwise go undetected; this includes large abnormal cells such as large cell lymphoma, acute promyelocytic leukemia and plasma cell myeloma. All cell types should subsequently be assessed with a ×40 or ×50 objective. Higher magnification review with oil immersion (×60–×100 objective) may be required for more detailed cellular analysis and specifically to assess intracellular (nuclear and cytoplasmic) detail.

This systematic and careful approach to blood film review, from low to high magnification, can be performed quickly and lead to the identification of specific abnormal cells which may be diagnostic of a malignancy. Other accompanying abnormalities may also be detected in the erythrocytes, leukocytes or platelets, be they in abnormal number, have abnormal morphology or be present in an abnormal pattern. These accompanying bystander features, or the "*company the cells keep*", can be extremely helpful in identifying an underlying abnormality and generating a provisional diagnosis. Some of the relevant accompanying features and the hematological malignancies with which they are associated are listed in Table 1.1. For some disorders, it may be a combination of these that may lead to a provisional diagnosis.

Blood film features of hematological malignancies

A general description of the most common blood film morphological abnormalities that are seen in hematological malignancies at diagnosis, including the "accompanying cells", will be presented. Details of the specific morphological appearances of the cells in individual neoplastic disorders are given in Chapters 7–15 in Section 2.

Cytopenias and pancytopenia

Cytopenias, which may be isolated, bi cytopenia or pancytopenia, occur as a consequence of reduced or ineffective hematopoiesis, increased peripheral cell destruction or splenic sequestration. There are some blood film abnormalities which occur in the presence of cytopenias that may give an indication of the underlying bone marrow pathology or diagnosis. These are listed below and will be discussed in more detail in subsequent sections:

1. Leukoerythroblastic blood film, i.e. the presence of erythroid and leukocyte precursors in the blood.

2. Leukocyte morphological abnormalities, e.g. blast cells, dysplastic neutrophils, abnormal lymphoid cells.
3. Red cell morphology, e.g. anisocytosis, rouleaux, tear-drop poikilocytes.
4. Platelet morphology, e.g. large or hypogranular platelets.

Leukoerythroblastic blood film

A leukoerythroblastic blood film can be seen with bone marrow infiltration (due to hematological malignancy or a metastatic infiltrate) or fibrosis, severe sepsis, cytokine administration and prolonged hypoxia. The presence of morphologically abnormal leukocytes, red cells or platelets may give an indication of the underlying diagnosis (e.g. myelofibrosis). If the etiology of the leukoerythroblastic film is not known or evident from the blood film, a bone marrow examination is indicated.

Leukocyte morphology

Abnormal leukocyte number and morphology are common at the initial diagnosis of a hematological malignancy. Close assessment of the following cellular features is therefore required:

1. Cell count.
2. Cell size and shape.
3. Nuclear : cytoplasmic ratio.
4. Nuclear size, shape, location and chromatin maturity.
5. Presence of nucleoli, their number, size and location.
6. Cytoplasmic shape, color, presence of inclusions or vacuoles.
7. Are there abnormal cells present? Are they monomorphic or pleomorphic?
8. The "*company the cells keep*".

Following is a description of the more common leukocyte abnormalities seen in blood films and which are features of hematological malignancies.

Neutrophils: Neutrophilia, neutropenia and qualitative neutrophil morphological abnormalities can all be seen as peripheral blood manifestations of hematological malignancies. Together with the accompanying blood film abnormalities, the neutrophil count and morphology may give an indication of the diagnosis.

Neutrophilia: Although neutrophilia is most commonly secondary to infection, inflammation,

Table 1.1. The "*company the cells keep*": blood film features associated with hematological malignancies.

Cell type	Blood film feature	Pathophysiology	Hematological malignancy
All	Pancytopenia	Bone marrow failure Bone marrow infiltration	Any hematological malignancy Metastatic bone marrow infiltrate
	Leukoerythroblastic blood film	Bone marrow infiltration	Any hematological malignancy Metastatic bone marrow infiltrate
		Marrow fibrosis	Primary myelofibrosis Metastatic bone marrow infiltrate
Red cells	Anisocytosis and/or poikilocytes	Dyserythropoiesis	Myelodysplastic syndromes Erythroleukemia
	Macrocytes	Dyserythropoiesis	Myelodysplastic syndromes
	Microcytes	Iron deficient erythropoiesis	Myeloproliferative neoplasms with iron deficiency
	Dimorphic red cells	Dyserythropoiesis	Myelodysplastic syndromes or Myelodysplastic/Myeloproliferative neoplasm with ring sideroblasts
	Dysplastic normoblasts	Dyserythropoiesis	Myelodysplastic syndromes Acute myeloid leukemia with myelodysplasia-related changes Erythroleukemia
	Tear-drop poikilocytes	Marrow fibrosis	Primary myelofibrosis Marrow fibrosis secondary to other hematological malignancies Metastatic bone marrow infiltrate
	Spherocytes	Immune hemolysis	Mature B-cell neoplasms, especially chronic lymphocytic leukemia
	Red cell agglutination	Cold hemagglutinins	Mature B-cell neoplasms
	Rouleaux	Proteinemia	Plasma cell myeloma Lymphoplasmacytic lymphoma/Waldenström macroglobulinemia
	Erythrocytosis	Erythroid hyperplasia	Polycythemia vera
Leukocytes	Dysplastic neutrophils	Dysgranulopoiesis	Myelodysplastic syndromes Myelodysplastic/Myeloproliferative neoplasms Acute myeloid leukemia
	Dysplastic promyelocytes	Leukemic promyelocytes	Acute promyelocytic leukemia
	Dysplastic monocytes	Abnormal monocytic differentiation	Myelodysplastic/Myeloproliferative neoplasms Acute myeloid leukemia (with monocytoid differentiation)
	Neutrophilia	Granulocytic hyperplasia	Myeloproliferative neoplasms Hodgkin lymphoma
	Eosinophilia	Eosinophilic hyperplasia	Myeloid neoplasms Mature B- or T-cell neoplasm Hodgkin lymphoma
	Basophilia	Basophilic hyperplasia	Myeloproliferative neoplasms, especially chronic myelogenous leukemia
	Monocytopenia	Marrow infiltration	Hairy cell leukemia
Platelets	Thrombocytosis	Megakaryocytic hyperplasia, normal or dysplastic	Myeloproliferative neoplasms Refractory anemia with ring sideroblasts associated with marked thrombocytosis Myelodysplastic syndrome associated with isolated del(5q)
	Thrombocytopenia	Reduced megakaryopoiesis, normal morphology	Any hematological malignancy
		Reduced megakaryopoiesis, dysplastic morphology	Myelodysplastic syndromes Primary myelofibrosis
	Platelet anisocytosis, hypogranular and/or agranular platelets	Megakaryocyte dysplasia	Myeloproliferative neoplasms Myelodysplastic syndromes Myelodysplastic/Myeloproliferative neoplasms
	Megakaryocyte nuclei or micromegakaryocytes	Megakaryocytic proliferation and/or dysplasia	Myeloproliferative neoplasms Myelodysplastic syndromes Myelodysplastic/Myeloproliferative neoplasms

hemorrhage or drugs, it can also be seen in neoplastic disorders, particularly those of myeloid origin. The extent of the neutrophilia, the presence of dysplasia, left shift or toxic granulation, and other blood count and film abnormalities (e.g. monocytosis, basophilia) can assist in distinguishing between entities (Figures 1.1 and 1.2). A mild reactive neutrophilia can be seen as part of the acute phase response in Hodgkin lymphoma and a neutrophilia of $50–100 \times 10^9$/L ("leukemoid reaction") in response to a non-hematopoietic malignancy (e.g. carcinoma of the lung; mesothelioma). Figure 1.1 gives an outline of an approach to use in the morphological assessment of a neutrophilia.

Neutropenia: At presentation neutropenia may be isolated, occur in conjunction with anemia or thrombocytopenia, or be part of a pancytopenia. The causes of neutropenia include:

1. Failure or suppression of granulopoiesis due to bone marrow failure, fibrosis or infiltration, drug therapy and toxins.
2. Abnormal granulopoiesis, i.e. myelodysplasia.

3. Consumption or destruction of mature neutrophils or their precursors from immune mechanisms as can occur in mature B-cell, T-cell or natural killer cell neoplasms or hypersplenism.

Hematological malignancies of both myeloid and lymphoid origin may present with neutropenia as a result of the above-mentioned mechanisms. It is therefore important that both neutrophil and lymphocyte morphology be evaluated to determine whether there are any hallmark features in any leukocytes that may give a guide to the underlying disorder. Figure 1.3 shows an approach to the morphological assessment of neutropenia utilizing the neutrophil morphology, presence of dysplasia, blast cells and other features which may lead to a provisional diagnosis.

Dysplastic neutrophils: The presence of circulating dysplastic neutrophils indicates marrow dysgranulopoiesis. The dysplastic features may be subtle and their detection requires careful review of excellent quality well-stained blood smears. Defining features of neutrophil dysplasia include (Figure 1.2b):

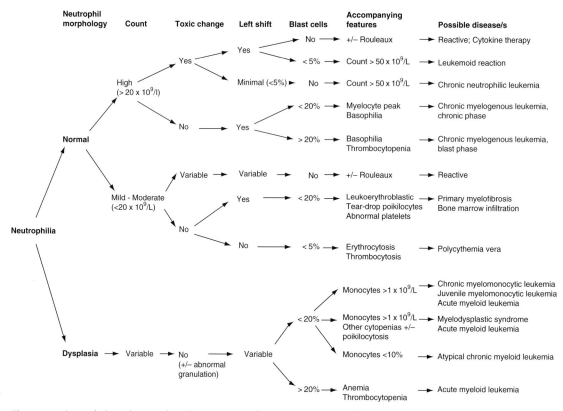

Figure 1.1. A morphological approach to the assessment of the cause of neutrophilia.

a

b

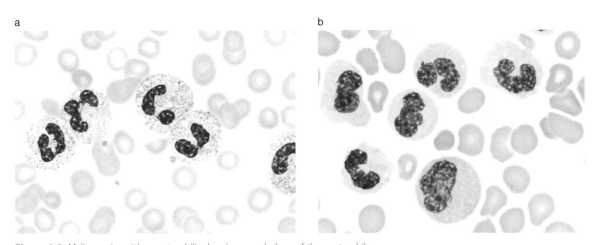

Figure 1.2. Malignancies with a neutrophilia showing morphology of the neutrophils.
a. Chronic neutrophilic leukemia showing a marked neutrophilia with increased cytoplasmic granulation and small vacuoles.
b. Myelodysplastic syndrome with dysplastic hypogranular and pseudo-Pelger neutrophils.

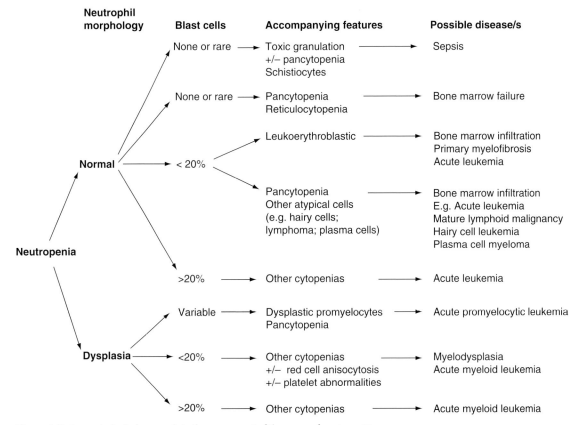

Figure 1.3. A morphological approach to the assessment of the cause of neutropenia.

1. Abnormal neutrophil size, e.g. large neutrophils.
2. Abnormal nuclear segmentation, including hypo-segmented (pseudo-Pelger forms or ring nuclei) or hypersegmented.
3. Abnormal nuclear chromatin condensation and nuclear karyorrhexis.
4. Abnormal cytoplasmic granulation including hypogranular or agranular neutrophils, small, fine eosinophilic granules or large granules (mimic Chediak–Higashi syndrome) and Döhle-like bodies.
5. Auer rods.

When dysplastic neutrophils are accompanied by left shift, the precursor forms are also commonly abnormal. Figures 1.1 and 1.3 list myeloid neoplasms

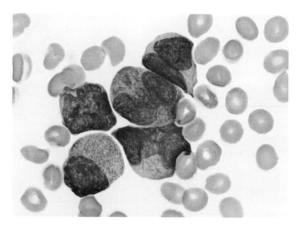

Figure 1.4. Blood film showing the morphology of acute promyelocytic leukemia.

in which peripheral blood neutrophil dysplasia may be the primary identifying feature.

Dysplastic promyelocytes: Of special importance is the presence of isolated dysplastic promyelocytes in the absence of other neutrophil precursors. This is highly suggestive of acute promyelocytic leukemia, which commonly presents with pancytopenia. The abnormal promyelocytes have an eccentrically located ovoid, reniform or bi-lobed nucleus and deeply azurophilic cytoplasmic granules with or without Auer rods (Figure 1.4). Due to their cell size (intermediate to large) the abnormal cells may be located at the edge or in the tail of the blood film. The abnormal cells can easily be overlooked; this highlights the importance of systematic low-power scanning of the entire blood film prior to detailed examination of individual cells. Confident identification of these atypical promyelocytes in the blood can lead to an early provisional diagnosis and instigation of specific therapy. The abnormal promyelocytes may be accompanied by blast cells.

Monocytes: Monocytosis ($> 1 \times 10^9$/L) is a defining feature of chronic myelomonocytic leukemia (CMML) and juvenile myelomonocytic leukemia (JMML). The monocytes may appear normal but more commonly have dysplastic features. The abnormalities include large cell size, increased cytoplasm, irregular nuclear morphology (e.g. nuclear folding, indentation or segmentation), abnormal chromatin pattern, fine azurophilic cytoplasmic granules and cytoplasmic vacuoles (Figure 1.5).

a

b

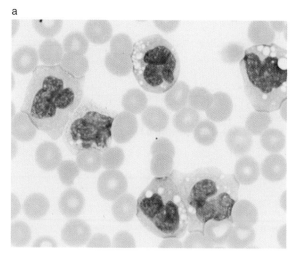

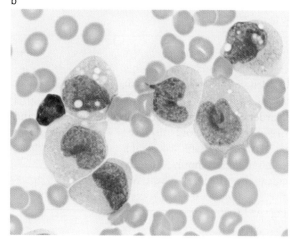

Figure 1.5. Chronic myelomonocytic leukemia (blood film).
a. Dysplastic monocytes.
b. Promonocytes and dysplastic monocytes.

a

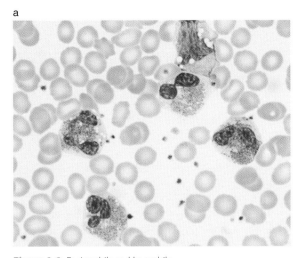

b

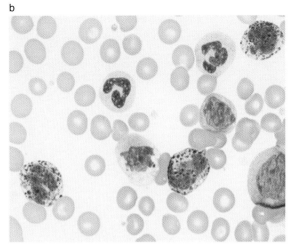

Figure 1.6. Eosinophils and basophils.
a. Abnormal eosinophils in chronic eosinophilic leukemia showing abnormal nuclear hypersegmentation and cytoplasmic granulation.
b. Peripheral blood film of chronic myelogenous leukemia showing basophilia. The basophils are hypogranular with small granules.

Promonocytes, monoblasts, other undifferentiated blast cells and dysplastic neutrophils may also be present [1]. Monocytosis with atypia and left shift can also be seen in acute leukemias with monocytoid differentiation and in atypical chronic myeloid leukemia. In chronic myelogenous leukemia (CML), *BCR-ABL1* positive, there may be a monocytosis but the monocytes generally have normal morphology and appear relatively indistinct amongst the background neutrophilia and left shift. Monocytosis can also be due to reactive causes; here the monocytes generally have normal morphology and promonocytes and blast cells are rarely seen. Monocytopenia is a rare abnormality in hematological malignancies but is a feature seen in hairy cell leukemia.

Eosinophils: A peripheral blood eosinophilia is most commonly secondary to allergy, parasitic infections and drugs, where the eosinophils generally have normal morphology. In contrast, primary eosinophil disorders (i.e. chronic eosinophilic leukemia and myeloid or lymphoid disorders with abnormalities of *PDGFRA*, *PDGFRB* or *FGFR1*) are rare, and the eosinophils commonly have one or more morphological abnormalities. These may assist in differentiating primary from reactive causes, such as (Figure 1.6a):

1. Cell size: large.
2. Nuclear segmentation: hyper- (mimic neutrophil nuclei) or hyposegmented.
3. Cytoplasmic vacuolation.

4. Granules: hypogranularity, small granules and patchy distribution with some clear areas of cytoplasm virtually devoid of granules.
5. Left shift: eosinophils accompanied by eosinophil myelocytes.

Other myeloid malignancies can also have an accompanying eosinophilia with morphological atypia, i.e. CML (e.g. eosinophils with basophilic granules or "baso-eosinophils"), acute myeloid and myelomonocytic leukemias (especially AML with inv(16)/t(16;16)) and systemic mastocytosis. Eosinophilia with normal morphology can occur in lymphoblastic leukemias, B- and T-cell lymphomas and Hodgkin lymphoma.

Basophils: Peripheral blood basophilia is rare, and, when present, should raise suspicion of a myeloproliferative neoplasm. This is particularly so in CML where the basophils tend to have abnormal granulation (i.e. hypogranular and small granules); these can easily be misinterpreted as dysplastic neutrophils (Figure 1.6b). Features that favor abnormal basophils are the slightly larger cell size and that any granules present are deep purple-black or violaceous and not azurophilic. The basophil count is important as it is a defining feature of accelerated phase CML (≥ 20%). In acute basophilic leukemia, mature basophils are rare in the blood but the blast cells contain basophilic granules.

Lymphoid cells: Abnormal lymphoid cells on a blood film may be reactive (e.g. secondary to viral infection) or neoplastic; careful morphological review is required

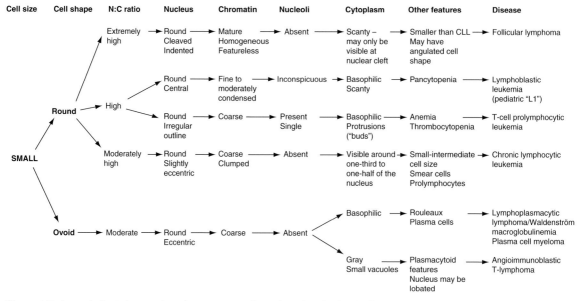

Figure 1.7. A morphological approach to the assessment of neoplastic lymphoid cells of small size.

to distinguish between these. The characteristics that should be assessed (with a ×40–×100 objective) include cell size, shape, nuclear and cytoplasmic features and whether they are pleomorphic or monomorphic. It is beyond the scope of this chapter to provide a detailed description of the appearances of individual reactive and neoplastic lymphoid cell types; more details are given in Chapters 9–11. Neoplastic lymphoid cells can have a wide range of morphologies, some of which may be diagnostic. Figures 1.7–1.11 show some of the important cellular features that can be used to distinguish between lymphoid entities. Once again, this is based on systematic and careful review of a range of cellular features commencing with cell size.

Despite careful assessment, there may be abnormal cells present that have clear neoplastic morphological features but cannot be precisely classified. This may be because the morphology is not characteristic, or because there are insufficient abnormal cells on the film to adequately assess and make a confident diagnosis. The "*company the cells keep*", e.g. rouleaux, spherocytes, neutropenia, may assist due to their associations with some specific lymphoid neoplasms. However, in the vast majority of settings lymphoid cell phenotyping is required to make a diagnosis with certainty. Phenotyping can assist in determining the cell lineage, assessing whether the lymphoid cells have a normal or atypical phenotype and, if B-cells, light chain restriction. This integrated morphology and cell phenotyping approach enables a distinction to be made between reactive and neoplastic lymphoid cells, and, may provide sufficient information to diagnose a specific lymphoid neoplasm. This is especially so for low-grade (small cell) lymphoid malignancies where the morphology may not be characteristic but there is a disease-associated phenotype.

Blast cells: Blast cells are not normally present in the blood. Their presence indicates recovery from bone marrow failure, severe sepsis, cytokine administration or underlying bone marrow pathology. Hematological malignancies which may present with circulating blast cells are:

1. Myelodysplastic syndromes and myelodysplastic/myeloproliferative neoplasms.
2. Acute leukemia, lymphoid or myeloid.
3. Chronic myelogenous leukemia.
4. Primary myelofibrosis.
5. Bone marrow infiltration by a non-hematopoietic malignancy, as part of a leukoerythroblastic blood film.

Blood film features that can aid in establishing the precise diagnosis are:

1. *Number of blast cells*: ≥ 20% circulating blast cells meets the WHO criteria for acute leukemia. When there are fewer than 20% circulating blast

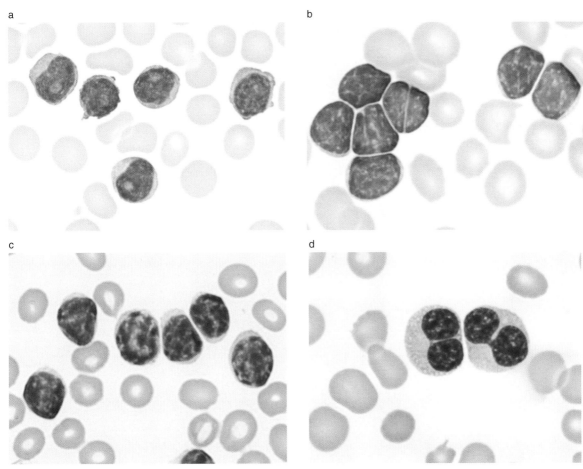

Figure 1.8. Morphology of small lymphoid cell neoplasms.
a. T-cell prolymphocytic leukemia.
b. Follicular lymphoma.
c. Chronic lymphocytic leukemia.
d. Angioimmunoblastic T-cell lymphoma.

cells a bone marrow examination is required to discriminate between myelodysplastic syndromes, myelodysplastic/myeloproliferative neoplasms, myeloproliferative neoplasms and acute leukemia.

2. *Blast cell morphology*: lymphoid or myeloid features (Table 1.2 and Figure 1.12). In some cases the blast cells do not have any specific morphological features that allow lineage assignment. These cases, which may be merely undifferentiated lymphoid or myeloid blasts, or be of ambiguous lineage, will always require phenotyping by flow cytometry to resolve (see Chapter 3).

3. *Accompanying cellular features*, for example:
   a. Leukoerythroblastic blood film: indicates bone marrow fibrosis or infiltration but not the cause.
   b. *Tear-drop poikilocytes*: marrow fibrosis.
   c. *Neutrophil dysplasia*: suggests myelodysplastic syndrome or acute myeloid leukemia.
   d. *Monocytosis*: suggests chronic or juvenile myelomonocytic leukemia or acute myeloid leukemia with monocytoid differentiation.
   e. *Thrombocytosis with abnormal morphology*: myeloproliferative neoplasm.
   f. *Dysplastic platelets* (e.g. large size, hypogranular): suggests a myelodysplastic syndrome, myeloproliferative neoplasm or acute megakaryoblastic leukemia.
   g. *Erythroblastosis with dyserythropoietic features*: suggests erythroleukemia or myelodysplasia.

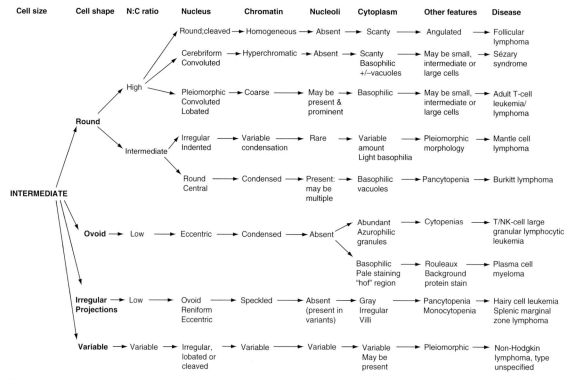

Figure 1.9. A morphological approach to the assessment of neoplastic lymphoid cells of intermediate size.

When there are circulating blast cells, a bone marrow examination is generally indicated to establish the precise diagnosis. In some situations (e.g. high blast cell count; delay in obtaining a bone marrow sample) it may be appropriate to perform flow cytometry on the circulating blast cells prior to the bone marrow examination to establish and/or confirm the diagnosis. This will give a clear indication of the type of blast cell (i.e. lymphoid or myeloid and subtype) and diagnosis.

Plasma cells: Plasma cells do not commonly appear in the circulation. Their presence indicates a florid B-cell response to infection or a B-cell neoplasm with plasmacytoid differentiation. The latter includes plasma cell myeloma, plasma cell leukemia and lymphoplasmacytic lymphoma / Waldenström macroglobulinemia. The morphology of circulating neoplastic plasma cells varies from well-differentiated, resembling those in bone marrow, to markedly pleomorphic with atypical features such as:

1. *Cell size*: vary from small plasmacytoid cells with minimal cytoplasm (lymphoplasmacytoid) to large plasma cells (which are commonly located at the edge of the film).

2. *Nuclei*: may be large, cleaved, indented or lobated.
3. *Nuclear chromatin*: less condensed than normal plasma cells.
4. *Nucleoli*: may be present.
5. *Cytoplasm*: this may be less basophilic than plasma cells in the marrow.

The number of circulating plasma cells discriminates between plasma cell myeloma ($< 2 \times 10^9$/L) and plasma cell leukemia ($\geq 20\%$ of leukocytes or $\geq 2 \times 10^9$/L).

Accompanying blood abnormalities that are commonly seen at presentation of myeloma are red cell macrocytosis (mean corpuscular volume (MCV) 100–105 fL), mild neutropenia and thrombocytopenia. Despite these features, it can, at times, still be difficult to distinguish between reactive and neoplastic plasma cells as both can be accompanied by cytopenias, a leukoerythroblastic film, rouleaux and background protein staining of the blood film. Additional investigations (e.g. serum protein analysis, bone marrow examination) are therefore often required.

Mast cells: The presence of circulating mast cells is pathological and defines mast cell leukemia ($\geq 10\%$

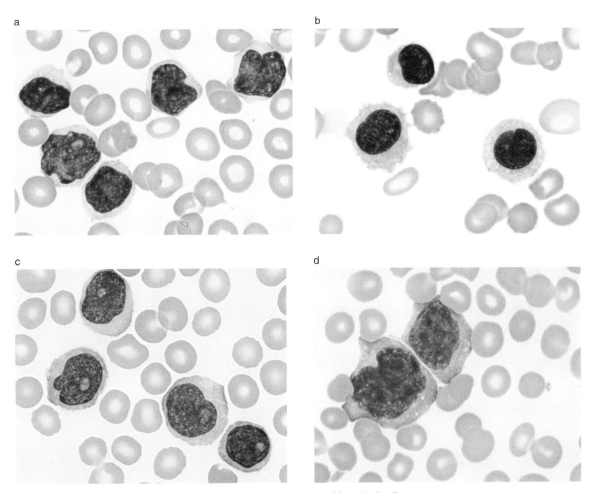

Figure 1.10. Examples of lymphoid cell neoplasms of intermediate (a, b) and large (c, d) cell size.
a. Mantle cell lymphoma.
b. Hairy cell leukemia.
c. B-cell prolymphocytic leukemia.
d. Diffuse large B-cell lymphoma.

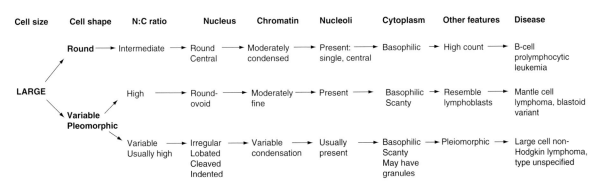

Cell size	Cell shape	N:C ratio	Nucleus	Chromatin	Nucleoli	Cytoplasm	Other features	Disease
	Round →	Intermediate →	Round Central →	Moderately condensed →	Present: single, central →	Basophilic →	High count →	B-cell prolymphocytic leukemia
LARGE		High ———→	Round-ovoid →	Moderately fine →	Present →	Basophilic Scanty →	Resemble lymphoblasts →	Mantle cell lymphoma, blastoid variant
	↘ **Variable Pleomorphic** ↗	Variable Usually high →	Irregular Lobated Cleaved Indented →	Variable condensation →	Usually present →	Basophilic Scanty May have granules →	Pleomorphic →	Large cell non-Hodgkin lymphoma, type unspecified

Figure 1.11. A morphological approach to the assessment of neoplastic lymphoid cells of large size.

Table 1.2. Morphological features that can be used to distinguish between lymphoblasts and myeloblasts.

Cytological feature	Lymphoblasts	Myeloblasts
Cell size	Small – intermediate	Intermediate – large
Nuclear:cytoplasmic ratio	Very high	Variable
Nuclear location	Central	Usually slightly eccentric
Nuclear shape	Round (usually) Irregular or convoluted (less common)	Round to oval May be indented or convoluted (monoblasts)
Nuclear chromatin structure	Fine to condensed or dispersed (small lymphoblasts)	Fine, delicate or granular
Nucleoli	If present, small and usually indistinct Absent in small lymphoblasts	Usually one or more, may be large Often prominent
Cytoplasm	Scanty Basophilic Cytoplasmic pseudopods: "hand-mirror" cells	Variable: moderate to abundant (monoblasts) Basophilic or blue/gray Cytoplasmic blebs (megakaryoblasts)
Cytoplasmic granules	Rare – coarse azurophilic granules (10%)	May be present: azurophilic
Auer rods	No	May be present
Cytoplasmic vacuoles	May be present	May be present, especially with monocytoid differentiation
Overall	Relatively homogeneous appearance	May be pleomorphic, especially with myeloid or monocytoid maturation
Accompanying myeloid cells	Normal	Dysplastic features may be present in maturing myeloid cells and neutrophils

of leukocytes) or its aleukemic variant (< 10% of cells). In the blood mast cells generally have atypical morphology such as angulated (rather than round) cell shape, hypogranularity, irregularly shaped or bi-lobed nuclei, or blast cell features with nucleoli and metachromatic granules.

Erythroid cell morphology

Erythrocytes: Anemia is a common presenting abnormality for hematological malignancies as a result of reduced erythropoiesis; the red cells are usually normochromic and normocytic. Macrocytic red cells are particularly seen with myelodysplasia, and dimorphic red cells with refractory anemia with ring sideroblasts. Other red cell abnormalities include rouleaux, red cell agglutination, tear-drop poikilocytes, spherocytes and hyposplenic features; Table 1.1 lists these abnormalities and their disease associations. Polycythemia vera, characterized by increased red cell production, presents with an elevated hemoglobin; the red cells may be normocytic, or, hypochromic and microcytic if there is iron depletion.

Nucleated red cells: Circulating nucleated red blood cells (erythroblasts) with normal morphology are commonly seen. They are one of the defining features of a leukoerythroblastic film and hence can be present with bone marrow infiltration due to any cause. Erythroblasts with abnormal morphology, such as cytoplasmic irregularity or vacuolation, megaloblastic chromatin pattern, nuclear budding, nuclear karyorrhexis or multinuclearity, imply bone marrow dyserythropoiesis. Circulating dysplastic erythroid progenitors are commonly accompanied by significant red cell anisocytosis, poikilocytosis, basophilic stippling and schistocytes. The presence of dyserythroid erythroblasts together with anisocytosis and poikilocytosis suggests myelodysplasia, acute myeloid leukemia with myelodysplasia-related changes or acute erythroid leukemia (Figure 1.13a).

Platelet morphology

Thrombocytopenia, common at presentation of a hematological malignancy, is usually due to reduced megakaryopoiesis and the platelet morphology is

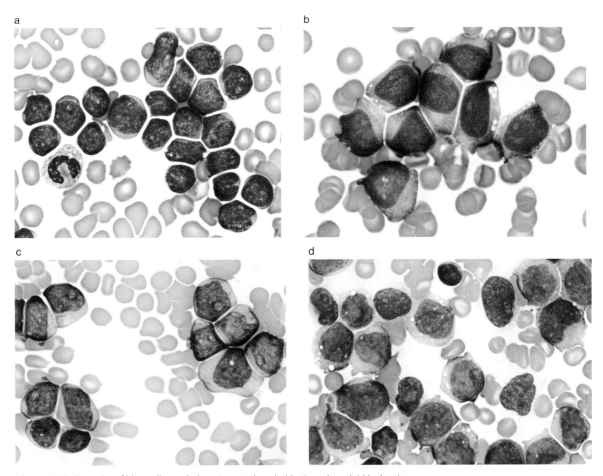

Figure 1.12. Examples of blast cell morphology in acute lymphoblastic and myeloid leukemias.
a. Lymphoblasts in a case of pediatric B lymphoblastic leukemia/lymphoma showing small lymphoblasts with a high nuclear : cytoplasmic ratio and inconspicuous nucleoli.
b. Larger lymphoblasts in a case of B lymphoblastic leukemia/lymphoma showing nucleoli and more abundant cytoplasm with some vacuoles. Immunophenotyping would be required to distinguish between lymphoblasts and myeloblasts in this case.
c. Myeloblasts in a case of acute myeloid leukemia. Auer rods are present in many of the blast cells.
d. Monoblasts and promonocytes in a case of acute monocytic leukemia. The nuclei show early monocytoid differentiation and the cytoplasm is gray with some vacuoles.

normal. Abnormal platelet morphology occurs with bone marrow dysmegakaryopoiesis such as seen in the myeloproliferative neoplasms and some myelodysplastic syndromes. The platelet abnormalities include (Figure 1.13b):

1. *Size*: large and giant platelets.
2. *Granulation*: hypogranular and agranular.
3. *Large fragments of megakaryocyte cytoplasm.*
4. *Circulating micro-megakaryocytes* (small mononuclear megakaryocytes the size of a large lymphoid cell, with coarse chromatin).
5. *Bare megakaryocyte nuclei.*

Thrombocytosis is seen in essential thrombocythemia, CML, some cases of primary myelofibrosis, and, at lower levels, in polycythemia vera. The platelet morphology can vary from normal (where the differential diagnosis is a reactive thrombocytosis) to significant platelet anisocytosis.

Role of the blood film

Blood film morphology has an important role in explaining blood count abnormalities at presentation, in disease monitoring and during and following therapy.

a
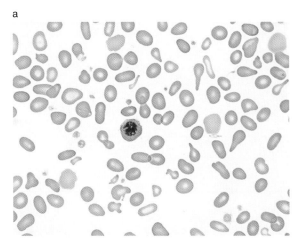

b
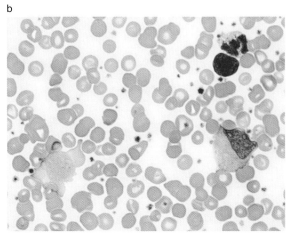

Figure 1.13. Blood films illustrating the *"company the cells keep"*.
a. Red cell abnormalities include a dysplastic nucleated red cell, anisocytosis and poikilocytosis (including tear-drop poikilocytes), and thrombocytopenia in a myelodysplastic syndrome.
b. Abnormal platelets, megakaryocyte fragment, micromegakaryocyte and a markedly hypogranular basophils in a case of primary myelofibrosis. Note the red cells are normochromic and do not show poikilocytosis.

At diagnosis: Blood film review may identify specific abnormal cells and/or accompanying features at presentation (as described above) which are sufficient to establish a definitive diagnosis or lead to a provisional diagnosis. In most circumstances one or more supplementary investigations will be required on the blood sample (e.g. flow cytometry) and a bone marrow examination to lead to a definitive diagnosis.

Disease monitoring and follow-up: Blood films should be reviewed during therapy, on completion of therapy and for disease monitoring to assess the number of abnormal cells in the blood and the effects of chemotherapy. Cytotoxic therapy can result in a number of blood film abnormalities including:

1. *Erythrocytes*: macrocytosis, anisocytosis, poikilocytosis, basophilic stippling and Howell–Jolly bodies.
2. *Neutrophils*: abnormalities of neutrophil nuclear segmentation and/or granulation.
3. *Platelets*: thrombocytopenia.

Marrow regeneration is evidenced by return of normal blood cells, initially with left shift (polychromatic erythrocytes and early myeloid cells) followed by mature cells. Toxic changes may be seen in neutrophils if therapy has been complicated by sepsis. Following normalization of counts and cell morphology, subsequent cytopenias or reappearance of neoplastic cells generally indicate morphological evidence of relapsed disease.

Reporting the blood film

The blood film report should include a description of the significant morphological findings, an interpretation of the features and give a provisional or differential diagnosis. The report should comment on:

1. The presence of abnormal cells and their cytological features, e.g. blast cells, smear cells, tear-drop poikilocytes.
2. Other accompanying features of significance (the *"company the cells keep"*).
3. An interpretation of the findings.
4. Definitive, provisional or differential diagnosis.
5. Supplementary investigations recommended be performed on the blood sample to reach a diagnosis, e.g. flow cytometry, serum protein analysis.
6. Other recommended investigations, e.g. bone marrow examination.

Bone marrow examination

The indications for performing a bone marrow examination have been formalized by the International Council for Standardization in Haematology (ICSH) and those specific for hematological malignancies are listed in Table 1.3 [9]. For details of bone marrow collection, staining and reporting procedures the reader is referred to other publications [9–11]. In general, a bone marrow examination is required whenever a hematological malignancy is suspected from the blood film. Bone

Table 1.3. Indications for bone marrow examination in the diagnosis and assessment of hematological malignancies from the ICSH standards [9].

Investigation of unexplained cytopenia/s or pancytopenia

Investigation of unexplained blood film morphological abnormalities

Investigation of a paraproteinemia

To confirm a diagnosis of a hematological malignancy made on peripheral blood

To classify a hematological malignancy

To determine the extent of bone marrow involvement by a hematological malignancy

Bone marrow staging of lymphoma

To obtain prognostic information based on the pattern of marrow infiltration

To obtain specimens for ancillary studies in the investigation of hematological malignancies

Post-therapy and post-transplant assessment of hematological malignancies

marrow aspirate and trephine biopsy specimens provide complementary information and both are therefore valuable in the initial assessment of a possible hematological malignancy. The aspirate gives detailed cytological detail, whereas the trephine biopsy provides more information about the overall marrow cellularity, architecture, cellular distribution and fibrosis. For some disorders the aspirate may provide sufficient information without the need for a trephine biopsy, e.g. acute leukemia. For others, the trephine biopsy is the prime diagnostic material, e.g. lymphoma staging (see Chapter 11) and myelofibrosis (see Chapter 14).

In addition to morphology, the marrow samples can be used for ancillary biological tests required to reach a diagnosis and WHO classification (i.e. flow cytometry, immunocytochemistry and genetics). Consideration should be given to the most appropriate specimen to use for these supplementary investigations (Table 1.4) [1,12]. For example, cytogenetic analysis by karyotyping and RT-PCR can only be performed on freshly aspirated marrow, whereas PCR can be performed on both aspirate and trephine biopsy specimens. A description of the principles of bone marrow examination follows together with some illustrative examples of their application. Chapters 7–15 give detailed descriptions of the morphological features of the bone marrow aspirate and trephine biopsy of individual neoplastic disorders.

Bone marrow aspirate

Aspirated marrow should routinely be prepared as both "squash" preparations and "smears" (Figure 1.14). After air-drying, these are fixed in methanol, stained with a Romanowsky stain (e.g. May–Grünwald Giemsa or Wright Giemsa) and a coverslip applied. Aspirated marrow can also be used to make particle clot preparations, for cytochemical stains, cell phenotyping, cytogenetics and molecular genetic analyses (Table 1.4).

Aspirate "squash" preparations: "Squash" preparations are imprints of bone marrow particles, and are particularly valuable for low-power (from ×4 up to ×20 objectives) assessment of marrow cellularity, megakaryocyte number, cell clumps and focal infiltrates (e.g. lymphoma, mastocytosis and plasma cell myeloma). Cells that may be encased in reticulin are more readily detectable in the "squash" preparation than smears (e.g. follicular lymphoma, Hodgkin lymphoma, neoplastic mast cells). Cytological detail is generally less well preserved than in smears.

Aspirate smears: The major roles of the bone marrow aspirate smear are to assess cytological detail and perform a nucleated differential cell count. Smears should first be scanned at low magnification (×4 and ×10 objectives) to assess the cellularity of the particles and trails and determine whether there are clumps of abnormal cells, particularly at the edge or in the tail of the smear. The cellular composition of the marrow should then be assessed in a representative trail behind a marrow particle using a ×40 or ×50 objective. Morphological review with a ×100 objective is used to assess fine cytological detail (e.g. nuclear folding; cytoplasmic inclusions) and for accurate cell identification. The number of individual

a
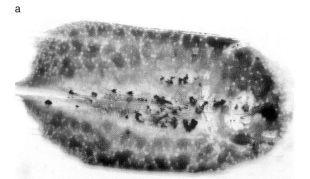

b
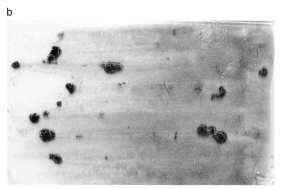

Figure 1.14. Bone marrow aspirate preparations.
a. "Squash" preparation: the marrow particles are in the middle of the slide and the hematopoietic elements are in close proximity having been "squashed".
b. "Smear" preparation: the marrow particles are in the tail of the smear and hematopoietic elements have trailed behind. Nucleated differential cell counts should be done in regions immediately behind the particles.

Table 1.4. Applications of bone marrow aspirate and trephine biopsies [9,12].

	Bone marrow aspirate		Bone marrow trephine biopsy
	"Squash" preparation	"Smear"	
Bone marrow morphological features			
Cellularity	+++	++	+++
Marrow topography	+	−	+++
Cytological detail	++	+++	+
Cell enumeration	++	+++	+
Megakaryocyte number	+++	+	+++
Megakaryocyte morphology	++	+++	+++
Cell clusters	+++	+	+++
Focal infiltrates	++	−	+++
Bone structure	−		+++
Marrow fibrosis	−		+++
Diagnostic techniques			
Flow cytometry	+++		−
Cytochemistry	+++		++
Immunocytochemistry	+++		+++
Karyotyping	+++		−
FISH	+++		++
FICTION ("immuno-FISH")	+++		++
PCR	+++		+ *
RT-PCR	+++		−

+++ = Excellent; ++ = Good; + = Limited role; − = Sample unsuitable; * limited DNA quality. FICTION: Fluorescence Immunophenotyping and Interphase Cytogenetics as a Tool for the Investigation of Neoplasms.

hematopoietic cell types and any abnormal cells should be determined from a count of at least 300 nucleated cells [9].

Particle "clot" preparations: Aspirated marrow can be clotted with thrombin, placed in fixative (e.g. neutral buffered formalin) and processed into paraffin. Sections of this clotted marrow are made (as for the trephine biopsy) and stained with hematoxylin and eosin (H&E) or other stains (e.g. Giemsa). Particle clot sections give comparable information to the trephine biopsy (i.e. marrow cellularity; detection of focal infiltrates) without the need for a trephine sample.

Cytochemical stains

Cytochemistry, when required, is usually performed on bone marrow aspirate smears but is also applicable to bone marrow trephine specimens. The principles of cytochemistry are that a chromogen localizes enzyme activity or non-enzymatic substrates within cells. Many cytochemical techniques are available with a wide range of applications (Table 1.5). The majority have now largely been replaced by cell phenotyping (i.e. flow cytometry and immunocytochemistry). This is because of the greater sensitivity and specificity of antibodies for individual cell types, the standardized methodology for all antigens, automation and faster turn-around-time than

Table 1.5. Cytochemical stains that can be used for the assessment of hematological malignancies [13,14].

Substrate type	Cytochemical test	Cellular component	Cell type	Hematological malignancy
Non-Enzyme	Perls' Prussian Blue	Iron (ferric)	Macrophages Late normoblasts	Iron status of all disorders Myelodysplastic syndromes Myelodysplastic/Myeloproliferative neoplasms
	Periodic acid-Schiff	Carbohydrate	Granulocytes	Precursor lymphoid neoplasms (block positivity)
			Megakaryocytes Plasma cells	Erythroleukemia Plasma cell myeloma
	Sudan Black B	Lipid	Myeloid cells	Acute myeloid leukemias (granulocytic differentiation)
	Oil Red O	Lipid	Neoplastic B-cells	Burkitt lymphoma
	Toluidine Blue	Metachromasia	Basophils Mast cells	Systemic mastocytosis Chronic myelogenous leukemia (basophils positive)
Enzyme	Alkaline phosphatase	Neutrophil alkaline phosphatase	Neutrophils (Score 0–400)	Polycythemia vera (high score) Chronic myelogenous leukemia (low score)
	Acid phosphatase	Lysosomes	Majority of normal hematopoietic cells	T-lymphoblastic leukemia/lymphoma Mature T-cell neoplasms Hairy cell leukemia (resistant to tartrate)
	Non-specific esterases	α-naphthyl acetate esterase	Monocytes (diffuse) Macrophages Lymphocytes (dot)	Acute monocytic and myelomonocytic leukemia Acute megakaryoblastic leukemia T-cell prolymphocytic leukemia
	Specific esterases	Chloroacetate esterase	Neutrophils	Acute myeloid leukemias (granulocytic differentiation)
			Mast cells	Systemic mastocytosis
	Lysozyme	Lysozyme (muramidase)	Monocytes	Acute monocytic and myelomonocytic leukemia
			Macrophages	Chronic myelomonocytic leukemia
	Myeloperoxidase	Primary granules	Myeloid cells	Acute myeloid leukemias (granulocytic differentiation)
	Sudan Black B	Myeloid cell granules	Myeloid cells Eosinophils	Acute myeloid leukemia

cytochemistry. Only the Perls' Prussian Blue reaction which utilizes potassium ferrocyanide to demonstrate ferric tissue iron, remains in common use. This is an important test of iron status and iron incorporation into developing erythroblasts; as such it should be performed in the initial assessment of hematological malignancies. For a full description of the principles and methods of cytochemical stains the reader is referred to other monographs [13–14].

Interpretation and reporting the bone marrow aspirate

The blood count and film should always be reviewed together with the bone marrow aspirate and the findings included in the marrow report. The cellularity of the bone marrow particles ("squash" preparation) and trails ("smears") should both be reported; these can differ, especially when there is significant fibrosis and the particles may be markedly hypercellular with hypocellular trails. In this situation the cellularity and morphology of the "squash" preparation may be more representative of overall hematopoietic activity and the presence of a neoplastic infiltrate. When there are no particles present (i.e. "blood tap") the sample may still be informative if there is a significant abnormal cell infiltrate. However if the sample is aparticulate, and there are no abnormal cells (a "blood tap"), the diagnosis will be dependent on the bone marrow trephine biopsy findings.

The number and the morphological appearances of all cell lineages, and any abnormal cells present in the marrow, should be reported. The results of the Perls' Prussian Blue reaction, flow cytometry and any other supplementary investigations should also be included in the report. A provisional report should be issued once the morphological assessment has been completed and whilst awaiting finalization of other investigations. The final conclusion should give a diagnosis or provisional diagnosis and indicate any additional investigations required. A final integrated report should include all bone marrow aspirate findings including the ancillary immunological and genotypic investigations (see Chapter 6). For follow-up and monitoring bone marrow the findings should be compared with previous marrow examinations.

Bone marrow trephine biopsy

Bone marrow trephine (BMT) biopsy specimens, in contrast to aspirates, have preserved bone marrow architecture which allows assessment of:

1. Overall marrow cellularity and topography.
2. Distribution of hematopoietic cellular elements within the inter-trabecular spaces and the relationship of cells to the bony trabeculae.
3. Pattern of involvement by abnormal cells, e.g. focal disease.
4. Stromal cell elements, marrow fibrosis and bone structure.

Bone marrow trephine biopsies are less sensitive than aspirates for assessing cytological detail, making it difficult to perform a nucleated differential count and enumerate the number of normal and abnormal cells in the marrow. It is generally recommended that a BMT be performed in the initial evaluation of a possible hematological malignancy. If it is anticipated that there may be focal disease, marrow fibrosis or where assessment of megakaryocyte number and location are required, a trephine biopsy is essential. Overall a BMT is indicated in the investigation of:

1. Leukoerythroblastic blood film.
2. Unexplained thrombocytosis.
3. Pancytopenia.
4. Paraproteinemia.
5. Lymphoma staging.
6. Diagnosis of mast cell disorders.
7. Inaspirable bone marrow (a "dry tap").

Bone marrow trephine biopsies are primarily used for histology and immunocytochemistry (see Chapter 2), but can also be used for cytochemistry and some genetic investigations as detailed in Table 1.4 [5,12,15–16].

Preparation and staining: The BMT biopsy is usually obtained from the posterior iliac crest and should be at least 2 cm in length; for some indications bilateral BMT may be required. Before placing into fixative, it is recommended that imprints be made by touching the core biopsy onto a glass slide. These can be fixed, stained and reviewed as for aspirate slides. The BMT biopsy is fixed by one of a number of methods to cross-link cellular proteins to maintain cellular integrity and morphology. Fixation methods available include neutral buffered formalin, mercury-containing fixatives (e.g. Zenker's fixative and B-5), Bouin's and zinc formaldehyde. Following fixation the BMT is decalcified to remove calcium from the cortical and trabecular bone using, for example, EDTA, picric, acetic, formic or nitric acids. Fixation and decalcification regimens are not standardized; they vary in their processing time and the resultant preservation of morphology and cellular antigens, and the integrity of DNA and RNA [9,17]. The most commonly used processing schedule utilizes neutral buffered formalin fixation and EDTA decalcification, a protocol which enables the full spectrum of ancillary tests (immunocytochemistry and genetic tests) to be performed without compromising morphological detail. Following fixation and decalcification the specimen is processed to paraffin wax, sectioned on a microtome at 2–4 μm and stained. Stains used include:

1. Hematoxylin and eosin ("H&E"): the standard stain.
2. Giemsa: highlights lymphoid cells, plasma cells and mast cells.
3. Gordon and Sweet or Gomori methenamine silver stains for reticulin.
4. Perls' Prussian Blue reaction: for the assessment of iron stores.
5. Various cytochemical stains, e.g. chloroacetate esterase, periodic acid-Schiff.

Resin (methyl-methacrylate) embedding can be used as an alternative to paraffin. This has the advantage of not requiring decalcification and semi-thin sections (1–2 μm) can be cut. Although this results in superb cytological detail, it takes time and experience to become familiar with the appearances as the morphology cannot be easily compared with paraffin sections. Other limitations of resin embedding are that it requires a separate method of preparation including a special heavy-duty microtome, there is some loss of cellular antigens and nucleic acids are poorly preserved [18–19].

Interpretation and reporting the bone marrow trephine biopsy

Systematic review of the BMT biopsy should commence at low magnification (×4 and ×10 objectives) to assess:

1. Adequacy of the biopsy, e.g. specimen length, sufficient inter-trabecular spaces, presence of crush artefact.
2. Marrow cellularity, i.e. the percent of inter-trabecular spaces occupied by cells.
3. Pattern of cell distribution.

4. Relationship of cellular elements to bony trabeculae.
5. Presence and location of any abnormal infiltrates.

The ×20 and ×40 objectives should then be used sequentially for an overall assessment of hematopoietic activity, including:

1. *Pattern* of normal hematopoiesis.
2. *Erythroid cells*: presence, location and size of erythroid islands; normally interstitial location.
3. *Granulocytic cells*: presence and location of immature and mature forms; normally immature forms are paratrabecular and migrate into the interstitium of the marrow with maturation.
4. *Megakaryocytes*: number, distribution and morphology; normally single and interstitial.
5. *Lymphoid cells*: normally scattered throughout the marrow and relatively inconspicuous.
6. *Plasma cells*: normally peri-vascular or scattered.
7. Macrophages, stromal cells and bony trabeculae (e.g. bone thickness; cement lines; osteoblasts; osteoclasts; osteocytes).
8. *Presence of abnormal infiltrates* and their cellular content:
    a. *Pattern*: diffuse, interstitial or focal (e.g. nodular, sinusoidal) (Figures 1.15a-d).
    b. *Location* of focal infiltrates: inter-trabecular or paratrabecular (Figure 1.15c,d).
    c. *Cell morphology*: size, shape and maturity (chromatin structure, nucleoli).
    d. Mitotic and apoptotic rate.
    e. The "*company the cells keep*" (e.g. macrophages, hemophagocytosis).

The reticulin pattern (fine, coarse, focal increase) and overall content should be quantified using a grading system [20]. Examples of some BMT morphological abnormalities and their disease associations are listed in Table 1.6. Immunocytochemistry may be performed on the trephine biopsy to confirm the number of normal hematopoietic cells of each lineage or to phenotype abnormal cells (see Chapter 2 for details). Cytochemical stains can be performed on the BMT, but are rarely required due to the widespread use of immunocytochemistry. Some genetic tests, (e.g. fluorescence *in situ* hybridization (FISH), polymerase chain reaction (PCR)) can be performed on the BMT biopsy (see Table 1.4).

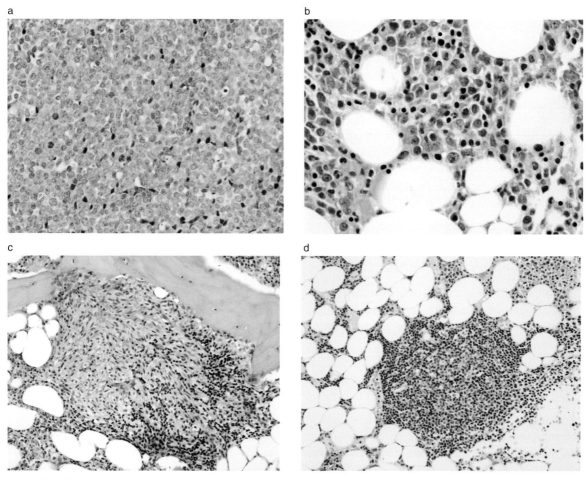

Figure 1.15. Patterns of bone marrow infiltration in bone marrow trephine biopsies.
a. Hypercellular marrow with a diffuse infiltrate in a case of B lymphoblastic leukemia.
b. Subtle interstitial infiltrate in a natural killer-cell lymphoma.
c. Paratrabecular infiltrate in systemic mastocytosis.
d. Nodular interstitial infiltrate in a case of chronic lymphocytic leukemia.

Integrated bone marrow reporting

The blood film, bone marrow aspirate and bone marrow trephine findings, together with results of ancillary tests, should all be included in a single integrated report (Table 1.7) [21]. This gives a complete interpretation of bone marrow function and a single WHO classification [1,9,21]. This ensures that all results are considered together and that any potential discrepancies which may, on occasion, arise with different samples are resolved prior to the final report. This should avert any misdiagnoses and result in *"one patient, one diagnosis and one report"*. Due to differences in turn-around times for the various test components, interim reports of individual analyses may be necessary prior to release

of the final integrated report. This concept is discussed in more detail in Chapter 6.

Applications of bone marrow aspirates and trephine biopsies

The bone marrow aspirate and trephine biopsy are taken from the same site, but are processed and stained differently and give different types of information about the state of the marrow. As a result they have different roles in the assessment of hematological malignancies. Examples are given of the relative merits of the aspirate and trephine for different indications at diagnosis, staging and for disease monitoring.

Table 1.6. Examples of bone marrow trephine (BMT) features seen in hematological malignancies.

BMT feature	Description	Abnormality	Hematological malignancies (examples)	Differential diagnosis
Marrow cellularity	Hypocellular	Reduced inter-trabecular hematopoiesis	Hypoplastic myelodysplastic syndromes Hypoplastic acute myeloid leukemia Acute leukemia	Aplastic anemia Drug therapy
	Hypercellular	Diffuse hypercellularity	Chronic myelogenous leukemia Extensive bone marrow infiltration	Reactive marrow
		Patchy hypercellularity	Non-Hodgkin lymphomas Myelodysplastic syndromes Systemic mastocytosis	Reactive marrow Metastatic malignancy Marrow regeneration
Marrow Architecture (Cellular distribution)	Paratrabecular	Infiltrates along bony trabeculae	Follicular lymphoma Systemic mastocytosis	
	Focal, nodular interstitial	Interstitial infiltrates surrounded by hematopoietic tissue and fat	Chronic lymphocytic leukemia Non-Hodgkin lymphoma, e.g. mantle cell lymphoma Hodgkin lymphoma Plasma cell myeloma	Reactive lymphoid nodules Granuloma Metastatic malignancy
	Interstitial infiltrates	Infiltrates between fat spaces	Chronic lymphocytic leukemia Hairy cell leukemia Mature T/NK-cell neoplasms	Reactive
	Diffuse infiltrates	Infiltrates that efface the bone marrow architecture	Acute leukemias (myeloid and lymphoid) Diffuse large B-cell lymphoma Extensive bone marrow infiltration	Reactive lymphocytosis Granulocytic hyperplasia Erythroid hyperplasia
	Sinusoidal or intravascular	Infiltrates in endothelial spaces	Intravascular large B-cell lymphoma Splenic marginal zone lymphoma Hepato-splenic T-cell lymphoma	
	"Starry sky" pattern	Abundant macrophages	Burkitt lymphoma Acute myeloid leukemia	Reactive histiocytosis
Cytological abnormalities	Megakaryocytes	Hyperplasia	Myeloproliferative neoplasms Myelodysplastic syndromes	Reactive marrow Immune thrombocytopenia
		Clustering	Myeloproliferative neoplasms	
		Pleomorphism	Polycythemia vera Primary myelofibrosis	Reactive marrow
		Small forms	Myelodysplastic syndromes (hypolobated or disrupted nuclei) Chronic myelogenous leukemia	Reactive marrow
		Large and giant forms	Essential thrombocythemia	
		Pyknotic forms and bare nuclei	Primary myelofibrosis	Drug therapy
	Granulocytic cells	Interstitial immature forms	Myelodysplastic syndromes Myelodysplastic/Myeloproliferative neoplasms Primary myelofibrosis Acute myeloid leukemia	
		Asynchronous maturation	Myelodysplastic syndromes Myelodysplastic/Myeloproliferative neoplasms	Cytokine therapy Drug effect
	Erythroid cells	Enlarged islands	Myelodysplastic syndromes Erythroleukemia	Erythroid hyperplasia Megaloblastic anemia

Table 1.6. (cont.)

BMT feature	Description	Abnormality	Hematological malignancies (examples)	Differential diagnosis
		Reduced erythropoiesis	Myelodysplastic syndromes Primary myelofibrosis	Drug therapy Parvovirus
		Asynchronous maturation	Myelodysplastic syndromes	Megaloblastic anemia
Cytological abnormalities (continued)	Progenitor cells	Interstitial location	Acute myeloid leukemia Myelodysplastic syndromes Accelerated phase of myeloproliferative neoplasms	
	Lymphoid cells	Small cells	Chronic lymphocytic leukemia Lymphoblastic leukemia/lymphoma T-cell prolymphocytic leukemia	Reactive lymphocytosis
		Large cells	Diffuse large B-cell lymphoma Anaplastic large cell lymphoma	Reactive lymphoid nodules
		Intermediate size, pleomorphic	Hairy cell leukemia Mantle cell lymphoma	
	Plasma cells	Plasmacytosis with pleomorphism	Plasma cell myeloma Lymphoplasmacytic lymphoma	Reactive marrow
	Macrophages	Hemophagocytosis	Anaplastic large cell lymphoma T/NK-cell lymphoma	Reactive marrow
		Pseudo-Gaucher cells	Plasma cell myeloma Chronic myelogenous leukemia	Gaucher disease
Reticulin	Increased	Fine	Acute leukemia Plasma cell myeloma Extensive bone marrow infiltration	Autoimmune disorders
		Coarse	Primary myelofibrosis	Metastatic carcinoma
		Focal	Focal infiltrates, including lymphomas, myeloma and systemic mastocytosis (random pattern)	Reactive lymphoid nodules ("organoid" pattern)
Bony trabeculae	Osteosclerosis	Thick trabeculae	Primary myelofibrosis Systemic mastocytosis	Paget's disease Osteopetrosis Metastatic disease
	Osteopenia Osteoporosis	Thin trabeculae	Plasma cell myeloma	Malnutrition Post-chemotherapy
Marrow necrosis	Marrow infarction	Necrotic cells	Acute leukemia Large cell non-Hodgkin lymphoma	Metastatic malignancy

Diagnosis and staging: examples

Circulating blast cells: A bone marrow aspirate is essential in the investigation of unexplained circulating blast cells. The aspirate is used to enumerate the blast cells, assess blast cell cytology (Figure 1.12) and assess for the presence of dysplasia in the other hematopoietic cells. In addition, aspirated marrow is the preferred specimen for blast cell phenotyping by flow cytometry, and for cytogenetic and molecular genetic analyses. A BMT biopsy is not essential as it generally shows diffuse marrow replacement by a monomorphic population of poorly differentiated cells and the cytology is often not discriminatory (Figure 1.15a); however, it is indicated if there are blood film features that suggest bone marrow fibrosis (i.e. tear-drop poikilocytes or leukoerythroblastic blood film) or myelodysplasia, or, if the marrow aspirate yields a "dry tap".

Lymphoma staging: As lymphomatous infiltrates in the marrow are commonly focal (nodular interstitial, para-trabecular, intravascular or sinusoidal), a BMT biopsy must be performed for lymphoma staging. Aspirated marrow may not include cells from the focal lesion, as there is commonly increased reticulin within the neoplastic infiltrates, and thereby give a false negative result.

Table 1.7. Information that should be included in a final integrated bone marrow report (see also Chapter 6).

Patient details	Surname, first name, date of birth, gender, unique patient number, specimen number
Clinical information	Indication for the bone marrow examination Relevant clinical findings Diagnosis, if known Recent drug therapy Procedure (i.e. aspirate and/or trephine biopsy) Anatomical site
Blood	Blood count and blood film morphology
Bone marrow aspirate	Samples evaluated (i.e. squash, smears, particle clot) Presence of particles Overall marrow cellularity Myeloid:erythroid ratio Cellularity and morphology of each cell lineage, i.e. erythroid, granulocytic, megakaryocyte, lymphocytes, macrophages, plasma cells Abnormal cells (e.g. blast cells): morphology and number Iron status and sideroblasts, i.e. number, pattern of siderotic granulation
Bone marrow trephine	Length of specimen Overall marrow cellularity and pattern Cellularity, location and morphology of each cell lineage: erythroid cells, granulocytic cells, megakaryocytes, lymphocytes, macrophages, plasma cells Presence of abnormal infiltrates: pattern, location and cellular composition Other abnormal findings: dyspoiesis, abnormal cells Bone structure and stromal cells Reticulin content Results of immunocytochemical and/or cytochemical stains
Ancillary tests	Flow cytometry Cytogenetics Molecular genetics
Other comments	Differences between the aspirate and bone marrow trephine Comparison with previous bone marrow examinations Correlation with clinical information
Diagnosis and WHO classification	Integrating results of blood, bone marrow aspirate and bone marrow trephine

Although the sensitivity of the aspirate can be increased with the addition of flow cytometry and molecular genetic analyses these analyses should not be performed in place of a BMT. For further details see Chapter 11.

Investigation of paraproteinemia: Bone marrow aspirate and trephine biopsies are both indicated in the investigation and monitoring of a paraproteinemia. The aspirate is useful to enumerate the plasma cells and to assess plasma cell morphology. The BMT biopsy is important to assess the disease burden as plasma cell infiltrates may be focal and, particularly in cases where there is increased reticulin (approximately 10% of myeloma). Aspirated marrow is commonly not representative and underestimates the disease burden. For further details see Chapter 12.

A "dry tap": Failure to aspirate bone marrow, or a "dry tap", is an absolute indication for a BMT biopsy. Causes of a "dry tap" include:

1. Marrow fibrosis: e.g. primary myelofibrosis, hairy cell leukemia, Hodgkin lymphoma and metastatic marrow infiltrates.
2. Markedly hypercellular bone marrow: e.g. acute leukemia, multiple myeloma.

Post-therapy assessment and disease monitoring: examples

Bone marrow examination is indicated following therapy for a hematological malignancy to assess:

1. Disease response.
2. Effects of therapy on normal hematopoiesis.
3. Marrow regeneration.

Table 1.8. Post-chemotherapy and regenerative bone marrow changes following myelosuppressive chemotherapy.

Morphological feature	Post-chemotherapy changes		Early bone marrow regeneration	
	Bone marrow aspirate	**Bone marrow trephine**	**Bone marrow aspirate**	**Bone marrow trephine**
Bone marrow structure	Hypocellularity Reduced erythroid, granulocytic and megakaryocytic activity	Aplasia or hypoplasia Absence of fat cells Serous atrophy/edema Sinusoidal expansion	Variable cellularity	Reappearance of fat cells Patchy cellularity Interstitial clusters of immature cells
Erythroid series	Dyserythropoiesis Megaloblastic differentiation	Disrupted erythroid islands	Left shift	Large erythroid islands Left shift
Granulocytic series	Dysgranulopoiesis Hypersegmented neutrophils Nuclear disruption Döhle bodies	Reduced	Left shift Increased granulation is common	Thickened band of paratrabecular myeloid precursors
Megakaryocytes	Disrupted nuclear lobes	Abnormal nuclear lobation	Delayed megakaryopoiesis compared to erythroid and granulocytic series Left shift, hypolobated nuclei	Interstitial clusters Left shift
Precursor cells	Reduced		Increased lymphoid progenitors ("hematogones")	Clusters of immature cells (may be CD34-positive)
Other	Necrotic tumor cells Relative increase in lymphocytes, plasma cells, macrophages and stromal cells			Mild reticulin increase

As at diagnosis, aspirated marrow is preferable to the trephine biopsy to assess cytological detail. Bone marrow trephine biopsies should be performed to monitor disorders that were previously involved, especially with focal infiltrates, and to assess overall hematopoietic regeneration. Some of the bone marrow features seen following myelosuppressive chemotherapy and in early marrow regeneration are given in Table 1.8.

Assessment of disease response: The extent of residual disease, is, for most disorders, best assessed on cytological detail in aspirated bone marrow. The post-chemotherapy marrow sample should always be reviewed alongside the diagnostic marrow to compare morphological features. The number of neoplastic cells requires accurate enumeration. Morphological response criteria and the definition of remission status vary by disease and according to the aims of therapy. Treatment with curative intent generally requires the demonstration of absence of neoplastic cells in the marrow, by all criteria, including morphology. Examples of complete morphological response are:

1. *Acute myeloid leukemia*: < 5% blast cells in the bone marrow aspirate [22–23].
2. *Myelodysplastic syndromes*: loss of dysplastic features and < 5% blast cells in the bone marrow (necessitating both an aspirate and BMT biopsy).
3. *Plasma cell myeloma*: ≤ 5% plasma cells in the bone marrow aspirate and BMT [24–25].
4. *Lymphoma*: no abnormal lymphoid infiltrate in the BMT.
5. *Chronic myelogenous leukemia*: no residual morphological features of CML in the aspirate or BMT biopsy [26].

The morphology should be reported in conjunction with other test modalities which may have greater sensitivity in disease monitoring, i.e. phenotyping, genetics.

a

b

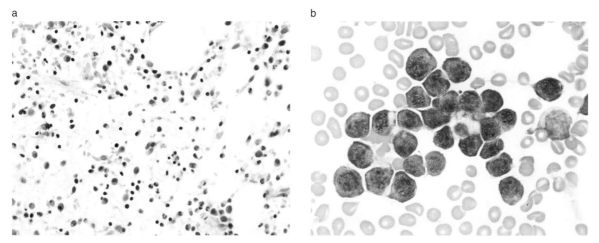

Figure 1.16. Effects of myelosuppressive chemotherapy on the bone marrow.
a. Hypocellular bone marrow trephine biopsy showing a marked reduction in normal hematopoiesis, marrow edema and sinusoidal expansion.
b. A regenerating erythroid island in a bone marrow aspirate. The erythroblasts show megaloblastic morphology.

Assessment of effect of therapy on normal hematopoiesis: The effects of therapy on the bone marrow depend on the type of drug/s, dose and duration, and the timing of the sample following therapy. Systemic myelosuppressive therapy generally causes ablation of normal hematopoietic activity within a week of administration. The major morphological changes are marrow aplasia, edema and sinusoidal expansion and are best seen in the trephine biopsy (Table 1.8 and Figure 1.16). Some cytotoxic drugs cause dysplasia of one or more hematopoietic cell lineages and this can be difficult to distinguish from primary myelodysplasia. Examples of drugs and the therapy-related morphological changes they cause are:

1. *Anti-metabolite drugs* (e.g. hydroxycarbamide; 6-mercaptopurine): megaloblastic erythropoiesis.
2. *CD20 immunotherapy*: nodular aggregates of reactive T-lymphocytes [27].
3. *Dasatinib therapy*: T-cell or natural killer cell large granular lymphocytosis, which may be clonal [28–29].
4. *Cytokine therapy*, e.g. G-CSF causes granulocytic hyperplasia, left shift and toxic granulation.

Evaluation of bone marrow regeneration: Hematopoietic regeneration usually commences 7–10 days after completion of myelosuppressive therapy and is best assessed in a BMT biopsy (Table 1.8). The first evidence of regeneration is interstitial erythroid islands and paratrabecular immature myeloid progenitors, followed later by megakaryocytes (Figure 1.16b). Interstitial clusters of progenitor cells in early regenerating marrows can be difficult to distinguish from residual neoplastic blast cells, especially in acute leukemia and myelodysplasia. Immunocytochemistry may be required to resolve whether these are leukemic cells or hematogones [30]. Normal hematopoiesis and marrow cellularity should be seen in 4–5 weeks.

Conclusion

Despite the explosion in our knowledge of the biology of hematological malignancies, the art of morphology using standard light microscopy continues to have a pivotal role in the diagnosis and ongoing assessment of hematological malignancies. Morphology is the first test performed and with careful and systematic analysis by a well-trained observer can be used to formulate a provisional diagnosis. This forms the foundation for informed decision-making regarding the need for and determining which ancillary immunological and genetic tests are required to reach a final diagnosis. Ignoring morphology will result in poor utilization of these newer more sophisticated investigations. Morphology is therefore the key starting point and is critical in the diagnosis of hematological malignancies.

References

1. Swerdlow SH, Campo E, Harris NL *et al.* (eds.). *WHO Classification of Tumours of Haematopoietic and Lymphoid Tissues*, 4th edn. Lyon: IARC; 2008.

2. Lewis SM, Bain BJ, Bates I. *Dacie and Lewis Practical Haematology*, 10th edn. Philadelphia, PA: Churchill Livingstone Elsevier; 2006.

3. Hoffbrand AV, Pettit JE, Vyas P. *Color Atlas of Clinical Hematology*, 4th edn. Philadelphia, PA: Mosby Elsevier; 2009.

4. Brown D, Gatter K, Natkunam Y, Warnke R (eds.). *Bone Marrow Diagnosis: An Illustrated Guide*, 2nd edn. Chichester: Wiley-Blackwell; 2006.

5. Bain BJ, Clark DM, Wilkins BS. *Bone Marrow Pathology*, 4th edn. Oxford: Wiley-Blackwell; 2010.

6. Barnes PW, McFadden SL, Machin SJ, Simson E. The international consensus group for hematology review: suggested criteria for action following automated CBC and WBC differential analysis. *Lab Hematol* 2005;**11**(2):83–90.

7. Briggs C, Longair I, Slavik M *et al.* Can automated blood film analysis replace the manual differential? An evaluation of the CellaVision DM96 automated image analysis system. *Int J Lab Hematol* 2009;**31**(1):48–60.

8. Simson E, Gascon-Lema MG, Brown DL. Performance of automated slidemakers and stainers in a working laboratory environment – routine operation and quality control. *Int J Lab Hematol* 2010;**32**(1 Pt 1):e64–76.

9. Lee SH, Erber WN, Porwit A, Tomonaga M, Peterson LC. ICSH guidelines for the standardization of bone marrow specimens and reports. *Int J Lab Hematol* 2008;**30**(5):349–64.

10. Bain BJ. Bone marrow aspiration. *J Clin Pathol* 2001;**54**(9):657–63.

11. Bain BJ. Bone marrow trephine biopsy. *J Clin Pathol* 2001;**54**(10):737–42.

12. Fend F, Tzankov A, Bink K *et al.* Modern techniques for the diagnostic evaluation of the trephine bone marrow biopsy: methodological aspects and applications. *Prog Histochem Cytochem* 2008;**42**(4):203–52.

13. Scott CS (ed.). *Leukaemia Cytochemistry and Diagnosis: Principles and Practice*. Chichester: Ellis Horwood; 1989.

14. Hayhoe FGJ, Quaglino D (eds.). *Haematological Cytochemistry*, 3rd edn. London: Churchill Livingstone; 1994.

15. Orazi A, O'Malley DP., Arber DA (eds.). *Illustrated Pathology of the Bone Marrow*. Cambridge: Cambridge University Press; 2006.

16. Brunning R, McKenna RW (eds.). *Tumors of the Bone Marrow, Atlas of Tumor Pathology*, 3rd series. Washington, DC: Armed Forces Institute of Pathology; 1994.

17. Torlakovic EE, Naresh K, Kremer M, van der Walt J, Hyjek E, Porwit A. Call for a European programme in external quality assurance for bone marrow immunohistochemistry; report of a European Bone Marrow Working Group pilot study. *J Clin Pathol* 2009;**62**(6):547–51.

18. Frisch B, Bartl R (eds.). *Biopsy Interpretation of Bone and Bone Marrow*. London: Edward Arnold; 1999.

19. Gatter KC, Heryet A, Brown DC, Mason DY. Is it necessary to embed bone marrow biopsies in plastic for haematological diagnosis? *Histopathology* 1987;**11**(1):1–7.

20. Thiele J, Kvasnicka HM, Facchetti F *et al.* European consensus on grading bone marrow fibrosis and assessment of cellularity. *Haematologica* 2005;**90**(8):1128–32.

21. Peterson LC, Agosti SJ, Hoyer JD. Protocol for the examination of specimens from patients with hematopoietic neoplasms of the bone marrow: a basis for checklists. *Arch Pathol Lab Med* 2002;**126**(9):1050–6.

22. Cheson BD, Bennett JM, Kopecky KJ *et al.* Revised recommendations of the International Working Group for Diagnosis, Standardization of Response Criteria, Treatment Outcomes, and Reporting Standards for Therapeutic Trials in Acute Myeloid Leukemia. *J Clin Oncol* 2003;**21**(24):4642–9.

23. de Greef GE, van Putten WL, Boogaerts M *et al.* Criteria for defining a complete remission in acute myeloid leukaemia revisited. An analysis of patients treated in HOVON-SAKK co-operative group studies. *Br J Haematol* 2005;**128**(2):184–91.

24. Durie BG, Harousseau JL, Miguel JS *et al.* International uniform response criteria for multiple myeloma. *Leukemia* 2006;**20**(9):1467–73.

25. Kyle RA, Rajkumar SV. Criteria for diagnosis, staging, risk stratification and response assessment of multiple myeloma. *Leukemia* 2009;**23**(1):3–9.

26. Dirnhofer S, Went P, Tichelli A. Diagnostic problems in follow-up bone marrow biopsies of patients treated for acute and chronic leukaemias and MDS. *Pathobiology* 2007;**74**(2):115–20.

27. Raynaud P, Caulet-Maugendre S, Foussard C *et al.* T-cell lymphoid aggregates in bone marrow after rituximab therapy for B-cell follicular lymphoma: a marker of therapeutic efficacy? *Hum Pathol* 2008;**39**(2):194–200.

28. Kim DH, Kamel-Reid S, Chang H *et al.* Natural killer or natural killer/T cell lineage large granular lymphocytosis associated with dasatinib therapy for

Philadelphia chromosome positive leukemia. *Haematologica* 2009;**94**(1):135–9.

29. Mustjoki S, Ekblom M, Arstila TP *et al.* Clonal expansion of T/NK-cells during tyrosine kinase inhibitor dasatinib therapy. *Leukemia* 2009;**23**(8):1398–405.

30. Rimsza LM, Larson RS, Winter SS *et al.* Benign hematogone-rich lymphoid proliferations can be distinguished from B-lineage acute lymphoblastic leukemia by integration of morphology, immunophenotype, adhesion molecule expression, and architectural features. *Am J Clin Pathol* 2000;**114**(1):66–75.

Immunocytochemistry

Wendy N. Erber

Immunocytochemistry, or immunohistochemistry, is the method by which antibodies are used to detect cellular antigens in clinical samples. This can be performed on all routine diagnostic samples, including blood and bone marrow smears and bone marrow trephine (BMT) biopsies, in the assessment of hematological malignancies. The methodology enables simultaneous assessment of antigen expression and cell morphology so that cells of interest can be identified by their appearance and their phenotype determined. The major role of immunocytochemistry is in the diagnosis and classification of hematological malignancies, but it also has applications in lymphoma staging, determining prognosis, detecting potential immuno-therapeutic targets and for disease monitoring. Immunocytochemistry is used routinely to determine the phenotype (lineage and stage of differentiation) of neoplastic cells and is essential for the classification of hematological malignancies according to WHO criteria. This chapter describes the principles and applications of immunocytochemistry in the analysis of hematological malignancies. It includes discussion of monoclonal antibodies, hematopoietic differentiation and technical considerations, and illustrates some applications with clinical examples.

Monoclonal antibodies

The majority of antibodies used in immunocytochemistry are monoclonal antibodies. These were first generated in 1975 by fusing an immortal myeloma cell line with splenic B-cells from an animal immunized with the desired antigen [1]. The resulting hybridoma (or hybrid cell) produces antibodies with unique heavy and light chains and hence binding site. They are therefore clonal, have a single specificity and are termed "monoclonal" antibodies. Many thousands of monoclonal antibodies are available covering a wide range of cellular antigens. "Polyclonal" antibodies, in contrast, are obtained from the serum of an animal that has been immunized with antigen and therefore consist of a mixture of immunoglobulins. Each polyclonal antibody has a range of specificities. In general, monoclonal antibodies are preferred to polyclonals for immunocytochemistry because of their greater specificity and lower level of non-specific background staining.

Hybridoma technology was such a significant breakthrough that by 1980 large numbers of monoclonal antibodies had been produced. These were initially named by the laboratory that developed them. It soon became clear that complex and internationally accepted standardized terminology was required to enable direct comparisons to be made between antibody clones. In 1981 the CD Nomenclature was introduced for antibodies to leukocyte differentiation-associated antigens. A CD or "cluster of differentiation" number refers to a group of monoclonal antibodies that recognize the same cellular antigen. Antibodies of the same CD cluster may however recognize different epitopes of the antigen (i.e. antigenic determinants) and consequently, antibodies with the same CD number may have slightly different reactivity patterns. There are now 350 CD numbers and many antibodies of these clusters have a role in the analysis of hematological malignancies [2].

Hematopoietic cell differentiation and antigen expression

The availability of monoclonal antibodies to leukocyte differentiation antigens has led to an explosion in our knowledge and understanding of normal hematopoietic cell differentiation. Through this we have learned that the antigenic profile of the majority of

---

Diagnostic Techniques in Hematological Malignancies, ed. Wendy N. Erber. Published by Cambridge University Press.
© Cambridge University Press 2010.

the malignancies mimics that of the normal equivalent cell. This phenotypic association between normal and malignant cells is the guiding principle of the WHO classification; it uses the antigen profile to classify neoplasms by cell lineage and their stage of differentiation [3]. As a consequence, knowledge of normal antigen expression during hematopoiesis is required so that informed decisions can be made about appropriate antibodies to be utilized in the asessment of hematological malignancies. A brief description follows of normal antigen expression during differentiation of B-cells, T-cells, natural killer cells and myeloid cells.

B-cell differentiation

Normal B-cells differentiate in the bone marrow from B-lymphoid progenitor cells (B-lymphoblasts) to become mature circulating B-lymphocytes. During this maturation process they acquire and lose antigens in a sequential fashion (Figure 2.1) and rearrange their immunoglobulin heavy and light chain genes. As the antigenic profile of malignant B-cells tends to mirror that of their normal

B-cell counterpart, antibodies to B-lymphoid differentiation-associated antigens can be used to determine the stage of development of a B-cell neoplasm. Normal precursor or progenitor B-cells have an immature B-cell phenotype expressing TdT, CD10, CD19, CD22 (initially within the cytoplasm and then on the cell membrane), CD79a and PAX5 antigens, and commonly CD34 antigen; this is also the phenotype of B lymphoblastic leukemia/lymphoma. As the early B-cell matures, CD10 and TdT antigens are lost and immunoglobulin (IgM) and CD20 antigen are gained. A fully mature B-lymphocyte expresses a number of pan-B cell antigens (including CD19, CD20, CD22, CD79a and PAX5) in addition to surface IgM and IgD and either kappa or lambda light chains. In a B-cell proliferation, the identification of restricted light chain expression (κ:λ ≥ 4:1 or ≤ 1:3) is an indicator of B-cell clonality [4]. However, it should be noted that it is difficult to detect kappa and lambda light chains on the surface of B-cells in cell smears and bone marrow sections

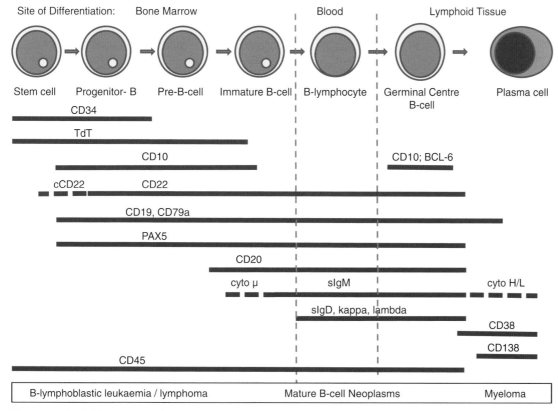

Figure 2.1. B-cell differentiation and antigen expression.

by immunocytochemistry due to the presence of plasma immunoglobulin causing background staining. Light chain analysis is more amenable to flow cytometry. When a naive mature B-cell is exposed to antigen in lymphoid tissue and undergoes transformation and proliferation to become a memory B-cell, other antigens are acquired. Many of these are useful in the diagnosis and classification of mature B-cell neoplasms, e.g. CD5 and CD23 in chronic lymphocytic leukemia, and BCL-6 in follicular lymphoma. Fully mature end-stage plasma cells have a different antigenic profile from mature B-cells, having lost pan-B-cell associated antigens CD20 and CD22, leukocyte common antigen CD45 and surface immunoglobulins, and acquired CD38, CD138 and MUM1 antigens and cytoplasmic immunoglobulin (heavy and light chains). CD19 antigen is expressed by normal plasma cells but is generally absent from neoplastic plasma cells.

T-cell differentiation

T-cell development occurs in the thymus with orderly acquisition of T-cell associated antigens and sequential rearrangement of the T-cell receptor α, β, γ and δ genes (Figure 2.2). Early thymocytes express CD3 (cytoplasmic), CD7 antigen (membrane) and TdT (nuclear) as well as CD45. Other T-cell associated antigens are acquired during further differentiation (cortical or intermediate thymocyte), specifically CD1a, CD2 and CD5, and both CD4 and CD8 antigens. CD3 is expressed on the cell membrane late in T-cell maturation (mature thymocyte) at the time of commitment to a helper/inducer CD4-positive T-cell or a suppressor/cytotoxic CD8 T-cell. The fully mature T-cell loses TdT, leaves the thymus and becomes a mature functional T-lymphocyte. The majority of mature T-cells express the αβ-T-cell receptor (TCR) and only 2% the γδ-TCR. The phenotypes of T-cell

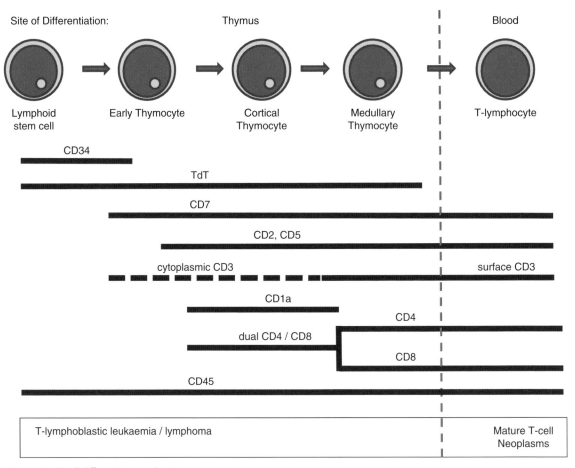

Figure 2.2. T-cell differentiation and antigen expression.

malignancies generally mimic these stages of T-cell development. T-cell clonality cannot be directly determined by phenotyping, but there are some useful phenotypic features that can be used as surrogate markers and which infer neoplasia, i.e.:

1. Aberrant loss of one or more T-cell antigen relative to normal T-cell populations, typically CD3, CD5 or CD7 antigens.
2. T-cell subset antigen restriction (i.e. restricted CD4 or CD8) or predominance of either CD4 or CD8 expressing T-cells.
3. Dual-positive or dual-negative CD4 and CD8 expression.
4. Loss or reduced intensity of CD45 expression.
5. Restricted T-cell receptor γδ-positive T-cells (rather than TCR αβ).
6. Restricted expression of the T-cell receptor β chain variable regions (Vβ repertoire) as each T-cell expresses only one of a restricted number of Vβ chains.
7. Expression of additional or aberrant antigens not expressed by normal T-cells (e.g. CD20, CD30).

Natural-killer cells

Natural-killer (NK) cells are derived from committed lymphoid progenitor cells in the bone marrow and express NK-cell-associated antigens CD16, CD56, CD57 and the killer-inducer receptor (KIR) CD158 antigen. There are a number of CD158 isoforms and restricted expression of one of these, or total lack of KIR antigens, are surrogates for NK-cell clonality (see Chapter 10) [5,6]. T-cell-associated CD2 and CD7 antigens, and both the ε and δ chains of the CD3 molecule, are also expressed by NK-cells. Surface CD3 is not expressed by NK-cells and the T-cell receptor is in germline configuration, enabling NK-cells to be distinguished from T-cells by both phenotype and genotype.

Myeloid differentiation and antigen expression

Myeloid cells undergo maturation within the bone marrow from the common myeloid progenitor (CD34, CD38 and HLA-DR positive) to fully mature end-stage cells of erythroid, granulocytic, monocytic and megakaryocytic lineages (Figure 2.3). As maturation proceeds, the differentiating cells lose CD34 and CD38 antigens and acquire lineage-associated antigens. CD13 and CD33 are the most ubiquitously expressed myeloid-associated antigens through myeloid differentiation to mature neutrophils and monocytes. Other antigens have more restricted expression and can be used to sub-classify cells of myeloid lineage, as follows:

1. Myeloid/granulocytic: CD15, CD65, myeloperoxidase (MPO), neutrophil elastase.
2. Monocyte: CD14, CD68, CD163 and lysozyme.
3. Erythroid: CD235a (glycophorin), hemoglobin A.
4. Megakaryocyte: CD31, CD41, CD42, CD61, Factor VIII-related antigen.

The phenotype of myeloid cell neoplasms, in general, reflects the normal counterpart, in a manner similar to lymphoid cells.

Antibodies for immunocytochemistry

There is an extensive range of diagnostically useful monoclonal antibodies available for the immunocytochemical analysis of hematological malignancies of both lymphoid and myeloid origin. These may be:

1. *Lineage-restricted*: antibodies that identify antigens that are restricted or specific to one lineage (e.g. Ig; TCR; myeloperoxidase; CD138).
2. *Lineage-associated*: antibodies to antigens associated with one lineage but which also react with others (e.g. CD7, CD11c, CD56).
3. *Differentiation stage-associated*: antibodies to antigens expressed at limited stages of hematopoietic cell differentiation (e.g. CD34; TdT).
4. *Pan-leukocyte*: e.g. leukocyte common antigen CD45.
5. Antibodies that recognize non-lineage-associated cellular components (e.g. sub-cellular organelles, cytoskeletal proteins or cell signaling molecules), cell cycle antigens (e.g. Ki67), apoptosis-related molecules and oncogenes.

In the majority of diagnostic settings a panel of antibodies is required as there are few, if any, disease-specific antigens. Antibodies that recognize lineage-restricted or associated antigens can be used to determine the lineage of a neoplasm (Table 2.1). Other antibodies are used to assess the stage of cell differentiation (e.g. CD34, TdT). Some malignant hematopoietic cells have inappropriate

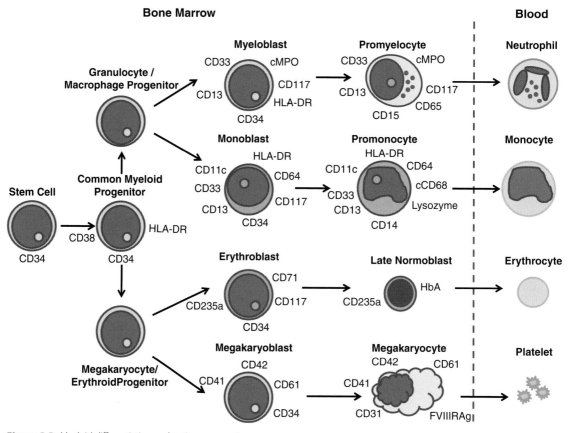

Figure 2.3. Myeloid differentiation and antigen expression.

expression of normal cellular antigens such that phenotyping can discriminate between normal and neoplastic cells. This includes aberrant loss of antigens expressed by a normal cell of that lineage or the acquisition of antigens not normally associated with that lineage ("lineage infidelity"). These aberrant phenotypes can support the diagnosis of malignancy without evidence of clonality.

The hematologist or pathologist must determine which of the enormous number of antibodies available to include in an immunocytochemistry panel when analyzing an individual case. This will depend on [7,8]:

1. The morphology of the cell population being analyzed.
2. The pattern of bone marrow infiltration.
3. The provisional diagnosis.
4. Antibodies which will discriminate between disorders.

5. The clinical question being asked, i.e. diagnosis, staging, monitoring, prognosis or detecting a potential therapeutic target.
6. Whether the phenotype of the abnormal population is already known, e.g. from flow cytometry or the phenotype from the primary tissue site (e.g. lymph node).
7. Sample type being analyzed (i.e. blood or bone marrow smears or fixed BMT biopsy).

Standard panels can be devised to cover common diagnostic problems, such as small lymphocytic or blast cell infiltrates. These panels can be formulated to address cell lineage, stage of differentiation and be able to identify disease-associated antigenic profiles. Both very large and extremely small focused panels should be avoided as these can be misleading. A structured two-panel approach is commonly utilized, especially for BMTs, as follows:

Table 2.1. Antibodies that recognize normal hematopoietic cells (see also Figures 2.1–2.3).

Lineage	Differentiation stage	Antibody
Leukocyte common	Leukocyte common antigen	CD45
	Hematopoietic stem cells	CD34, CD38
B-cells	Precursor B-cells	CD10, CD19, CD22, CD34, CD79a,b, PAX5, HLA-DR, TdT
	Mature B-cells	CD19, CD20, CD22, CD79a,b, PAX5, Igμ, Igδ, kappa, lambda, HLA-DR
	Germinal center B-cells	CD10, BCL-6
	Mantle zone B-cells	CD5, CD23
	Plasma cells	CD19, CD38, CD138, VS38c, cytoplasmic kappa / lambda, MUM1, PAX5
T-cells	Precursor T-cells	CD1a, CD2, cCD3, CD4, CD5, CD7, CD8, CD34, CD99 TdT
	Mature T-cells	CD2, CD3, CD4, CD5, CD7, CD8, CD43, CD45RO, TCRαβ, TCRγδ
NK-cells		CD2, CD7, CD8, CD16, CD56, CD57, CD158
Myeloid cells	Myeloid precursors	CD13, CD33, CD34, CD38, CD117, MPO, neutrophil elastase, HLA-DR
	Mature granulocytes	CD11c, CD13, CD15, CD16, CD33, MPO, neutrophil elastase
	Mature monocytes/macrophages	CD4, CD11c, CD13, CD14, CD33, CD64, CD68, CD163, lysozyme, HLA-DR
	Eosinophils	CD9, CD68
	Basophils	CD9, CD68
	Mast cells	CD9, CD68, CD117, mast cell tryptase
Erythroid cells	Proerythroblasts	CD71, CD235a
	Late normoblasts	CD235a, hemoglobin A
Megakaryocytes	Megakaryoblasts	CD41, CD42, CD61
	Mature megakaryocytes	CD31, CD41, CD42, CD61, Factor VIII-related antigen

1. A primary comprehensive antibody panel to determine the cell lineage and stage of differentiation, and,
2. A more focused secondary panel to distinguish between entities to reach a definitive classification.

This two-panel approach, which is also commonly utilized in flow cytometry (see Chapter 3), averts the need for a large number of possibly inappropriate antibodies being used up-front. Tables 2.2 and 2.3 give examples of this two-panel approach for blast or immature cell proliferations and small lymphocytic infiltrates, respectively. Although practical, strategy is not universally applicable, and especially not for unusual or atypical cases where individualized antibody panels are commonly required. Details of the phenotypes of specific malignancies will not be discussed here but are described in Chapters 7–15 in Section 2.

Immunocytochemical techniques

Immunocytochemical techniques are used to determine whether the antibody that has been applied to a sample has bound to cellular antigen. The antigen–antibody reaction is visualized by the use of a "label,"

such as a fluorescent dye or enzyme, which is linked to the antibody. This technology dates back to 1941 when Albert Coons first demonstrated the use of a fluorescently labeled antibody to localize cellular antigens in tissue sections [9]. This immunofluorescent method became widely used on fresh frozen tissue sections in the 1950s, and in the 1970s began to be used for leukemia diagnosis. However, because of the requirements for fluorescent microscopy this was not applicable to routine diagnostic laboratories. Staining techniques utilizing enzyme labels such, as horseradish peroxidase and alkaline phosphatase, were subsequently developed in the 1970s and 1980s and largely replaced fluorescence as the label of choice. Immunoenzyme methods are now used routinely in diagnostic haemato-pathology [10,11].

Antibody labels

Fluorescent labels

Immunofluorescent labeling is now only used in a few applications (see below). The most commonly used fluorescent labels (fluorochromes) are fluorescein

Table 2.2. Example of two-panel approach for the investigation of a blast cell or immature cell bone marrow infiltrate.

				Blast or immature cells			
1° Panel			CD3, CD7, CD10, CD19/PAX5, CD34, CD45, CD117, Myeloperoxidase, TdT				
	B-cell CD45 + CD19 / PAX5 + CD10 +/−			**T-cell** CD45 + CD3 + CD7 + TdT + CD10 −/+ CD34 −/+	**Myeloid** CD45 + CD117 + Myeloperoxidase +/− CD34 +/−	**Plasma cell** CD45 − CD19 − PAX5 −/+	**Non-hemato-poietic** CD45 − All −
	TdT+ and/or CD34 +	TdT − and CD34 −					
2° Panel (based on results of 1° Panel)	CD20 CD79a	CD20 BCL-6 Cyclin D1 Ki67		CD1a CD2 CD4 CD5 CD8	CD11c CD15 CD33 CD61 CD68 CD235	CD38 CD56 CD138 Kappa Lambda	Cytokeratin CD56
Diagnosis/ differential diagnosis	B-lymphoblastic leukemia/ lymphoma	Mantle cell lymphoma, blastoid variant Diffuse large B-cell lymphoma Burkitt lymphoma		T-lymphoblastic leukemia / lymphoma	Acute myeloid leukemia and subtypes	Anaplastic myeloma	Metastatic malignancy

Table 2.3. Example of two-panel approach for the assessment of small lymphocytic infiltrates in bone marrow.

					Small lymphocytic infiltrate		
1° Panel				CD2, CD3, CD5, CD10, CD19/PAX5, CD20			
			B-cell CD19 / PAX5 + CD20 +			**T-cell** CD2 + CD3 + CD5 +	**NK-cell** CD2 + CD3 − CD5 −
	CD5 +	CD5 − / CD10 +	CD5 − / CD10 −				
2° Panel (based on results of 1° Panel)	CD23 Cyclin D1	BCL-2 BCL-6	BCL-6 CD11c CD123			CD4 CD7 CD8 CD30 TCR αβ TCR γδ	CD8 CD16 CD56 CD57
Diagnosis/differential diagnosis	Chronic lymphocytic leukemia Mantle cell lymphoma	Follicular lymphoma	Hairy cell leukemia Extranodal marginal zone lymphoma Other B-cell non-Hodgkin lymphoma			Mature T-cell neoplasm	Mature NK-cell neoplasm

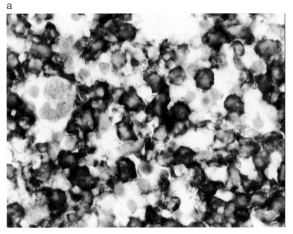

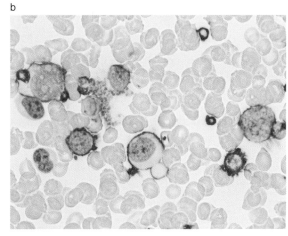

Figure 2.4. Examples of immunocytochemical staining.
a. Immuno-peroxidase staining of a bone marrow trephine of hairy cell leukemia stained with CD11c (DAB substrate).
b. Immuno-alkaline phosphatase staining of a blood smear of acute megakaryoblastic leukemia stained with CD61 antibody (Fast red substrate).

isothiocyanate (FITC), rhodamine and Texas red. The fluorescent compound is the label which is deposited at the site of antigen expression when antibody is bound. Cells or tissue are counterstained, commonly with 4',6-diamidino-2-phenylindole (DAPI) or propidium iodide which bind to DNA, to enable cell nuclei to be visualized. Antigen labeling and cell nuclei are viewed with a fluorescent microscope. The *advantages* of immunofluorescent staining are:

1. Sub-cellular localization of an antigen can be detected (e.g. membrane, nuclear, nucleolar, organelle).
2. Multiple antigens can be detected on a single cell when antibodies with different fluorochromes are used and in association with appropriate analytical filter combinations.
3. Immunofluorescent labeling can be combined with fluorescence *in situ* hybridization (FISH) in the FICTION (Fluorescence Immunophenotyping and Interphase Cytogenetics as a Tool for the Investigation of Neoplasms) method [12,13].

The major *disadvantages* of immunofluorescent labeling are:

1. The requirement for a fluorescent microscope.
2. Cell and tissue morphology cannot be easily visualized.
3. The staining reaction is not permanent and must be recorded photographically.
4. Background auto-fluorescence of the sample can interfere with interpretation.

5. Hematologists and pathologists are not familiar with fluorescent microscopy.

Despite these limitations, there are some specific applications where immunofluorescent staining is the most appropriate test (see below: PML protein).

Enzyme labels

Horseradish peroxidase and alkaline phosphatase are the most common enzyme labels used in immunocytochemistry. Presence of the enzyme, which is detected by the application of a chromogenic substrate, indicates that antigen–antibody binding has occurred. Bound enzyme catalyzes the substrate to produce a color reaction and this is identifiable by light microscopy. Presence of the color deposit therefore indicates expression of the antigen in question. Both peroxidase and alkaline phosphatase enzymes occur naturally in hematopoietic cells. Any endogenous enzyme activity present in the sample must be blocked to avoid non-specific or background staining which could otherwise interfere with the interpretation of true positive staining.

Horseradish peroxidase: Immuno-peroxidase techniques utilize horseradish peroxidase as the enzyme label [10]. The high levels of endogenous peroxidase activity in hematopoietic cells (especially erythroid cells, neutrophils and eosinophils) must be blocked, commonly by pre-treatment with hydrogen peroxide, to prevent non-specific staining. The most commonly used chromogenic substrate is 3,3'-diaminobenzidine (DAB), which generates a brown color reaction (Figure 2.4a). The intensity of this reaction product

Table 2.4. Outline of immunoenzyme labeling procedures.

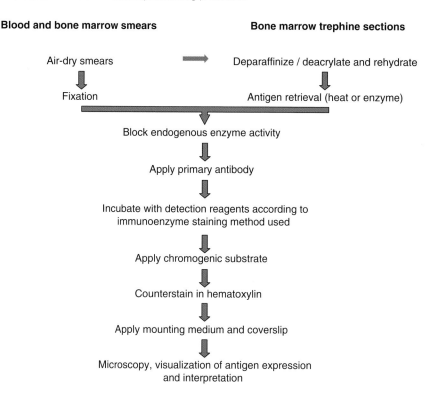

can be enhanced by the addition of cobalt chloride, nickel sulfate or copper sulfate to the DAB substrate.

Alkaline phosphatase: Immuno-alkaline phosphatase techniques were developed in the 1980s and use calf intestinal alkaline phosphatase as the enzyme label [11]. Endogenous alkaline phosphatase is present in neutrophils but as this survives poorly in fixed tissue and cell smears it rarely causes problems of non-specific background staining. However any residual endogenous enzyme activity can be selectively inhibited by levamisole without interfering with the alkaline phosphatase enzyme label. This ability to completely block endogenous enzymatic activity makes immuno-alkaline phosphatase methods preferable to peroxidase-based techniques for hematological samples and particularly blood and bone marrow smears. The chromogenic substrate for alkaline phosphatase methods utilizes naphthol-phosphate and a dye, most commonly Fast red or new fuchsin. These generate a vivid red reaction product and provide clear contrast from negative cells and

background erythrocytes in blood and bone marrow (Figure 2.4b).

Technical aspects of immunocytochemistry

A number of immunocytochemical techniques are available and in common use. These vary in their complexity and sensitivity (Table 2.4 and Figure 2.5). *Direct method*: This is a simple, rapid but insensitive one-step method that uses a directly labeled primary antibody (i.e. the label is directly conjugated to the primary antibody). This is rarely used for immunocytochemistry but is the most common technique for flow cytometry (see Chapter 3).

Indirect method: This is a two-step procedure that uses an unlabeled primary antibody (yellow) followed by a labeled secondary antibody (red) (Figure 2.5a). The secondary antibody is directed against the immunoglobulin of the animal species in which the first antibody was raised and has the label (red circle) directly conjugated to it. For example, a primary

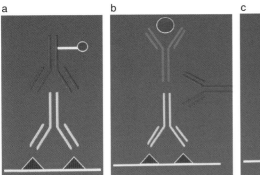
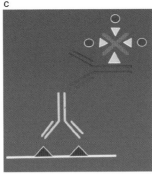

Figure 2.5. Immunocytochemical techniques (see text for explanation).
a. Indirect method.
b. Unlabeled "antibody bridge" method.
c. Avidin-biotin Complex (ABC) method.

mouse anti-human CD3 antibody is followed by a labeled anti-mouse immunoglobulin raised in another species such as rabbit or goat. This method is more sensitive than the "direct" method because several secondary antibodies bind to different antigenic sites on the primary antibody. This results in a greater number of labels and therefore increased signal intensity. Further amplification can be achieved with a three-stage indirect method: the two-stage method is performed followed by a third stage, consisting of a labeled antibody directed against the second antibody. Again, signal amplification is achieved by the greater number of labels.

Polymer methods: Polymer-based methods are very simple and sensitive two-stage procedures. The secondary antibody is conjugated with a large number of enzyme molecules attached to a polymer backbone (e.g. dextran or other macromolecule). This increase in the number of enzyme labels amplifies the signal intensity.

Unlabeled antibody bridge method: This is a 3-stage method whereby the primary antibody is applied, followed by an anti-species antibody which is added in excess. The third stage is immune complexes formed between an enzyme (the "label") and its anti-enzyme antibody (blue-Figure 2.5b). The anti-enzyme antibody is of the same species as the primary antibody. Hence both the primary antibody and the anti-enzyme antibody are bound to the second layer, the unlabeled "antibody bridge." This can be performed with peroxidase (peroxidase anti-peroxidase or "PAP") and alkaline phosphatase (alkaline phosphatase anti-alkaline phosphatase or "APAAP") as the enzyme label [10,11,14]. These are reported to be 100–1000 times more sensitive than the two-stage indirect method.

Avidin-biotin complex (ABC) methods: This is a sensitive staining method that uses avidin (greenX), a large glycoprotein extracted from egg white, and biotin (yellow triangle) with which it has high affinity. In the ABC method, the primary antibody is applied, followed by a biotinylated (i.e. biotin-conjugated) secondary antibody (Figure 2.5c). The third layer is an avidin-biotin complex labeled with an enzyme. Background staining can be a problem due to:

1. Non-specific binding of avidin to tissue lectins: this can be reduced by replacing avidin with streptavidin.
2. Endogenous biotin which is present in many cells and exposed by antigen retrieval (see below).

Regardless of which of these techniques is used, the chromogenic substrate must be applied on completion of the immunocytochemical procedure. The sample is then counterstained, most commonly with hematoxylin. This gives a blue nuclear counterstain which is distinct from the red or brown substrate reaction product and enables cell identification. A coverslip is then applied to allow light microscopy review. The stained slide can be stored permanently and reviewed at a later date.

Double and triple staining

Double and triple immunocytochemical staining can be performed to detect antigens on more than one cell population (e.g. T-cells and B-cells) in a specimen. With immuno-enzyme methods, this is usually performed by sequential application of immuno-peroxidase and immuno-alkaline phosphatase methods. The chromogen for each must be carefully chosen to ensure maximal discrimination between the colors for the two antigen labels. Detection of two antigens on the same cell is much more difficult to interpret because of the problem in discriminating mixed colors. Practically this can only be achieved when the antigens are present in different cellular compartments (e.g. surface membrane and nuclear); it is virtually impossible to interpret when both antigens are in the same part of the cell. For these applications immuno-fluorescent methods are preferable.

Samples

Cell smears: Immunocytochemistry can be performed on directly prepared air-dried cell smears or cytocentrifuged preparations of blood, bone marrow, fine needle aspirates or body fluids (e.g. cerebrospinal fluid, pleural fluid). The smears can be retained at room temperature for up to 7 days without any loss of cellular antigens; alternatively the slides can be wrapped and stored at −20 °C, indefinitely, without loss of immuno-reactivity. Prior to application of the primary antibody, the smears must be at room temperature. They are then fixed to stabilize antigens and enable antibodies to access intracellular (as well as surface membrane) antigens. A variety of fixatives can be used and these have different effects on morphology and antigen expression. A compromise must be reached between optimizing antigen expression without distorting morphology; the preferred fixative is a combination of acetone, methanol and formalin [14]. Following fixation, endogenous enzyme activity is blocked and then the immuno-enzymatic staining procedure performed, as described above and detailed in Table 2.4 [14]. Despite the applicability of immunocytochemical stains to cell smears, in general, flow cytometry is the preferred method for analysing blood and bone marrow aspirates. This is because of the ability to analyze large numbers of cells rapidly and assess the expression of multiple antigens simultaneously. However, there are some situations where immunocytochemical staining of cell smears is preferable. The advantages and disadvantages of the two approaches are listed in Table 2.5.

Bone marrow trephines: Immunocytochemistry of BMT biopsy specimens is a widely used routine diagnostic procedure. However development of this technology for BMT had lagged behind cell smears and other tissue specimens. This was because of concerns that sample processing, especially decalcification and plastic embedding in methyl-methacrylate, had destroyed, denatured or "masked" cellular antigens,

preventing their binding by antibodies. These technical issues have now been overcome by:

1. Development of antibodies raised against epitopes that survive tissue processing.
2. Improvements in bone marrow decalcification, reducing the denaturation of antigens.
3. Improvements in antigen retrieval (see below).
4. Development of highly sensitive immunocytochemical detection methods, as described above.

As a result, immunocytochemistry can now be performed on both formalin-fixed, decalcified paraffin-embedded and plastic (methyl-methacrylate)-embedded BMT biopsies, yielding excellent results [15]. The procedure for immunocytochemistry of BMT biopsies is as follows. Sections of 1–4 μm thickness are cut on a microtome and placed onto 3-aminopropyl methoxysilane (APES) coated slides, to aid adhesion. Paraffin sections are dewaxed, and plastic sections deacrylated, and then rehydrated prior to antigen retrieval. Antigen retrieval is the method by which antigens that may have been "masked" or modified during fixation, decalcification or embedding of the bone marrow trephine can be "recovered." Two main methods are used [16]:

1. *Enzyme digestion*: Proteolytic enzymes such as proteinase K, protease, pepsin or pronase are used to restore immuno-reactivity. Enzyme digestion is time-dependent, with under-digestion resulting in poor antigen exposure, and, over-digestion destroying some epitopes and resulting in poor morphology.
2. *Heat-induced antigen (epitope) retrieval*: Heating tissue sections in a microwave oven, pressure cooker, steamer, waterbath or autoclave in a buffer solution (e.g. citrate, Tris; pH from 3–10) to expose masked tissue antigens [17]. Heat-induced antigen retrieval is, in general, more reliable than enzyme digestion, increases the intensity of immuno-staining and gives consistent high quality staining.

Following antigen retrieval, endogenous enzyme activity is blocked (as described above) and the primary antibody applied. Due to the above-mentioned technical advances, the range of antigens that can be assessed in BMTs is now virtually the same as for fresh cells and flow cytometry. However, care must be taken when selecting the antibody clone to be used. Different clones may be required for fixed tissue (i.e. BMT) from those

Table 2.5. Advantages and disadvantages of immunocytochemistry and flow cytometry.

	Immunocytochemistry	Flow cytometry
Hematological specimens	Air-dried smears of blood and bone marrow aspirate Formalin-fixed decalcified paraffin BMT specimens Resin-embedded BMT specimens	Fresh cells or tissue biopsy
Antibodies[*]	Air-dried smears: unlimited Paraffin sections: more limited Resin-embedded: fewer antibodies available	Unlimited
Morphology	Preservation of tissue architecture Direct morphological identification of cells	No direct morphological correlation
Cell types	All cell types can be analyzed	Unsuitable for fragile and large cells
Cell viability	Non-viable cells can be analyzed	Requires viable cells Loss of antigen viability with transport > 24 hours
Simultaneous detection of multiple antigens	Same cell: difficult to interpret Different cell populations: yes	Routine Multiple antigen analysis using multiple fluorochromes
B-cell clonality	Difficult to interpret due to background staining from plasma immunoglobulin	Light chain restriction
Quantify antigen density	No	Yes
Interpretation	Manual: subjective and semi-quantitative Automated analysis methods available	Objective and quantitative Depends on gating correct cell population
Value for rare cell analysis	Yes: cell identification by morphology and antigen expression	Requires knowledge of cell phenotype Large numbers of cells must be analyzed
Minimal residual disease assessment	Increased sensitivity over morphology alone	Routine especially if the neoplastic cells have a specific phenotype
Automation	Automated immunostainer Automated image capture analysis	Flow cytometer and software
Turn-around time	3 hours (usually performed after microscopy review)	< 3 hours
Permanent record	Yes: stained slides can be stored	Listmode analysis for re-analyzing data

[*] Some antibody clones are specific for fresh cells and others for formalin-fixed tissue.

used for fresh cells; this is because some antibodies can only detect formalin-resistant epitopes and vice versa. The immuno-enzymatic staining procedure performed is the same as for cell smears (Table 2.4).

Positive and negative controls

Both positive and negative controls should be included with all immunocytochemical analyses as this guarantees the quality of the procedure. Positive controls contain cells known to express the antigen under investigation and these should be fixed and processed using the same protocol as the test sample. Usually there are normal cells in the blood or marrow sample being analyzed that will show clear positive staining of the relevant antigen. These "internal" positive controls are the best indicator of the integrity of the antigen and the sample being studied. Absence of expected staining in the positive control means that the staining in the test sample cannot be interpreted. Normal bone marrow, normal tonsil or normal blood can also be used as positive controls.

A negative control is a slide in which either the primary antibody has been omitted or an irrelevant antibody, unreactive with hematopoietic cells, is substituted for the primary antibody. Any staining on the negative control indicates non-specific staining or endogenous enzyme activity which has been inadequately quenched. For most specimens there are internal negative control cells, i.e. cells that lack the antigen being assessed.

Interpretation of immunocytochemistry

Immunocytochemistry must be interpreted together with the cellular morphology, and for bone marrow trephines, the marrow architecture. The cells of interest are identified by their morphology and location and the presence (or absence) of the color reaction determines whether the antigen in question is expressed. Interpretation therefore requires:

1. Morphological expertise so that the correct population of cells is analyzed.
2. Knowledge of the antigens being assessed (i.e. cell expression pattern; sub-cellular localization).
3. Knowledge of the specificity of the antibodies that have been used.
4. The question being asked, e.g. cell lineage, diagnosis, prognosis, staging, residual disease or detection of a potential therapeutic target.

Some scenarios are straightforward, e.g. an antigen expressed (i.e. positive staining) by an abnormal cell population may be diagnostic, or, an immunocytochemical stain may positively identify neoplastic cells that are not visible on standard microscopy, e.g. Hodgkin cells. Other cases may be more difficult, e.g. equivocal staining patterns or the results of a panel of antibodies do not fit neatly into a diagnostic entity. These need careful consideration and may require a further panel of antibodies to resolve.

For some diseases there may be a need to enumerate positively stained cells, e.g. percent CD34-positive cells in myelodysplasia or CD138-positive plasma cells. For cell smears, counting the number of positive cells is generally straightforward and is analogous to performing a nucleated differential cell count. However cell enumeration is more difficult to perform on BMT sections with wide inter-observer variability. More accurate objective counts can be obtained with automated methods that use a digital camera and computer-assisted image analysis to quantify antigen-positive cells. This is more rapid, reliable and re-producible than semi-quantitative manual interpretation [18,19]. If the percent positive cells is to be used for clinical decision-making, standardized protocols should be used for sample preparation (fixation, decalcification, processing into paraffin), section thickness and the immunocytochemical procedure.

Pitfalls and limitations of immunocytochemistry

A number of technical or procedural problems can interfere with the quality of immunocytochemical staining and can potentially result in the incorrect interpretation of positive and negative staining reactions; common technical problems are listed in Table 2.6. The most common are smears or sections lifting from the slide, poor morphological preservation, background staining, no staining, weak staining and patchy staining.

Some limitations remain despite the enormous advances that have been made and the wide acceptability of immunocytochemistry in diagnostic practice. These include:

1. Relatively slow turn-around-time, especially for BMTs, if only performed after the morphology has been assessed.
2. The inability to detect more than one antigen on a cell, as can be achieved by flow cytometry.
3. The inability to quantify antigen expression, i.e. to discriminate weak from strong.
4. Limited sample size limits the number of antibodies that can be used.
5. The inability to detect surface membrane immunoglobulin and thereby assess clonality of B-cells due to background plasma immunoglobulin.

Standardization and automation

Immunocytochemical staining is a technically demanding, laborious, time-consuming procedure that is not currently standardized and lacks reproducibility between laboratories [20,21]. This lack of standardization is because of the many variables involved in the process, including tissue fixation (method and time), decalcification (reagent and time) and processing, antigen retrieval (method), choice of primary antibody, immunocytochemical detection method and the overall interpretation of staining. As increasing importance is being placed on immunocytochemistry results in the assessment of hematological malignancies, it is critical that there be better standardization of methodology and interpretation to ensure reproducibility. Approaches being used to address this are automated tissue processing, automated immunocytochemical staining, automated image analysis (as above) and external quality assurance programs. Automation of immunocytochemistry has been introduced, primarily to cope with workload, and shown to produce more reliable, reproducible, higher quality and standardized staining than manual methods [16]. These machines can perform the entire immunocytochemical process, including dewaxing of paraffin-embedded tissues, antigen retrieval, dilution and application of antibodies, applying the chromogenic substrate and counterstaining; automation is applicable to both tissue biopsies and cell smears [22].

Applications of immunocytochemistry to hematological malignancies

Immunocytochemistry has an established and critical role in the diagnosis and classification of hematological malignancies. It can also be used to provide considerable information regarding prognosis and disease staging, to detect antigens of potential therapeutic significance and to monitor residual disease (Table 2.7). Some illustrative examples are given.

Blood and bone marrow smears

Although the majority of cell phenotyping of blood and bone marrow aspirates is performed by flow cytometry, there are some specific situations where immunocytochemistry on cell smears is preferred:

1. Morphology is required to identify the cell in question.
2. Flow cytometry is unsuitable.
3. There is a need to assess antigen localization within the cell.
4. Combined phenotype and genotype analyses.

Table 2.6. Pitfalls in the interpretation of immunocytochemical staining.

Specimen	Staining defect	Cause
All specimen types (smears and sections)	Stain too weak or no staining	Antibody concentration too low Inadequate incubation time Specimen dried out during staining
	Stain too strong	Incorrect antibody concentration Incorrect incubation time
	Background staining (inter-cellular stain)	Incorrect antibody concentration Inadequate washing steps Endogenous enzyme activity Section or smear dried during staining Detecting cellular antigens that are present in high concentration in plasma (i.e. kappa and lambda light chains)
	Non-specific staining (false positive staining)	Incorrect antibody concentration Endogenous enzyme activity, i.e.: • Peroxidase methods: erythrocytes, eosinophils, mast cells • Alkaline phosphatase: neutrophils
	Unstained areas	Poor fixation Air bubbles in the applied solutions
Air-dried smears	No staining Non-specific neutrophil staining Poor morphology Smears lifted from the slide	Smears kept at room temperature for > 7 days Smears kept at room temperature for > 7 days Inadequate quenching of endogenous alkaline phosphatase Poor fixation, e.g. smears not air-dried adequately prior to fixation Smears not air-dried adequately prior to fixation Smears too thick (especially bone marrow) Fatty bone marrow aspirate sample
Bone marrow trephine biopsies	Poor tissue morphology	Poor fixation and/or decalcification Problems with antigen retrieval: incorrect time, pH or concentration
	Sections detached from slide	Excess antigen retrieval Sections not bound to slide surface
	Edge of section stain artefact	Incorrect tissue fixation time especially with small biopsies Non-specific staining of the edge of tissues with some mercury-based fixatives

Table 2.7. Applications of immunocytochemistry and clinical examples.

Application	Principles	Examples
Diagnosis and classification	Determine cell type	Lymphoid, myeloid or other
	Determine cell lineage	Lymphoid: T, B, NK-cell Myeloid: granulocytic, monocytic, erythroid or megakaryoblastic
	Determine stage of differentiation	Precursor or mature cell
	Detect disease-associated phenotype	Assist in differential diagnosis, e.g. small B-cell neoplasms • Chronic lymphocytic leukemia: CD5, CD23 • Hairy cell leukemia: CD11c, CD25, CD103, CD123
	Clonality assessment: restricted expression of molecules	Plasma cells: cytoplasmic kappa / lambda T cells: restricted CD4 / CD8 NK-cells: restricted CD158 isoforms
	Detect phenotype-genotype-association	PML-1 pattern in APML t(15;17); *PML-RARA* Cyclin D1 in mantle cell lymphoma t(11;14); *IgH-CCND1* CD10, TdT-negative in B-lymphoblastic leukemia with chromosome 11(q23); *MLL* abnormalities
	WHO-Classification	Determine by integration of phenotype with morphology and genetic data
Disease staging	Detect bone marrow involvement by lymphoma	Non-Hodgkin lymphoma Hodgkin lymphoma
Rare event analysis	Determine the phenotype of morphologically abnormal cells present in small numbers	Establish cell lineage and stage of differentiation
	Enumeration of cells based on phenotype	CD34-positive stem cells, e.g. myelodysplastic syndromes CD138-positive plasma cells, e.g. plasma cell myeloma
Detect potential immuno-therapeutic targets	Detect leukocyte surface antigens that may be targets for therapy	B-cell neoplasms: CD20, CD40, CD122 T-cell neoplasms: CD3, CD52 Acute myeloid leukemia: CD33 Anaplastic large cell lymphoma: CD30
Detect prognostic markers	Detect antigens associated with disease prognosis	Acute myeloid leukemia: cytoplasmic NPM Chronic lymphocytic leukemia: CD38, ZAP70, p53 Plasma cell myeloma: CD27, CD28, CD33
Minimal residual disease detection/monitoring therapeutic response	Detect disease associated or aberrant phenotype Detect small numbers of cells Localize cell clusters	Acute myeloid leukemia: monitor known blast cell phenotype Myelodysplastic syndromes: monitor CD34-positive cells Plasma cell myeloma: CD56, CD138, light chain restriction Follicular lymphoma: distinguish reactive from neoplastic lymphoid cells (e.g. paratrabecular infiltrates or nodules)
Assess bone marrow regeneration	Detect regenerating hematopoiesis	CD10, CD34, CD61, CD117, CD235, myeloperoxidase, TdT
Internal quality assurance	Utilize antibodies and immunocytochemistry to confirm morphological findings	All disorders and antibodies

Morphology is required to identify the cells of interest: Immunocytochemistry of cell smears is the preferred test when morphology is essential to identify the cells of interest and determine their phenotype, e.g.:

1. There are only few abnormal cells present in the sample.
2. The cells have a particular appearance requiring simultaneous visualization of morphology and

a

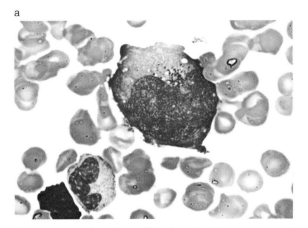

b

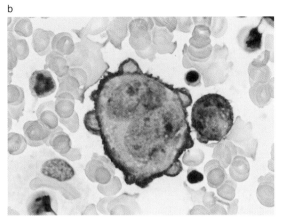

Figure 2.6. Anaplastic large cell lymphoma in a bone marrow aspirate.
a. Romanowsky stain showing a single large anaplastic cell with an eccentric indented nucleus and azurophilic cytoplasmic granules.
b. CD30 staining (APAAP method) showing the large neoplastic cell, which has the same morphological features as (a) and a smaller cell to be positive.

antigen expression, e.g. large anaplastic cells (Figure 2.6).

3. The cells of interest are present in clusters precluding analysis by flow cytometry.
4. The abnormal cells cannot be identified with certainty on flow cytometry. For example platelets can adhere to the surface of blast cells and, on flow cytometry, the phenotype can be misinterpreted as that of megakaryoblasts and give a false diagnosis. Immunocytochemistry averts this as there is morphological identification of the positive events (see Figure 2.4b).

Flow cytometry is unsuitable: There are situations when flow cytometry cannot be performed but air-dried smears are available which are suitable for immunocytochemical analysis. For example:

1. There is no or insufficient bone marrow aspirate sample available for flow cytometry, e.g. when a neoplasm was not a diagnostic consideration, but air-dried smears are available.
2. Presence of large abnormal cells in the sample which are unsuitable for flow cytometry.
3. Non-viable cells in the sample.
4. Technical reasons, e.g. availability of resource, appropriate antibodies, machine.

Cellular localization of antigen: Immunocytochemical staining of cell smears can be used to assess the cellular localization and pattern of an intracellular protein. For example, in acute myeloid leukemia

immunofluorescent staining of blood or bone marrow aspirate smears can be used to assess PML protein expression. A micro-granular speckled nuclear pattern resulting from disruption of PML bodies is a surrogate marker of the chromosomal translocation t(15;17); *PML-RARA* and can only be assessed by immunofluorescent staining (Figure 2.7) [23]. Flow cytometry is non-discriminatory in this situation and would yield a positive signal irrespective of the number and cellular distribution of PML bodies.

Combined phenotyping and genotyping: Phenotyping and genotyping can be integrated in a single analysis using FICTION (Fluorescence Immunophenotyping and interphase Cytogenetics as a Tool for the Investigation of Neoplasms). FICTION combines immuno fluorescent labeling and Interphase fluorescence *in situ* hybridization and can be performed on cell smears or bone marrow biopsy sections [24]. This integrated phenotypic–genotypic fluorescent method enables specific genetic abnormalities (e.g. gene translocations; numerical abnormalities) to be assessed in cells that have been identified by their phenotype. Figure 2.8 illustrates FICTION in a bone marrow aspirate of a case of multiple myeloma; CD138 reactivity identifies the plasma cells and FISH shows del(17p). FICTION has applications at diagnosis and for the assessment of residual disease post-therapy and can be performed on cell smears and tissue sections [12,13].

a

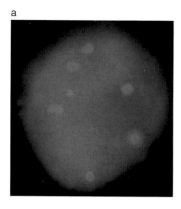

b

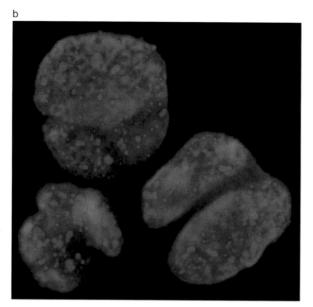

Figure 2.7. Immunofluorescent staining for PML protein using an anti-PML antibody and DAPI counterstain (blue).
a. Normal pattern with few large PML bodies in acute myeloid leukemia.
b. Abnormal micropunctate speckled pattern in acute promyelocytic leukemia.

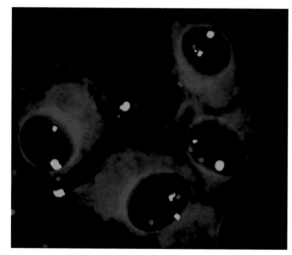

Figure 2.8. FICTION on a bone marrow smear of multiple myeloma. Immunofluorescence with CD138-Alexa Fluor 350 (blue surface antigen expression) identifies the plasma cells and interphase FISH with *TP53* (red; R) and chromosome 17 centromere (green; G) probes. Four CD138-positive plasma cells are present, two of which have a normal signal (2R2G pattern) and two with deletion of TP53 (1R2G).

Bone marrow trephines

Immunocytochemistry of the BMT is essential in the following situations:

1. Bone marrow is inaspirable.
2. Focal bone marrow lesions.
3. Lymphoma staging.

4. To meet specific WHO diagnostic criteria.
5. Only few abnormal cells are present in the marrow ("rare events").

In other situations, immunocytochemistry of the trephine biopsy may not be required as the cell phenotype may already be known from phenotyping (e.g. flow cytometry) of blood or the bone marrow aspirate. In these settings it can still be beneficial to have a baseline phenotype on the trephine biopsy which can subsequently be used to monitor disease following therapy. Illustrative examples of the role of BMT immunocytochemistry are given.

Inaspirable bone marrow: A BMT biopsy must be performed when bone marrow cannot be aspirated (a "dry tap"). This most commonly occurs due to marrow fibrosis, significant hypercellularity or because of technical issues. When marrow is inaspirable and an abnormal population is present, cell phenotyping must be performed on the trephine biopsy to reach a diagnosis. The antibodies to be used on the BMT will be analogous to those that would have been applied to the aspirate and flow cytometry to:

1. Determine the lineage, stage of differentiation and phenotype of an abnormal cell infiltrate (Figure 2.9). Appropriate antibodies should be

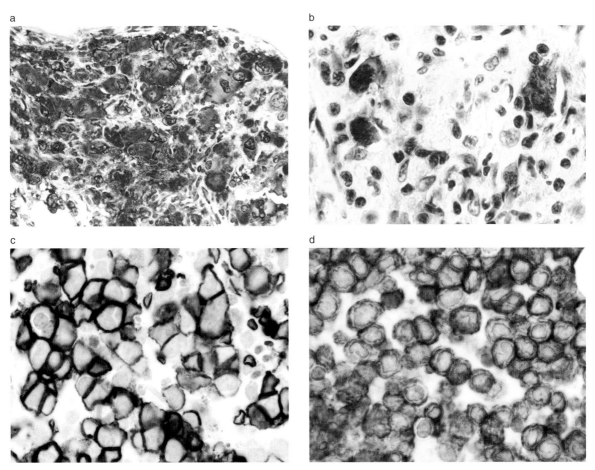

Figure 2.9. Immunocytochemistry of bone marrow trephine biopsies. In all cases illustrated bone marrow was inaspirable ("dry tap").
a. Acute megakaryoblastic leukemia stained with a CD61 antibody showing extensive bone marrow infiltration by neoplastic cells of megakaryocytic origin (immuno-alkaline phosphatase and Fast red).
b. Hodgkin lymphoma stained with CD30 antibody highlighting the neoplastic Hodgkin cells (immuno-alkaline phosphatase and Fast red).
c. Erythroleukemia (pure erythroid leukemia) stained with CD235 (glycophorin A) showing extensive bone marrow infiltration by blast cells of erythroid lineage (immuno-peroxidase and DAB).
d. Acute myeloid leukemia stained with CD33 showing the blast cells to be positive (immuno-peroxidase and DAB).

selected based on the marrow histology and cytological features. A non-hematopoietic malignancy should be considered if CD45 (leukocyte common antigen) is negative.
2. To enumerate antigen-positive cells, e.g. CD34-positive cells in primary myelofibrosis.

Focal bone marrow infiltrates: Focal bone marrow lesions may be paratrabecular, interstitial, intravascular or sinusoidal. The cells within these foci may be encased in a reticulin network and consequently aspirated bone marrow may not contain the abnormal cells and phenotypic analysis of the aspirate may be misleading. Immunocytochemistry of the bone marrow trephine is therefore the only method that can be used to characterize the cells within these focal cell infiltrates. This is demonstrated in Figure 2.10 which shows the role of immunocytochemistry in phenotyping the paratrabecular infiltrates of follicular lymphoma (Figure 2.10a, b) and systemic mastocytosis (Figure 2.10c, d). The antibodies to use will depend on the clinical history, marrow architecture, cytology of the cells within the focal lesions and whether it is a staging marrow (hence, known phenotype) or a diagnostic sample (unknown phenotype).

One of the most common and important questions that can be addressed is whether interstitial lymphoid

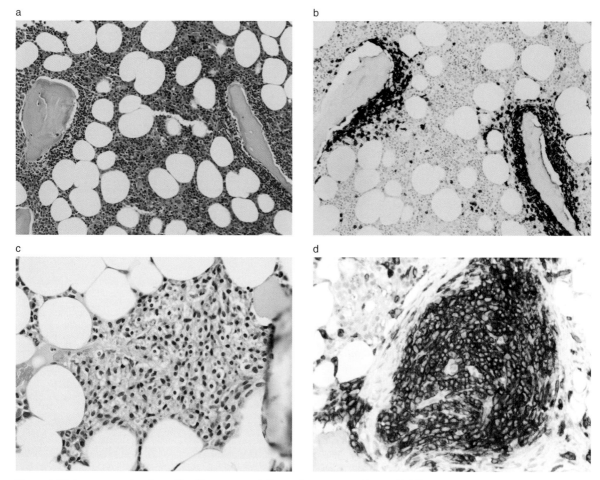

Figure 2.10. Immunocytochemistry of focal bone marrow infiltrates (immunoperoxidase and DAB).
a. Follicular lymphoma showing a paratrabecular lymphoid infiltrate (H&E). In (b) the neoplastic B cells are highlighted with a CD20 antibody.
c. Systemic mastocytosis with a paratrabecular infiltrate (H&E). In (d) the neoplastic cells mast cells are CD117 positive.

nodules are benign or malignant. Although some morphological features are helpful (e.g. location, polymorphous or monotonous, presence of germinal centers, organized or disordered reticulin pattern), immunocytochemistry is generally required. Features that would favor malignancy are a monomorphic B- or T-cell infiltrate, expression of an abnormal lymphoid phenotype and plasma cell monotypia. A clinical history of lymphoma would also suggest residual marrow involvement by lymphoma; however this is not necessarily the case as benign lymphoid infiltrates can mimic residual disease.

Particular care must be taken when assessing lymphoid lesions following CD20 immunotherapy since these may be interpreted as false negative or false positive for lymphoma (Figure 2.11):

1. *False negative*: The CD20 antigen expression may be lost or weak and B-cells may be undetectable. Persistent bone marrow infiltration by the B-cell neoplasm may therefore be CD20-negative. Alternative B-cell antibodies (e.g. CD79a, PAX5) must be used to monitor B-cell lymphomas [25].
2. *False positive*: Reactive nodular T-cell infiltrates in the marrow can mimic residual lymphoma [26].

Lymphoma staging and monitoring: Immunocytochemistry on the bone marrow trephine can be used to highlight low levels of neoplastic infiltration (e.g. single cells or small foci of disease) and thereby increases the sensitivity and accuracy for the detection of marrow involvement by lymphoma [27]. This is for all types of

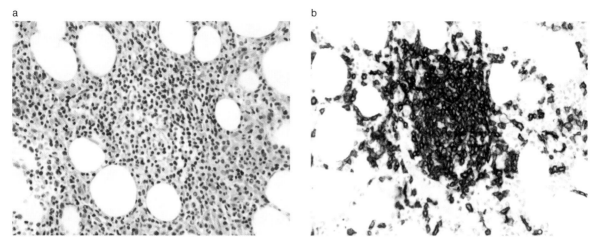

Figure 2.11. Reactive nodular T-cell infiltrate in the marrow following CD20 immunotherapy for chronic lymphocytic leukemia.
a. The interstitial lymphoid nodule showing predominantly small lymphoid cells. On H&E the differential diagnosis is between nodular CLL and a
   reactive lymphoid nodule.
b. Immuno-peroxidase staining for CD3 shows the lymphoid nodule to be comprised of T-cells and is therefore reactive and not residual
   leukemia (DAB substrate).

lymphoma, and is irrespective of the pattern of marrow involvement. The antibodies to use will be determined by the known phenotype of the neoplastic cells (i.e. from the primary diagnostic material, e.g. lymph node). Immunocytochemistry is of particular importance for staging mature T/NK-cell neoplasms as marrow infiltrates of these diseases are commonly subtle (interstitial or sinusoidal pattern) and can go undetected on routine hematoxylin and eosin staining. Since bone marrow involvement by these lymphomas has poor prognostic significance, it is critical that immunocytochemistry be performed. For suspected intravascular or sinusoidal infiltrates double immunocytochemical staining may be useful to identify and localize the abnormal cells (Figure 2.12).

Immunocytochemistry to meet diagnostic criteria: Some diseases require bone marrow immunocytochemistry to meet the disease definition. For example, for systemic mastocytosis one of the diagnostic criteria required to meet the WHO definition is the expression of CD2 and/or CD25 by the mast cells in the bone marrow trephine biopsy. Other examples are Burkitt lymphoma which is associated with nearly 100% Ki67 positivity, a measure of cells in cell cycle, and in suspected hairy cell leukemia where absence of CD11c expression virtually excludes the diagnosis.

Rare event analysis: Immunocytochemistry of the bone marrow trephine can be used to identify rare events, such as:

1. To determine the phenotype of morphologically identifiable abnormal cells that are only present in the marrow in low numbers.
2. To identify malignant cells that are not readily detected in the aspirate and hence cannot be analyzed by flow cytometry. Examples include the identification of Reed–Sternberg and Hodgkin cells in Hodgkin lymphoma (CD30-, CD15-and MUM1-positive, CD45-negative – see Figure 2.9b), and, metastatic infiltrates (e.g. carcinoma) that may mimic a hematopoietic neoplasm.
3. To highlight specific cells or cell types which may not be evident on H&E staining but can be identified based on their phenotype (see Figure 2.12).

This application increases the sensitivity and accuracy of assessing small numbers of cells, their location and pattern (e.g. clusters; paratrabecular; sinusoidal) within the marrow.

Detection of antigens of clinical significance: New emphasis is being placed on immunocytochemistry to provide information to guide clinical decision-making. This is for the following applications:

1. Detection of antigens associated with prognosis. For example, the identification of aberrant cytoplasmic nucleophosmin in bone marrow trephines of acute myeloid leukemia associated with *NPM1* mutations and good prognosis (Figure 2.13) [3,28].
2. To detect antigens that may be potential therapeutic targets. For example, CD20 positivity

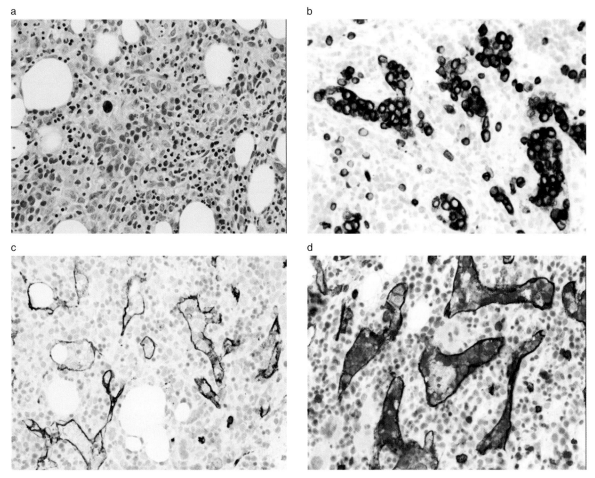

Figure 2.12. Diffuse large B-cell lymphoma staging bone marrow showing an intravascular pattern of involvement.
a. The neoplastic infiltrate is subtle and difficult to identify on H&E stain.
b. CD20 highlights clusters of B-cells in the marrow (immuno-peroxidase and DAB).
c. CD34 staining of endothelial cells highlights the expanded vascular spaces (immuno-peroxidase and DAB).
d. Double immunocytochemical staining for the B-cells (CD20 – immuno-alkaline phosphatase; Fast red) and the endothelium (CD34 immuno-peroxidase and DAB; brown) shows the neoplastic B-cell infiltrate to be intravascular.

in B-cell neoplasms or CD52 in mature T-cell neoplasms.

3. To detect phenotypes associated with specific genetic abnormalities. Products of up- or dysregulated genes resulting from genetic aberrations (e.g. mutations or translocations) can be detected by immunocytochemistry e.g. Cyclin D1 in neoplasms with t(11;14); *CCND1-IGH*. Other examples are given in Table 2.8.

Disease monitoring: Residual disease monitoring is, in general, more amenable to flow cytometry on the bone marrow aspirate than immunocytochemical analysis on the trephine biopsy. If, however, a disease-associated phenotype was established at diagnosis, then this can be used to monitor disease in the BMT following therapy. This increases the sensitivity over morphology alone for the detection of low-level residual disease and to discriminate between malignant cells and regenerating marrow. However if the neoplastic cell does not have a unique phenotype it can be very difficult to determine the presence or extent of residual disease. For example, regenerating B-lymphoid cells and residual B-lymphoblastic leukemia/lymphoma have the same phenotype (CD10-, CD19-, TdT-positive)-making it virtually impossible to discriminate between regeneration and residual

Table 2.8. Examples of some hematological malignancies and their phenotype–genotype correlations [3,23,28,29].

Diagnosis	Antigen expression	Genotype	Genes involved
Acute myeloid leukemia	Cytoplasmic NPM	*NPM1* mutation	*NPM1*
Acute myeloid leukemia with maturation	CD19, CD79a, CD56	t(8;21)(q22;q22)	*RUNX1-RUNX1T1*
B Lymphoblastic leukemia/lymphoma with t(v;11q23)	NG2-positive-CD10, TdT; negative	t(v;11q23)	*MLL*
Lymphoblastic leukemia/lymphoma, *BCR-ABL1* positive	CD13, CD33 commonly positive	t(9;22)(q34;q11.2)	*BCR-ABL1*
Mantle cell lymphoma	Cyclin D1	t(11;14)(q13;q32)	*CCND1-IGH@*
Anaplastic large cell lymphoma	ALK1, CD30	t(2;5)(q23;q35)	*NPM-ALK*
Plasma cell myeloma	CD20	t(11;14) (q13;q32)	*CCND1-IGH@*
Myeloproliferative neoplasms	pAkt	*JAK2* V617F	*JAK2*

a
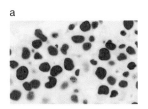
b
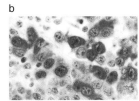

Figure 2.13. Bone marrow trephine biopsies of acute myeloid leukemias stained for NPM1 (immuno-alkaline phosphatose; Fastred). a. Nuclear positivity in a case with wildtype *NPM1*. b. Nuclear and cytoplasmic positivity in a case with *NPM1* mutation.

leukemia. The pattern of infiltration by the cells may be helpful as normal regenerating B-lymphoid cells are usually scattered throughout the marrow, whereas residual leukemic cells may be present in small foci.

Conclusion

Immunocytochemistry, in conjunction with morphology, has an established and essential role in the assessment of hematological malignancies. The antibody repertoire and techniques available enable immunocytochemistry to be performed on all routine diagnostic blood and bone marrow biopsy specimens. Applications of the technology extend beyond diagnosis with an expanding role for the assessment of residual disease, predicting prognosis and identifying potential therapeutic targets. Developments in automation, new antibodies, refinement and standardization of the methodology, incorporation with FISH, and automation of analysis and interpretation will result in further new applications for immunocytochemistry in diagnostic practice.

Acknowledgments

The author wishes to thank Lisa Happerfield for her critical review of the manuscript and Dr Gary Hoffman for his masterful editorial assistance.

References

1. Kohler G, Milstein C. Continuous cultures of fused cells secreting antibody of predefined specificity. *Nature* 1975;**256**(5517):495–7.

2. Zola H, Swart B, Banham A *et al.* CD molecules 2006 – human cell differentiation molecules. *J Immunol Methods* 2007;**319**(1–2):1–5.

3. Swerdlow SH, Campo E, Harris NL (eds.). *WHO Classification of Tumours of Haematopoietic and Lymphoid Tissues*, 4th edn. Lyon: IARC; 2008.

4. Iancu D, Hao S, Lin P *et al.* Follicular lymphoma in staging bone marrow specimens: correlation of histologic findings with the results of flow cytometry immunophenotypic analysis. *Arch Pathol Lab Med* 2007;**131**(2):282–7.

5. Morice WG. The immunophenotypic attributes of NK cells and NK-cell lineage lymphoproliferative disorders. *Am J Clin Pathol* 2007;**127**(6):881–6.

6. Epling-Burnette PK, Painter JS, Chaurasia P *et al.* Dysregulated NK receptor expression in patients with lymphoproliferative disease of granular lymphocytes. *Blood* 2004;**103**(9):3431–9.

7. Garcia CF, Swerdlow SH. Best practices in contemporary diagnostic immunohistochemistry: panel approach to hematolymphoid proliferations. *Arch Pathol Lab Med* 2009;**133**(5):756–65.

8. Olsen RJ, Chang CC, Herrick JL, Zu Y, Ehsan A. Acute leukemia immunohistochemistry: a systematic diagnostic approach. *Arch Pathol Lab Med* 2008; **132**(3):462–75.

9. Coons AH, Creech HJ, Jones R. Immunological properties of an antibody containing a fluorescent group. *Proceedings of the Society of Experimental Medicine* 1941;**47**:2.

10. Sternberger LA, Hardy PH, Jr., Cuculis JJ, Meyer HG. The unlabeled antibody enzyme method of immunohistochemistry: preparation and properties of soluble antigen-antibody complex (horseradish peroxidase-antihorseradish peroxidase) and its use in identification of spirochetes. *J Histochem Cytochem* 1970;**18**(5):315–33.

11. Cordell JL, Falini B, Erber WN *et al.* Immunoenzymatic labeling of monoclonal antibodies using immune complexes of alkaline phosphatase and monoclonal anti-alkaline phosphatase (APAAP complexes). *J Histochem Cytochem* 1984;**32** (2):219–29.

12. Fend F, Tzankov A, Bink K *et al.* Modern techniques for the diagnostic evaluation of the trephine bone marrow biopsy: methodological aspects and applications. *Prog Histochem Cytochem* 2008; **42**(4):203–52.

13. Mattsson G, Tan SY, Ferguson DJ *et al.* Detection of genetic alterations by immunoFISH analysis of whole cells extracted from routine biopsy material. *J Mol Diagn* 2007;**9**(4):479–89.

14. Erber WN, Mason DY. Immuno-alkaline phosphatase labelling of haematological samples: technique and applications. *Leuk Res* 1985;**9**(6):829–30.

15. Kunze E, Middel P, Fayyazi A, Schweyer S. Immunohistochemical staining of plastic (methyl-methacrylate)-embedded bone marrow biopsies applying the biotin-free tyramide signal amplification system. *Appl Immunohistochem Mol Morphol* 2008;**16** (1):76–82.

16. Taylor CR, Shi S-R, Barr NJ, Wu N. Techniques of immunohistochemistry: principles, pitfalls and standardisation. In Dabbs DJ (ed.). *Diagnostic Immunohistochemistry*, 2nd edn. Philadelphia, PA: Churchill Livingstone; 2002, 343.

17. Shi SR, Liu C, Taylor CR. Standardization of immunohistochemistry for formalin-fixed, paraffin-embedded tissue sections based on the antigen-retrieval technique: from experiments to hypothesis. *J Histochem Cytochem* 2007;**55**(2):105–9.

18. Taylor CR, Levenson RM. Quantification of immunohistochemistry – issues concerning methods, utility and semiquantitative assessment II. *Histopathology* 2006;**49**(4):411–24.

19. Cualing HD, Zhong E, Moscinski L. "Virtual flow cytometry" of immunostained lymphocytes on microscopic tissue slides: iHCFlow tissue cytometry. *Cytometry B Clin Cytom* 2007;**72**(1):63–76.

20. Cregger M, Berger AJ, Rimm DL. Immunohistochemistry and quantitative analysis of protein expression. *Arch Pathol Lab Med* 2006;**130**(7):1026–30.

21. Torlakovic EE, Naresh K, Kremer M *et al.* Call for a European programme in external quality assurance for bone marrow immunohistochemistry; report of a European Bone Marrow Working Group pilot study. *J Clin Pathol* 2009;**62**(6):547–51.

22. Happerfield LC, Saward R, Grimwade L, Bloxham D, Erber WN. Automated immunostaining of cell smears: an alternative to flow cytometry. *J Clin Pathol* 2008; **61**(6):740–3.

23. Villamor N, Costa D, Aymerich M *et al.* Rapid diagnosis of acute promyelocytic leukemia by analyzing the immunocytochemical pattern of the PML protein with the monoclonal antibody PG-M3. *Am J Clin Pathol* 2000;**114**(5):786–92.

24. Weber-Matthiesen K, Winkemann M, Muller-Hermelink A, Schlegelberger B, Grote W. Simultaneous fluorescence immunophenotyping and interphase cytogenetics: a contribution to the characterization of tumor cells. *J Histochem Cytochem* 1992;**40**(2):171–5.

25. Hiraga J, Tomita A, Sugimoto T *et al.* Down-regulation of CD20 expression in B-cell lymphoma cells after treatment with rituximab-containing combination chemotherapies: its prevalence and clinical significance. *Blood* 2009;**113**(20):4885–93.

26. Raynaud P, Caulet-Maugendre S, Foussard C *et al.* T-cell lymphoid aggregates in bone marrow after rituximab therapy for B-cell follicular lymphoma: a marker of therapeutic efficacy? *Hum Pathol* 2008; **39**(2):194–200.

27. Talaulikar D, Dahlstrom JE, Shadbolt B, Broomfield A, McDonald A. Role of immunohistochemistry in staging diffuse large B-cell lymphoma (DLBCL). *J Histochem Cytochem* 2008;**56**(10):893–900.

28. Falini B, Mecucci C, Tiacci E *et al.* Cytoplasmic nucleophosmin in acute myelogenous leukemia with a normal karyotype. *New Engl J Med* 2005; **352**(3):254–66.

29. Grimwade LF, Happerfield L, Tristram C *et al.* Phospho-STAT5 and phospho-Akt expression in chronic myeloproliferative neoplasms. *Br J Haematol* 2009;**147**(4):495–506.

Flow cytometry

Maryalice Stetler-Stevenson and Constance M. Yuan

Introduction

Flow cytometry immunophenotyping (FCI) is invaluable in the diagnosis and classification of hematolymphoid neoplasms, in determining prognosis and monitoring therapy. It is especially suited for the immunophenotypic analysis of blood, body fluids (e.g. cerebrospinal fluid, pleural fluid), bone marrow aspirates and cells extracted from lymphoid tissue. Flow cytometry is ideal for small samples; its multiparametric nature allows concurrent staining of cells with multiple antibodies conjugated with different fluorochromes, thus maximizing the data that can be obtained from a few cells. Flow cytometry can characterize surface and intra-cellular (cytoplasmic and nuclear) antigen expression, and can provide highly accurate quantitation of cellular antigen expression. Flow cytometry identification of potential therapeutic targets on the surface of malignant cells is an expanding application due to the increasing use of antibody-based therapies. Flow cytometry analysis also provides high sensitivity in the detection of minimal disease (on the order of 1 in 10^{4-6}), to monitor disease progression and/or the impact of prior therapy. This chapter will describe the principles and applications of FCI in the diagnosis and analysis of hematological malignancies.

Principles of flow cytometry

In a flow cytometer, cells in fluid suspension rapidly pass in single-file through a finely focused laser beam at an appropriate wavelength. The cell momentarily breaks the laser beam, simultaneously scattering light and, if fluorochrome-conjugated antibody is bound, emitting light from the fluorochromes. The light is detected by an intricate combination of filters, mirrors and detectors, collected and saved as digital information (Figure 3.1). Computer analysis of these data allows characterization of each individual cell for a number of parameters.

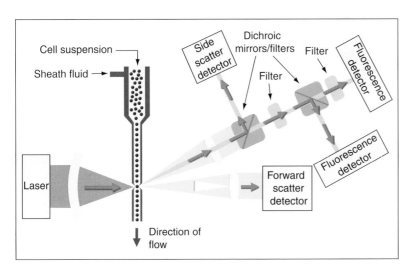

Figure 3.1. Schematic diagram of a flow cytometer. The signals received by the forward scatter detector reflect cell size. Side scatter gives an indication of cell internal complexity. The fluorescence detectors detect the light signals emitted from each fluorescent label (fluorochromes).

Labels in figure: Cell suspension; Sheath fluid; Side scatter detector; Dichroic mirrors/filters; Filter; Filter; Fluorescence detector; Fluorescence detector; Forward scatter detector; Laser; Direction of flow

Diagnostic Techniques in Hematological Malignancies, ed. Wendy N. Erber. Published by Cambridge University Press.
© Cambridge University Press 2010.

Table 3.1. Characteristics of common fluorochromes used in clinical flow cytometry.

Fluorochrome	Absorption (Maximum nm)	Emission (Maximum nm)
Pacific Blue	405	455
AmCyan	457	491
FITC (fluoroscein)	494	519
Alexa Fluor 488	495	519
PE (phycoerythrin)	496, 564	578
ECD (PE-Texas Red tandem)	496, 564	615
APC (allophycocyanin)	650	660
Alexa Fluor 647	650	668
PE-Cy5 (PE-cyanine dye tandem)	496, 564	667
PerCP (peridinin-chlorophyll)	482	678
PerCP-Cy5.5 (PerCP-cyanine dye tandem)	482	695
PE-Cy7 (PE-cyanine dye tandem)	496, 564	785
APC-Cy7 (APC-cyanine dye tandem)	650	785

Light scatter

As each cell passes through the laser, it scatters light at a low angle (*forward scatter*), almost like casting a shadow. This forward scatter (FSC) is reflective of the cell volume. Laser light is simultaneously scattered at a high angle (*side scatter*, SSC) which is proportional to the cell's complexity. This is determined by a number of cellular features including the type and amount of cytoplasmic granularity and the nuclear characteristics. These physical scatter properties can be used to define various cell types, and are the basis for the automated leukocyte differential count in many commercial hematology blood count analyzers [1].

Fluorochromes

Cells can be further characterized by using fluorescent markers, such as fluorochrome-conjugated antibodies or DNA-binding dyes. Fluorochrome-conjugated antibodies are used to assess the expression of a cellular antigen. If a cell expresses an antigen that binds to a fluorochrome-conjugated antibody, fluorescent light is emitted by the fluorochrome and this can be measured. If used in combination with DNA binding dyes, the DNA content can also be determined.

Lasers of various wavelengths in the visible spectra and in the UV spectra excite the fluorochromes and the emitted light is measured by the detectors. In this way signals from each antibody bound to a single cell can be recorded. A variety of fluorochromes ("colors") are available with unique excitation and emission characteristics depending upon the types of lasers used (Table 3.1) [2]. Light emitted from each fluorochrome has uniquely identifiable spectral characteristics, enabling multiple combinations to be measured simultaneously with multiple detectors. The fluorochromes also differ in the amount or intensity of emitted fluorescence. Consequently the most appropriate fluorochrome must be selected for each antibody to maximize antigen detection (i.e. bright fluorochrome such as phycoerythrin for a dimly expressed antigen). Multiple fluorochromes can be used simultaneously and 3-color analysis is regarded as the minimal acceptable standard for reliable discrimination of neoplastic cell populations in a broad range of sample types [2,3]. Most clinical laboratories utilize 4- to 6-color FCI, and protocols are being developed for more than 8-color analyses.

Compensation

The advantage of using multiple fluorochromes is the increased number of parameters that can be measured simultaneously [4]. The disadvantage is that the emission spectra from the varying fluorochromes will inevitably exhibit some overlap (i.e. signal spilling from one channel into an adjacent channel) resulting in a degree of false signal positivity in that adjacent channel [2,4]. Using fluorochromes with narrow emission spectra can help overcome this.

When the emission spectra of fluorochromes overlap the proportion of overlapping signal needs to be subtracted from the adjacent channel, a process called "compensation" [2]. Compensation is unique to each combination of fluorochromes utilized in a single tube. To perform compensation, each antibody-fluorochrome is acquired on the machine individually, and the spillage between channels is subtracted. Traditionally compensation has been performed manually, by visual inspection. Appropriate training is required to perform compensation, as under-compensation can result in weak false positivity while over-compensation can result in false negativity [2]. Compensation has become more complex with the use of increasingly large combinations of fluorochromes and digital instead of analog flow cytometers. Multi-parameter FCI in a digital machine necessitates compensation through the use of a software compensation matrix for optimal results [2,4]. The software mathematically creates a matrix from single fluorochrome controls, to optimize compensation. It is strongly recommended that this approach be used as visual inspection and manual compensation will undoubtedly produce errors of over- or under-compensation when there are so many parameters.

Number of events

It is critical that sufficient events are acquired to ensure even small populations of cells can be identified. Inadequate data acquisition may result in significant populations (e.g. small numbers of neoplastic cells) being undetectable. A minimum of 10 000 total events (cells) per collection tube should be acquired as ungated listmode data [2]. This is generally adequate to represent both normal (for internal positive and negative controls) and malignant cells (for disease characterization). When testing for minimal residual disease, the number of events acquired should be sufficient to yield at least 200 tumor cells; this may require the analysis of 50 000 or more events.

Gating

Analysis software facilitates the identification of specific cell populations of interest from within a mixed population. This is performed by "gating" or the electronic selection of events that meet certain criteria [2]. For example, gating on events with low SSC and CD20 positivity identifies B-lymphocytes. Sequential gates can also be created, which enables highly selected populations of interest to be identified; these can ultimately be quite small populations. Gates can also serve as "boundary lines," designed to surround normal populations; any atypical populations falling outside of these can then be easily identified. This approach is particularly useful in distinguishing between neoplastic cells and their normal counterparts, e.g. normal B-cell precursors/hematogones and neoplastic B-lymphoblastic leukemia/lymphoma cells [5].

The choice of gating strategies is vital and the use of criteria that are too restrictive or too inclusive may prevent the detection and isolation of an abnormal cell population. Examples are:

1. Ungated analysis: is sufficient when the majority of cells in a sample are abnormal, e.g. peripheral blood with 90% leukemia cells.
2. FSC versus SSC: a commonly used analysis gating strategy (Figure 3.2A). Neoplastic cells may be detected as a population with distinctly different FSC or SSC properties relative to the normal cells present.
3. Combination of light scatter (FSC or SSC) and fluorescence, useful for analyzing mixed cell populations not resolved by light scatter alone. An example is CD45 versus SSC gating (Figure 3.2B), useful in examination of bone marrow aspirates, immature hematolymphoid cells and specimens with non-hematolymphoid elements.

Most software products allow subpopulations to be assigned different colors, permitting these populations to be followed through multiple successive dual display scatter plots thereby facilitating the detection and immunophenotypic characterization of abnormal populations (Figure 3.2C).

Interpretation of flow cytometry

Flow cytometry interpretation has evolved from a simple "positive" or "negative" for a given antigen, to an assessment of the number of cells and the degree or intensity of antigen expression [2]. The latter is highly reliable in discriminating between cell types, and can be useful in identifying characteristic features and patterns unique to certain malignancies. Since the antigen expression of many hematological malignancies overlaps with their normal counterparts, the ability of FCI to highlight subtle temporal patterns and differences in antigen intensity can be discriminatory, making it a powerful diagnostic tool. Examples are the differential expression of CD20 antigen in normal B-cells and chronic lymphocytic leukemia (weak), CD7 expression in T-cell prolymphocytic leukemia (strong) and CD45 in hairy cell leukemia (strong).

Reporting flow cytometry

The flow cytometry report should include the flow cytometry results together with an overall interpretation. The following information should be reported:

1. Patient information: demographics (at least two unique patient identifiers) and, clinical history,

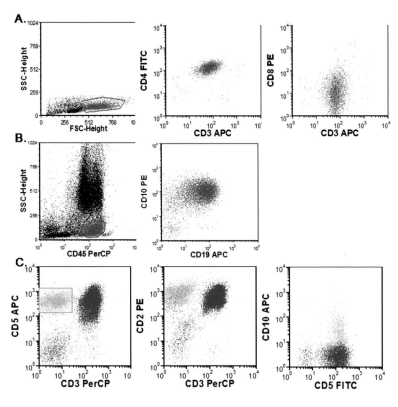

Figure 3.2. Examples of gating strategies that can be used in flow cytometry.

A. FSC versus SSC gating: Abnormal T-cells with abnormally high FSC (red) are large, CD3 positive, CD4 positive and dim to negative for CD8.

B. CD45 versus SSC gating of a bone marrow aspirate: A population with dim CD45 and low SSC cells are gated (red) and shown to be CD19 and CD10 positive leukemic cells.

C. Gating on cells with an abnormal phenotype: An abnormal CD5-positive and CD3-negative T cell population (green) is gated and analyzed further. These abnormal T-cells express CD2 and CD10, the phenotype of angioimmunoblastic T cell lymphoma.

prior therapy and previous flow cytometry results, if available.

2. Sample details: sample type and date of collection.
3. Sample viability.
4. Region (cell type) analyzed: gating strategy used, population analyzed and the number of events acquired.
5. Results: an estimate of the percentage of abnormal cells in the speciman; the phenotype of the cell population analyzed (antigens expressed and unexpected loss or down-regulation), including fluorescence intensity for relevant antigens. relevant negatively for appropriate antigens, disease-associated phenotype and/or descriptive text [6].
6. Data interpretation or conclusion: descriptive summary of the findings, correlation with morphology, overall diagnosis, WHO classification, genotype association, prognostic indicators or extent of residual disease.

Indications for flow cytometry of hematological malignances

Historically, the indications for FCI had been based upon final diagnosis; for example FCI in the analysis of "acute leukemia" but not the chronic phase of chronic myelogenous leukemia. This approach is, however, not practical as one must decide whether or not to perform FCI based upon the presenting clinical features and morphology and not the final diagnosis; the diagnosis is often reached using FCI data. To address this anomaly the 2006 Bethesda International Consensus Conference on Flow Cytometric Immunophenotyping of Hematolymphoid Neoplasia developed a set of recommended medical indications for FCI based upon the patient's clinical scenario [6].

Identification of blast cells or atypical mononuclear cells in a specimen is an absolute indication for FCI [6,7]. Flow cytometry plays an important role in the diagnosis as well as classification of acute leukemia and can assist in the appropriate interpretation of proliferations of maturing blasts in normal bone marrow. When atypical mononuclear cells are detected in body fluids, FCI is useful to differentiate hematolymphoid neoplasia from reactive activated lymphoid cells. Furthermore, FCI is more sensitive than morphology alone in the detection of neoplastic cells in body fluids, and, as such, FCI is indicated when hematolymphoid neoplasia is suspected in the evaluation of serous effusions, CSF and aqueous or vitreous

Table 3.2. Indications for flow cytometry.

Indication	Applications
Lymphocytosis	B-, T- or NK-cell lineage Stage of differentiation Normal or aberrant lymphoid phenotype Restricted populations of lymphoid cells Clonality Disease-associated phenotype and disease classification Detection of potential therapeutic targets Detection of prognostic markers
Cytopenias	To detect abnormal hematopoietic cell type To establish a diagnosis
Leukocytosis for investigation	Distinguish between normal/ reactive and neoplastic cells
Plasmacytosis	Normal or aberrant plasma cell phenotype and enumeration Clonality assessment Detection of prognostic markers Detection of circulating plasma cells Enumerating neoplastic plasma cells Residual disease assessment in plasma cell myeloma
Blast cells	Determining lymphoid or myeloid lineage B- or T-cell origin of lymphoblasts Subtyping myeloblasts Enumerating neoplastic blast cells Evaluation of disease progression of MDS, MDS/ MPN and MPN Detection of potential therapeutic targets Detecting phenotype/ genotype associations Detection of prognostic markers Assessing therapeutic response Residual disease monitoring and detect disease relapse
Other atypical cells in blood, marrow, fluids or tissue where there is a clinical suspicion of a hematological malignancy	Determining cell lineage Differentiate between reactive and neoplastic cells Determining stage of differentiation

Table 3.2. (cont.)

Indication	Applications
	Determining clonality, if lymphoid Disease classification
Lymphoma staging	To document extent of disease Detecting and enumerating lymphoid cells with the disease-associated phenotype
Diagnosis of MDS	Identification of abnormal antigen expression during myeloid maturation Enumerating blast cells Identification of cells with the phenotype of paroxysmal nocturnal hemoglobinuria

humor [6,8]. Flow cytometry is also extremely useful in the diagnosis and subclassification of non-Hodgkin lymphoma and leukemic infiltration of tissues. This testing is therefore indicated in lymphadenopathy, organomegaly (especially splenomegaly and hepatomegaly) and tissue infiltrates (e.g. skin, mucosal sites and bone) [6,9,10].

Table 3.2 lists the most common indications for flow cytometry. Peripheral blood and bone marrow abnormalities (numerical or morphological) are common indications for FCI, as follows.

Cytopenias: Flow cytometry is indicated in the evaluation of patients with cytopenias [6,11–14] once non-neoplastic causes (e.g. nutritional deficiencies, systemic illness, infection and drug suppression) have been excluded. Leukemia, lymphoma and myelodysplastic syndromes can all present with pancytopenia and therefore FCI may be indicated after blood film review [6,11–14]. Because cytopenias can be a presenting abnormality in many hematological malignancies, both lymphoid and myeloid cells should be evaluated.

Leukocytosis: Peripheral blood leukocytosis, especially lymphocytosis, monocytosis and eosinophilia, may indicate the presence of an underlying hematolymphoid neoplasm. Flow cytometry is indicated in the evaluation of lymphocytosis and is helpful in the diagnosis and classification of neoplastic disorders of lymphocytes [6,15]. In the setting of a monocytosis,

FCI is helpful in distinguishing malignant monocytes (in chronic myelomonocytic leukemia and other myeloproliferative neoplasms) from reactive monocytes [6,11,15]. Eosinophilia can be a presenting blood film feature of acute myeloid leukemia, mastocytosis, lymphoblastic leukemia/lymphoma or T-cell lymphoproliferative disorders and FCI testing may be diagnostically useful. Neutrophilia, polycythemia, thrombocytosis and basophilia are generally not indications for FCI testing in the absence of other suspicious signs or symptoms as they are often.

Abnormal hematopoietic cells: Flow cytometry is particularly helpful in establishing the lineage and stage of differentiation of morphologically abnormal cells in blood and bone marrow. This includes blast cells, abnormal lymphoid cells and other abnormal cells of unknown type. For lymphoid cells, FCI can establish clonality of B-cells, using kappa and lambda light chain restriction.

Plasma cells: Flow cytometry is useful in the evaluation of plasma cells in bone marrow or other specimens (e.g. unexplained plasmacytosis) [6,16,17]. This is due to the ability to detect aberrant plasma cell phenotypes and clonality (cytoplasmic light chain restriction). Flow cytometry assists in the differential diagnosis between myeloma and monoclonal gammopathies of undetermined significance by determining the percentage of aberrant or clonal plasma cells of all bone marrow plasma cells [17].

Disease staging: Flow cytometry may be useful in staging a patient with a diagnosis of a hematolymphoid neoplasm. Tissue biopsies, fine needle aspirates, serous effusions or other body fluids from a patient with leukemia or lymphoma can all be evaluated. Specifically, FCI is indicated in the evaluation of CSF in patients with hematolymphoid malignancies that are known to have a high frequency of central nervous system involvement as it increases the diagnostic accuracy and has greater prognostic significance over morphology alone [1,4]. Due to its sensitivity, FCI is extremely useful for detection of low levels of disease. It is therefore highly efficacious in bone marrow staging of non-Hodgkin lymphoma to document the presence and extent of involvement. For example FCI of bone marrow increases the sensitivity of detection of stage IV lymphoma over morphology alone [8,16,18]. Flow cytometry analysis of peripheral blood can also be used, for example, to detect leukemic spread of a lymphoma, potentially eliminating the need for a bone marrow aspirate.

Disease prognosis: Testing directed specifically at identifying prognostic indicators may be integrated into initial diagnostic immunophenotyping; alternatively it can be performed once the diagnosis has been established. Flow cytometry analysis of ZAP-70 and CD38 antigen expression is useful for prognostication in chronic lymphocytic leukemia (CLL) [6,19,20]. Antigen expression profiles, as determined by FCI, are predictive in acute leukemia [6,21]. Flow cytometry is also of prognostic utility in plasma cell dyscrasias: detection of circulating plasma cells, enumeration of plasma cells and assessment of plasma cell proliferative rate within the total bone marrow plasma cell compartment can all be used to predict survival in myeloma [6,16].

Therapeutic targets: Due to the increased usage of antibody-based therapies such as Rituximab and Alemtuzumab, FCI has become vital in the detection of potential therapeutic targets [6,22,23]. Pretreatment evaluation of the malignant cells may aid in guiding patient management and limit unnecessary exposure. Therapeutic antibodies directed against antigens expressed by normal leukocytes can result in substantial toxicity and increased risk of viral and other opportunistic infections due to attendant immunosuppression associated with its use.

Residual disease detection: The ability to detect low-level involvement by hematological malignancies makes FCI useful in assessment of response to therapy, including "minimal residual disease" (MRD) testing. Persistence of FCI-detectable MRD following therapy is an adverse prognostic factor in a number of diseases [6,24,25]. Due to the high sensitivity, quantitative and qualitative nature of the data, FCI is efficient for documentation of disease progression, relapse, acceleration (e.g. CML blast phase) or transformation (e.g. diffuse large B-cell lymphoma in CLL) [6].

Specimens and processing

Specimen types

Flow cytometry can be performed on blood, bone marrow, body fluids (e.g. cerebrospinal fluid, pleural fluid), fine needle aspirates and single cell suspensions prepared from tissue biopsies. Cells must be viable and in solution. Specimen integrity is dependent on appropriate anticoagulation, storage conditions (time and temperature) and the procedure used for sample preparation.

Anticoagulation

Specimens containing blood must be anticoagulated and this may be with:

1. Ethylene-diaminetetraacetic acid (EDTA): stable for 12 to 24 hours.
2. Acid citrate dextrose (ACD): stable for 72 hours.
3. Sodium heparin: the preferred anticoagulant for bone marrow samples stable for 48 to 72 hours.

Specimen storage

Sample storage time is a critical variable in FCI and especially for tumors with a high proliferation rate (e.g. Burkitt lymphoma) and following recent cyto-toxic therapy. Although a 48–72-hour sample cutoff is generally applied, irreplaceable specimens should not be rejected if they exceed this. All specimens can be maintained at room temperature (18–22 °C) if they are to be processed immediately. Blood samples can be maintained at room temperature for up to 72 hours in sodium heparin and ACD anticoagulants. Bone marrow aspirates in sodium heparin anticoagulant may be maintained at room temperature for up to 24 hours. Fresh tissue samples should be kept moist throughout transport to the laboratory and cell suspensions placed in tissue culture media (if the specimen is kept for any period of time). Cold (4 °C) storage may be useful for prolonged storage of some specimens, such as pleural fluids and cell suspensions prepared from tissue samples [2]. As cellular viability in cerebrospinal fluid decreases rapidly, these specimens should be immediately placed into a stabilization media (e.g. RPMI with 5% fetal bovine serum giving up to 18 hours stability at 4 °C) [26].

Cell viability

Non-viable cells may non-specifically bind antibodies making FCI difficult to interpret. Cell viability should therefore be assessed in all tissue samples, and blood and bone marrow specimens which have been stored for more than 48 hours, prior to staining. Viability can be assessed by including fluorescent viability dyes in a FCI antibody panel. Alternatively manual methods (e.g. trypan blue exclusion) can be performed prior to staining [2]. Guidelines are to reject samples with < 75% viability, unless it is an irreplaceable sample (e.g. lymph node biopsy); in the latter case any identified abnormal populations should be reported with a disclaimer statement about suboptimal viability [2].

Specimen processing

Specimens should be manipulated as little as possible during processing. If significant numbers of erythrocytes are present in the sample, whole blood lysis should be performed. Lysing reagents include water, Tris-buffered ammonium chloride and hypotonic buffer. Red cell lysis can be performed either prior to or following antibody labeling. Washing with phosphate-buffered saline (PBS) is required before staining with antibodies to immunoglobulins to remove residual plasma or cytophilic immunoglobulin that can interfere with immunophenotypic analysis.

Membrane permeabilization

If intracellular antigens (e.g. cytoplasmic IgM, CD3 or myeloperoxidase, or nuclear TdT) are being studied the cell membrane must be permeabilized prior to antibody labeling. The optimal permeabilization reagent is dependent on the antigen being studied. If it is necessary to simultaneously stain surface and intracellular antigens, the surface markers are usually stained first followed by cell fixation, membrane permeabilization, and then intracellular staining. It is critical that the surface marker fluorochrome not be affected by the subsequent fixation and permeabilization steps [2].

Antibody incubation

Antibodies to be used should be added to the sample according to the manufacturers' recommendations. The incubation time is affected by temperature, cell count, amount of cellular antigen present, antibody–antigen affinity and antibody concentration. In general, incubation is in the dark and at room temperature (18–22 °C) and times vary from 10 to 30 minutes. When panels contain antibodies with different recommended incubations, the longest time period should be applied, or, intra-laboratory validation performed to ensure optimum performance is achieved. Of note, some antigens, such as CD3 and CD19, begin to modulate after 10 minutes at room temperature; this may

Table 3.3. Primary and secondary antibody panels for the assessment of cell lineage by flow cytometry.

Lineage	Primary Panel	Secondary Panel
B-cells	CD5, CD10, CD19, CD20, CD45, Kappa, Lambda	CD9, CD11c, CD15, CD22, cCD22, CD23, CD25, CD13, CD33, CD34, CD38, CD43, CD58, cCD79a, CD79b, CD103, FMC7, Bcl-2, cKappa, cLambda, cMPO, TdT, ZAP-70, cIgM
T-cells and NK-cells	CD2, CD3, CD4, CD5, CD7, CD8, CD45, CD56	CD1a, cCD3, CD10, CD16, CD25, CD26, CD30, CD34, CD45RA, CD45RO, CD57, CD158 isoforms, TCR αβ, TCR γδ, cMPO, cTIA-1, TCR Vβ-chain isoforms, TdT
Myelomonocytic cells	Regular: CD7, CD11b, CD13, CD14, CD15, CD16, CD33, CD34, CD45, CD56, CD117, HLA-DR Limited: CD13, CD33, CD34, CD45	CD2, cCD3, CD4, cCD22, CD25, CD36, CD38, CD41, CD61, cCD61, CD64, CD71, cCD79a, cMPO, CD123, CD163, CD235a
Plasma cells	CD19, CD38, CD45, CD56, CD138	CD10, CD27, CD28, CD117, cKappa, cLambda

give false negative results. Most commercial reagents recommend the amount of antibody to be added per fixed unit of blood or cells. These have been determined to provide maximal separation between positive and negative populations [2].

Controls

Internal negative (i.e. normal cells in the sample that lack the antigen) and positive (i.e. normal cells in the sample that express the antigen) controls for the antibodies and staining procedure are usually sufficient to control the flow cytometric procedure. For example, CD3-negative lymphoid cells (i.e. the B-cells) in a specimen are a negative reagent control for CD3, whereas the CD3-positive T-cells serve as positive controls for both the reagent and process. If there is no appropriate internal control cell in the sample (i.e. positive and negative), control cells of known reactivity with the antibody should be used. Antibodies with broad reactivity with hematopoietic target cells (e.g. CD45) should be included in every panel for use as a positive process control. Results should be interpreted with caution if there is no reactivity of any cells in the sample as this may be due to an error in processing or a problem due to lack of sample integrity [2].

Antibody panels

Antibody panels for FCI detection of hematologic malignancies depend upon the clinical history, morphological evaluation of the sample and whether the neoplastic cell phenotype is already known from prior testing. This information enables a well-designed and focused antibody panel to be utilized. When this information is unavailable the antibody panel must be sufficient to detect any possible hematolymphoid malignancy while being as efficient and cost effective as possible [2,27]. To accomplish this goal the 2006 Bethesda International Consensus Conference on Flow Cytometric Immunophenotyping of Hematolymphoid Neoplasia guidelines recommend using an initial short primary panel followed by a more focused secondary panel to further characterize abnormal populations identified (Table 3.3) [27]. These panels should be based upon the indication for FCI and allow the final analysis to detect all major cell populations present in the specimen. Furthermore, the "flow cytometric testing performed should be comprehensive enough to identify all major categories of hematopoietic neoplasia relevant to the clinical circumstances, including but not limited to the submitted medical indication(s)" [27]. For less specific indications (e.g. anemia for investigation) and when no specific morphologically abnormal cell can be identified by microscopy, more extensive panels may be required to assess B-cell, T/NK-cells, myelomonocytic and plasma cell lineages. Flow cytometry testing in the setting of a lymphocytosis, on the other hand, is more straightforward and assessment of B-cell and T/NK-cell lineages is sufficient [27].

Antibody panels should be designed to be able to assess cell lineage and stage of differentiation of the cell of interest, and enable disease subclassification (e.g. of leukemia or lymphoma). As discussed in Chapter 2, the antibody panel design therefore requires in-depth knowledge of antigen expression patterns in normal and neoplastic cells. Most antibodies are not cell lineage-specific and neoplastic cells may lack one or more antigens of a particular lineage. Multiple antibodies are therefore required for lineage assignment [2,27]. In addition to selecting the most appropriate antibodies, the fluorochrome label must be chosen for each to maximize antigen detection (i.e. bright fluorochrome such as phycoerythrin for weakly expressed antigens). Antibodies that identify lineage sub-populations should be used in combination with a broadly expressed lineage-associated marker (e.g. CD23 with a pan-B-cell lineage antibody such as CD19). Antigens that are expressed at a particular maturational stage are useful to identify specific sub-populations (e.g. CD34, CD10 and CD20 in B-cell maturation, or, CD11b, CD13 and CD16 in granulocytic differentiation) and should be used in combinations that optimize assessment of maturation [2,27].

Flow cytometric analysis of hematological malignancies

Acute leukemia

Comprehensive FCI panels can be used to establish the lineage of blast cells and to distinguish acute lymphoid from myeloid leukemias. This can be achieved even when there is aberrant expression of lymphoid antigens by a true myeloid leukemia, and vice versa [3,28]. Flow cytometry can also be used to identify phenotypic features associated with specific genetic alterations. Other important applications of FCI in acute leukemia are the identification of potential therapeutic targets and detection of minimal residual disease; the latter has important prognostic implications and may guide further therapeutic options.

Precursor lymphoid neoplasms

Correct determination that blast cells are of lymphoid origin (i.e. lymphoblastic leukemia/lymphoma (ALL)) is essential for correct therapy. B- or T-lineage of the blast cells can have impact on therapy. ALL cells characteristically have normal, decreased or absent CD45 expression with low side scatter and intracellular TdT is usually expressed [29]. The co-expression of lymphoid and myeloid antigens (such as CD13, CD33) in ALL, can, at times, cause diagnostic difficulty and necessitates a thorough FCI evaluation to exclude acute myeloid leukemia (AML).

B lymphoblastic leukemia/lymphoma (B-ALL): B-ALL typically expresses CD10, CD19, CD22, TdT, CD34, HLA-DR and CD45 (dim to negative) antigens, and is negative for surface immunoglobulin. Some cases have a more differentiated-appearing immunophenotype with slightly increased CD45 intensity and diminished CD34, and express cytoplasmic immunoglobulin heavy chains (cμ). Rare cases show aberrant surface immunoglobulin; of these, 20–25% are associated with the t(1;19)(q23;p13.3) translocation fusing the *PBX* and *E2A* genes [30,31]. B-ALL lacking expression of CD10 and CD24 are associated with 11q23 abnormalities involving the *MLL* gene, a prognostically unfavorable subtype. In contrast, intense expression of CD10 with dim CD9 and CD20 is typical of the prognostically favorable translocation t(12;21)(p13; q22); *ETV6-RUNX1* [28,29]. Initial FCI identification of these phenotypic features provides the first clue to these significant genetic abnormalities.

Flow cytometry can be used to monitor B-ALL despite normal B-lymphoblasts (hematogones) being present in the bone marrow and having phenotypic similarities. Flow cytometry is still highly sensitive in detecting MRD for the following reasons (see also Table 7.5) [32,33]:

1. The immunophenotypic patterns of normal B-cell maturation are synchronized, and regulated, based on the timing and intensity of expression of CD19, CD34, CD10, CD45, CD22, CD20 and CD58 antigens.
2. Residual B-ALL cells do not have the defined normal antigen expression pattern. Differences include unusually bright, homogeneous expression of CD10, persistence of CD34 with temporally aberrant co-expression of CD22 or CD20, or arrest in the progression of CD45 expression. Also, CD58 is usually more intensely expressed in residual B-ALL than hematogones.

Interpretation of these data requires extensive knowledge and familiarity with normal FCI patterns of B-cell maturation (Figures 2.1 and 3.3).

T lymphoblastic leukemia/lymphoma (T-ALL): Compared with B-ALL, T-ALL usually has brighter CD45 expression, with the blast population positioned more closely to the location of normal mature lymphocytes on the CD45 versus SSC data plot [29]. Detection of intra-cytoplasmic CD3 (cCD3) is key to determining T-cell lineage, since T-ALL may lack

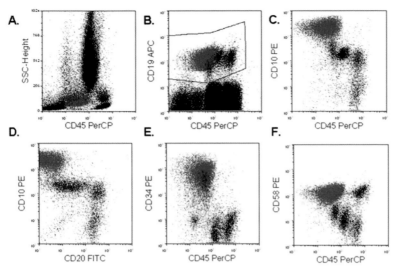

Figure 3.3. Flow cytometric analysis of ALL cells (red) in a bone marrow aspirate.
A. The ALL cells have abnormally dim CD45 expression (x-axis) and low side scatter (y-axis) characteristics.
B. CD19-positive cells are gated and utilized for further examination. This includes the ALL cells.
C– F. CD19-positive gate: The All cells (red) are bright CDl0-PE positive, CD34-PE postive CD58-PE postive (y axes) and CD20-FITC negative. Residual normal CD19-postive B cells (black) have normal antigen expression.

surface CD3 antigen. T-cell lymphoblasts typically express TdT (intra-nuclear) with variable expression of surface T-cell associated antigens CD1a, CD2, CD3, CD4, CD5, CD7 and CD8. CD10 can also be expressed (40–45% of cases) [34]. Although CD4 and CD8 may be expressed separately, co-expression is a distinct diagnostic feature, recapitulating the "common thymocyte" stage of T-cell maturation. Aberrant myeloid antigen expression (CD13 and CD33) has been observed [29], and may prompt the consideration of an AML; utilization of a comprehensive panel should resolve lineage discrepancies.

A recognized pitfall in the flow cytometric analysis of mediastinal tumors or pleural effusions is the identification of a CD4+/CD8+/TdT+ common thymocyte phenotype. This is not diagnostic of T-ALL as it is also seen in normal thymus, thymic hyperplasia and lymphocyte-rich thymoma. Flow cytometry can be used to distinguish between neoplastic T-ALL and non-neoplastic T-lymphoblasts with this phenotype [35,36]. Detection of normal synchronized patterns of T-cell maturation, based on the timing and intensity of expression of CD2, CD3, CD5, CD7, CD4, CD8, CD34, CD10 and CD45 antigens indicates normal progressively developing sub-populations of T-cells. In contrast, asynchronous maturation of the T-lymphoblasts or maturation arrest favors T-ALL.

Acute myeloid leukemia

Flow cytometry information is a key component in the WHO classification for the diagnosis and sub-typing of acute myeloid leukemia (AML). In the assessment of AML, FCI can be used to:

1. Establish the myeloid lineage of blast cells and thereby differentiate AML from ALL.
2. Identify granulocytic, monocytic, erythroid and megakaryocytic differentiation.
3. Assist in differentiating *de novo* AML from one arising from myelodysplasia.
4. Detect potential therapeutic targets, such as CD33 [37].
5. Monitor MRD which has important prognostic implications and may guide further therapeutic options.

Generally, AML blasts express dim CD45, CD34, HLA-DR, CD117 (with some variation, such as lack of CD34 or HLA-DR), in combination with myeloid antigens, such as CD13, CD33, CD15, CD11b and myeloperoxidase. AML blast cells tend to have higher SSC than lymphoblasts, and, the more granulated the blast cells (e.g. acute promyelocytic leukemia) the greater the SSC. Certain AML subtypes have characteristic genetic features and associated immunophenotypic characteristics. For example, AML blasts with t(8;21)(q22;q22); *RUNX1-RUNXT1* are usually CD34+, CD13+, CD33+ with expression of B-lymphoid marker CD19 and the NK-associated marker CD56 (on a subset of the blast cells) [38–40]. Acute promyelocytic leukemia (APML) with translocation t(15;17) (q22;q12);*PML-RARA* also has a characteristic immunophenotype:

1. CD33 expression is usually homogeneously positive and bright.
2. CD13 is positive but with heterogeneous expression.
3. HLA-DR and CD34 are usually absent or dimly expressed in a minor subset of the leukemic promyelocytes.
4. CD15 is negative.
5. Co-expression of CD2, typically in the microgranular variant [41,42].

This classic phenotype, if obtained quickly by FCI, can be used in combination with morphology, to make a rapid diagnosis of APML and specific treatment commenced (see also Chapter 8).

The blast cells in AML with a monocytic component (e.g. myelomonocytic, monoblastic or monocytic) exhibit brighter CD45 expression than pure myeloblastic AML. On the CD45 versus SSC plot, the blast "pocket" is positioned close to or overlapping with normal monocytes. In acute myelomonocytic leukemia, the blast population may have bimodal CD45 expression, with a subset of blasts exhibiting slightly more intense CD45. Blast cells with monocytic differentiation initially express HLA-DR, CD64 and CD36 antigens and, with further monocytoid differentiation, express CD14. The leukemic cells in acute monoblastic and monocytic leukemia can also express CD4, CD11b, CD11c and lysozyme. Monocytic and myeloid cells express some common antigens (such as CD13 and CD33), but they differ in the timing and intensity of expression of these antigens compared with normal maturation patterns [43,44]. AML with inv(16)(p13.1q22); *CBFB-MYH11* is characterized by CD2 expression [29,34].

Pure erythroid leukemia is a rare entity. The erythroid blast cells can be identified by expression of CD71, CD36 and CD235 (glycophorin A) [28,29]. Both CD71 and CD235 antigens are expressed at lower levels than normal erythroid progenitors. CD117 may be positive but other myeloid markers, including myeloperoxidase, HLA-DR and CD34 are generally negative. Because CD36 and CD71 are not lineage-specific, and unlysed glycophorin-positive red blood cells can contribute technical artefacts, care should be taken in interpretation of the blast cell phenotype.

Blast cells of acute megakaryoblastic leukemia (AMKL) characteristically exhibit high FSC, corresponding to the larger size and volume of the leukemic cell relative to typical myeloblasts. The blast cells may express one or more platelet glycoproteins, CD41, CD61 and (to a lesser extent) CD42, as well as CD36. Platelets adhering to the surface of blast cells may give a false positive result for CD41 and CD61 and thereby mimic the phenotype of AMKL [28,29]. Myeloid antigens CD13 and CD33 may be expressed but CD34 and HLA-DR are commonly negative. This entity represents less than 5% of all AML; therefore, an AML or ALL needs to be excluded in the immunophenotypic work-up [28].

Acute leukemias of ambiguous lineage

This WHO-defined entity includes acute leukemias that do not show clear evidence of lymphoid or myeloid differentiation. These are rare (< 5% of acute leukemias) and occur in both children and adults. They may have t(9;22); *BCR-ABL1* or t(v;11q23); *MLL* rearranged chromosomal translocations. There are two main types:

1. Acute undifferentiated leukemias, which do not express lineage-specific antigens.
2. Mixed phenotype acute leukemias (MPAL), express antigens of more than one lineage such that lymphoid or myeloid origin cannot definitively determined. These may express a combination of B-cell and myeloid-associated antigens ("B/myeloid") or T-cell and myeloid antigens ("T/myeloid"). This category includes cases historically referred to as "bilinear" or "bilineage" (two or more blast populations of differing lineages) and "biphenotypic" (one blast population expressing antigens of more than one lineage).

The diagnosis of acute leukemias of ambiguous lineage necessitates immunophenotyping, and flow cytometry is the preferred method. This is because of the need to specifically identify co-expression of mixed lineage antigens on the blast cells. Antigens that must be expressed by the blast cells to meet the definition of MPAL are:

1. B lineage: CD19, plus one or more of CD79a, cytoplasmic CD22 or CD10. One additional B-cell-associated antigen is required with strong CD19, and at least two when CD19 expression is weak.
2. T lineage: CD3 (cytoplasmic or surface expression).

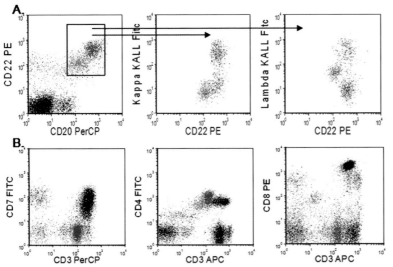

Figure 3.4. Abnormal antigen intensity in detecting lymphoproliferative disorders.
A. Identification of CLL/SLL cells among normal polyclonal B-cells. CLL/SLL cells (red) have lower CD20 and CD22 expression than normal B-cells (blue). Gating on CD20 and CD22-positive B-cells shows the CLL/SLL cells (red) to be negative for kappa and positive for lambda (i.e. monoclonal). The B-cells with normal CD20 and CD22 levels (blue) express both kappa and lambda light chains.
B. Cutaneous T-cell lymphoma cells with abnormally dim CD3 (red). These T-cells are CD7-negative, CD4-positive and CD8-negative, an aberrant phenotype consistent with a neoplastic process.

3. Myeloid lineage: myeloperoxidase or, two or more of CD11c, CD14, CD64 and lysozyme monocyte-associated antigens. Note that the myeloid-associated antigens CD13, CD33 and CD117 are *not* sufficiently specific to meet the definition of "ambiguous" lineage.

The phenotype of ambiguous lineage cases can become more clear-cut following therapy or at relapse. At follow-up the phenotype may "change" to lymphoblastic or myeloid and no longer show the ambiguous phenotype seen at diagnosis.

Mature B-cell neoplasms

Flow cytometry immunophenotyping can identify mature B-cell neoplasms, by evidence of their B-cell lineage, light chain restriction, abnormal levels of antigen expression, absence of normal antigens and presence of antigens not normally present on mature B-cells [45].

Monoclonality: Monoclonality is the expression of a single surface immunoglobulin by a population of B-cells. Typically restricted expression of surface kappa or lambda light chains is utilized as a surrogate for B-cell clonality [46]. A monoclonal B-cell population is (with rare exception) considered a B-cell neoplasm. Occasionally monoclonal B-cell populations are detected in patients with no evidence of lymphoma [47,48]; however, this may represent early, pre-clinical detection of a B-cell malignancy [49]. In normal/

benign lymphoid tissue and blood the ratio of kappa to lambda light chain-expressing B-cells ranges from 4:1 to 1:1 [50]. A deviation from this suggests an underlying monoclonal B-cell population, prompting further immunophenotypic search for such a population. Flow cytometry can successfully identify monoclonal B-cells even when there is B-cell lymphopenia, due to the sensitivity of the method through analysis of large numbers of cells.

Aberrant B-cell phenotypes: Neoplastic B-cells can be found in a background of normal polyclonal B-cells when "aberrant" antigens are expressed by the neoplastic cells, such as CD5 in mantle cell lymphoma or CD10 in follicular lymphoma [46,50]. B-cell antigen intensity can also be used to distinguish normal from neoplastic B-cells (Figure 3.4). Gating on B-cell populations with varying intensities of B-cell antigens (e.g. CD19, CD20 or CD22) may highlight a monoclonal B-cell population [46,51]. If there is only minimal involvement by a neoplastic monoclonal B-cell population this may not be evident from the kappa : lambda ratio of the entire B-cell population (i.e. a skewed kappa: lambda ratio would not be detected). Gating should be performed specifically on B-cells with an aberrant phenotype (e.g. CD20 bright+ B-cells) and assessing the kappa and lambda expression of this population; this will assess the light chain profile within that particular B-cell population. The complexity of some of these analyses to detect relevant neoplastic populations illustrates the need for multi-parametric flow cytometry; single dimension histogram displays are not sufficiently sensitive for these analyses.

Absence of surface immunoglobulin may also indicate the presence of a mature B-cell neoplasm [52,53]. However this can also be seen in some normal or reactive lymphoid tissues. For example, reactive germinal center cells may have B-cells with dim surface immunoglobulin expression and these are increased in reactive follicular hyperplasia. They can be identified and distinguished from follicular lymphoma by virtue of their expression of high levels of CD20, co-expression of CD10 and lack of intracellular Bcl-2 [54,55]. Kappa and lambda expression is typically dim, and is best appreciated when compared to immunoglobulin- negative T-cells within the sample [56].

A laboratory's ability to assess surface light chain expression can be affected by antibody choice and artefact [46]. False positivity may result from passively absorbed immunoglobulin bound to Fc receptors on natural killer cells, activated T-cells, monocytes, granulocytes, and even some B-cells. Washing the cells in PBS prior to staining, sometimes at 37 °C, and using CD20 or CD19 for B-cell selection prior to FCI analysis can eliminate this artefact [46]. Occasionally, a neoplastic B-cell population may express light chain epitopes not readily detected by a single set of monoclonal antibodies; using two sets of light chain reagents will increase the sensitivity of monoclonal B-cell detection [46].

Disease-associated phenotypes: The phenotype of some B-cell lymphoproliferative disorders is characteristic, making FCI a useful diagnostic tool (see also Chapter 9). Chronic lymphocytic leukemia (CLL) is characterized by abnormally decreased or dim CD20 and CD22 expression, and positivity for CD5 and CD23 antigens (Figure 3.5). Hairy cell leukemia exhibits abnormally intense, or bright expression of CD20 and CD22 antigens and the cells are positive for CD11c, CD25 and CD103 antigens [57]. Follicular lymphoma is characterized by dim expression of CD19 and co-expression of CD10 antigen [58]. Aberrant expression of T-cell markers such as CD2, CD4, CD7 and CD8 can occur, albeit rarely, in CLL, hairy cell leukemia, and other B-cell non-Hodgkin lymphomas [59,60]. Light scatter characteristics can also be helpful, such as abnormally increased FSC in large cell lymphomas or increased SSC in hairy cell leukemia. Loss of mature B-cell antigens is also an important feature. With the exception of plasma

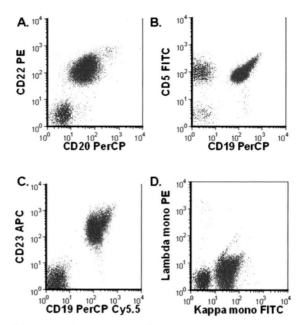

Figure 3.5. Flow cytometry of chronic lymphocytic leukemia in peripheral blood (red).
A. The CLL cells have abnormally dim CD20-PerCP (x-axis) and CD22-PE (y-axis) positivity.
B. CLL cells are positive for CD19-PerCP (x-axis) and CD5-FITC (y-axis).
C. The CD19-PerCP (x-axis) positive B-cells are CD23-APC-positive.
D. The CLL cells show light chain restriction ("clonal"), positive for kappa FITC and are negative for lambda PE.

cells, the absence of CD19, CD20, and/or CD22 on mature B-cells is abnormal. An important caveat is a history of monoclonal antibody therapy, as the therapeutic antibody may mask detection of the targeted antigen. After treatment with Rituximab, B-cells (both normal and malignant) will have weak or absent CD20 expression; this may persist for 6 months or longer after Rituximab therapy has ceased [61].

Plasma cell disorders

Flow cytometry can be used to distinguish normal from neoplastic plasma cells based on the type and intensity of surface antigen expression, presence of aberrant antigens and monoclonal cytoplasmic immunoglobulin [62]. Flow cytometry however, is not routinely utilized in plasma cell enumeration within bone marrow. This is because plasma cells are usually significantly underrepresented in the marrow sample due to hemodilution, sampling artefact, or plasma cell fragility. Nevertheless, detection of MRD where abnormal plasma cells are expressed as a percentage of total plasma cells is prognostically relevant but this necessitates good quality bone marrow aspirates being available [62].

Normal plasma cells are characterized by intense expression of CD38, CD138, polyclonal cytoplasmic immunoglobulin light chain, CD27 and low levels of CD45 and CD19. Surface immunoglobulin, CD20, CD22 and CD56 are absent. In contrast, neoplastic plasma cells express monoclonal cytoplasmic immunoglobulin, aberrant antigens such as CD56, CD20, CD28 or CD117, diminished CD38, CD27, and absence of CD19 and CD45 [62–64]. These phenotypic differences enable multi-parametric flow cytometric analysis to distinguish normal from malignant plasma cells in the majority of cases [17,64–66]. Flow cytometry can evaluate neoplastic plasma cells below the level of morphological assessment, even when obscured by a background of polyclonal plasma cells. As such, it is useful in the investigation of bone marrow plasmacytosis of unknown etiology [6]. Flow cytometry can also be used to differentiate monoclonal gammopathy of uncertain significance from early plasma cell myeloma, as normal (polyclonal) residual plasma cells are present in the former, and not the latter [63]. Furthermore, studies suggest a role for FCI monitoring in myeloma, both in the detection of minimal residual disease and prognosis [62,67,68].

Mature T-cell neoplasms

Flow cytometry is useful in the diagnosis and subclassification of mature T-cell neoplasms [45], and identifying targets of potential antibody therapy, such as CD52 (see also Chapter 10) [22]. Malignant T-cells can be identified by subset restriction (i.e. restricted CD4 or CD8 expression), abnormal expression of T-cell antigens (absent, diminished or increased), presence of aberrant antigens and/or expansion of normally rare T-cell populations [45,69]. The light scatter properties and antigen expression profile of the T-cell populations in question can be compared with normal T-cells within the same sample to detect any deviation. Additionally, T-cell clonality can be assessed by FCI analysis of the β-chain variants of the T-cell receptor (Vβ). All of these phenotypic features should be integrated in the interpretation; individual "abnormalities" may represent variations found in benign activated T-cell populations or reactive expansions of minor T-cell subsets and do not necessarily imply a neoplasm.

CD4/CD8 expression: Normal T-lymphoid populations contain a mixture of CD4-and CD8-positive cells (generally CD4 > CD8). Clonal T-cells will express either CD4 or CD8 antigens, or both, or neither. Co-expression of CD4 and CD8 is unusual and is most frequently seen in T-cell prolymphocytic leukemia and T-lymphoblastic leukemia/lymphoma (TdT+). If the specimen is from the mediastinum neoplastic T-cells must be distinguished from normal cortical thymocytes (i.e. thymoma or thymic hyperplasia) [35,36]. Dual CD4+/CD8+ T-cells may also be a technical artefact in the staining of unwashed blood [70]; care should be exercised in interpretation. Some T-cell neoplasms lack both CD4 and CD8 antigens; however, some normal TCRγδ and TCRαβ+ T-cells are also dual CD4/CD8-negative and their presence should not be interpreted as a T-cell lymphoproliferative disorder [71]. The differential diagnosis of a mature T-cell neoplasm may include viral infections as these can cause a CD8+ T-cell lymphocytosis; these usually show other indicators of T-cell activation, such as increased CD2, decreased CD7 or the presence of activation markers [72].

Minor T-cell subset expansion: Significant expansion of a normally minor T-cell subset may represent a T-cell malignancy. For example, increased CD8+ T-cells co-expressing CD57, CD56 or CD16 raises the possibility of a T-cell large granular lymphocytic (LGL) leukemia, and, increased numbers of TCRγδ T-cells raises the suspicion of a hepatosplenic T-cell lymphoma. T-cell receptor gene rearrangement studies would be helpful in demonstrating T-cell clonality in these situations.

Abnormal antigen expression: Mature T-cell neoplasms frequently lack expression of at least one T-cell antigen (i.e. negative for CD3, CD5, CD7, or less commonly, CD2); a more useful finding this can be than CD4/CD8 subset restriction [69,73]. This demonstrates the value of the inclusion of antibodies to multiple T-cell-associated antigens in a diagnostic panel. It is important to note that not all T-cell antigens are universally expressed by mature T-cells. For example, a minor proportion of normal blood T-cells lack CD7 and a subset of normal TCRγδ T-cells lack CD5. However, if this finding is noted on a significant proportion of T-cells, a neoplastic T-cell process should be considered.

Differential intensity of antigen expression: Neoplastic T-cells may be identified as a homogeneous population with an abnormal level of antigen expression (e.g. abnormal levels of CD2, CD3, CD5, CD7 or CD45 antigens) [69,73]. For example, CD3 may be

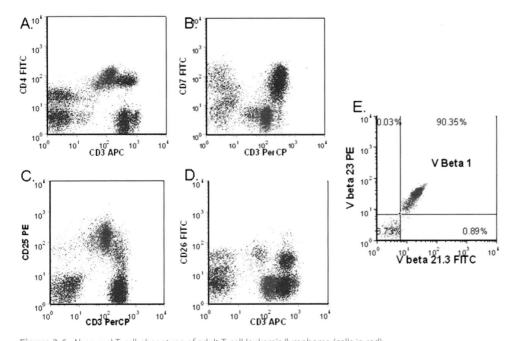

Figure 3.6. Abnormal T-cell phenotype of adult T-cell leukemia/lymphoma (cells in red).
A. Abnormal T-cells have dim CD3-APC (x-axis) and all are CD4-FITC (y-axis) positive.
B–D. T-cells with dim CD3-PerCP (x-axis) are CD7-FITC (y-axis) negative (B), have homogeneously bright CD25-PE (y-axis) (C) and are CD26-FITC (y-axis) negative (D).
E. The cells with abnormally dim CD3 and which are CD4-positive (see A), have VBeta1 restriction, indicating it is a clonal T-cell process.

expressed at a higher or lower level on neoplastic T-cells than on normal T-cells (Figure 3.6) [74,75]. Weak CD5 expression is typically present in T-cell large granular lymphocytic leukemia and strong CD7 in T-cell pro-lymphocytic leukemia. Some normal T-cell subpopulations also have differential antigen intensity, such as upregulated CD2 in reactive T-cells [45], and intense CD3 in normal TCRγδ T-cells. Keeping these normal variations in mind will prevent misinterpretation of a normal or reactive T-cell subset for a T-cell neoplasm.

TCR Vβ repertoire: Since the vast majority of normal and neoplastic T-cells express the TCR αβ chain, T-cell subpopulations can be assessed for a restricted TCR Vβ repertoire [76]. A wide variety of Vβ classes are utilized by normal T-cells and the distribution (proportion) on normal CD4+ or CD8+ T-cells is well defined [77]. In contrast, a clonal T-cell population will have the same VDJ segment and therefore identical ("monoclonal") Vβ protein expression. Expansion of a single Vβ population (i.e. restricted Vβ repertoire) is consistent with a clonal T-cell population; this is analogous to light chain restricted B-cells in a monoclonal B-cell population. TCR Vβ antibodies can be used to determine clonality

of a phenotypically abnormal T-cell population at diagnosis and to monitor MRD [78,79].

Mature natural-killer (NK)-cell neoplasms

Flow cytometry can identify neoplasms of NK-cell lineage as these are characterized by expression of CD2, CD16, CD56, CD57 and CD122 antigens. CD7 and CD8 antigens may also be expressed but surface CD3, CD4 and CD5 are usually negative (see also Chapter 10) [28,80]. Phenotyping can be used to identify NK-cell leukemias and NK/T-cell lymphomas, even in the typical background of extensive necrosis and inflammation. Although there are no specific immunophenotypic markers that can definitively distinguish between reactive and neoplastic NK-cells there are some helpful features: the number and proportion of NK-cells, and increased FSC compared with normal lymphocytes due to the cytoplasmic granulation.

NK-receptor expression: There is no reliable method to confirm the clonality of NK-cells. Unlike B- and T-cell neoplasms, NK-cells have germline configuration of the Ig and T-cell receptor genes, respectively. Antibodies to NK-receptors such as the NK-cell killer inhibitory receptor repertoire (CD158-KIR) and the NK-cell expression of CD94-NKG2 heterodimers can be used as surrogates of NK-cell clonality. Normal NK-cell populations will express a diverse set of these NK-receptors [81], whereas a clonal NK-cell population will show a skewed or restricted NK-receptor expression repertoire. This approach bears resemblance to that of TCR Vβ repertoire analysis in T-cells. It is important to note that skewed NK-receptor expression is not specific to malignant NK-cells as this has also been detected in viral processes and EBV-driven lymphoproliferations [82–84].

Myeloproliferative neoplasms and myelodysplastic syndromes

In recent years, the role of FCI has expanded to assist in the diagnosis and assessment of myeloproliferative neoplasms and myelodysplastic syndromes. Flow cytometry can be used to quantify immature precursors or blast cells and is now being further developed to detect qualitative maturation abnormalities within a cell lineage.

Myeloproliferative neoplasms

In chronic phase chronic myelogenous leukemia (CML) there is little indication for FCI. However, FCI can provide accurate blast cell enumeration and characterize the blast cells in the accelerated and blast phases of the disease. Flow cytometry has an emerging role in the identification of other myeloproliferative neoplasms (i.e. polycythemia vera, essential thrombocythemia, primary myelofibrosis). A combination of myeloid, monocytic and hematopoietic precursor markers can be used to identify recurring FCI abnormalities in myeloid antigen expression and which correlate with cytogenetic abnormalities [43].

Myelodysplastic syndromes

Although bone marrow aspirate and biopsy morphology are the "gold standard" for the diagnosis of myelodysplastic syndromes (MDS), FCI is increasingly being used (see also Chapter 15). Multiple phenotypic abnormalities are seen [11,43,85], which can contribute to the diagnosis of MDS even in the absence of overt morphological dysplasia or increased blast cells [13]. However, no single MDS-specific immunophenotype exists. The success of FCI requires the use of large numbers of antibodies in a carefully controlled multi-parameter panel (four or more colors),

evaluating multiple cellular features and cautious interpretation. The abnormalities that can be seen in MDS include:

1. Abnormally decreased SSC properties in granulocytes (due to hypogranularity).
2. Absence of normal antigens.
3. Asynchronous antigenic expression patterns during maturation.
4. Abnormal intensity of antigen expression.
5. Non-myeloid (i.e. lymphoid) antigens on myeloid precursors [11,14,43,85,86].

Asynchronous myeloid cell maturation is often detected by examining the relationship and patterns of expression of CD13, CD33, CD16, CD11b, CD34, CD117 and HLA-DR antigens in maturing cells [85,86]. This is also relevant in the assessment of acute leukemia: asynchronous antigen expression in the maturing myeloid cells suggests the leukemia may have arisen from preceding myelodysplasia. It is important to note that there are a number of factors that can confound the interpretation of FCI for the assessment of aberrant expression of myeloid antigens. These include technical factors such as machine and protocol standardization, careful gating of the cell population of interest, definitions of "normal" and strict quality control. Clinical factors include knowing the effects of drugs and cytokines on antigen expression, changes in antigen expression during marrow regeneration following myelosuppressive therapy and the effects of sample storage and anticoagulation on antigen expression. If these issues are addressed, FCI analysis can be used to add diagnostic and prognostic information to the evaluation of MDS. The follwing prognostic information can be provided by FCI:

1. Certain immunophenotypic profiles and FCI abnormalities are associated with a poor IPSS score and risk category.
2. A high number of FCI abnormalities are associated with post-transplantation relapses and poor overall survival, which is independent of the IPSS and survival prediction [14].

Conclusion

Flow cytometry is one of the most important diagnostic techniques in the diagnosis and ongoing analysis of hematological malignancies. Its prime roles are to establish the cell lineage, stage of differentiation and disease-association (and thereby diagnosis and classification) by virtue of the antigens expressed by the neoplastic cells. However, the applications of FCI now also extend to detecting potential therapeutic targets, genetic associations, prognostic predictors and residual disease post-therapy. Flow cytometry is also pivotal in diagnostic algorithms; the results of immunophenotyping can be used to allow rational choice of the most appropriate genetic tests required to further delineate the molecular basis of the disease and for clinical management.

Acknowledgments

The authors wish to acknowledge Dr. Raul C. Braylan for his pioneering work in the field of clinical flow cytometry, and its positive impact in improving the diagnosis of lymphoproliferative disorders.

References

1. Bourner G, Dhaliwal J, Sumner J. Performance evaluation of the latest fully automated hematology analyzers in a large, commercial laboratory setting: a 4-way, side-by-side study. *Lab Hematol* 2005; **11**(4):285–97.

2. Stetler-Stevenson MAE, Barnett D, Braylan RC *et al. Clinical Flow Cytometric Analysis of Neoplastic Hematolymphoid Cells; Approved Guideline, 2nd Edn. CLSI document H43-A2*. Wayne, PA: Clinical and Laboratory Standards Institute; 2005.

3. Braylan RC, Orfao A, Borowitz MJ, Davis BH. Optimal number of reagents required to evaluate hematolymphoid neoplasias: results of an international consensus meeting. *Cytometry*. 2001; **46**(1):23–7.

4. Wood B. Nine-color and 10-color flow cytometry in the clinical laboratory. *Arch Pathol Lab Med* 2006; **130**(5):680–90.

5. Weir EG, Cowan K, LeBeau P, Borowitz MJ. A limited antibody panel can distinguish B-precursor acute lymphoblastic leukemia from normal B precursors with four-color flow cytometry: implications for residual disease detection. *Leukemia* 1999; **13**(4):558–67.

6. Davis BH, Holden JT, Bene MC *et al.* 2006 Bethesda International Consensus recommendations on the flow cytometric immunophenotypic analysis of hematolymphoid neoplasia: medical indications. *Cytometry B Clin Cytom* 2007;**72** Suppl. 1:S5–13.

7. Orfao A, Ortuno F, de Santiago M, Lopez A, San Miguel J. Immunophenotyping of acute leukemias and myelodysplastic syndromes. *Cytometry A* 2004; **58**(1):62–71.

8. Hegde U, Filie A, Little RF *et al.* High incidence of occult leptomeningeal disease detected by flow cytometry in newly diagnosed aggressive B-cell lymphomas at risk for central nervous system involvement: the role of flow cytometry versus cytology. *Blood* 2005;**105**(2):496–502.

9. Almasri NM, Zaer FS, Iturraspe JA, Braylan RC. Contribution of flow cytometry to the diagnosis of gastric lymphomas in endoscopic biopsy specimens. *Mod Pathol* 1997;**10**(7):650–6.

10. Mourad WA, Tulbah A, Shoukri M *et al.* Primary diagnosis and REAL/WHO classification of non-Hodgkin's lymphoma by fine-needle aspiration: cytomorphologic and immunophenotypic approach. *Diagn Cytopathol* 2003;**28**(4):191–5.

11. Stetler-Stevenson M, Arthur DC, Jabbour N *et al.* Diagnostic utility of flow cytometric immunophenotyping in myelodysplastic syndrome. *Blood* 2001;**98**(4):979–87.

12. Truong F, Smith BR, Stachurski D *et al.* The utility of flow cytometric immunophenotyping in cytopenic patients with a non-diagnostic bone marrow: a prospective study. *Leuk Res* 2009;**33**(8):1039–46.

13. Valent P, Horny HP, Bennett JM *et al.* Definitions and standards in the diagnosis and treatment of the myelodysplastic syndromes: Consensus statements and report from a working conference. *Leuk Res* 2007; **31**(6):727–36.

14. Wells DA, Benesch M, Loken MR *et al.* Myeloid and monocytic dyspoiesis as determined by flow cytometric scoring in myelodysplastic syndrome correlates with the IPSS and with outcome after hematopoietic stem cell transplantation. *Blood* 2003;**102**(1):394–403.

15. DiGiuseppe JA, Borowitz MJ. Clinical utility of flow cytometry in the chronic lymphoid leukemias. *Semin Oncol* 1998;**25**(1):6–10.

16. Nowakowski GS, Witzig TE, Dingli D *et al.* Circulating plasma cells detected by flow cytometry as a predictor of survival in 302 patients with newly diagnosed multiple myeloma. *Blood* 2005;**106**(7):2276–9.

17. Ocqueteau M, Orfao A, Almeida J *et al.* Immunophenotypic characterization of plasma cells from monoclonal gammopathy of undetermined significance patients. Implications for the differential diagnosis between MGUS and multiple myeloma. *Am J Pathol* 1998;**152**(6):1655–65.

18. Duggan PR, Easton D, Luider J, Auer IA. Bone marrow staging of patients with non-Hodgkin lymphoma by flow cytometry: correlation with morphology. *Cancer* 2000;**88**(4):894–9.

19. Del Poeta G, Maurillo L, Venditti A *et al.* Clinical significance of CD38 expression in chronic lymphocytic leukemia. *Blood* 2001;**98**(9):2633–9.

20. Wiestner A, Rosenwald A, Barry TS *et al.* ZAP-70 expression identifies a chronic lymphocytic leukemia subtype with unmutated immunoglobulin genes, inferior clinical outcome, and distinct gene expression profile. *Blood* 2003;**101**(12):4944–51.

21. Borowitz MJ, Shuster J, Carroll AJ *et al.* Prognostic significance of fluorescence intensity of surface marker expression in childhood B-precursor acute lymphoblastic leukemia. A Pediatric Oncology Group Study. *Blood* 1997;**89**(11):3960–6.

22. Jiang L, Yuan CM, Hubacheck J *et al.* Variable CD52 expression in mature T cell and NK cell malignancies: implications for alemtuzumab therapy. *Br J Haematol* 2009;**145**(2):173–9.

23. Perz J, Topaly J, Fruehauf S, Hensel M, Ho AD. Level of CD20-expression and efficacy of rituximab treatment in patients with resistant or relapsing B-cell prolymphocytic leukemia and B-cell chronic lymphocytic leukemia. *Leukemia Lymphoma* 2002;**43**(1):149–51.

24. Coustan-Smith E, Sancho J, Hancock ML *et al.* Clinical importance of minimal residual disease in childhood acute lymphoblastic leukemia. *Blood* 2000;**96**(8):2691–6.

25. Rawstron AC, Kennedy B, Evans PA *et al.* Quantitation of minimal disease levels in chronic lymphocytic leukemia using a sensitive flow cytometric assay improves the prediction of outcome and can be used to optimize therapy. *Blood* 2001;**98**(1):29–35.

26. Kraan J, Gratama JW, Haioun C *et al.* Flow cytometric immunophenotyping of cerebrospinal fluid. *Curr Protoc Cytom* 2008;Chapter 6:Unit 6.25.

27. Wood BL, Arroz M, Barnett D *et al.* 2006 Bethesda International Consensus recommendations on the immunophenotypic analysis of hematolymphoid neoplasia by flow cytometry: optimal reagents and reporting for the flow cytometric diagnosis of hematopoietic neoplasia. *Cytom B Clin Cytom* 2007;**72** Suppl. 1:S14–22.

28. Jaffe ES, Harris NL, Stein H, Vardiman JW. *Pathology and Genetics of Tumours of Haematopoietic and Lymphoid Tissues.* Kleihues PSL (ed.). Lyon: IARC Press; 2001.

29. Weir EG, Borowitz MJ. Flow cytometry in the diagnosis of acute leukemia. *Semin Hematol* 2001;**38**(2):124–38.

30. Borowitz MJ, Rubnitz J, Nash M, Pullen DJ, Camitta B. Surface antigen phenotype can predict TEL-AML1 rearrangement in childhood B-precursor ALL: a Pediatric Oncology Group study. *Leukemia* 1998;**12**(11):1764–70.

31. De Zen L, Orfao A, Cazzaniga G *et al.*Quantitative multiparametric immunophenotyping in acute lymphoblastic leukemia: correlation with specific genotype. I. ETV6/AML1 ALLs identification. *Leukemia* 2000;**14**(7):1225–31.

32. Lee RV, Braylan R C, Rimsza LM. CD58 expression decreases as nonmalignant B cells mature in bone marrow and is frequently overexpressed in adult and pediatric precursor B-cell acute lymphoblastic leukemia. *Am J Clin Pathol* 2005;**123**(1):119–24.

33. Davis RE, Longacre TA, Cornbleet PJ. Hematogones in the bone marrow of adults. Immunophenotypic features, clinical settings and differential diagnosis. *Am J Clin Pathol* 1994;**102**:202–11.

34. Dunphy CH. Comprehensive review of adult acute myelogenous leukemia: cytomorphological, enzyme cytochemical, flow cytometric immunophenotypic, and cytogenetic findings. *J Clin Lab Analysis* 1999;**13**(1):19–26.

35. Li S, Juco J, Mann KP, Holden JT. Flow cytometry in the differential diagnosis of lymphocyte-rich thymoma from precursor T-cell acute lymphoblastic leukemia/lymphoblastic lymphoma. *Am J Clin Pathol* 2004;**121**(2):268–74.

36. Gorczyca W, Tugulea S, Liu Z *et al.* Flow cytometry in the diagnosis of mediastinal tumors with emphasis on differentiating thymocytes from precursor T-lymphoblastic lymphoma/leukemia. *Leukemia Lymphoma* 2004;**45**(3):529–38.

37. Raza A, Jurcic JG, Roboz GJ *et al.* Complete remissions observed in acute myeloid leukemia following prolonged exposure to lintuzumab: a phase 1 trial. *Leukemia Lymphoma* 2009; **50**:1336–44.

38. Hurwitz CA, Raimondi SC, Head D *et al.* Distinctive immunophenotypic features of t(8;21)(q22;q22) acute myeloblastic leukemia in children. *Blood* 1992;**80**(12):3182–8.

39. Baer MR, Stewart CC, Lawrence D *et al.* Expression of the neural cell adhesion molecule CD56 is associated with short remission duration and survival in acute myeloid leukemia with t(8;21)(q22;q22). *Blood* 1997;**90**(4):1643–8.

40. Kita K, Nakase K, Miwa H *et al.* Phenotypical characteristics of acute myelocytic leukemia associated with the t(8;21)(q22;q22) chromosomal abnormality: frequent expression of immature B-cell antigen CD19 together with stem cell antigen CD34. *Blood* 1992;**80**(2):470–7.

41. Orfao A, Chillon MC, Bortoluci AM *et al.* The flow cytometric pattern of CD34, CD15 and CD13

expression in acute myeloblastic leukemia is highly characteristic of the presence of PML-RAR alpha gene rearrangements. *Haematologica* 1999;**84** (5):405–12.

42. Lin P, Hao S, Medeiros LJ *et al.* Expression of CD2 in acute promyelocytic leukemia correlates with short form of PML-RARalpha transcripts and poorer prognosis. *Am J Clin Pathol* 2004;**121**(3):402–7.

43. Kussick SJ, Wood BL. Using 4-color flow cytometry to identify abnormal myeloid populations. *Arch Pathol Lab Med* 2003;**127**(9):1140–7.

44. Kussick SJ, Wood BL. Four-color flow cytometry identifies virtually all cytogenetically abnormal bone marrow samples in the workup of non-CML myeloproliferative disorders. *Am J Clin Pathol* 2003;**120**(6):854–65.

45. Stetler-Stevenson M, Schrager JA. Flow cytometric analysis in the diagnosis and prognosis of lymphoma and chronic leukemias. In McCoy JP, Carey JL, Keren DF (eds.), *Flow Cytometry in Clinical Diagnosis*, 4th edn. Chicago: ASCP Press; 2006: 129–67.

46. Fukushima PIN, Nguyen PKT, O'Grady P, Stetler-Stevenson M. Flow cytometric analysis of kappa and lambda light chain expression in evaluation of specimens for B-cell neoplasia. *Cytometry* 1996;**26**:243–52.

47. Kussick S, Kalnoski M, Braziel R, Wood B. Prominent clonal B-cell populations identified by flow cytometry in histologically reactive lymphoid proliferations. *Am J Clin Pathol* 2004;**121**:464–72.

48. Marti G, Rawstron, AC, Ghia, P *et al.* Diagnostic criteria for monoclonal B-cell lymphocytosis. *Br J Haematol* 2005;**130**:325–32.

49. Rawstron A, Green MJ, Kuzmicki A *et al.* Monoclonal B lymphocytes with the characteristics of indolent chronic lymphocytic leukemia are present in 3.5% of adults with normal blood counts. *Blood* 2002;**100**:635–9.

50. Maiese RL, Segal GH, Iturraspe JA, Braylan RC. The cell-surface antigen and DNA content distribution of lymph-nodes with reactive hyperplasia. *Modern Pathol* 1995;**8**(5):536–43.

51. Huang J, Fan, G, Zhong, Y *et al.* Diagnostic usefulness of aberrant CD22 expression in differentiating neoplastic cells of B-cell chronic lymphoproliferative disorders from admixed benign B cells in four-color multiparameter flow cytometry. *Am J Clin Pathol* 2005;**123**:826–32.

52. Kaleem Z, Zehnbauer BA, White G, Zutter MM. Lack of expression of surface immunoglobulin light chains in B-cell non-Hodgkin lymphomas. *Am J Clin Pathol* 2000;**113**(3):399–405.

53. Li S, Eshleman JR, Borowitz MJ. Lack of surface immunoglobulin light chain expression by flow cytometric immunophenotyping can help diagnose peripheral B cell lymphoma. *Am J Clin Pathol* 2002;**118**:229–34.

54. Cornfield DB, Mitchell DM, Almasri NM *et al.* Follicular lymphoma can be distinguished from benign follicular hyperplasia by flow cytometry using simultaneous staining of cytoplasmic bcl-2 and cell surface CD20. *Am J Clin Pathol* 2000;**114**(2):258–63.

55. Almasri NM, Iturraspe JA, Braylan RC. CD10 expression in follicular lymphoma and large cell lymphoma is different from that of reactive lymph node follicles. *Archives Pathol Lab Med* 1998; **122**(6):539–44.

56. Chen X, Jensen PE, Li S. HLA-DO – A useful marker to distinguish florid follicular hyperplasia from follicular lymphoma by flow cytometry. *Am J Clin Pathol* 2003;**119**(6):842–51.

57. Ginaldi L, De Martinis M, Matutes E, Farahat N, Morilla R. Levels of expression of CD19 and CD20 in chronic B cell leukaemias. *J Clin Pathol* 1998; **51**:364–9.

58. Yang W, Agrawal N, Patel J *et al.* Diminished expression of CD19 in B-cell lymphomas. *Cytom B Clin Cytom* 2005;**63**B:28–35.

59. Kingma DW, Imus, P, Xie, XY *et al.* CD2 is expressed by a sub-population of normal B cells and is frequently present in mature B-Cell neoplasms. *Clin Cytom* 2002;**50**:243–8.

60. Kaleem Z, White G, Zutter, MM. Aberrant expression of T-cell-associated antigens on B-cell non-Hodgkin lymphoma. *Am J Clin Pathol* 2001;**115**:396–403.

61. Foran J, Norton AJ, Micallef INM *et al.* Loss of CD20 expression following treatment with rituximab (chimaeric monoclonal anti-CD-20): a retrospective cohort analysis. *Br J Haematol* 2001;**114**:881–3.

62. Rawstron AC, Orfao A, Beksac M *et al.* Report of the European Myeloma Network on multiparametric flow cytometry in multiple myeloma and related disorders. *Haematologica* 2008;**93**(3):431–8.

63. Ocqueteau M, Orfao A, Almeida J *et al.* Immunophenotypic characterization of plasma cells from monoclonal gammopathy of undetermined significance patients. Implications for the differential diagnosis between MGUS and multiple myeloma. *Am J Pathol* 1998;**152**:1655–65.

64. Almeida J, Orfao A, Ocqueteau M *et al.* High-sensitive immunophenotyping and DNA ploidy studies for the investigation of minimal residual disease in multiple myeloma. *Br J Haematol* 1999;**107**:121–31.

65. Konoplev S, Medeiros LJ, Bueso-Ramos CE, Jorgensen JL, Lin P. Immunophenotypic profile of

lymphoplasmacytic lymphoma/Waldenström macroglobulinemia. *Am J Clin Pathol* 2005;**124**:414–20.

66. Lin P, Owens R, Tricot G, Wilson CS. Flow cytometric immunophenotypic analysis of 306 cases of multiple myeloma. *Am J Clin Pathol* 2004;**121**:482–8.

67. Rawstron AC, Davies FE, DasGupta R *et al.* Flow cytometric disease monitoring in multiple myeloma: the relationship between normal and neoplastic plasma cells predicts outcome after transplantation. *Blood* 2002;**100**(9):3095–100.

68. Mateo G, Montalban MA, Vidriales MB *et al.* Prognostic value of immunophenotyping in multiple myeloma: a study by the PETHEMA/GEM cooperative study groups on patients uniformly treated with high-dose therapy. *J Clin Oncol* 2008;**26**(16):2737–44.

69. Gorczyca W, Weisberger J, Liu Z *et al.* An approach to diagnosis of T-cell lymphoproliferative disorders by flow cytometry. *Clinical Cytometry* 2002;**50B**: 177–90.

70. Nicholson JK, Rao PE, Calvelli T *et al.* Artifactual staining of monoclonal antibodies in two-color combinations is due to an immunoglobulin in the serum and plasma. *Cytometry* 1994;**18**(3):140–6.

71. McClanahan J, Fukushima PI, Stetler-Stevenson M. Increased peripheral blood gamma delta T-cells in patients with lymphoid neoplasia: A diagnostic dilemma in flow cytometry. *Cytometry* 1999; **38**(6):280–5.

72. Lima M, Teixeira MD, Queiros ML *et al.* Immunophenotype and TCR-V beta repertoire of peripheral blood T-cells in acute infectious mononucleosis. *Blood Cells Molecules Diseases* 2003;**10**:1–12.

73. Jamal S, Picker LJ, Aquino DB *et al.* Immunophenotypic analysis of peripheral T-cell neoplasms. A multiparameter flow cytometric approach. *Am J Clin Pathol* 2001;**116**:512–26.

74. Edelman J, Meyerson HJ. Diminished CD3 expression is useful for detecting and enumerating Sézary cells. *Am J Clin Pathol* 2000;**114**(3):467–77.

75. Yokote T, Akioka T, Oka S *et al.* Flow cytometric immunophenotyping of adult T-cell leukemia/ lymphoma using CD3 gating. *Am J Clin Pathol* 2005;**124**(2):199–204.

76. Li Y, Braylan RC, Al-Quran SZ. Flow-cytometric assessment of T-cell clonality in clinical specimens. *LabMed* 2007;**38**(8):477–82.

77. van den Beemd RB, Boor PPC, van Lochem EG *et al.* Flow cytometric analysis of the V beta repertoire in healthy controls. *Cytometry* 2000;**40**(4):336–45.

78. Ferenczi K, Yawalkar N, Jones D, Kupper TS. Monitoring the decrease of circulating malignant T cells in cutaneous T-cell lymphoma during photopheresis and interferon therapy. *Archives of Dermatology* 2003;**139**(7):909–13.

79. Morice WG, Katzmann JA, Pittelkow MR *et al.* A comparison of morphologic features, flow cytometry, TCR-V-beta analysis, and TCR-PCR in qualitative and quantitative assessment of peripheral blood involvement by Sezary syndrome. *Am J Clin Pathol* 2006;**125**(3):364–74.

80. Lima M, Almeida J, Montero AG *et al.* Clinicobiological, immunophenotypic, and molecular characteristics of monoclonal CD56-/+dim chronic natural killer cell large granular lymphocytosis. *Am J Pathol* 2004;**165**(4):1117–27.

81. Husain Z, Alper CA, Yunis EJ, Dubey DP. Complex expression of natural killer receptor genes in single natural killer cells. *Immunology* 2002;**106**(3):373–80.

82. Epling-Burnette PK, Painter JS, Chaurasia P *et al.* Dysregulated NK receptor expression in patients with lymphoproliferative disease of granular lymphocytes. *Blood* 2004;**103**(9):3431–9.

83. Pascal V, Schleinitz N, Brunet C *et al.* Comparative analysis of NK cell subset distribution in normal and lymphoproliferative disease of granular lymphocyte conditions. *European J Immunol* 2004;**34**(10):2930–40.

84. Sawada A, Sato E, Koyama M *et al.* NK-cell repertoire is feasible for diagnosing Epstein-Barr virus-infected NK-cell lymphoproliferative disease and evaluating the treatment effect. *Am J Hematol* 2006;**81**(8):576–81.

85. Kussick SJ, Fromm JR, Rossini A *et al.* Four-color flow cytometry shows strong concordance with bone marrow morphology and cytogenetics in the evaluation for myelodysplasia. *Am J Clin Pathol* 2005;**124**(2):170–81.

86. Maynadie M, Picard F, Husson B *et al.* Immunophenotypic clustering of myelodysplastic syndromes. *Blood* 2002;**100**(7):2349–56.

4 Cytogenetics

Christine J. Harrison and Claire Schwab

Introduction

For many years cytogenetic analysis has provided the gold standard tool for basic genetic diagnosis in hematological malignancies. Although resolution is somewhat limited, it provides a global analysis of the entire genome. In recent years a range of fluorescence *in situ* hybridization (FISH) and high resolution array-based techniques have become integrated into the broader field of cytogenetics, which have provided complementary rather than replacement approaches. They have identified novel and submicroscopic genetic changes, which need to be considered alongside the traditional karyotype.

A number of chromosomal abnormalities provide the definitive diagnosis of a specific type of leukemia. The best known examples include the association of the Philadelphia chromosome (Ph), arising from the translocation, t(9;22)(q34;q11), with chronic myelogenous leukemia (CML) and the translocation, t(15;17)(q22;q21), with acute promyelocytic leukemia (APL). Of particular interest is the strong link between certain abnormalities and outcome, which are used to determine the risk stratification of patients for treatment. For example, the Ph and near haploidy (< 30 chromosomes) are associated with a poor prognosis in childhood acute lymphoblastic leukemia (ALL) and patients with these abnormalities are treated as high risk. Other genetic abnormalities are associated with a favorable outcome, e.g. core binding acute myeloid leukemias (AML) with chromosomal rearrangements t(8;21)(q22;q22) and inversion of chromosome 16, inv(16)(p13q22)/t(16;16)(p13;q22), and childhood ALL with hyperdiploidy (51–65 chromosomes) and t(12;21)(p13;q22). An increasing number of specific gene mutations are being described in the acute leukemias and myeloproliferative neoplasms. In AML these have been shown to have an impact on outcome and treatment protocols are beginning to be modified to incorporate these findings. Cytogenetic analysis and related procedures may be useful in relapse to confirm the presence of the original clone and identify clonal evolution.

The classification of hematological malignancies follows the definition of the World Health Organization (WHO) that "a classification should contain diseases that are clearly defined, clinically distinctive, non-overlapping (mutually exclusive) and together comprise all known entities" [1]. The recently updated *WHO Classification of Tumours of Haematopoietic and Lymphoid Tissues* builds on the understanding that there is no one "gold standard" by which a disease is defined. It relies on the combination of cellular morphology, immunophenotype and genetic features, with variable input within each entity. For example, many malignancies have a specific immunophenotype, while in others the defining criterion is provided by the genetic abnormality. WHO recognizes that genetic changes may be highly characteristic of a single disease type or determine prognosis in a range of diseases. The WHO therefore recommends that chromosomal analysis should be carried out at the time of diagnosis to establish the cytogenetic picture. However, how genetics fits into current diagnosis based on WHO criteria can be difficult to decipher. This chapter will focus on the description of those genetic abnormalities defined by WHO which identify significant disease entities within the hematological neoplasms. The principles of the main techniques used in their detection are provided. Data interpretation using clinical examples is given to illustrate how they are incorporated into the overall diagnosis.

Diagnostic Techniques in Hematological Malignancies, ed. Wendy N. Erber. Published by Cambridge University Press.
© Cambridge University Press 2010.

Principles of methods

Cytogenetics

In acute leukemia and other hematological malignancies, a bone marrow sample taken at diagnosis provides the material for all genetic diagnostic tests. Sometimes, if it is known that the cells of interest are present in the peripheral blood, a blood sample may be appropriate for cytogenetic analysis, for example in CML. For cytogenetic analysis, bone marrow is set up in short-term culture, usually overnight, to stimulate cells into division while maintaining them as close to the *in vivo* situation as possible. Cells are exposed to the spindle poison, colcemid, for one to 16 hours to maximize the arrest of cells in metaphase. A hypotonic solution is applied, which weakens the plasma membrane, then cells are fixed and washed in Carnoy's fixative (3 : 1 methanol : acetic acid). After cooling, a drop of this suspension, adjusted to the optimum cell density, is dropped onto a glass slide. As the fixative evaporates, the surface tension ruptures the plasma membrane and the cells flatten onto the slide. In a good preparation the chromosomes from the same metaphase will be maintained within close proximity to each other without overlapping. A short and controlled enzymatic treatment with dilute trypsin, followed by Giemsa staining, produces banding patterns along the chromatids. These patterns are specific to each chromosome pair and, in association with chromosome size and centromere position, are used to identify the chromosomes. This procedure is termed karyotyping and the chromosomes are ordered into pairs within a karyogram (Figure 4.1a). Diagrammatic representation of the individual chromosomal banding patterns is depicted in idiograms in which each chromosomal band is assigned a number radiating outwards from the centromere (Figure 4.1b). This classification allows chromosomal abnormalities to be accurately described according to international guidelines produced by the member committee of the International System for Human Cytogenetic Nomenclature (ISCN) [2]. In the ISCN a clone is defined as two cells with the same chromosomal gain or structural change or three cells with the same chromosomal loss. For a karyotype to be defined as normal requires the full analysis of 20 normal cells. If fewer than 20 are available, the cytogenetic analysis is regarded as "failed." Table 4.1 details the cytogenetic nomenclature used in reporting hematological

malignancies. Cytogenetic analysis may be used to monitor minimal residual disease if an abnormal karyotype is present at diagnosis. However, its low specificity and the risk of analyzing metaphases from normal cells represent major obstacles for its routine use for disease monitoring.

Fluorescence *in situ* hybridization (FISH)

Cytogenetic analysis (karyotyping) depends on the presence of dividing cells within the sample. This limitation has been overcome to a certain extent by the development of FISH techniques, for which one major advantage is the ability to visualize abnormalities in the non-dividing cells. This is particularly important in those hematological malignancies with a low proliferative index when chromosome morphology is poor and cytogenetic analysis is unsuccessful. The ability to analyze non-dividing cells also gives the capability to perform FISH on directly prepared samples. Another significant advantage of FISH techniques is that, in addition to aspirated bone marrow and peripheral blood, it may be carried out on sections of paraffin-embedded tissue, and for hematological malignancies, specifically on bone marrow trephine (BMT) biopsies. In tissue biopsies, although care must be taken to analyze complete cells, excellent results have been obtained with the locus-specific probe approaches (described below). In some clinical scenarios it may be necessary to carry out FISH on specific cell types (e.g. plasma cells). One approach used to achieve this is FICTION (Fluorescence Immunophenotype and Interphase Cytogenetics as a Tool for Investigation of Neoplasms). This involves simultaneous application of FISH and immunofluorescent staining to intact cells, usually in cytospin preparations, but it has also been achieved on paraffin-embedded sectioned material (see also Chapter 2 and Figure 2.8). FICTION therefore enables specific genetic abnormalities to be assessed in cells identified by their phenotype (e.g. CD138-positive plasma cells).

FISH is essentially a molecular technique which has greatly enhanced the accuracy of chromosomal analysis by bringing together cytogenetics and molecular biology. FISH is based on single-stranded DNA probe annealing to its complementary sequence in a target genome. It is able to detect and localize the presence or absence of specific DNA sequences on metaphases which are spread onto a glass slide. FISH uses fluorescent probes (whole chromosome paints or

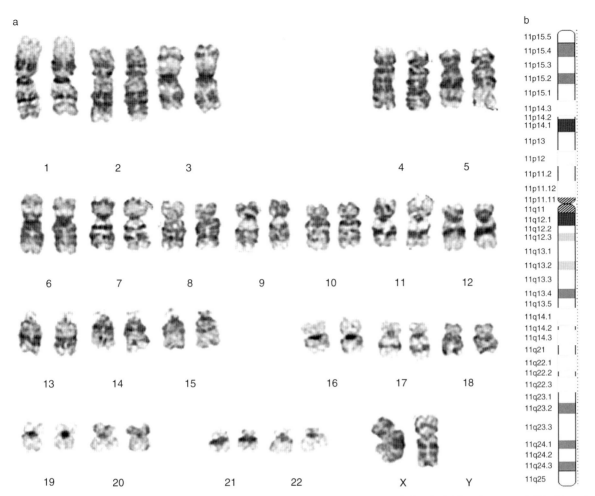

Figure 4.1. a. A karyogram from a metaphase from a leukemic cell found in the bone marrow of a female childhood patient with ALL. Although the chromosomes appear normal, the cell has a t(12;21)(p13;q22), which is cryptic by cytogenetic analysis.
b. An idiogram of chromosome 11 depicting the numbering system of the chromosome bands.

locus-specific probes) that bind only to those parts of the chromosome with which they show a high degree of sequence homology. Fluorescence microscopy is used to examine the location of the fluorescent probe bound to the chromosomes.

There are two main types of probe for FISH, chromosome paints and locus-specific probes. **Whole chromosome paints** are generated from chromosome-specific probe libraries. They may be hybridized to metaphases in various combinations using different fluorochromes to visualize different chromosomes at the same time. They are used to determine the origin of structural abnormalities. Techniques have been developed using differentially labeled multiple paints to visualize all chromosome pairs simultaneously.

These multiplex FISH techniques (M-FISH) have greatly improved the interpretation of complex chromosomal rearrangements and characterization of previously unidentified chromosomal changes.

Locus-specific probes are most frequently used to target genes of interest in order to identify rearrangements, deletions, and gains in both interphase and metaphase cells. Centromere-specific probes may be directed to the alpha (or beta) satellite repeat sequences within the centromeric regions specific for each chromosome. FISH using locus-specific probes may be used to monitor minimal residual disease if a distinctive abnormality is present. However, many probes have a relatively high false positive detection rate due to the chance localization of probes close together within the

Table 4.1. Cytogenetic nomenclature with illustrative examples.

Symbol	Definition	Example	Interpretation
add	Additional material of unknown origin	46,XY,**add**(9)(q22)	Unknown chromosomal material attached to the long arm of chromosome 9 at band q22
brackets, angle (< >)	Surround the ploidy level	26<1n>,XY,+14,+21	Karyotype with 26 chromosomes and gain of chromosomes 14 and 21 onto the haploid chromosome set
brackets, square ([])	Surround the number of cells	46,XY[20]	Normal male karyotype seen in 20 cells analyzed
c	Constitutional abnormality	48,XX,+21,+21**c**	Karyotype with a constitutional and an acquired gain of chromosome 21
comma (,)	Separates chromosome numbers, sex chromosomes and chromosomal abnormalities	45,X,-Y,t(8;21)(q22;q22)	
cp	Composite karyotype	45~48,XY,del(5)(q15)[3],-7[4],+8[3][**cp**7]	Composite karyotype of seven cells, each has at least one of the abnormalities listed, number of cells with each abnormality is shown in the square brackets. Some of the cells have more than one of the abnormalities
decimal point (.)	Denotes chromosomal subbands	46,XX,t(9;22)(q34;q11.2)	
del	Deletion	46,XY,**del**(9)(p13p22)	Deletion of the short arm of chromosome 9 between the bands p13 and p22
der	Derivative chromosome: structurally rearranged chromosome arising from a rearrangement of two or more chromosomes. The derivative chromosome has an intact centromere.	46,XY,**der**(9)del(9)(p13)t(9;22)(q34;q11.1)	Derivative chromosome 9 with a deletion of the short arm at 9p13 and a translocation of the same chromosome 9 with chromosome 22
dic	Dicentric chromosome: replaces one or two chromosomes and has two centromeres	45,XY,**dic**(9;20)(p13;q11)	Dicentric chromosome of the long arm of chromosome 9 and the short arm of chromosome 20, the breakpoints are in the short and long arms, respectively
dmin	Double minutes: acentric structures	49,XY, ...~15**dmin**	A cell with approximately 15 double minutes, written at the end of the karyotype
dup	Duplication	46,XY,**dup**(21)(q21q22)	The segment of chromosome 21 between bands q21 and q22 is duplicated
hsr	Homogeneously staining region	46,XX,**hsr**(2)(q31)	hsr inserted into the long arm of chromosome 2 at band q31
i	Isochromosome: breakpoints are assigned to the centromeric bands	46,XY,**i**(17)(q10)	Isochromosome comprising the long arms of chromosome 17
idem	Denotes the stemline karyotype in a subclone	46,XX,t(9;22)(q34;q11.2)[6]/47,**idem**,+8[12]	Clone with 46 chromosomes and translocation between chromosomes 9 and 22 in six cells, the subclone has the same translocation but has gained a chromosome 8 in 12 cells
inc	Incomplete karyotype with unidentifiable abnormalities	46,XY,del(9)(p13),**inc**	It has only been possible to identify a deletion of the short arm of chromosome 9, but there are additional abnormalities which cannot be identified

Table 4.1. (cont.)

Symbol	Definition	Example	Interpretation
ins	Insertion	46,XY,**ins**(8;21)(q22; q21q22)	An insertion of bands q21 to q22 from chromosome 21 into 8 at band q22
inv	Inversion: paracentric inversion, the breakage and reunion occurs in the same chromosome arm; pericentric, occurs in both arms	46,XX,**inv**(3)(q21q26)	The region between the bands q21 and q26 is inverted within the long arm of chromosome 3
mar	Marker or unidentified chromosome	47,XX,t(9;22)(q34;q11.2), +**mar**	An unidentified chromosome in addition to the translocation between chromosomes 9 and 22, written at the end of the karyotype
minus sign (−)	Loss	45,XY,−7	Loss/monosomy of chromosome 7
multiplication sign (x)	Multiple copies of re-arranged chromosomes	46,XY,del(6)(q15q21)**x**2	Karyotype with two copies of the deleted chromosome 6
p	Chromosome short arm	46,XY,del(9)(**p**13**p**22)	Denoting the breakpoints on the short arm of chromosome 9 at which the deletion occurs
parentheses ()	Surround structurally altered chromosomes and breakpoints	46,XY,der(9)del(9)(p13)t (9;22)(q34;q11.1)	
plus sign (+)	Gain	47,XY,**+**8	Gain/trisomy of chromosome 8
q	Chromosome long arm	46,XX,t(9;22)(**q**34;**q**11.2)	Denoting the breakpoints on the long arm of chromosomes 9 and 22 at which the translocation occurs
question mark	Questionable identifica-tion of a chromosome or chromosome structure	45,XX,inv(3)(q21q2**?**6),-**?**7	Breakpoint on the long arm of chromosome 3 is in the region 3q2, probably in band 3q26 but this is uncertain, there is loss of a chromosome, probably 7, but this is uncertain
r	Ring chromosome	46,XY,**r**(7)(p22q36)	Ring chromosome in which breakage and reunion has occurred at bands p22 and q36 to form a ring
sdl	Sideline: lines deviating from the stem line (see below)	46,XX,t(9;22)(q34;q11.2)[6]/ 47,sl,+8[12]/48,**sdl1**,+9	47,sl,+8 is the side line (see below), the population with 48 chromosomes has the abnormalities of the stem line plus the side line replaced by sideline number 1 (sdl1) with the gain of chromosome 9
semicolon (;)	Separates altered chromo-somes and breakpoints in structural rearrangements involving more than one chromosome	46,XX,t(9;22)(q34;q11.2),t (4;11)(q21;q23)	
sl	Stem line: the most basic population	46,XX,t(9;22)(q34;q11.2)[6]/ 47,**sl**,+8[12]	The stem line is 46,XX,t(9;22)(q34;q11.2), the popula-tion with 47 chromosomes has the abnormalities of the stem line replaced by sl with gain of chromo-some 8
slant line (/)	Separates cell populations	46,XX,t(9;22)(q34;q11.2)[6]/ 47,idem,+8[12]	
t	Translocation	46,XX,**t**(9;22)(q34;q11.2)	Indicates a translocation between chromosomes 9 and 22

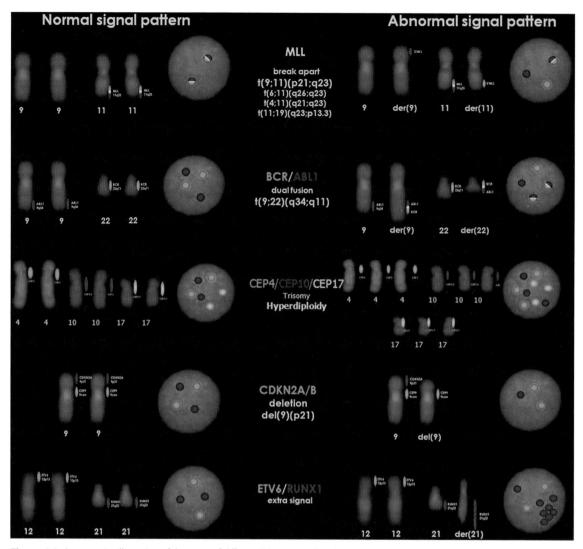

Figure 4.2. A composite illustration of the types of different FISH approaches (breakapart, dual fusion, copy number) and applications with specific abnormalities as examples.
Left shows the normal configurations of the probes on metaphase chromosomes and in interphase cells.
The right depicts the expected corresponding abnormal signal patterns.

nucleus, thus reducing its sensitivity. Therefore FISH is not recommended for accurate detection of low-level clones for minimal residual disease monitoring. The three main types of probe design for the locus-specific probes are described below.

Dual color breakapart probes

Spectrum red (R) and spectrum green (G) labeled probes are located 3′ and 5′ to a gene of interest. When the probe is hybridized to normal cells, the red and green signals are juxtaposed and appear as a yellow fusion (F) signal. A 0R0G2F signal pattern is produced in interphase, representing the intact locus on two normal homologous chromosomes. If as a result of a chromosomal rearrangement, a break occurs in the chromosome at this locus, the red and green signals become separated and appear as individual signals. The resulting signal pattern is a "split" of one fusion signal into the component red and green parts (1R1G1F). This type of probe is particularly useful when the partner gene in a rearrangement is unknown, or when the target gene has multiple partners. The example of the breakapart probe given in Figure 4.2 is the *MLL* locus located to chromosome band 11q23, which has more than 40 partner genes.

Dual color, dual fusion probes

In dual color, dual fusion, both probes are localized to and extend beyond the breakpoints of both chromosomes. Thus, when a translocation occurs, two fusions are formed, one on each derived chromosome as shown in the example given in Figure 4.2 of the translocation, t(9;22)(q34;q11), which gives rise to the *BCR-ABL1* fusion gene. The standard abnormal signal pattern is 1R1G2F. Dual fusion probes have a very low false-positive rate as dual fusion signal patterns rarely arise by chance.

Copy number probes

Centromeric probes are used to detect loss or gain of whole chromosomes and ploidy changes. They are used to identify the origin of chromosomes in metaphase and enumerate specific chromosomes in interphase cells, providing a rapid and accurate method to ascertain chromosome copy number. They may be purchased labeled with different fluorochromes and should be applied in dual or triple color combinations as shown for the determination of high hyperdiploidy in Figure 4.2. Unique sequence probes may also identify deletion or gain of a particular gene. To detect the deletion of a gene of interest, a probe is selected to cover the gene (R). This is tested in a dual color hybridization with another probe which identifies the chromosome on which this gene is localized, usually a centromeric probe (G). Two copies of the red and green probes (2R2G) indicate normal copy number, whereas 1R2G indicates a deletion of the gene of interest as shown in Figure 4.2 for the deletion of *CDKN2A*. Similarly extra copies of a specific gene may be identified. In the example given in Figure 4.2, *ETV6* acts as the control probe and multiple copies of *RUNX1* indicate copy number gain of this gene.

High resolution array-based analysis

Array-based comparative genomic hybridization (aCGH) has recently been developed and is a valuable complementary tool in genetic analysis of hematological malignancies. It is based on established FISH technology. DNA from the leukemic sample (test DNA) is labeled with one fluorescent reporter molecule. This is mixed with a differentially labeled control DNA (reference DNA) and competitively hybridized to a microarray containing genome sequences as

oligonucleotides which acts as the target. This procedure allows copy number changes to be mapped to the genome at high resolution (Figure 4.3). The fluorescence ratio between test and reference DNA is measured and plotted using sophisticated software packages.

Alternatively, single nucleotide polymorphism (SNP) arrays, represented by oligonucleotides, may be used to characterize SNPs in lymphoblasts from patients with leukemia. Recent SNP arrays feature almost two million genetic markers, including equal numbers of SNPs and probes for the detection of copy number variation. In conjunction with conventional cytogenetics, the application of FISH and aCGH/SNP arrays has facilitated the identification of novel chromosomal abnormalities as well as improved the understanding of the molecular genotype underlying established rearrangements. These technologies are important in research; however, they have not yet been integrated into clinical practice.

Multiplex ligation-dependent probe amplification (MLPA)

Multiplex ligation-dependent probe amplification (MLPA) is a rapid, high-throughput multiplex PCR method which can detect abnormal copy numbers of up to 50 different genomic DNA or RNA sequences. It targets very small sequences and can distinguish those differing in a single nucleotide. Thus MLPA is able to identify the frequent, single gene aberrations which are too small to be detected by FISH. One advantage over PCR is that although well-characterized deletions and amplifications can be detected by PCR, the exact breakpoint site of most deletions is unknown. Compared to aCGH and SNP arrays, MLPA is a low-cost simple method. Although it is not suitable for genome-wide research screening, it is a good alternative to array-based techniques for many routine applications.

Real-time quantitative polymerase chain reaction

Depending on the chromosomal abnormality, real-time quantitative PCR performed at diagnosis, may provide a baseline against which response to therapy in the form of minimal residual disease may be measured at specific time points (see Chapter 5 for the principles and applications). This is relevant as cytogenetics and FISH are not sufficiently sensitive to monitor response to therapy, except in CML (see below).

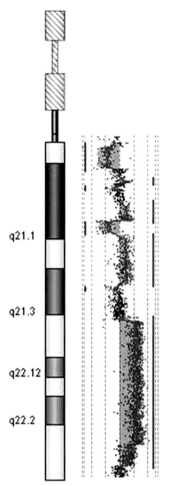

q21.1

q21.3

q22.12

q22.2

Figure 4.3. An example of an aCGH profile. The idiogram of chromosome 21 is shown on the left. On the right is an aCGH profile of an abnormal chromosome 21 from a patient with intrachromosomal amplification of chromosome 21 (iAMP21). The profile is based on the ratio of test DNA (from the leukemic cells of the patient with the abnormality) compared to the reference (control) DNA. A shift to the left (green dots) indicates chromosomal loss, a shift to the right (red dots) indicates chromosomal gain, while the midline (black dots) indicates no genomic imbalance. Thus it is apparent that this copy of chromosome 21 is highly unbalanced with multiple genomic gains and losses. Such a profile gives no indication of where these abnormalities may be located within the karyotype.

Examples of the role of cytogenetics in hematological malignancies

B-cell precursor acute lymphoblastic leukemia

Acute lymphoblastic leukemia (ALL) is primarily a disease of childhood, with more than 75% of cases reported in children between the ages of 2–5 years,

and, of these the majority (85%) are B-cell precursor ALL (BCP-ALL). Many important chromosomal abnormalities have been reported in both B- and T-lineage ALL. It is of interest that a number have been shown to arise prenatally, long before the onset of leukemia is diagnosed [3]. BCP-ALL is generally associated with a good outcome in children, with a cure rate of approximately 85%, while in adults the overall survival is less than 50% (see Chapter 7 for more details). Those features associated with an adverse outcome in ALL are infancy, age > 10 years, high white blood cell count, slow response to initial therapy and the presence of minimal residual disease after first therapy. In BCP-ALL, many non-random chromosomal abnormalities have been described [4]. According to the WHO classification, genetic entities are included in the classification if they:

a. are associated with distinctive clinical or phenotypic features,
b. are biologically distinct, or,
c. have important prognostic implications.

Although the first two categories are of interest in terms of accurate diagnosis, the third is of greatest importance in ALL as this is used in risk stratification for treatment. Thus the accurate detection of these abnormalities at the time of diagnosis is essential. In this section these abnormalities and the best methods for their detection are discussed.

MLL gene rearrangements

Approximately 3% of children with ALL have re-arrangements of the *MLL* (mixed lineage in leukemia) gene. The majority of these occur in infants and children under the age of 2 years; particularly in infants, the prognosis is poor. The *MLL* gene has many chromosomal partners in ALL. The most frequent is the translocation, t(4;11)(q21;q23), which gives rise to the *MLL-MLLT2* (*MLL-AF4*) fusion. Also important in ALL are the translocations t(11;19)(q23;p13.3), t(9;11)(p21;q23), t(6;11)(q27;q23) and t(10;11)(p12; q23), producing the *MLL-MLLT1* (*MLL-ENL*), *MLL-MLLT3* (*MLL-AF9*), *MLL-MLLT4* (*MLL-AF6*) and *MLL-MLLT10* (*MLL-AF10*) fusions, respectively. The formation of the *MLL-MLLT10* fusion arises from heterogeneous and complex rearrangements of chromosomes 10 and 11 due to the opposite orientation of the genes. Two breaks, as seen in a simple reciprocal translocation, are insufficient to produce an in-frame fusion. The t(4;11) has been reported to have the worst prognosis, although the prognosis of the other partners is uncertain due to their relative rarity.

The t(4;11) is clearly visible by cytogenetics; however, it is recommended that FISH be performed to confirm *MLL* involvement. A dual color breakapart probe specific for *MLL* will detect translocations involving all *MLL* partner genes (Figure 4.2). In interphase the involvement of *MLL* is confirmed, while in metaphase the origin of the partner gene is indicated. For example, the translocations t(6;11)(q27;q23) and t(11;19)(q23;p13) may be difficult to detect by cytogenetic analysis, particularly in poor quality preparations, while in cases with abnormalities of chromosomes 10 and 11, the presence of the *MLL-MLLT10* fusion may need to be confirmed. FISH also provides a simple approach to screen cases in which the cytogenetic analysis has failed. RT-PCR is a less effective method as it is only informative in a multiplex approach including all fusion transcripts.

t(9;22)(q34;q11); *BCR-ABL1*

Ph-positive ALL has the translocation, t(9;22)(q34;q11), which gives rise to the *BCR-ABL1* fusion. This fusion is diagnostic for CML, while in ALL the incidence varies considerably according to age, occurring rarely in childhood (~3%) and more frequently in adult ALL (~25%). In all age groups it is associated with an adverse outcome. Accurate identification of the fusion is vital as patients with Ph-positive ALL are treated with specific protocols including imatinib treatment (as described for CML, see below), which has been shown to improve early event-free survival.

Cytogenetic detection of t(9;22) is reliable; however a number of cryptic insertions and three-way translocations have been described which may be difficult to interpret. FISH using the dual color, dual fusion approach as shown in Figure 4.2 provides a rapid and accurate detection method. RT-PCR for the *BCR-ABL1* fusion transcript offers a good alternative method. With the appropriate primers this PCR approach will distinguish between the major (M-BCR) and minor (m-BCR) breakpoint cluster regions within the *BCR* gene (see Chapter 5 for technical details and Chapter 13 for clinical details). The most sensitive method to monitor response to treatment is real-time quantitative PCR.

t(12;21)(p13;q22); *ETV6-RUNX1*

This translocation is common in childhood BCP-ALL, occurring at an incidence of ~25%, with a peak at 2–5 years of age. It is not found in infants and is rarely seen

in adults. There is strong evidence that the translocation arises *in utero* [5]. It is associated with a good prognosis in children, with a cure rate of > 95% if they possess other favorable clinical features. In spite of its relatively high incidence, this translocation was not discovered until the mid 1990s because it is cryptic by cytogenetic analysis. FISH using chromosome paints specific for chromosomes 12 and 21 initially identified the abnormality (Figure 4.4a). The translocation gives rise to a fusion between *ETV6* and transcription factor, *RUNX1*, and is readily detected by FISH using the dual color approach with probes targeting these two genes, as described for *BCR-ABL1* (Figure 4.4b). The fusion transcript can also be identified by RT-PCR. One advantage of FISH is that it will simultaneously identify those secondary chromosomal changes associated with the translocation, for example, deletion of the normal homolog of *ETV6*, gain of chromosome 21 and an additional copy of the derived chromosome 21.

Screening with the *ETV6-RUNX1* probe led to the identification of the abnormality described as intrachromosomal amplification of chromosome 21 (iAMP21) [6]. Although this abnormality is noted by the WHO classification, it is not identified as a separate entity. This is likely to change as patients have distinctive clinical features and the presence of the abnormality has prognostic significance. Patients are older children (median age 9 years) with a low white cell count. It is associated with a poor prognosis when children are treated on standard therapy [7]. These patients have one grossly abnormal copy of chromosome 21, which has a highly complex aGCH profile (Figure 4.3). Although negative for the *ETV6-RUNX1* fusion, all patients have at least three additional copies of the *RUNX1* gene located to the abnormal chromosome 21; this feature defines the abnormality. To confirm the presence of iAMP21 in interphase, a *RUNX1* probe is applied in a dual color hybridization with a probe specific for the sub-telomeric region of chromosome 21. Patients with iAMP21 show normal or loss of copy number for this sub-telomeric region. Therefore a higher *RUNX1* : sub-telomere ratio will distinguish iAMP21 from patients with multiple copies of intact chromosome 21 as found in high hyperdiploidy. Currently this FISH approach provides the only reliable detection method for iAMP21.

t(1;19)(q23;p13.3); *TCF3-PBX1*

This translocation occurs in approximately 6% of ALL across all age groups. It is usually associated

a 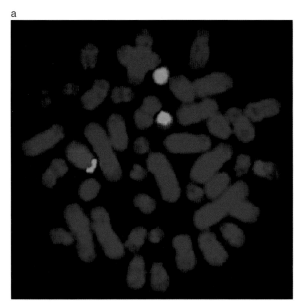 b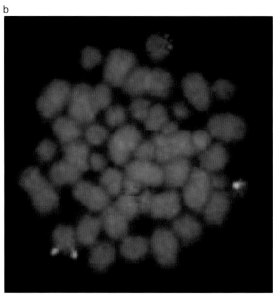

Figure 4.4. a. Chromosome painting of a metaphase from a child with ALL showing the translocation, t(12;21)(p13;q22). Although cryptic by cytogenetic abnormality, painting shows the translocation from one copy of chromosome 12 (red) with one copy of chromosome 21 (green). The normal chromosomes can also be identified.
b. FISH with specific probes for *ETV6* (green) and *RUNX1* (red). There is one normal copy of *ETV6* (green signals on the two chromatids of chromosome 12), one normal copy of *RUNX1* on the normal chromosome 21 (red signal in center). There is a second red signal on the derivative chromosome 12 (top) and a yellow (red-green) fusion signal on the derivative chromosome 21 (on the right-hand side of the picture), indicating the presence of the *ETV6-RUNX1* fusion.

with a pre-B immunophenotype with blasts expressing CD10 and cytoplasmic immunoglobulin. The t(1;19) leads to the fusion of the *TCF3* gene (transcription factor 3, previously known as *E2A* immunoglobulin enhancer binding factor) at 19p13 with the *PBX1* (pre-B-cell leukemia homeobox 1) gene at 1q23 to form the *TCF3-PBX1* fusion. The fusion protein has an oncogenic role as a transcriptional activator. An unbalanced form of the translocation exists in which the derivative chromosome 1 is lost; interestingly this is the most frequent form of the translocation, accounting for 75% of cases. In early studies, the prognosis for patients with this translocation was poor, but this has now been overcome by treatment with modern therapies. In 5–10% of cases with visible translocations, no apparent molecular involvement of *TCF3* and *PBX1* is found [8]. These are usually translocations found in high hyperdiploid karyotypes. A rare variant, t(17;19)(q22;p13), involving *TCF3* and *HCF* has also been described. The prognosis associated with this translocation is extremely poor, with all reported patients having died [9]. Screening by FISH with a breakapart probe specific for *TCF3*, as described for *MLL* above (Figure 4.2)

has provided the opportunity to accurately detect cases with the *TCF3-PBX1* fusion as well as the rare variants [10].

(5;14)(q31;q32); *IGH@-IL3*

This rare translocation has been classified by the WHO as it represents a clinical entity with increased levels of circulating eosinophils. Interestingly, it involves the immunoglobulin heavy chain locus (*IGH@*) and the *IL3* receptor. The translocation juxtaposes the *IGH@* promoter with *IL3*, leading to its over-expression [11]. This type of translocation is commonly described in mature B-cell malignancies, the best known example being the t(8;14)(q24;q32) in which *MYC* is deregulated by *IGH@* in Burkitt lymphoma. The description here of the t(5;14) is one of the early examples of *IGH@* translocations in BCP-ALL, which can now be substantially added to by recent discoveries. These include: translocations of *IGH@* with five members of the *CEBP* (CCAAT enhancer binding-proteins) gene family [12], *ID4* (one of the bHLH family of transcription factors) [13], *EPOR* (the cytokine receptor for erythropoietin) [14] and the cytokine receptor type II, *CRLF2*

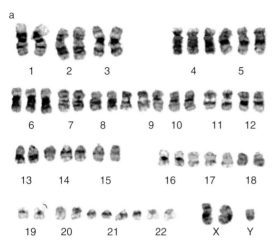

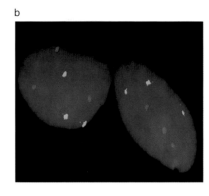

Figure 4.5. a. A karyogram from the leukemic cells of a male with high hyperdiploid ALL. Note the extra copies of chromosomes 4, 5, 6, 10, 14, 17 and X, with two extra copies of chromosome 21. The red signals indicate the location of centromeric probes specific for chromosome 4 and the green signals for chromosome 17.
  b. FISH red and green signals specific for chromosomes 4 and 17, respectively, can be clearly enumerated in interphase cells.

(otherwise known as *TSLPR*, thymic stromal derived lymphopoietin) [15]. Although these over-expressed genes show no similarities in function they clearly share the same mechanism of deregulation by *IGH@*. The other common feature is that they are most frequent in teenagers and adults. These *IGH@* translocations are initially detected using a breakapart FISH approach as described for *MLL* translocations (Figure 4.2), followed by FISH mapping with specific probes to identify the partner gene.

In addition to the translocation *IGH@-CRLF2*, a fusion between *CRLF2* and the *P2RY8* (purinergic receptor P2Y) gene, occurring as a result of a deletion from the pseudo-autosomal region (PAR1) of both sex chromosomes, also leads to over-expression of CRLF2 [15]. This deletion is readily detected at the genomic level by a specifically designed FISH probe, or by increased cell surface protein expression using an antibody to CRLF2. It is of interest to note that this deletion is common in Down syndrome patients with ALL where it is strongly associated with mutations of the *JAK2* pseudokinase domain [16]. The cooperation between *JAK2* mutations and CRLF2 expression interrupts the JAK-STAT pathway and provides potential targets for therapy in high-risk ALL.

High hyperdiploidy (51–65 chromosomes)

Patients with high hyperdiploidy are characterized by non-random chromosomal gains. Those most

frequently gained include trisomies of chromosomes 4, 6, 10, 14, 17, 18, 21 and gain of an X chromosome in both males and females. Multiple copies of chromosome 21 are often present [17]. Patients with high hyperdiploidy have a good prognosis. However, there is controversy as to whether this is determined by the number or the specificity of chromosomes gained. In UK trials the good prognosis has been associated with the gain of chromosome 18 [17], whereas in US childhood ALL trials the simultaneous gains of chromosomes 4, 10 and 17 have been linked to the most favorable outcome [18].

Cytogenetic analysis can readily detect the presence of high hyperdiploidy in relation to chromosome number, although poor chromosome morphology often prevents the accurate identification of the gained chromosomes (Figure 4.5a). This can be overcome by FISH using selected centromeric probes and triple (Figure 4.2) or dual (Figure 4.5b) color hybridization. There are no molecular techniques appropriate for the reliable detection of high hyperdiploidy. Flow cytometry can be used to detect hyperdiploidy; a DNA index of > 1.16 using flow cytometry indicates the presence of a high hyperdiploid clone, but gives no indication of the specific chromosomes gained.

Hypodiploidy

The WHO defines "hypodiploidy" as ALL cases with less than 44 chromosomes. This is in spite of karyotypes with 45 or less chromosomes being truly hypodiploid. This is largely because karyotypes with 44 and 45 chromosomes occur within the entities of other well-defined chromosomal abnormalities. Hypodiploidy of 45 chromosomes or less accounts for approximately 5% of ALL, while 44 chromosomes or less comprises only about 1%. The main group of hypodiploid cases in childhood ALL is "near-haploidy" (< 30 chromosomes). This is a rare and unique entity associated with an adverse outcome. In these patients the haploid chromosome set is observed with non-random gains, typically of chromosomes X, 14, 18 and 21 [19]. It is interesting to note the similarity between these gains and those gained in high hyperdiploidy. Structural abnormalities are rare in this group.

Near-haploidy is frequently associated with a hyperdiploid population of cells with doubling of the near-haploid chromosome number, producing tetrasomies of the gained chromosomes. The presence of these tetrasomies distinguishes this abnormality from the classical form of high hyperdiploidy. This is important because of the different prognosis associated with the two groups. Cytogenetic analysis is reliable for detection of the near-haploid population; however accurate identification of the gained chromosomes is particularly important for the associated doubled population. FISH with carefully selected centromeric probes may be helpful for this purpose. DNA indexing may be necessary for the detection of both the near-haploid and the doubled population.

Another rare but distinctive hypodiploid entity is low hypodiploidy (31–39 chromosomes). This abnormality occurs more frequently in adults than children. They show chromosomal gains onto the haploid chromosome set as for near-haploidy, with additional gains of chromosomes 1, 11 and 19. Chromosomes 3, 4, 7, 13, 15 and 17 are rarely gained [19]. Structural abnormalities are more frequent in this group than in near-haploidy. However, in common with near-haploidy, they often show a population with doubling of the low hypodiploid chromosomes, known as near-triploidy. The same technical approaches for the accurate detection of the numerical changes as used for near-haploidy may be applied.

Other abnormalities in BCP-ALL

Childhood B-lineage ALL has been the focus of study by SNP arrays. A revolutionary discovery was the finding that approximately 40% of childhood BCP-ALL had mutations (most often deletions) involving the B-cell differentiation genes [20]. The main targets are *PAX5* and *IKZF1* (Ikaros). Further studies demonstrated a strong association of *IKZF1* deletions in *BCR-ABL1*-positive ALL patients, known to have a poor prognosis [21]. *BCR-ABL1*-negative, high-risk BCP-ALL patients were also shown to have *IKZF1* deletions and a poor outcome using this approach [22]. A specifically designed MLPA kit can detect deletions of the B-cell differentiation genes, *PAX5* and *IKZF*, *PAR1* and *CDKN2A* (inhibitor of cyclin-dependent kinase gene, involved in cell cycle control) in the same hybridization (Figure 4.6). Homozygous and heterozygous deletions of *CDKN2A*, although common in BCP-ALL, appear to have no prognostic association when investigated in isolation, although they are known to be associated with high-risk features. FISH has provided an appropriate method for their detection, as shown in Figure 4.2 [23]. However, some of the focal deletions of *CDKN2A*, as well as *PAX5* and *IKZF1*, are too small for accurate detection by FISH. MLPA provides a reliable approach for simultaneous detection of these deletions regardless of size.

T-cell precursor acute lymphoblastic leukemia

T-cell precursor ALL (T-ALL) accounts for approximately 15% of childhood (most frequently found in adolescents) and 25% of adult ALL. In general, the prognosis of T-ALL is inferior to BCP-ALL, due to the presence of high-risk features. Gene expression studies have shown that the genes involved in normal T-cell development are rearranged or deregulated in T-ALL. Almost all cases show clonal rearrangements of the T-cell receptor genes (*TCR*). An abnormal karyotype is seen by cytogenetic analysis in between 50–70% of patients. The most common abnormalities involve *TCR* alpha/delta (*TRA@/TRD@*) at 14q11.2, *TCR* beta (*TRB@*) at 7q35 and the *TCR* gamma (*TRG@*) locus at 7p14, each with a range of partner genes. These translocations lead to deregulated transcription of the partner gene by juxtaposition with the promoter of the *TCR* locus. Abnormalities of this type involve transcription factors, the best known being *TLX1* (*HOX11*) at 10q24, found in 7% of childhood and 30% adult T-ALL. Other transcription factors upregulated in T-ALL include *TLX3* (*HOX11L2*) (5q35), *TAL1* (1p32), *MYC* (8q24.1), *LMO1* (11p15), *LMO2* (11p13), *LYL1* (19p13), and the cytoplasmic tyrosine kinase, *LCK* (1p34.3~35). In a large number of cases the

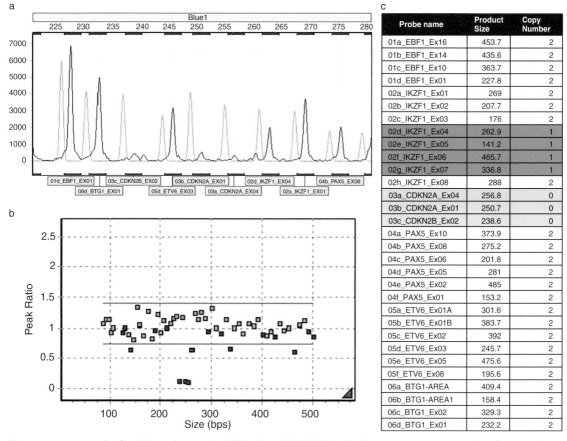

a

Probe name	Product Size	Copy Number
01a_EBF1_Ex16	453.7	2
01b_EBF1_Ex14	435.6	2
01c_EBF1_Ex10	363.7	2
01d_EBF1_Ex01	227.8	2
02a_IKZF1_Ex01	269	2
02b_IKZF1_Ex02	207.7	2
02c_IKZF1_Ex03	176	2
02d_IKZF1_Ex04	262.9	1
02e_IKZF1_Ex05	141.2	1
02f_IKZF1_Ex06	465.7	1
02g_IKZF1_Ex07	336.8	1
02h_IKZF1_Ex08	288	2
03a_CDKN2A_Ex04	256.8	0
03b_CDKN2A_Ex01	250.7	0
03c_CDKN2B_Ex02	238.6	0
04a_PAX5_Ex10	373.9	2
04b_PAX5_Ex08	275.2	2
04c_PAX5_Ex06	201.8	2
04d_PAX5_Ex05	281	2
04e_PAX5_Ex02	485	2
04f_PAX5_Ex01	153.2	2
05a_ETV6_Ex01A	301.6	2
05b_ETV6_Ex01B	383.7	2
05c_ETV6_Ex02	392	2
05d_ETV6_Ex03	245.7	2
05e_ETV6_Ex05	475.6	2
05f_ETV6_Ex08	195.6	2
06a_BTG1-AREA	409.4	2
06b_BTG1-AREA1	158.4	2
06c_BTG1_Ex02	329.3	2
06d_BTG1_Ex01	232.2	2

Figure 4.6. An example of a MLPA result using the MRC Holland P335-IKZF1 ALL kit. Results are taken as screen shots from GeneMarker V1.85 analysis software (SoftGenetics).
Panel A shows a normalized electropherogram trace for a test sample (blue) with the control sample trace (red). The exon names are displayed below their corresponding peaks. The ratio of normalized peaks between the test and control samples is used to calculate copy number, which is shown in the ratio plot in Panel B. The three lowest red points indicate the presence of a homozygous deletion of *CDKN2A* and the higher red points a heterozygous deletion of *IKZF1*. The blue (references probes) and green (test probes) points, located between the green lines, are within the normal range. Panel C shows the copy number for the different exons of each gene. The heterozygous deletion of *IKZF1* (blue boxes with copy number 1) covers exons 4–7 inclusive, while the whole of *CDKN2A* with 0 copy number (yellow boxes), has a homozygous deletion.

abnormalities are cryptic by cytogenetic analysis; these include upregulation of *TLX3* in the translocation, t (5;14)(q35;q32) (Figure 4.7). Juxtaposition to the Krüppel-like zinc finger gene, *BCL11B*, at 14q32 (rarely *TCR*) leads to the upregulation of *TLX3* in approximately 20% of childhood and 10–15% of adult ALL. The *TAL1* gene is upregulated by *TRA/D* in the rare translocation, t(1;14)(p32;q11). *TAL1* is deregulated in approximately 20% of T-ALL as a result of a submicroscopic deletion within 1p32, involving *STIL* (SCL/TAL1-interrupting locus) which leads to the formation of the *STIL-TAL1* fusion gene. These cryptic abnormalities can be clearly visualized by FISH using a breakapart approach [24]. Over-expression of all these genes has been observed in the absence of detectable rearrangements at the DNA level, providing evidence that the expression of such genes provides the significant leukemogenic event.

Two important fusion genes in T-ALL have been described:

a. *PICALM-MLLT10* (*CALM-AF10*) arising from the translocation, t(10;11)(p13;q14) and which occurs in ~10% of cases.

b. *MLL-ENL* resulting from t(11;19)(q23;p13) and seen in ~8% T-ALL cases.

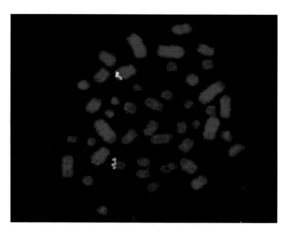

Figure 4.7. A breakapart FISH approach demonstrating the cryptic translocation, t(5;14)(q35;q32). The yellow (red-green) signal on chromosome 5 indicates that the *TLX3* gene is intact. The split of the red (remaining on the derivative chromosome 5) and the green signals (translocated to the derivative chromosome 14) indicates that the translocation has moved *TLX3* onto chromosome 14 to juxtapose *BCL11B*.

The genetic abnormalities described above that occur in T-ALL are usually mutually exclusive. However they are often accompanied by a number of other abnormalities, as shown by genetic and gene expression studies, which provide strong evidence to support a multi-step process of pathogenesis of T-ALL [25]. One frequently occurring additional change is deletion of *CDKN2A*, either in heterozygous or homozygous form as seen in BCP-ALL. Mutations seen in association with all other abnormalities are those involving the extracellular hetero-dimerization domain and/or c-terminal PEST domain of the *NOTCH1* gene. This gene encodes a protein which is critical for early T-cell development. *MYC* is a direct downstream target of *NOTCH1*, which contributes to the growth of the leukemic cells. In addition to *NOTCH1* mutations, about 30% of T-ALL cases have missense mutations of *FBXW7*, a negative regulator of *NOTCH1*.

Acute myeloid leukemia with recurrent genetic abnormalities

The WHO defines this AML subgroup according to the genetic changes which have prognostic significance. Detailed coverage of the chromosomal abnormalities found in AML is described in Chapter 8 and other references [26]. In describing these abnormalities it must be taken into consideration that multiple aberrations cooperate in a multistep process to initiate the leukemic phenotype. These somatically acquired mutations belong to two defined groups: Class I and Class II. Class I promote proliferation and/or produce a survival advantage, but do not have an effect on differentiation. They include mutations of *FLT3*, *KIT*, *RAS*, *PTPN11* and *JAK2*. Class II mutations are linked to impaired hematopoietic differentiation and subsequent apoptosis. In this group are *RUNX1-RUNX1T1*, *CEBP-MYH11*, *PML-RARA* and *MLL* fusions, as well as mutations of *CEBPA* and *NPM1*. *FLT3*, *CEBPA* and *NPM1* mutations are common in patients with otherwise normal karyotypes, although they are also important considerations within the classification of AML with recurring genetic abnormalities. These are described in more detail below. The presence of these mutations is increasing in importance in the routine diagnosis of hematological neoplasms as an indicator of outcome.

Mutations of FMS-like tyrosine kinase 3, *FLT3*, occur within a number of different entities and the WHO recommends that this mutation be tested for in all AML patients because of its prognostic significance. For example, *FLT3* ITD (internal tandem duplication), but not activating point mutations of the tyrosine kinase domain of the gene, *FLT3* TKD, have been associated with a poor outcome. Copy number neutral loss of heterozygosity (LOH) is a mechanism responsible for a "double hit" producing *FLT3* ITD of both alleles. These homozygous deletions appear to correlate with a worse prognosis. In view of the strong link between a poor outcome and *FLT3* ITD, *FLT3* tyrosine kinase inhibitors are being evaluated within AML clinical trials. On the other hand, the presence of mutations in the nucleophosmin gene, *NPM1*, in the absence of *FLT3* ITD or mutations of CCAAT enhancer binding protein, alpha, *CEBPA*, has a favorable prognosis, particularly in AML with a normal karyotype [27].

t(8;21)(q22;q22); *RUNX1-RUNX1T1*

This translocation occurs in approximately 10% of AML, predominantly in younger patients (see Figure 8.4b). It is included within the AML entity regardless of blast count and is associated with a favorable prognosis. It involves the *RUNX1* gene, which encodes the core-binding alpha subunit, giving the name of "core binding factor leukemia" to this entity. A number of translocation variants have been described [28]. Therefore for accurate detection, FISH using probes directed to *RUNX1* and *RUNX1T1* (*ETO*) in a dual color approach, as described for *BCR-ABL1*

(Figure 4.2), or RT-PCR for the fusion transcript should be applied (see Chapter 5 for details). This is particularly relevant in cases in which abnormalities of chromosomes 8 or 21 are observed, as well as those with a normal karyotype or failed cytogenetic result. The majority of cases also show additional chromosomal changes, typically loss of a sex chromosome or deletion of chromosome 9, del(9q), with no effect on outcome. Mutations of *RAS* or *KIT* have been identified as the cooperating class I mutations in 30% and 25% respectively of patients with the *RUNX1-RUNX1T1* fusion class II mutation.

inv(16)(p13q22) or t(16;16)(p13;q22); *CBFB-MYH11*

These rearrangements define the second core binding factor leukemia and also have a good outcome. Characteristically, patients with these abnormalities have an abnormal eosinophil component in the bone marrow. The gene, *CBFB* (core binding factor subunit beta), fuses with *MYH11*, a gene which encodes a smooth muscle myosin heavy chain. This is a subtle rearrangement which may be difficult to identify in poor quality preparations, therefore dual color FISH with probes directed to the genes involved in the fusion (as shown for the *BCR-ABL1* fusion; Figure 4.2) or RT-PCR are recommended for accurate detection and appropriate risk stratification (see Chapter 5 for details). Trisomy 22 is a secondary chromosomal abnormality highly specific for this leukemia subtype, while trisomy 8 is also common. As for t(8;21), the class I mutations of *RAS* and *KIT* are commonly associated with inv(16). These abnormalities define AML regardless of the blast cell count.

t(15;17)(q22;q21); *PML-RARA*

The translocation, t(15;17) or more precisely the *PML-RARA* gene fusion, is diagnostic for APL, and has not been reported in any other disease entity. APL comprises approximately 5% of AML cases and, on current therapy, these patients have a good prognosis. The *RARA* (retinoic acid receptor alpha locus) at 17q22 regulates myeloid differentiation. As a result of the translocation it fuses with the *PML* (promyelocytic leukemia) gene, which encodes a growth-suppressing transcription factor. The resultant chimeric protein causes maturation arrest at the promyelocytic stage, with increased proliferation of neoplastic promyelocytes. APL is a paradigm for the successful treatment of leukemia using targeted therapy to the responsible molecular mechanism. The interruption of the *RARA*

locus in the formation of this fusion led to the discovery that APL cells underwent differentiation in the presence of retinoic acid and successful treatment with all-*trans* retinoic acid in combination with chemotherapy (see Chapter 8 for details). The monitoring of APL for the presence of the molecularly detectable *PML-RARA* transcript enables early identification of patients at risk of relapse; in recent years this has become established as a routine procedure [29]. A number of rare variant translocations have been reported in fusions with *RARA*. Trisomy 8 is a frequent secondary chromosomal change. The class I mutations, *FLT3* ITD and *FLT3* TKD occur in 20–40% and 10–20% of APL, respectively. The presence of such mutations in APL has been associated with high white blood cell counts but has not been shown to impact on the favorable outcome.

t(9;11)(p21;q23); *MLL-MLLT3*

This translocation is the most prevalent of the *MLL* translocations in AML, constituting approximately 3% of AML cases. There is a higher frequency in children (10%) due to the frequency of occurrence in infant AML. It predominantly occurs in AML with monocytoid differentiation, although it has been reported within other morphological types. In acute monoblastic/monocytic leukemia in children this translocation has been associated with a good outcome, in contrast to other *MLL* translocations [30]. FISH using the breakapart approach on metaphases (as shown in Figure 4.2) or RT-PCR is recommended to distinguish t(9;11) from other *MLL* translocations.

More than 80 rearrangements involving the *MLL* gene have been reported in AML, of which more than 50 have been molecularly characterized. Although *MLL-MLLT3* predominates in AML and *MLL-MLLT2* predominates in ALL, the same translocations are reported to occur in both disease entities (see above). An exception is the *MLL-ELL* fusion arising from the translocation, t(11;19)(q23;p13.1), which has only been reported in AML. Due to the diversity of *MLL* partners FISH may be necessary to confirm the involvement of *MLL*. Previously all *MLL* translocations were categorized together as AML with 11q23 abnormalities. The WHO now recommends that the AML diagnosis should specify the specific abnormality and should be limited to cases with balanced translocations involving *MLL*. As an example, cases with an *MLL-MLLT2* fusion should be described as AML with t(4;11)(q21;q23); *MLL-MLLT2*. AML cases in which the *MLL* gene is deleted are excluded.

t(6;9)(p22;q34); *DEK-NUP214*

This is a rare AML entity accounting for approximately 1% of cases and is associated with a poor outcome in both childhood and adult AML. The gene *DEK* at 6p22 fuses to the gene coding for nucleoporin 214 kDa, *NUP214*. The nucleoporin fusion protein acts as an aberrant transcription factor which impacts on nuclear transport. The translocation is usually the sole karyotypic change, although the class I mutation, *FLT3* ITD is common in this subgroup.

inv(3)(q21q26.2) or t(3;3)(q21;q26.2); *RPN1-EVI1*

A range of abnormalities involving 3q have been described in myeloid hematological malignancies. Of these inv(3)(q21q26.2) and t(3;3)(q21;q26.2); *RPN1-EVI* are the most common and these are often associated with monosomy 7. They mainly occur in adults and account for about 1% of AML cases. They are associated with aggressive disease and short survival. Both abnormalities involve the *EVI1* gene at 3q26.2, which encodes a zinc finger transcription factor. FISH using a breakapart probe targeting *EVI1*, confirms the presence of the abnormality and detects cryptic rearrangements not seen by cytogenetic analysis. EVI1 (or MDS1-EVI1) is highly expressed in these cases, most likely as a result of juxtaposition to the enhancer elements of the *RPN1* gene, located to 3q21. Interestingly, approximately 20% of AML over-express EVI1 without evidence of chromosomal rearrangement. This may be explained in part by the presence of cryptic rearrangements of the gene or indicate that *EVI1* is activated by alternative mechanisms.

t(1;22)(p13;q13); *RBM15-MKL1*

AML with this translocation is extremely rare. The patients are usually infants, show maturation of the megakaryocytic lineage and are usually classified as acute megakaryoblastic leukemia. The *RBM15* (RNA binding motif protein 15 or *OTT*) gene fuses to *MKL1* (megakaryocyte leukemia 1 or *MAL*). The prognosis was originally reported to be poor but this has now been revised due to an improved response to intensive therapy.

Complex karyotypes

Although not defined as a distinct disease entity by WHO, AML with complex karyotypes is noteworthy due to the association with an adverse outcome. The number of chromosomal abnormalities required to define a complex karyotype is controversial. It has been variously defined as having equal to or more than three or five unrelated aberrations [31,32]. A recent large UK study has conclusively defined complexity as four or more unrelated abnormalities in patients lacking any of those abnormalities known to have independent adverse risk, those with *PML-RARA* fusion, core binding factor leukemia or t(9;11). The important chromosomal changes that are most commonly identified in complex karyotypes are abnormalities of 5q, monosomy 7, deletions of 17p, as well as mutations of *TP53* [31].

Myeloproliferative neoplasms

The myeloproliferative neoplasms are clonal hematopoietic stem cell disorders of one or more myeloid lineages, primarily found in adults, and are described in detail in Chapters 13 and 14. Examples of the genetic associations are described.

Chronic myelogenous leukemia, *BCR-ABL1* positive

Chronic myelogenous leukemia (CML) is a distinctive disease in which the presence of the Ph chromosome arising from the translocation, t(9;22)(q32;q11.2), or more precisely the *BCR-ABL1* fusion, defines this myeloid disease entity (see Figure 13.1). The detection methods are the same as described for ALL above, using FISH (see Figures 13.2 and 13.3) or RT-PCR (see Figure 13.4). CML is highly responsive to the tyrosine kinase inhibitor, imatinib mesylate. Tyrosine kinase inhibitors act by competitively binding to the kinase domain (ATP binding site) of bcr-abl, inhibiting the enzyme activity of the protein by preventing binding and phosphorylation of the substrate. One major problem of imatinib therapy has been the development of resistance in a small but significant number of patients. The most common type of resistance is the acquisition of point mutations in the BCR-ABL1 kinase domain that interfere with optimal drug target interactions [33]. The mutations show different susceptibilities to alternative kinase inhibitors, so detection of the specific mutation is necessary so that the patient can be transferred to a more appropriate alternative therapy. The response to imatinib therapy has traditionally been monitored by cytogenetics and interphase FISH focused on the blood granulocytes, although real-time quantitative PCR offers a more sensitive approach (for details see Chapter 13) [34].

Other *BCR-ABL1* negative myeloproliferative neoplasms

This includes chronic neutrophilic leukemia (CNL), polycythemia vera (PV), primary myelofibrosis (PMF), essential thrombocythemia (ET), chronic eosinophilic leukemia (CEL), mastocytosis, MPN unclassified (see Chapter 14 for details). These diseases are characterized by a range of clonal chromosomal abnormalities, including trisomies of chromosomes 8, 9 and 21, del(20q), del(11q) and del(12p), as well as those involving activating protein tyrosine kinases. The latter include translocations and point mutations which activate signal transduction pathways leading to abnormal proliferation. The presence of a clonal abnormality in these patient groups provides evidence that the myeloid proliferation is indeed neoplastic.

The most common mutation found in MPN is *JAK2* V617F, which results in activation of the STAT (signal transducer and activator of transcription), MAPK (mitogen activated protein kinase) and PI3K (phosphotidylinositol 3-kinase) signaling pathways which promote transformation and proliferation of hematopoietic progenitors. These *JAK2* mutations are found in almost all cases of PV and approximately 50% of those with PMF and ET. Mutations of *MPL* and *TET2* have recently been found to occur in MPN. *TET2* mutations can be in association with or independent of *JAK2* mutations [35].

Myeloid0 and lymphoid neoplasms with eosinophilia and abnormalities of *PDGFRA*, *PDGFRB* and *FGFR1*

Patients with these characteristics are now defined as a distinct entity in the WHO classification. Characteristically they have rearrangements of genes that encode the alpha or beta chains of the receptor protein tyrosine kinases, *PDGFR* (platelet derived growth factor receptors): alpha at 4q21 and beta at 5q33, or *FGFR1* (fibroblast growth factor receptor 1) at 8p11. Abnormalities of *PDGFR* were first described in CEL or chronic myelomonocytic leukemia (CMML), although they are now found to be more widespread in association with idiopathic eosinophilic syndrome. The most common MPN in this group is that associated with the *FIP1L1-PDGFRA* fusion resulting from a cryptic deletion of chromosome 4, del(4)(q12), or rarely translocations involving the breakpoint 4q12.

FISH probes directed to the gene *CHIC2* are effective as this gene is uniformly deleted. The fusion gene can also be detected by RT-PCR. Those with *FGFR1* abnormalities are a more heterogeneous group with prominent eosinophilia. They involve a range of translocations of 8p11. Depending on the partner, a variety of fusion genes involving *FGFR1* are produced, all of which encode an aberrant tyrosine kinase.

Myelodysplastic syndromes

The genetic abnormalities of the myelodysplastic syndromes (MDS) correlate with the morphology and clinical features (see Chapter 15 for details) and determine clonality and prognosis of the disease. However clonal abnormalities, which include monosomy 5/del(5q), monosomy 7/del(7q), trisomy 8, del(11q), monosomy 13/del(13q), del(17q) and del(20q), are seen in only approximately 5% of patients.

5q- syndrome

One subtype of MDS defined by the WHO is characterized by isolated del(5q), in which the deletion encompasses chromosomal bands 5q31–q33. The patients are usually women with specific morphological features and indolent disease. Del(5q) is detectable by cytogenetics and FISH (see Figures 15.2b, c).

Juvenile myelomonocytic leukemia

Childhood patients within this MDS/MPN category generally have a normal karyotype although about 25% have monosomy 7. JMML has a high incidence (80%) of the mutually exclusive mutations of *PTNPN11*, *NRAS*, *KRAS* or *NF1*, all of which encode signaling proteins in *RAS*-dependent pathways.

Conclusion

Although the chromosomal and genetic abnormalities described in this chapter are by no means exhaustive, they relate to the entities of hematological malignancies currently defined by WHO. The continuing discovery of novel abnormalities and mutations by array-based technologies and now whole genome sequencing is highlighting novel abnormalities of prognostic significance which either alone or in combination are likely to define novel disease entities and molecular targets for therapy in the future. However, until these become available for routine use, cytogenetic analysis and FISH remain the gold standard techniques of genetic analysis in hematological malignancies for diagnosis and prognosis.

References

1. World Health Organization. *WHO Classification of Tumours of Haematopoietic and Lymphoid Tissue.* Lyon: IARC Press; 2008.

2. ISCN. *An International System for Human Cytogenetic Nomenclature.* Shaffer LG, Slovak ML, Campbell LJ (eds.). Basel: S. Karger; 2009.

3. Greaves M. In utero origins of childhood leukaemia. *Early Hum Dev* 2005;**81**:123–9.

4. Harrison CJ, Johansson B. Acute lymphoblastic leukaemia. In Heim S, Mitelman F (eds.), *Cancer Cytogenetics*, 3rd edn. Hoboken, NJ: John Wiley and Son Inc.; 2009.

5. Hong D, Gupta R, Ancliff P *et al.* Initiating and cancer-propagating cells in *TEL-AML1*-associated childhood leukemia. *Science* 2008;**319**:336–9.

6. Harewood L, Robinson H, Harris R *et al.* Amplification of *AML1* on a duplicated chromosome 21 in acute lymphoblastic leukemia: a study of 20 cases. *Leukemia* 2003;**17**:547–53.

7. Moorman AV, Richards SM, Robinson HM *et al.* Prognosis of children with acute lymphoblastic leukemia (ALL) and intrachromosomal amplification of chromosome 21 (iAMP21). *Blood* 2007;**109**:2327–30.

8. Privitera E, Kamps MP, Hayashi Y *et al.* Different molecular consequences of the 1;19 chromosomal translocation in childhood B-cell precursor acute lymphoblastic leukemia. *Blood* 1992; **79**:1781–8.

9. Hunger SP. Chromosomal translocations involving the *E2A* gene in acute lymphoblastic leukemia: clinical features and molecular pathogenesis. *Blood* 1996;**87**:1211–24.

10. Barber KE, Harrison CJ, Broadfield ZJ *et al.* Molecular cytogenetic characterization of *TCF3* (*E2A*)/19p13.3 rearrangements in B-cell precursor acute lymphoblastic leukemia. *Genes Chromosomes Cancer* 2007;**46**:478–86.

11. Grimaldi JC, Meeker TC. The t(5;14) chromosomal translocation in a case of acute lymphocytic leukemia joins the interleukin-3 gene to the immunoglobulin heavy chain gene. *Blood* 1989;**73**:2081–5.

12. Akasaka T, Balasas T, Russell LJ *et al.* Five members of the CEBP transcription factor family are targeted by recurrent *IGH* translocations in B-cell precursor acute lymphoblastic leukemia (BCP-ALL). *Blood* 2007;**109**:3451–61.

13. Russell LJ, Akasaka T, Majid A *et al.* t(6;14)(p22;q32): a new recurrent *IGH@* translocation involving *ID4* in B-cell precursor acute lymphoblastic leukemia (BCP-ALL). *Blood* 2008;**111**:387–91.

14. Russell LJ, De Castro DG, Griffiths M *et al.* A novel translocation, t(14;19)(q32;p13), involving *IGH@* and the cytokine receptor for erythropoietin. *Leukemia* 2009;**23**:614–17.

15. Russell LJ, Capasso M, Vater I *et al.* Deregulated expression of cytokine receptor gene, *CRLF2*, is involved in lymphoid transformation in B-cell precursor acute lymphoblastic leukemia. *Blood* 2009;**114**:2688–98.

16. Hertzberg L, Vendramini E, Ganmore I *et al.* Down syndrome acute lymphoblastic leukemia: a highly heterogeneous disease in which aberrant expression of *CRLF2* is associated with mutated *JAK2*: a report from the iBFM Study Group. *Blood* 2010; **115**(5):1006–17.

17. Moorman AV, Richards SM, Martineau M *et al.* Outcome heterogeneity in childhood high-hyperdiploid acute lymphoblastic leukemia. *Blood* 2003;**102**:2756–62.

18. Sutcliffe MJ, Shuster JJ, Sather HN *et al.* High concordance from independent studies by the Children's Cancer Group (CCG) and Pediatric Oncology Group (POG) associating favorable prognosis with combined trisomies 4, 10, and 17 in children with NCI Standard-Risk B-precursor Acute Lymphoblastic Leukemia: a Children's Oncology Group (COG) initiative. *Leukemia* 2005;**19**:734–40.

19. Harrison CJ, Moorman AV, Broadfield ZJ *et al.* Three distinct subgroups of hypodiploidy in acute lymphoblastic leukaemia. *Br J Haematol* 2004;**125**:552–9.

20. Mullighan CG, Goorha S, Radtke I *et al.* Genome-wide analysis of genetic alterations in acute lymphoblastic leukaemia. *Nature* 2007;**446**:758–64.

21. Mullighan CG, Miller CB, Radtke I *et al.* BCR-ABL1 lymphoblastic leukaemia is characterized by the deletion of *Ikaros*. *Nature* 2008;**453**:110–14.

22. Mullighan C, Downing J. *Ikaros* and acute leukemia. *Leuk Lymphoma* 2008;**49**:847–9.

23. Sulong S, Moorman AV, Irving JA *et al.* A comprehensive analysis of the *CDKN2A* gene in childhood acute lymphoblastic leukemia reveals genomic deletion, copy number neutral loss of heterozygosity, and association with specific cytogenetic subgroups. *Blood* 2009;**113**:100–7.

24. van der Burg M, Poulsen TS, Hunger SP *et al.* Split-signal FISH for detection of chromosome aberrations

in acute lymphoblastic leukemia. *Leukemia* 2004;**18**:895–908.

25. De Keersmaecker K, Marynen P, Cools J. Genetic insights in the pathogenesis of T-cell acute lymphoblastic leukemia. *Haematologica* 2005;**90**:1116–27.

26. Johansson B, Harrison CJ. Acute myeloid leukaemia. In Heim S, Mitelman F (eds.). *Cancer Cytogenetics*, 3rd edn. Hoboken, NJ: John Wiley and Son Inc.; 2009.

27. Gale RE, Green C, Allen C *et al.* The impact of *FLT3* internal tandem duplication mutant level, number, size, and interaction with *NPM1* mutations in a large cohort of young adult patients with acute myeloid leukemia. *Blood* 2008;**111**:2776–84.

28. Harrison CJ, Radford-Weiss I, Ross F *et al.* Fluorescence in situ hybridization of masked t(8;21) (q22;q22) translocations. *Cancer Genet Cytogenet* 1999;**112**:15–20.

29. Grimwade D, Jovanovic JV, Hills RK *et al.* Prospective minimal residual disease monitoring to predict relapse of acute promyelocytic leukemia and to direct pre-emptive arsenic trioxide therapy. *J Clin Oncol* 2009;**27**:3650–8.

30. Balgobind BV, Raimondi SC, Harbott J *et al.* Novel prognostic subgroups in childhood 11q23/*MLL*-rearranged acute myeloid leukemia: results of an international retrospective study. *Blood* 2009;**114**:2489–96.

31. Schoch C, Kern W, Kohlmann A *et al.* Acute myeloid leukemia with a complex aberrant karyotype is a distinct biological entity characterized by genomic imbalances and a specific gene expression profile. *Genes Chromosomes Cancer* 2005; **43**:227–38.

32. Grimwade D, Walker H, Oliver F *et al.*, on behalf of the Medical Research Council Adult and Children's Leukaemia Working P. The importance of diagnostic cytogenetics on outcome in AML: analysis of 1,612 patients entered into the MRC AML 10 trial. *Blood* 1998;**92**:2322–33.

33. Jabbour E, Koscielny S, Sebban C *et al.* High survival rate with the LMT-89 regimen in lymphoblastic lymphoma (LL), but not in T-cell acute lymphoblastic leukemia (T-ALL). *Leukemia* 2006;**20**:814–19.

34. Baccarani M, Saglio G, Goldman J *et al.* Evolving concepts in the management of chronic myeloid leukemia: recommendations from an expert panel on behalf of the European LeukemiaNet. *Blood* 2006;**108**:1809–20.

35. Tefferi A, Pardanani A, Lim KH *et al.* TET2 mutations and their clinical correlates in polycythemia vera, essential thrombocythemia and myelofibrosis. *Leukemia* 2009;**23**:905–11.

5 Molecular genetics

Ken Mills

Introduction

Molecular genetic-based methods are now an integral component in the diagnostic workup of hematological malignancies. This will be evident in the clinical Chapters 7–15, each of which includes discussion of the use of molecular diagnostic methods in the analysis of acute and chronic lymphoid and myeloid neoplasms. This is a major change which has taken place over the past 10 years. Molecular genetics has moved from research-based applications and the simple amplification and detection of an abnormal gene to highly sensitive and reproducible monitoring of minimal residual disease. This chapter describes some of the types of PCR-based assay methods commonly used in the analysis of hematological malignancies, demonstrates their strengths and gives some clinical applications.

Polymerase chain reaction

Principles of PCR amplification

Polymerase chain reaction (PCR) is the method by which DNA is amplified to generate thousands of copies of the same sequence [1,2]. The principle is the utilization of repeated cycles of heating and cooling (thermal cycling) and a thermostable DNA polymerase to replicate DNA. The heat physically separates the double strands of DNA and replication occurs at the cooler temperatures. The cycles of heating and cooling are repeated over and over, allowing primers to bind to the original DNA sequences of interest and to newly synthesized sequences (Figure 5.1). The enzyme, *Taq* polymerase, will again extend primer sequences. This cycling of temperatures results in copying and then copying of copies, and so on, leading to an exponential increase in the number of copies of specific DNA sequences.

PCR has rapidly become one of the most widely used techniques in molecular biology and for good reason: it is a rapid, inexpensive and simple means of producing relatively large numbers of copies of DNA molecules from minute quantities of source DNA material. In addition, it does not necessarily require the use of radioisotopes or toxic chemicals. PCR is also very versatile, enabling nucleic acids from many different types of samples to be analyzed, including blood, bone marrow and fixed tissue. PCR can be performed even when the source DNA is of relatively poor quality (e.g. extracted from paraffin-embedded material or air-dried smears scraped from glass slides).

There are several steps in the PCR procedure and also several important components to ensure a reproducible reaction, as will be described below. The method is largely automated with large-scale PCR machines available in 48-, 96- and 384-well formats. This combined with the use of multichannel pipettes, means that large numbers of reactions can be done simultaneously.

The DNA template

Most PCR uses DNA as a target because of the stability of the DNA molecule and the ease with which DNA can be isolated from clinical samples. DNA is first extracted from the test sample and this is the template for amplification. Any impurities must be sufficiently diluted so as not to inhibit the polymerization step of the PCR reaction. PCR can also be performed using cDNA as the template; cDNA is generated after reverse transcription from RNA and then amplified (see the next section of this chapter).

DNA polymerase

PCR requires a DNA polymerase to synthesize the new DNA strand from the sample DNA template. The DNA polymerase used in PCR, known as "*Taq* polymerase,"

Diagnostic Techniques in Hematological Malignancies, ed. Wendy N. Erber. Published by Cambridge University Press.
© Cambridge University Press 2010.

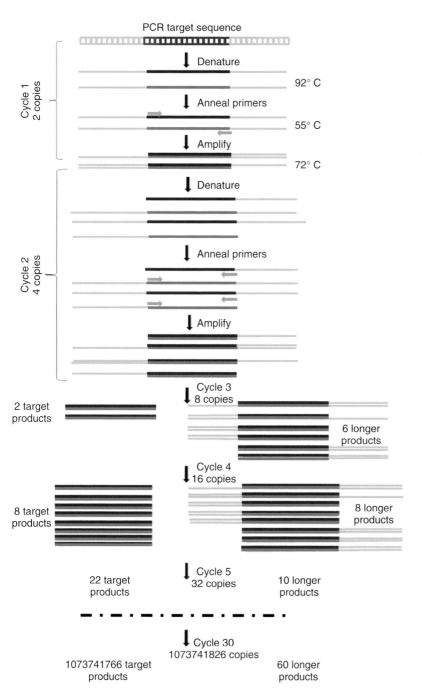

Figure 5.1. The processes involved in PCR. The DNA strands, including the target region, are denatured, primers are annealed at either end of the target region which is copied by *Taq* polymerase to produce two copies of the target region flanked by the non-target DNA. The extension, annealing and extension phases are repeated. It is not until cycle 3 that two of the eight PCR products are of the target sequence size. The longer products increase by two copies each cycle, whilst the number of target products double each cycle. After 30 cycles there are more than 1 000 0000 000 specific target PCR products.

is named after the hot-spring bacterium *Thermus aquaticus* from which it was originally isolated. This enzyme can withstand the high temperatures needed for DNA-strand separation, and can be left in the reaction tube. Higher *Taq* polymerase concentrations than needed may cause synthesis of non-specific products. Other thermostable polymerases have also been isolated although *Taq* is by far the commonest used.

Primers

A primer is a short segment of nucleotides (20–30 bases) which is complementary to the target section of the DNA (template) which is to be amplified in the PCR reaction. Two primers that flank the region of DNA to be amplified anneal to the denatured DNA template to provide an initiation site for the elongation of the new DNA molecule. Primers can either be specific to a particular DNA nucleotide sequence or they can be "universal." The vast majority of PCR reactions use specific primers to amplify a particular target region. Universal primers, in contrast, are complementary to nucleotide sequences which are very common in a particular set of DNA molecules. Thus they are able to bind to a wide variety of DNA templates. The selected primers bind to the DNA template allowing *Taq* polymerase to initiate incorporation of the deoxynucleotides (dNTPs).

The primers should be designed to follow a set of rules to ensure specific amplification. The GC content should be 40–60%. The primer should not be self-complementary or complementary to any other primer in the reaction mixture, to prevent primer-dimer and hairpin formation. Melting temperatures of primer pairs should not differ by more than 5 °C, so that the GC content and length must be chosen accordingly. The annealing temperature should be about 5 °C lower than the melting temperature.

MgCl$_2$ concentration

Divalent cations such as MgCl$_2$ are required in the PCR reaction mixture for two reasons:

a. They promote DNA/DNA interactions which are essential between the target DNA and PCR primers.
b. They form complexes with dNTPs that are the substrates for *Taq* polymerase.

The concentration of MgCl$_2$ must be optimized for each type of PCR experiment because Mg^{2+} ions form complexes with dNTPs, primers and the DNA template. Too few Mg^{2+} ions results in a low yield of PCR product and too many increases the yield of non-specific products. The dependence of the PCR yield on MgCl$_2$ is a bell-shaped curve with a broad maximum. At a low MgCl$_2$ concentration the primers fail to anneal to the target DNA. When the MgCl$_2$ concentration is too high, the base pairing becomes too strong and during the PCR cycles, the amplicon (i.e. the pieces of DNA formed as a result of PCR amplification) fails to denature completely when heated to 94 °C. The recommended range of MgCl$_2$ concentration is 1 to 3 mM, under the standard reaction conditions specified [3].

Deoxynucleoside triphosphates

Deoxynucleoside triphosphates (dNTPs) are the "building blocks" used by *Taq* polymerase to synthesize new strands of DNA. The concentration of each dNTP (dATP, dCTP, dGTP, dTTP) in the reaction mixture is usually 200 μM.

The PCR method

There are three main steps in the PCR reaction and these are repeated to achieve the amplification of a specific region of DNA. The steps are denaturation, annealing and extension.

Denaturation (about 1 minute at 95 °C): During this phase the DNA is heated at a high temperature to melt the DNA double helix to single strands. The resulting single strands of DNA become accessible to primers. Complete denaturation of the DNA template is essential; incomplete denaturation will result in the inefficient use of the template in the first amplification cycle and, consequently, poor yield of PCR product.

Annealing (about 1 minute at temperatures ranging between 45 °C and 60 °C): During this phase the primers anneal to the complementary regions of single stranded DNA. Double strands of DNA are formed between primers and complementary sequences. The annealing temperature may be estimated as 5 °C lower than the melting temperature of the primer–template DNA duplex. If non-specific PCR products are obtained in addition to the expected product, the annealing temperature can be optimized by increasing it stepwise by 1–2 °C. When the second cycle of PCR commences, there are effectively two types of template:

a. The original DNA strands.
b. The newly synthesized DNA strands, consisting of the target region and variable lengths of the flanking region at the 3′ end. When the latter template is used in this cycle, only the target region is replicated.

Extension (about 1 minute at 72 °C): In this phase *Taq* polymerase synthesizes a complementary strand. The enzyme reads the opposing strand sequence and extends the primers by adding nucleotides in the order in which they can pair. Usually, the extension step is performed at 72 °C and a 1 minute extension is sufficient to synthesize PCR fragments as long as 2 kb (kb = kilobase = 1000 bp). When larger DNA fragments are amplified, the extension time is usually increased by 1 minute per 1000 bp. In this extension phase of the PCR cycle, the newly synthesized target region DNA (i.e. without flanking regions) acts as the template. The original DNA molecule is still present, and will be until the end of the reaction. However, after a few cycles, the newly synthesized DNA fragment quickly establishes itself as the predominant template.

These three PCR steps are carried out, one after the other, in bouts of cycling, typically repeated 25 to 45 times. The number of PCR cycles will depend on the expected yield of the PCR product. After the last cycle, samples are usually incubated at 72 °C for 5 minutes to fill in the protruding ends of newly synthesized PCR products. There are a number of variants of this basic PCR technique and some of these are listed in Table 5.1.

Avoiding contamination

PCR is a very sensitive technique which allows the amplification of millions of copies of a target DNA sequence from only a few molecules of starting DNA; this is an essential feature for disease diagnosis or monitoring of hematological malignancies. However, this level of PCR sensitivity means that it is essential that the sample must not be contaminated with any other genomic DNA or previously amplified PCR products that may reside in the laboratory environment. Steps that should be taken to eliminate any potential contamination and false positive results are:

a. DNA (or RNA) extraction and PCR reaction mixing and processing should be performed in separate areas to avoid sample contamination. PCR analysis procedures should be done in a third area, separate and distinct, from the nucleic acid extraction and the PCR set up areas.

b. Separate pipettes and sole-purpose vessels should be used in the DNA (or RNA) extraction area to those used for PCR set up and analysis areas. Pipette tips with aerosol filters allow the prevention of micro-droplets being injected into the PCR mixture, and thus prevent contamination of PCR reaction mixtures.

c. Ideally, a laminar flow cabinet should be used. This should be equipped with a UV lamp to prevent bacterial growth.

d. Sterile microtubes and autoclaved solutions (where possible) should be used.

e. Fresh gloves should be worn at all times when PCR is performed.

f. All solutions, except dNTPs, primers and *Taq* polymerase, should be autoclaved or UV

Table 5.1. Commonly used variations of the PCR technique.

PCR method	Principle	Clinical example
Allele-specific PCR (AS-PCR)	Primers include a known single nucleotide polymorphism or mutations	*JAK2* V617F *KIT* D816V
Methylation-specific PCR	Assesses the methylation status of CpG sites within a CpG island. Sodium bisulphite is used to chemically modify DNA so that unmethylated cytosines are converted to uracil. Subsequent amplification is specific for methylated DNA and analyzed by sequence detection methods, e.g. AS-PCR, pyrosequencing	
Microsatellite PCR	PCR amplification using primers that surround a di-, tri-, tetra- or penta-nucleotide repeat. The number of each building block of the repeat is polymorphic hence there are a large number of alleles possible	Chimerism studies: to discriminate between two individuals
Multiplex PCR	Multiple primer sets are used in a single PCR reaction to target multiple regions simultaneously	*IG* or *TCR* gene rearrangement assays
Nested PCR	Two sets of primers are used in two successive PCR amplifications First PCR generates DNA products which are used as the template for the second PCR Sensitive method for MRD detection but not quantitative	*BCR-ABL1* *PML-RARA* *FIP1L1-PDGFRA*
Reverse transcription PCR (RT-PCR)	Convert RNA to cDNA which is then a substrate for PCR amplification	t(8 ;21); *AML1-ETO*
Real-time quantitative PCR (RQ-PCR)	Used to measure absolute or relative amount of a cDNA or DNA molecule within a sample	t(15;17); *PML-RARA* monitoring *BCR-ABL1* in CML

irradiated. Where possible, solutions should be aliquoted in small quantities and stored in designated PCR areas.

g. A good practice, to confirm absence of contamination, is to add a control reaction without template DNA. Negative controls should be performed, in which the reaction mixture does not have the DNA template. If bands are seen after PCR, they are either contaminants or primer dimers.

h. Never open or return vials containing amplified PCR products to the nucleic acid extraction area or the PCR set up area.

Data interpretation

The usual method of detection of the end-point of the PCR reaction is by measurement of the size of the amplified DNA product generated. There are many ways in which end-point analysis can be performed and the most common methods are described.

Gel electrophoresis

a. *Agarose gel electrophoresis*: The easiest way of separating and analyzing PCR products is by identifying their size following migration through an agarose gel. The sample taken from the PCR reaction product, along with appropriate molecular-weight markers, is loaded onto an agarose gel. Shorter DNA molecules migrate further through the agarose than those which are larger. Most agarose gels are between 0.7% and 2%; the lower concentrations of agarose will show good resolution of large DNA fragments (5–10 kb) whilst higher gel concentrations will show good resolution for small fragments (0.2–1 kb range). The purpose of the gel might be to look at the DNA, to quantify it or to isolate a particular band. The DNA is visualized in the gel by addition of ethidium bromide. This binds strongly to DNA by intercalating between the bases and fluoresces under ultraviolet trans-illumination. By comparing the product bands with those of the known molecular weight markers, PCR product fragments of the appropriate molecular weight can be identified.

b. *Polyacrylamide gel electrophoresis* (PAGE): Polyacrylamide gels separate PCR products by size but have higher resolution than agarose which is helpful for the following reasons:

i. Amplified products that differ by only a few bases can be detected. This is especially useful for lymphoid cell clonality assessment or detection of small insertions/deletions (e.g. *NPM1* mutations)

ii. Smaller PCR products can be detected than on agarose gels (i.e. to < 100 bp).

Polyacrylamide is formed by the polymerization of the monomer molecule acrylamide crosslinked by N,N'-methylene-bis-acrylamide (BIS). The advantage of polyacrylamide gel systems is that the initial concentrations of acrylamide and BIS control the hardness and degree of crosslinking of the gel. The hardness of a gel in turn controls the friction that PCR products, or other macro-molecules, experience as they move through the gel in an electric field, and therefore affects the resolution of the components to be separated. Hard gels (12–20% acrylamide) retard the migration of large PCR products more than smaller ones.

c. *Capillary gel electrophoresis*: Capillary gel electrophoresis uses narrow bore fused-silica capillaries to separate a complex array of large and small molecules. High electric field strengths are used to separate the molecules by differences in charge, size and hydrophobicity. The sample is introduced into the system by immersing the end of the capillary into a sample vial and applying pressure, vacuum or voltage. PCR products are identified by a laser as they pass the detection point. This method has the highest resolution potential to single base differences. It is therefore applicable for the detection of small insertions, clonality using *IGH* or *TCR* rearrangements (see below) or chimerism studies (microsatellites).

d. *Other methods*: Alternative methods of electrophoresis are available which utilize micro-fluidics matrix-filled channels such as used by the Bioanalyser 2100 system. The advantages of these systems are that the results can be stored and compared electronically, and the size and amount of PCR product can be determined.

Pyrosequencing

Pyrosequencing is a "sequencing by synthesis" method in which a single strand of the DNA to be sequenced and then its complementary strand are synthesized enzymatically [4]. The pyrosequencing method is based on detecting the activity of DNA polymerase

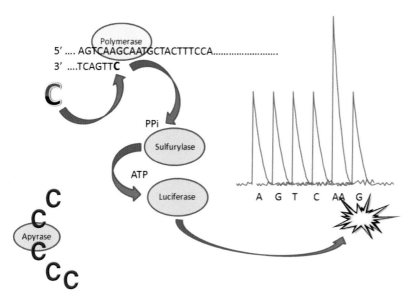

Figure 5.2. Pyrosequencing technology is sequencing by synthesis which enables mutations and SNPs to be easily detected for accurate and quantitative analysis of DNA sequences.

with another chemi-luminescent enzyme (Figure 5.2). Essentially, the method allows sequencing of a single strand of DNA by synthesizing the complementary strand along it, one base pair at a time, and detecting which base was actually added at each step. The template DNA is immobilized, and solutions of A, C, G and T nucleotides are added and removed after the reaction, sequentially. Light is produced only when the nucleotide solution complements the first unpaired base of the template [5]. The size of the light peak is proportional to the number of those bases in sequence, i.e. a GG will give a light peak height twice that of a single G. The sequence and height of the chemi-luminescent signals allows the determination of the sequence of the template [6]. Unincorporated NTP are degraded from the reaction by apyrase prior to the next bases in sequence being added to the reaction.

Melting curve analysis

Melting curve analysis is another method for analyzing PCR products. This assesses the dissociation characteristics of DNA as the strands transition from double to single stranded with increasing temperature. High resolution melt analysis is simple, sensitive and rapid and allows detection to the level of single base pair differences. It also allows direct assessment without the need for any additional manipulation of the PCR product by the user. This can be used for the detection of a number of acquired mutations in hematological malignancies, such as *JAK2* exon 12, *FLT3* ITD and

NPM1 exon 12. See Figure 8.6e for an example of melting curve analysis for *NPM1* mutation detection.

Other gel-based techniques

There are many other gel-based methods that are based on sequence differences for the interpretation of the end-point of PCR, some of which are used in the diagnosis and assessment of hematological malignancies (Table 5.2.) These include, but are not restricted to:

a. *Denaturing gradient gel electrophoresis* (DGGE): a molecular fingerprinting method that separates polymerase chain reaction (PCR)-generated DNA products [7]. DGGE separates PCR products based on sequence differences that result in differential denaturing characteristics of the DNA. During DGGE, PCR products encounter increasingly higher concentrations of chemical denaturant as they migrate through a polyacrylamide gel [8].

b. *Single strand conformational polymorphism* (SSCP): In this approach, rapid chilling of denatured PCR products generates base pairing within the single stranded DNA molecule. The folding and hence shape of this molecule depends upon the sequence of the PCR product. Sequences that differ by a single nucleotide (such as point mutation compared to normal sequence) migrate at different rates through a polyacrylamide gel.

c. *Temperature gradient electrophoresis* (TGGE): This is an electrophoretic method which separates

Table 5.2. Commonly used mutation detection methods.

Method	Principle	Clinical example
PCR followed by restriction endonuclease digestion	Restriction enzymes are used to cut the amplified DNA product into fragments at specific sequences	*FLT3* TKD
High resolution melt	Melting profile differs between wildtype and mutant sequences	*JAK2* exon 12 mutations
Capillary gel electrophoresis	Separates PCR products based on size	*NPM1* exon 12 mutation
Direct sequencing	Sanger sequencing useful to confirm a mutation that has been detected by other methods	Any unknown mutation, e.g. *CEBPA*, *TET2*
Pyrosequencing	Addition of individual nucleotides. Incorporation detected by chemi-luminescence	*JAK2* V617F

DNA based on melting characteristics. It uses a temperature gradient across the gel to analyze the movement of the DNA based on its structure. The most common application is in mutation analysis.

d. *Heteroduplex analysis*: Heteroduplex analysis is a method for identifying sequence differences between a reference and a test sample. The reference and test DNA samples are mixed, heated to denature the double strands and then cooled to reanneal the duplex. If reannealing occurs between test and reference DNA, and these have different sequences as a result of a mutation, "heteroduplexes" are formed. Heteroduplexes migrate more slowly through the gel than their "homoduplex" counterparts. The heteroduplex can therefore be seen as an additional band and signifies the presence of a mutation.

Limitations of end-point analysis for interpretation of PCR

There are some limitations in the analysis of the PCR end-product (i.e. end-point analysis) which vary by the analysis method used. However the major limitation which is applicable to all the above-mentioned methods is that the results are qualitative and cannot be quantified. This can be addressed by using real-time quantitative PCR which quantifies the end product (detailed later in this chapter).

Clinical examples of the application of PCR

PCR is widely used in the diagnosis and molecular monitoring of a number of hematological malignancies. Two of the most common applications, the assessment of lymphoid cell clonality and the analysis

of *JAK2* in myeloproliferative neoplasms, will be described.

Lymphoid cell clonality

PCR is used for the assessment of clonality of lymphoid cell proliferations (see Chapters 7, 8 and 11 for details of applications). B-cell clonality can be determined by *IG* heavy and light chain gene rearrangement and T-cell clonality by rearrangements of the T-cell receptor (*TCR*) gene. During differentiation of B and T progenitor cells, DNA rearrangements of immunoglobulin (*IG*) and T-cell receptor (*TCR*) genes result in a massive diversity of genotypically different cells with the ability to recognize different antigens. This process of gene rearrangement of the V, D and J domains can be utilized for the detection of clonal lymphoid cells since all the neoplastic cells will have undergone the same *TCR* and/or *IG* gene rearrangement. By contrast, a polyclonal population of lymphoid cells will have undergone different rearrangements and each will be unique. Because of the large number of V, D and J domains that exist, multiplex PCR assays have been developed using primers that bind to the most widely used domains. The BIOMED-2 PCR protocols can be applied to the assessment of *IG* and *TCR* gene rearrangements in the investigation of lymphoid proliferations in fresh and formalin-fixed paraffin-embedded tissue. All malignant lymphocytes will have a common clonal origin whereas reactive lymphocytes are polyclonal [9–12].

B-cells and IG gene rearrangements: More than 90% of lymphoid malignancies are of B-cell origin. During B-cell development, the immunoglobulin genes undergo a complex rearrangement process to produce diverse antibody coding sequences. Rearrangement of Ig heavy chain (*IGH*) and Ig light chain genes (*IGK* and *IGL*) can be detected by PCR. In the case of *IGH* rearrangement, primers are designed to conserved regions of the V domain, so-called Framework (FR) regions, so that one primer may anneal to several V_H domains. DNA is amplified with a series of consensus primers that are complementary to sequences of variable regions FR1, FR2 and FR3, and to joining regions of the IGH gene (Figure 5.3). Using this assay on DNA from a polyclonal population of cells, PCR products differ in both sequence and size. By contrast, within a clonal population of

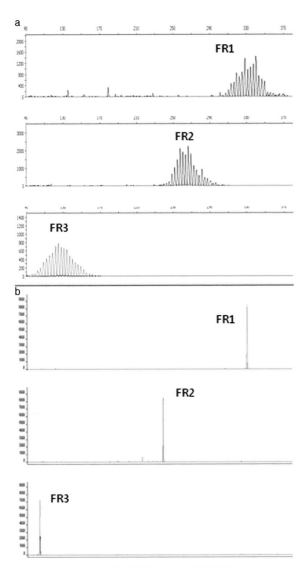

Figure 5.3. Example of *IGH* PCR using the BIOMED2 primers.
a. Polyclonal B-cells showing a polyclonal ladder of peaks for FR1, FR2 and FR3 from a normal individual.
b. Well-defined peaks for FR1, FR2 and FR3 in a clonal B-cell disorder.

B-cells, the majority of PCR products will be identical. The PCR products can be analyzed using a number of techniques to determine their size and sequence differences. Capillary gel electrophoresis can be used to separate the products at very high resolution. If a significant population of cells contains the same *IGH* rearrangement, this appears as a well-defined peak. In contrast, polyclonal B-cells yield a ladder of peaks. Heteroduplex analysis can be used in combination with polyacrylamide gel electrophoresis to detect polyclonal or clonal populations. Heteroduplex analysis for the assessment of clonal *IG* or *TCR* gene rearrangements relies on the presence of multiple different sequences within a polyclonal population (due to junctional diversity and multiplex amplifications). Hence a polyclonal template (many different sequences) gives many heteroduplexes which form the polyclonal smear at a different position within the gel as compared with the homoduplex "clonal" fragment even though the sizes may be similar. It is not necessary to add wild-type DNA to force the generation of heteroduplexes.

This PCR technique for *IGH* rearrangements is fast and only requires a small amount of DNA, can be performed on fresh, frozen or paraffin-embedded specimens, and has a relatively good sensitivity for low-level clones. However, false positive PCR results ("pseudo-clonality") may be a problem if the assay is poorly designed or if interpretation criteria are inadequate for discriminating monoclonal from polyclonal products. False negative *IGH* PCR results are a problem when primer design is suboptimal to detect all possible rearrangements. False negative can also be seen with somatic hypermutation of the *IGH* variable region, which leads to improper annealing of consensus primers to the rearranged *IGH* gene segment, with post-germinal center lymphomas or if the *IG* rearrangement is uncommon. For post-germinal center lymphomas it is important to assess other *IG* gene loci, e.g. *IGH* D-J and *IGK* and *IGL* loci. The BIOMED-2 study shows the promise that standardization of PCR primers and protocols for detecting IGH gene rearrangements can achieve [10].

T-cells and TCR gene rearrangements: PCR amplification of DNA for *TCR* gene rearrangement analysis is commonly used for the diagnostic evaluation of T-cell proliferations to assess clonality [10,12,13]. Primers to a number of *TCR* genes can be used to amplify different *TCR* loci (i.e. *TCRB*, *TCRG* and *TCRD*). PCR products are analyzed in a similar way to IGH, i.e. polyacrylamide or capillary gel

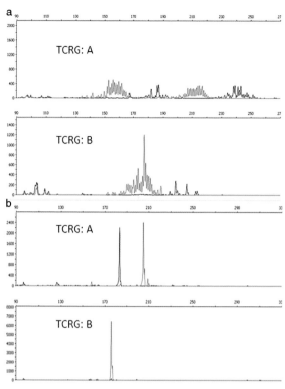

Figure 5.4. Example of *TCRG* PCR using the BIOMED2 primers.
a. Polyclonal patterns for *TCRG* associated for a normal individual.
b. A monoclonal pattern from a patient with a T-cell lymphoproliferative disease.

electrophoresis. Agarose gels are not recommended due to their low resolution.

The specificity of each T lymphocyte *TCR* comes from the characteristic rearrangement of antigen-receptor genes in T-cells. The germline TCR genes consist of variable (V), diversity, joining (J) and constant regions. The number of genes for each region varies for each locus. During T-cell maturation, genes coding for the TCR undergo rearrangement. T-cell receptor delta (*TCRD*) is the first gene rearranged during development, followed by rearrangement of TCR genes coding for gamma (*TCRG*), beta (*TCRB*) and alpha (*TCRA*). The DNA fragments from each polyclonal lymphocyte or a monoclonal population of lymphoid cells of T-cell lineage will show a different mobility compared to the other fragments (Figure 5.4). This allows easy identification of a monoclonal T-cell population and unique identification of each tumor [12].

JAK2 V617F mutation analysis

Another commonly performed PCR technique is detection of the *JAK2* V617F mutation in the diagnostic assessment of possible myeloproliferative neoplasms. *JAK2* V617F is a somatic mutation in the regulatory pseudokinase JH2 domain of JAK2, in which a missense mutation changes the amino acid at position 617 of the JAK2 protein from a valine to a phenylalanine residue. This leads to cytokine-independent activation of downstream signaling molecules. The mutation is detectable in over 95% of patients with polycythemia vera, and 50–60% of those with essential thrombocythemia and primary myelofibrosis (see also Chapter 14) [14–16]. It is also present in refractory anemia with ring sideroblasts associated with marked thrombocytosis, and a small percent of patients with acute myeloid leukemia and other myeloproliferative and myelodysplastic disorders. A number of PCR-based methods can be used to test for the *JAK2* V617F mutation. These include allele-specific PCR (AS-PCR), real-time quantitative PCR, melting curve analysis, pyrosequencing and restriction enzyme digestion (Table 5.1). AS-PCR of peripheral blood DNA has a sensitivity of 1–3% and a low false positive rate; the sensitivity is further increased if performed on purified granulocyte DNA. Real-time quantitative PCR (see below) has a sensitivity of 0.5% [17–20].

Reverse transcription PCR (RT-PCR)

Principles of RT-PCR

PCR can also be performed using mRNA as the starting point in a process called reverse transcription PCR (RT-PCR). RT-PCR can be used to determine the expression of a gene or to identify the sequence of an RNA transcript. It is particularly applicable in hematological malignancies for mutation detection and for the detection of chimeric mRNA resulting from chromosomal translocations. In RT-PCR RNA is first reverse transcribed to complementary DNA (cDNA); the cDNA is then amplified by conventional PCR techniques [21].

cDNA is made from RNA with the use of reverse transcriptase, an enzyme originally isolated from retroviruses. Using an RNA molecule as a template, reverse transcriptase synthesizes a single-stranded DNA molecule that can then be used as a template for PCR. The primers for initiating cDNA synthesis can be either a collection of random hexamers that cover the entire range of different base sequences that could be present in six bases or it can be a specific 3' primer that will allow the cDNA production only from a specific mRNA subtype. Some genetic assays may be applicable to analysis of either DNA or RNA (e.g. *FLT3*, *NPM1* mutations) whereas others require mRNA (e.g. *BCR-ABL1* and *AML1-ETO*). RT-PCR can be performed on fresh material (i.e. blood and bone marrow aspirates). Due to poor preservation of RNA in fixed tissue it is not applicable to fixed bone marrow biopsies.

Data interpretation

RT-PCR products can be analyzed using similar methodologies to conventional end-point PCR, such as agarose gel electrophoresis.

Clinical examples of the application of RT-PCR

RT-PCR is the preferred molecular genetic method for the assessment of chromosomal translocations. The chimeric mRNA which results from translocations is preferred to genomic DNA as the template for PCR amplification. Examples include *BCR-ABL1* in chronic myeloid leukemia (CML) and Ph-positive lymphoblastic leukemia/lymphoma with t(9;22)(q34;q11), and *RUNX1-RUNXT1* (*AML1-ETO*) in acute myeloid leukemia with (8;21)(q22;q22). RT-PCR can also be used as an alternative to PCR, such as in the assessment of mutations, such as in *FLT3* and *NPM1* mutations.

Detection of *BCR-ABL1*

The t(9;22)(q34;q11) translocation occurs in CML and a subset of patients with lymphoblastic leukemia/lymphoma [22]. The *BCR-ABL1* fusion gene is formed by rearrangement of the breakpoint cluster region (*BCR*) on chromosome 22 with the c-*ABL1* proto-oncogene on chromosome 9. The *BCR-ABL1* rearrangement causes production of an abnormal tyrosine kinase molecule with increased activity, postulated to be responsible for the development of leukemia. Three common fusion transcripts can result from the *BCR-ABL1* rearrangement, depending on the breakpoint on chromosome 22. These involve the fusion of *BCR* exons e12-e16 and exon a2 of the *ABL1* gene. Most patients with CML have breakpoints in the M-BCR resulting in the generation of e13a2 or e14a2 transcripts. Patients with lymphoblastic leukemia/lymphoma generally have e1a2 transcripts [23]. Due to

the variations in the genomic breakpoints and the large breakpoint regions, RT-PCR is preferred to PCR for the detection of *BCR-ABL1*. Transcripts coding for both the p190 and p210 variants of *BCR-ABL1* can easily be detected by RT-PCR using *BCR*-specific primers upstream of the breakpoint. *BCR-ABL1* transcript levels can be monitored as a measure of residual disease; it is recommended that real time quantitative PCR be used for this (see Chapter 14 for details).

Detection of t(8;21); *RUNX1-RUNX1T1* and inv(16); *CBFB-MYH11* in acute myeloid leukemia

Balanced reciprocal translocations are a feature of acute myeloid leukemia (AML) and in particular those involving a translocation of chromosomes 8 and 21 and internal translocation of chromosome 16. The t(8;21)(q22;q22) involves the *RUNX1-RUNX1T1* genes (also known as *AML1-ETO*) whilst the inv(16) (p13q22) and t(16;16)(p13;q22), the *CBFB-MYH11* genes. Due to the variable nature of genomic breakpoints spread over a wide region, both of these translocations are detected by RT-PCR from the fusion or chimeric RNA resulting from the chromosomal translocation [24–27]. The presence of the fusion transcript is used in conjunction with morphology, cytogenetics and flow cytometry results for a definitive diagnosis. Nested RT-PCR increases the sensitivity of the assay for the detection of minimal residual disease.

NPM1 and *FLT3* mutations in acute myeloid leukemia

Mutations of the nucleophosmin (*NPM1*) gene have been reported as the most frequent mutation in AML, especially in the presence of a normal karyotype. In this subgroup of intermediate-risk AML, the identification of other gene mutations (e.g. *FLT3* and CCAAT/enhancer-binding protein-alpha [*CEBPA*]) has helped to refine the prognosis. In particular, *NPM1* mutant with wild type *FLT3* within normal cytogenetics identifies a group of AML patients with a relatively favorable prognosis. *NPM1* mutations involve a four or eight base pair insertion at a specific site of the gene sequence. Although there are several variations of the insertion, Type A (TCTG) is the most common insertion seen in around 50% of cases [28–32]. The *NPM1* mutation can be easily detected by a number of PCR- or RT-PCR-based methods including capillary gel electrophoresis, sequencing, high resolution melting curve analysis and pyrosequencing (Figure 5.5).

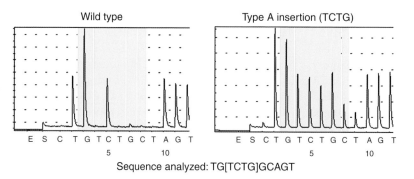

Sequence analyzed: TG[TCTG]GCAGT

Figure 5.5. An example pyrosequencing for the detection of a Type A insertion in the *NPM1* gene. Left is the wildtype pattern and on the right the pattern for the Type A insertion in the *NPM1* gene.

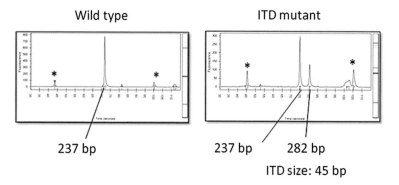

ITD size: 45 bp

Figure 5.6. Detection of an ITD mutation in the *FLT3* gene using the Agilent 2100 Bioanalyser.
Left is the wild type RNA peak detected at 237 base pairs. On the right is the ITD peak at 282 base pairs, resulting in a duplication of 45 base pairs. The two peaks marked * are the top and bottom markers used for size calibration. If any DNA contamination was present, using these primers, a peak would have been seen at 325 base pairs (a very small peak around 82 in the wild type pattern is from DNA).

Internal tandem duplications (ITD) of the juxtamembrane domain-coding sequence and missense mutation of D835 within the kinase domain of the *FLT3* gene occurs in 15–35% and 5–10% of adults with AML, respectively. In addition, point mutations, deletions, and insertions have been found in the juxtamembrane domain (exons 14 and 15) and in the other codons within the kinase domain, though these are less common. *FLT3* ITDs can be detected in DNA or RNA from diagnostic samples by PCR using primers within exon 14 and 15. The D835 TKD mutation can be detected by restriction endonuclease digestion of the exon 20 PCR product followed by agarose or polyacrylamide gel electrophoresis. Multiplex PCR methods can be used to detect both *FLT3* ITD and D835 TKD mutations. Several large-scale studies in well-documented patients have demonstrated that *FLT3* mutations are strongly associated with a poor prognosis and a high leukemia cell count in patients with AML, suggesting that *FLT3* mutations are involved in disease progression. *FLT3* ITD mutations can be detected by a size change using gel or capillary electrophoresis [33–41] (Figure 5.6).

Real-time quantitative PCR

Principles of the technique

Real-time quantitative PCR (RQ-PCR) allows the "real-time" monitoring and quantitation of amplified products during PCR and can be applied to DNA and RNA. RQ-PCR measures the kinetics of the PCR reaction during the early phases of amplification. This provides a distinct advantage over conventional end-point PCR analysis using gel electrophoresis or other detection methods and is specifically applicable to monitoring changes in the level of gene expression. The principles of RQ-PCR are based on the three phases of PCR:

i. Exponential phase: a doubling of product occurs with every cycle (assuming 100% reaction efficiency). The reaction is very specific and precise.

ii. Linear phase: During this phase the PCR reaction components are consumed as a result of amplification and the reaction rate is slowing.

iii. Plateau phase: At this stage the amplification reaction has stopped, no more products are being made and if left long enough, the PCR products will begin to degrade. This is the end-point phase in conventional PCR when the product is detected (e.g. by gel electrophoresis).

RQ-PCR is based on the rate of consumption and depletion of PCR reagents as these will occur at different rates for each replicate. During cycling the reactions start to slow down and the PCR product is no longer being doubled at each cycle. Eventually the reactions stop all together or plateau. Each tube or reaction will plateau at a different point due to the different reaction kinetics for each sample. As there are different amounts of starting DNA in each sample, these will reach the plateau at a different cycle, but at the end of the run when the measurement is taken, there will be no obvious difference between the samples. RQ-PCR is a major development of PCR technology that enables reliable detection and measurement of products generated during each cycle of the PCR process.

Two main variations are available for real-time PCR. TaqMan assay (named after *Taq* DNA polymerase) was one of the earliest methods introduced for real-time PCR reaction monitoring and has been widely adopted for the quantification of mRNAs. The method uses the $5'$ endonuclease activity of *Taq* DNA polymerase to cleave an oligonucleotide probe during PCR, thereby generating a detectable signal. The probes are fluorescently labeled at their $5'$ end and are non-extendable at their $3'$ end by chemical modification. Specificity is conferred at three levels: via two PCR primers and the probe. This probe is a sequence-specific oligonucleotide with a reporter dye attached to the $5'$ end and a quencher dye attached to the $3'$ end. If the quencher and fluorophore remain close to each other, separated only by the length of the probe, this will be sufficient to quench the fluorescence of the reporter dye. However, during PCR, the polymerase will extend the PCR primer and the $5'$ exonuclease activity of the *Taq* polymerase will cleave the probe, releasing the fluorescence reporter molecule away from the effect of the quencher. The fluorescence intensity of the reporter dye increases, as the PCR cycle and product numbers increase. This process repeats in every cycle and does not interfere with the accumulation of PCR product. Variations on this method are also reported including those with quencher/probe combinations that are on different primers or probes.

Other methods use dyes that bind to DNA to measure the total amount of double stranded DNA present at the end of each reaction. Ethidium bromide is a dye that binds to double stranded DNA by interpolation (intercalation) between the base pairs. Here it fluoresces when irradiated in the UV part of the spectrum. However, the fluorescence is not very bright. Other dyes such as SYBR green are much more fluorescent than ethidium bromide. SYBR green binds the Minor Groove of double stranded DNA, and as more dye binds the intensity of the fluorescent emissions increases. Therefore as more double stranded PCR products are produced the SYBR green signal will increase stoichiometrically. Use of SYBR green eliminates the need for product expensive specific probes. However, it is important to prevent primer-dimer formation since these will also bind SYBR green.

Data interpretation

RQ-PCR gives a precise measurement of the amount of a specific DNA or RNA present in a sample. Quantitation is usually performed by comparing the expression with that of a control ("normalized") gene. The normalized gene may be a housekeeping gene whose level does not change between samples, e.g. 18S ribosomal RNA, beta-2-microglobulin or GAPDH. Alternatively, the normalization gene may be associated with the test gene; for example *ABL1* as the normalization gene for the *BCR-ABL1* test gene. The normalized data can then be expressed in terms of:

a. Copy number of transcripts comparing control and experimental data, or
b. Changes in cycle threshold (Ct) values between the normalization target and the test target.

Different applications have different methods of determining levels of test RNA expression depending on the normalization gene.

Clinical examples of the application of RQ-PCR

RQ-PCR is used to quantify gene expression. It is particularly useful to monitor changes in the level of expression during and following therapy (e.g. *BCR-ABL1* in chronic myeloid leukemia) and as an early warning system to predict disease relapse (e.g. *PML-RARA* in acute promyelocytic leukemia). These examples will be described in more detail.

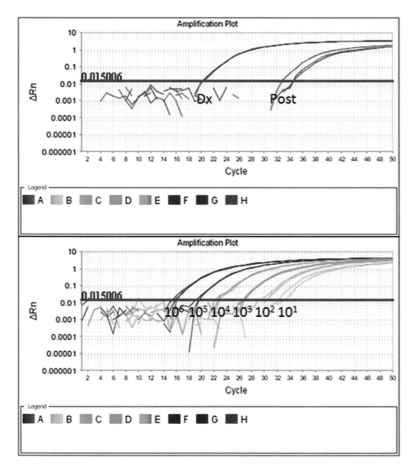

Figure 5.7. Real-time quantitative PCR for *BCR-ABL1* fusion. The lower panel shows a dilution standard curve with each set of paired colored curves representing the amplification of 10^6, 10^5, 10^4, 10^3, 10^2 and 10^1 copies of *BCR-ABL1*. In the upper panel the patient diagnostic (labeled "Dx") and 1-year post-therapy ("Post") curves are shown. At diagnosis, the patient had nearly 10^5 copies of *BCR-ABL1*, whilst after therapy less than 10 copies are detectable.

BCR-ABL1 quantitation in chronic myeloid leukemia

Real-time quantitative polymerase chain reaction (RQ-PCR) of *BCR-ABL1* hybrid transcripts is now the standard method for monitoring the response to treatment in patients with chronic myeloid leukemia (CML) who have been induced into complete cytogenetic remission. Differences still exist between laboratories in the methodology and timing of molecular monitoring in CML, however, they are becoming increasingly standardized (see Chapter 14 for details) [42–45]. *BCR-ABL1* transcripts present at extremely low levels can be accurately detected and quantitated by RQ-PCR which is capable of detecting a single chronic myeloid leukemia cell in a population of 10^5–10^6 normal cells (Figure 5.7).

Treatment of CML is mainly using ATP-competitive kinase inhibitors that block BCR-ABL kinase activity, particularly imatinib mesylate (Glivec) which can induce durable responses in the vast majority of patients [46]. However, the re-emergence of the CML

cells which may be associated with the emergence of resistant leukemia clones bearing mutations in the *BCR-ABL1* kinase domain are a major challenge. These may be treated with alternative therapeutic options, if these cells can be detected early enough.

Currently there is an international attempt to standardize the assessment and reporting of the results from MRD monitoring. An International Scale (IS) has been proposed that defines a 3-log reduction in the transcript ratio from the IRIS trial baseline as 0.10% and the baseline as 100% [47–49]. In addition, the level of molecular response or the complete molecular response (CMR) has been defined as the achievement of undetectable *BCR-ABL1* transcripts. The finding of CMR must be based on RQ-PCR methodology that is capable of reliably detecting transcripts at the 0.001% (10^{-5}) level. In addition, a new response, the major molecular response (MMR), was defined as being a $\geq$ 3-log reduction in the *BCR-ABL1/BCR* ratio from the diagnostic baseline obtained [47]. Therefore, a 3-log reduction in transcript levels represents a reduction from a standard baseline, rather than an individual patient baseline, and indicates an absolute, and not a relative, value for residual disease. Achievement of at least a MMR has been correlated with a good outcome in CML [50]. A continued decline in BCR-ABL transcript level should be interpreted as continued response, while increasing BCR-ABL transcript levels have been correlated with imatinib-resistant *BCR-ABL1* mutations and relapse. However, because of inherent variability in RQ-PCR reliability, confirmation with a second test is more predictive of mutational resistance than a single finding. RQ-PCR detection of an increase in BCR-ABL transcripts should trigger more stringent RQ-PCR evaluation, rather than an immediate change in treatment.

PML-RARA quantitation in acute promyelocytic leukemia

Acute promyelocytic leukemia (APL) cells contain a fusion gene comprising the downstream sequences of the retinoic acid receptor alpha gene (*RARA*) fused to the promoter region and upstream sequences of one of several genes, the most common (> 80%) being the promyelocytic leukemia gene (*PML*). The fusion gene, *PML-RARA*, may be seen in a karyotype as t(15;17)(q22;q12). Messenger RNA (PML-RARA) produced from the fusion gene can be detected by RT-PCR and indicates the presence of neoplastic cells. The PCR-based assay has greater sensitivity than standard methods such as morphology review, karyotyping, or fluorescence *in situ* hybridization (FISH) [51]. Approximately 40% of t(15;17)-positive

cases demonstrate a breakpoint within intron 3 of the *PML* gene (Figure 5.8); this is referred to as *bcr3* and results in the fusion of *PML* exon 3 with *RARA* exon 3. The *bcr1* is detected in approximately 45–55% of positive cases and results in the fusion of *PML* exon 6 and *RARA* exon 3 as the breakpoint occurs in intron 6. The *bcr2* is involved in 8–10% of t(15;17)-positive cases and unlike *bcr1* and *bcr3*, the breakpoint of *bcr2* occurs at inconsistent sites within exon 6 of the *PML* gene, resulting in the fusion of a variable portion of *PML* exon 6 with exon 3 of the *RARA* gene. The location of *bcr1*, *bcr2* and *bcr3* produces fusion transcripts of varying lengths that are referred to as the long, variant and short forms, respectively. It is important to identify the *PML-RARA* fusion gene and type at diagnosis, since this group of patients is highly likely to benefit from targeted therapies and can be monitored by RQ-PCR during therapy. Therefore, for the assay to be used for ongoing monitoring after treatment, the *PML-RARA* transcript type must be established at the time of diagnosis.

Recent studies have clearly demonstrated that sensitive RQ-PCR monitoring is important during and following therapy, just as for *BCR-ABL1* monitoring in chronic myeloid leukemia. This is because the majority of patients who remain PCR-positive, or revert to PCR-positivity following therapy, will relapse. It is important to identify these patients as they are likely to benefit from early intervention for residual or recurrent disease (see also Chapter 8) [52]. RQ-PCR allows *PML-RARA* levels to be regularly monitored rather than simply detecting the presence or absence of disease and at a single timepoint [53–55]. For disease monitoring, the MRD assay is reported in the form

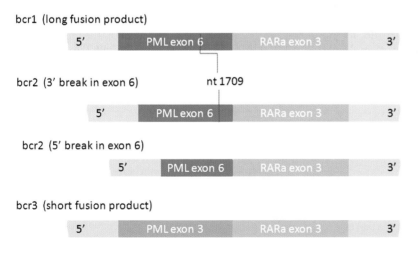

bcr1 (long fusion product)

bcr2 (3′ break in exon 6)

nt 1709

bcr2 (5′ break in exon 6)

bcr3 (short fusion product)

Figure 5.8. Diagram showing the different *PML-RARA* fusion transcripts in acute promyelocytic leukemia with the t(15;17) translocation.

of a normalized ratio, an estimate of the level of *PML-RARA* RNA present in the specimen, expressed in relation to the level of RNA from an internal control gene to give a measure of sensitivity [53]. The RQ-PCR normalized ratio at each time point is compared with the previous values for the patient. Critical results, such as increased transcript levels, should be repeated on another specimen to verify the result. As a word of caution, *PML-RARA* levels can only be compared reliably if tested in the same laboratory using the same procedure each time. The assay will only detect *PML-RARA* RNA and will not detect RNA from the less common *RARA* fusion genes.

Gene expression analysis

Microarray-based gene expression profiling technology was introduced over a decade ago. This powerful technology allows the simultaneous assessment of the expression of many thousands of genes, and, potentially, every gene within a cell. Gene expression arrays can be used to detect DNA or RNA and have been used to characterize neoplastic cells, including leukemias. The technology enables gene expression profiles of normal and malignant cells or between subtypes of diseases (e.g. AML subtypes) to be compared [56]. Gene expression profiling has been evaluated as a potential diagnostic tool for hematological malignancies as well as for characterizing cellular pathways. It has successfully identified gene expression patterns that segregate between leukemia subtypes.

Principles of gene expression arrays

The principle of gene expression arrays is that there is hybridization between the nucleotides in a test sample (target) and gene-specific nucleotides (probes) that are spotted or directly synthesized on a solid support ("array"), e.g. glass. The arrayed nucleotides may be oligonucleotides or PCR products and these may represent entire genes. The test sample is labeled (e.g. fluorochrome) and, if complementary sequences are present, the target hybridizes with the relevant sequence on the array. Hybridization or binding results in a detectable signal (e.g. fluorescent signal) which can be measured. Signal intensity correlates with the amount of target present in the sample for each gene sequence. Data analysis is complex due to the large amount of information generated from a single array. However, the test enables the full nucleic acid composition of the sample to be determined.

Many commercial arrays on a variety of platforms are now available for clinical and research applications. These vary in their resolution and technical performance.

Gene expression arrays can be used to assess the gene expression profile of a sample, e.g. leukemic cells. The first study utilizing microarray technology demonstrated the power of this tool to classify and predict human acute leukemia [56]. This array-based classification was performed solely on gene expression and was independent of previous biological knowledge. It has since been shown that, although morphology, complemented by cytogenetics or molecular markers, is still the gold standard in diagnosis and prognosis, gene expression profiling has proven to be a capable alternative. Recent microarray studies in a number of malignancies indicate that this technology may supplant the labor-intensive "gold standard" methods [57–60]. This could be in the form of whole transcriptome arrays (i.e. 30–100 000 transcripts) or with leukemia-specific "chips." Microarrays can even further magnify the precision of diagnosis and prognosis, as well as provide a single standardized platform. Furthermore, gene expression profiling revealed several molecularly distinct subtypes of diseases, which were formerly considered the same disease, based on morphological diagnosis. Indeed, this stratification was in correlation with the response to treatment and prognosis. Notably, prediction of outcome was based on gene expression profiling of samples taken at the time of diagnosis [61–65]. Therefore, genomic large-scale gene expression profiling should be included in designing clinical trials, in order to refine the diagnosis and matching treatment of each malignancy. In conclusion, although not currently widely utilized in clinical practice, microarray technology is destined to eventually enable physicians to tailor-fit therapies for malignant hematological disorders.

Data interpretation

Regardless of the platform used, each microarray experiment produces a data set containing tens to hundreds of thousands of values of gene expression. This overwhelming abundance of data requires the use of powerful statistical and analytical tools. There are two basic approaches to analyze a gene expression data set:

a. "Supervised" approach: This is based on determining genes that fit a predetermined pattern.

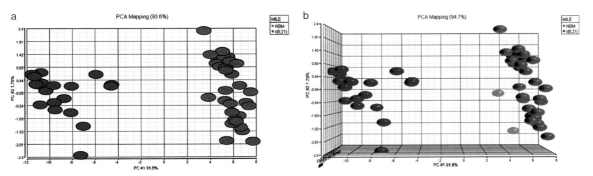

Figure 5.9. Gene expression array data. Principal component analysis (PCA) plots using 30 normal bone marrow (NBM; red) and 19 AML samples from patients with t(8;21) translocation (blue) based on the 64 most differentially expressed genes between the two sample types.
a. A two-dimensional representation of the principal component axes.
b. A three-dimensional representation of the same data.

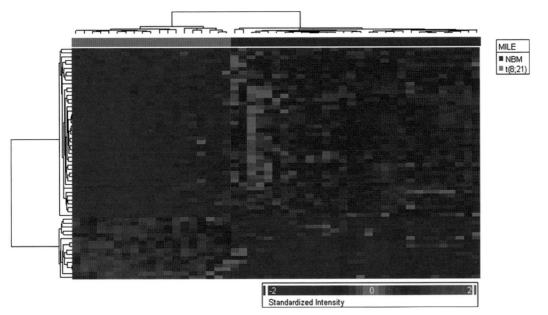

Figure 5.10. A hierarchical clustering heatmap of the samples and genes shown in Figure 5.9. High gene expression is in red and low expression in blue. The normal bone marrow samples (blue bar under the top dendrogram) cluster together and separately from the AML t(8;21) samples (green). The dendrogram on the y-axis shows the clustering of the genes; the top cluster shows genes more highly expressed in the normal marrow compared with the t(8;21), and the lower cluster those higher in the t(8;21) patients.

This is usually used to correlate gene expression and clinical data [66]. The two most common supervised techniques are nearest neighbor analysis and support vector machines [67,68].

b. "Unsupervised" approach: This is based on characterizing the components of the data set without the a priori input or knowledge of a training signal. This is usually used to identify a distinct subgroup of tumors that share similar gene expression profiles. The four most common

unsupervised techniques are hierarchical clustering [69,70] (Figure 5.10), principal-component analysis (PCA)[71–74] (Figure 5.9), self-organizing maps and relevance networks.

Clinical examples of gene expression arrays

Leukemia classification

Hierarchical cluster analysis is traditionally used in phylogenetic research and has been adapted to microarray analysis. The goal of cluster analysis in microarray technology is to group genes or experiments into clusters with similar profiles. These types of analyses are often seen to show relationships between patient samples or between different groups of genes. Several studies in 2004 showed that AML could be clustered into different subgroups; each subgroup had different cytogenetics or mutations predominating in the subgroups [59,75]. More recently, the MILE study group profiled over 3200 leukemia samples to produce a molecular classifier for up to 18 different types of leukemia, both chronic and acute [57]. In a subsequent assessment, a focused group of 14 classes of acute leukemia showed high diagnostic classification accuracy (95.6% median sensitivity and 99.8% median specificity) when compared with the current "gold standard" diagnostic approach. A review of the discordant results in this analysis showed that the microarray results were in fact correct and had outperformed the standard diagnostic methods in 75% of these discrepant cases. This and other similar studies demonstrate that gene expression profiling can be used to diagnose and classify hematological malignancies with extremely high accuracy.

Prediction of prognosis and therapeutic response

Information obtained from gene expression microarrays can also be used to predict disease prognosis and therapeutic response. Gene expression profiling of cytogenetically normal AML, for example, has identified both previously known subgroups and novel classes with distinct expression clusters that were associated with prognosis [76]. Other studies have examined two groups of AML patients (good-prognosis group and poor-prognosis group) to identify differences in treatment responses [63]. These studies have been able to identify candidate genes with differential levels of expression between good- and poor-prognosis AML groups. This approach may, in future, be used clinically to allow better determination of prognosis of AML.

The MILE study also assessed myelodysplasia with the following findings:

a. Gene expression patterns in myelodysplasia were highly predictive of time to AML transformation. This was further enhanced when a gene expression-based prognostic classifier was constructed [61].

b. The expression profile of CD34-positive bone marrow cells from myelodysplasia patients differed from normal individuals.

c. Gene expression profiles could identify differing clinical outcomes, such as therapy-related myelodysplasia versus secondary myelodysplasia or with different cytogenetics [77].

d. Molecular criteria could be used for refining prognostic categorization in myelodysplasia.

Other molecular genetic test types

Over the past decade there has been a tremendous explosion in the number and range of genetic tests available for the assessment of specific chromosomal changes and the perturbed genes in hematological malignancies. Many of these (as described above) are now in routine practice for diagnosis, determining prognosis and for disease monitoring. Other molecular genetic techniques are also available but either only have a limited role in clinical practice or are yet to be introduced. Some of the newer techniques involve genome-wide molecular strategies and include:

a. Whole genome DNA sequencing: to detect acquired mutations specific for a malignancy.

b. Oligonucleotide arrays to analyze single-nucleotide polymorphisms and identify regions of genomic loss or amplification, and loss of heterozygosity or uniparental disomy.

Conclusion

There is a vast array of molecular genetic techniques available for the identification of genes involved in mutations, rearrangements or translocations in hematological malignancies. Many of these are now essential in the diagnostic armamentarium of hematological malignancies. As well as increasing knowledge about disease development they have been shown to have clinically useful beneficial consequences for both diagnosis and management such as:

a. Confirming clonality.
b. Detecting disease-associated genotypes.
c. Determining prognosis.
d. Monitoring residual disease following therapy.
e. Predicting imminent relapse.

Reliable and accurate molecular-based diagnostic tests have also contributed to ensuring subsets of patients have the most beneficial therapies for their disease. New genetic testing strategies continue to be developed and their roles will require assessment in clinical trials. Whole genome sequencing is currently in its infancy and it remains to be seen whether this may become a clinically useful tool in the future. The rational use of these genomic tests will become ever more important as we move towards personalized therapies.

References

1. Saiki RK, Gelfand DH, Stoffel S *et al*. Primer-directed enzymatic amplification of DNA with a thermostable DNA polymerase. *Science* 1988;**239**(4839):487–91.

2. Erlich HA. Polymerase chain reaction. *J Clin Immunol* 1989;**9**(6):437–47.

3. Williams JF. Optimization strategies for the polymerase chain reaction. *Biotechniques* 1989;**7**(7):762–9.

4. Ronaghi M, Karamohamed S, Pettersson B, Uhlen M, Nyren P. Real-time DNA sequencing using detection of pyrophosphate release. *Anal Biochem* 1996;**242**(1):84–9.

5. Alderborn A, Kristofferson A, Hammerling U. Determination of single-nucleotide polymorphisms by real-time pyrophosphate DNA sequencing. *Genome Res* 2000;**10**(8):1249–58.

6. Ahmadian A, Ehn M, Hober S. Pyrosequencing: history, biochemistry and future. *Clin Chim Acta* 2006;**363**(1–2):83–94.

7. Hovig E, Smith-Sorensen B, Uitterlinden AG, Borresen AL. Detection of DNA variation in cancer. *Pharmacogenetics* 1992;**2**(6):317–28.

8. Righetti PG, Gelfi C. Capillary electrophoresis of DNA for molecular diagnostics. *Electrophoresis* 1997;**18**(10):1709–14.

9. Deane M, McCarthy KP., Wiedemann LM, Norton JD. An improved method for detection of B-lymphoid clonality by polymerase chain reaction. *Leukemia* 1991;**5**(8):726–30.

10. Evans PA, Pott Ch, Groenen PJ *et al*. Significantly improved PCR-based clonality testing in B-cell malignancies by use of multiple immunoglobulin gene targets: report of the BIOMED-2 Concerted Action BHM4-CT98-3936. *Leukemia* 2007;**21**(2):207–14.

11. Potter MN, Steward CG, Maitland NJ, Oakhill A. Detection of clonality in childhood B-lineage acute lymphoblastic leukaemia by the polymerase chain reaction. *Leukemia* 1992;**6**(4):289–94.

12. van Dongen JJ, Langerak AW, Bruggemann M *et al*. Design and standardization of PCR primers and protocols for detection of clonal immunoglobulin and T-cell receptor gene recombinations in suspect lymphoproliferations: report of the BIOMED-2 Concerted Action BMH4-CT98-3936. *Leukemia* 2003;**17**(12):2257–317.

13. Langlands K, Craig JI, Anthony RS, Parker AC. Clonal selection in acute lymphoblastic leukaemia demonstrated by polymerase chain reaction analysis of immunoglobulin heavy chain and T-cell receptor delta chain rearrangements. *Leukemia* 1993;**7**:1066–70.

14. Jones AV, Kreil S, Zoi K *et al*. Widespread occurrence of the *JAK2* V617F mutation in chronic myeloproliferative disorders. *Blood* 2005;**106**(6):2162–68.

15. Scott LM, Campbell PJ, Baxter EJ *et al*. The *JAK2* V617F mutation is uncommon in cancers and in myeloid malignancies other than the classic myeloproliferative disorders. *Blood* 2005;**106**(8):2920–1.

16. Levine RL, Wadleigh M, Cools J *et al*. Activating mutation in the tyrosine kinase *JAK2* in polycythemia vera, essential thrombocythemia, and myeloid metaplasia with myelofibrosis. *Cancer Cell* 2005;**7**(4):387–97.

17. Campbell PJ, Green AR. The myeloproliferative disorders. *New Engl J Med* 2006;**355**(23):2452–66.

18. Tan AY, Westerman DA, Dobrovic A. A simple, rapid, and sensitive method for the detection of the *JAK2* V617F mutation. *Am J Clin Pathol* 2007;**127**(6):977–81.

19. Ma W, Kantarjian H, Zhang X *et al*. Mutation profile of *JAK2* transcripts in patients with chronic myeloproliferative neoplasias. *J Mol Diagn* 2009;**11**(1):49–53.

20. Jones AV. Cross NCP. White HE, Green AR, Scott LM. Rapid identification of *JAK2* exon 12 mutations using high resolution melting analysis. *Haematologica* 2008;**93**(10):1560–4.

21. Dvorak Z, Pascussi JM, Modriansky M. Approaches to messenger RNA detection – comparison of methods. *Biomed Pap Med Fac Univ Palacky Olomouc Czech Repub* 2003;**147**(2):131–135.

22. Vardiman JW. Chronic myelogenous leukemia, *BCR-ABL1+*. *Am J Clin Pathol* 2009;**132**(2):250–60.

23. Hughes TP, Ambrosetti A, Barbu V *et al*. Clinical value of PCR in diagnosis and follow-up of leukemia and lymphoma: Report of the third workshop of the molecular biology/BMT study group. *Leukemia* 1991;**5**:448–51.

24. Liu Yin JA. Minimal residual disease in acute myeloid leukaemia. *Best Pract Res Clin Haematol* 2002;**15**(1):119–35.

25. Fujimaki S, Funato T, Harigae H *et al*. A quantitative reverse transcriptase polymerase chain reaction method for the detection of leukaemic cells with t(8;21) in peripheral blood. *Eur J Haematol* 2000;**64**(4):252–8.

26. Tobal K, Newton J, Macheta M *et al*. Molecular quantitation of minimal residual disease in acute myeloid leukemia with t(8;21) can identify patients in durable remission and predict clinical relapse. *Blood* 2000;**95**(3):815–19.

27. Tobal K, Liu Yin JA. Molecular monitoring of minimal residual disease in acute myeloblastic leukemia with t(8;21) by RT-PCR. *Leuk Lymphoma* 1998; **31**(1–2):115–20.

28. Papadaki C, Dufour A, Seibl M *et al*. Monitoring minimal residual disease in acute myeloid leukaemia with *NPM1* mutations by quantitative PCR: clonal evolution is a limiting factor. *Br J Haematol* 2009;**144**(4):517–23.

29. Schnittger S, Kern W, Tschulik C *et al*. Minimal residual disease levels assessed by *NPM1* mutation specific RQ-PCR provide important prognostic information in AML. *Blood* 2009; **114**(11):2220–31.

30. Barragan E, Pajuelo JC, Ballester S *et al*. Minimal residual disease detection in acute myeloid leukemia by mutant nucleophosmin (*NPM1*): comparison with WT1 gene expression. *Clin Chim Acta* 2008;**395** (1–2):120–3.

31. Scholl S, Mugge LO, Landt O *et al*. Rapid screening and sensitive detection of *NPM1* (nucleophosmin) exon 12 mutations in acute myeloid leukaemia. *Leukemia Research* 2007;**31**(9):1205–11.

32. Chen W, Rassidakis GZ, Medeiros LJ. Nucleophosmin gene mutations in acute myeloid leukemia. *Arch Pathol Lab Med* 2006;**130**(11):1687–92.

33. Kiyoi H, Naoe T, Nakano Y *et al*. Prognostic implication of *FLT3* and *N-RAS* gene mutations in acute myeloid leukemia. *Blood* 1999; **93**(9):3074–80.

34. Abu-Duhier FM, Goodeve AC, Wilson GA *et al*. *FLT3* internal tandem duplication mutations in adult acute myeloid leukaemia define a high-risk group. *Br J Haematol* 2000;**111**(1):190–5.

35. Abu-Duhier FM, Goodeve AC, Wilson GA *et al*. Identification of novel *FLT-3* Asp835 mutations in adult acute myeloid leukaemia. *Br J Haematol* 2001; **113**(4):983–8.

36. Griffin JD. Point mutations in the *FLT3* gene in AML. *Blood* 2001; **97**(8): 2193A–22193.

37. Schnittger S, Schoch C, Dugas M *et al*. Analysis of *FLT3* length mutations in 1003 patients with acute myeloid leukemia: correlation to cytogenetics, FAB subtype, and prognosis in the AMLCG study and usefulness as a marker for the detection of minimal residual disease. *Blood* 2002;**100**(1):59–66.

38. Kottaridis PD, Gale RE, Linch DC. *Flt3* mutations and leukaemia. *Br J Haematol* 2003;**122**(4):523–38.

39. Reilly JT. *FLT3* and its role in the pathogenesis of acute myeloid leukaemia. *Leuk Lymphoma* 2003; **44**(1):1–7.

40. Whitman SP, Ruppert AS, Radmacher MD *et al*. *FLT3* D835/I836 mutations are associated with poor disease-free survival and a distinct gene-expression signature among younger adults with de novo cytogenetically normal acute myeloid leukaemia lacking FLT3 internal tandem duplications. *Blood* 2008; **111**(3):1552–9.

41. Meshinchi S, Appelbaum FR. Structural and functional alterations of *FLT3* in acute myeloid leukaemia. *Clinical Cancer Research* 2009;**15**(13):4263–9.

42. Deininger MW. Milestones and monitoring in patients with CML treated with imatinib. *Hematol Am Soc Hematol Educ Program* 2008;**2008**(1):419–26.

43. Faderl S, Hochhaus A, Hughes T. Monitoring of minimal residual disease in chronic myeloid leukemia. *Hematol Oncol Clin N Am* 2004;**18**(3):657–70.

44. Hughes T, Hochhaus A. Clinical strategies to achieve an early and successful response to tyrosine kinase inhibitor therapy. *Semin Hematol* 2009;**46**(2 Suppl. 3): S11–15.

45. Radich JP. Monitoring treatment results in patients with chronic myelogenous leukemia. *Clin Adv Hematol Oncol* 2008;**6**(8):577–8, 586.

46. John AM, Thomas NS, Mufti GJ, Padua RA. Targeted therapies in myeloid leukemia. *Semin Cancer Biol* 2004;**14**(1):41–62.

47. Cross NC, Hughes TP, Hochhaus A, Goldman JM. International standardisation of quantitative real-time RT-PCR for *BCR-ABL*. *Leuk Res* 2008;**32**(3):505–6.

48. Hughes T, Saglio G, Branford S *et al*. Impact of baseline *BCR-ABL* mutations on response to nilotinib in patients with chronic myeloid leukemia in chronic phase. *J Clin Oncol* 2009;**27**(25):4204–10.

49. Hughes TP, Branford S. Measuring minimal residual disease in chronic myeloid leukemia: fluorescence in situ hybridization and polymerase chain reaction. *Clin Lymphoma Myeloma* 2009;**9**(Suppl. 3):S266–71.

50. Giles FJ, DeAngelo DJ, Baccarani M *et al*. Optimizing outcomes for patients with advanced disease in chronic myelogenous leukemia. *Semin Oncol* 2008;**35**(1 Suppl. 1):S1–17.

51. Grimwade D. The pathogenesis of acute promyelocytic leukaemia: Evaluation of the role of molecular diagnosis and monitoring in the management of the disease. *Br J Haematol* 1999;**106**:591–613.

52. Grimwade D, Lo-Coco F. Acute promyelocytic leukemia: a model for the role of molecular diagnosis and residual disease monitoring in directing treatment

approach in acute myeloid leukemia. *Leukemia* 2002;**16**(10):1959–73.

53. Sanz MA, Grimwade D, Tallman MS *et al.* Guidelines on the management of acute promyelocytic leukemia: Recommendations from an expert panel on behalf of the European LeukemiaNet. *Blood* 2008;**113**:1875–91.

54. Testi AM, Biondi A, Lo-Coco F *et al.* GIMEMA-AIEOPAIDA protocol for the treatment of newly diagnosed acute promyelocytic leukemia (APL) in children. *Blood* 2005;**106**(2):447–53.

55. Diverio D, Rossi V, Avvisati G *et al.* Early detection of relapse by prospective reverse transcriptase-polymerase chain reaction analysis of the *PML/RARalpha* fusion gene in patients with acute promyelocytic leukemia enrolled in the GIMEMA-AIEOP multicenter "AIDA" trial. GIMEMA-AIEOP Multicenter "AIDA" Trial. *Blood* 1998;**92**(3):784–9.

56. Golub TR, Slonim DK, Tamayo P *et al.* Molecular classification of cancer: class discovery and class prediction by gene expression monitoring. *Science* 1999;**286**(5439):531–7.

57. Haferlach T, Kohlmann A, Wieczorek L *et al.* The clinical utility of microarray-based gene expression profiling in the diagnosis and sub-classification of leukemia: report on 3248 cases from the international MILE study group. *J Clin Oncol* in press.

58. Goswami RS, Sukhai MA, Thomas M, Reis PP, Kamel-Reid S. Applications of microarray technology to acute myelogenous leukemia. *Cancer Inform* 2009;**7**:13–28.

59. Bullinger L, Dohner K, Bair E *et al.* Use of gene-expression profiling to identify prognostic subclasses in adult acute myeloid leukemia. *New Engl J Med* 2004;**350**(16):1605–16.

60. Valk PJ, Delwel R, Lowenberg B. Gene expression profiling in acute myeloid leukemia. *Curr Opin Hematol* 2005;**12**(1):76–81.

61. Mills KI, Kohlmann A, Williams PM *et al.* Microarray-based classifiers and prognosis models identify subgroups with distinct clinical outcomes and high risk of AML transformation of myelodysplastic syndrome (MDS). *Blood* 2009;**114**:1063–72.

62. Willman CL. Has gene expression profiling improved diagnosis, classification, and outcome prediction in AML? *Best Pract Res Clin Haematol* 2008;**21**(1):21–8.

63. Park MH, Cho SA, Yoo KH *et al.* Gene expression profile related to prognosis of acute myeloid leukemia. *Oncol Rep* 2007;**18**(6):1395–402.

64. Dunphy CH. Gene expression profiling data in lymphoma and leukemia: review of the literature and extrapolation of pertinent clinical applications. *Arch Pathol Lab Med* 2006;**130**(4):483–520.

65. Bullinger L, Valk PJ. Gene expression profiling in acute myeloid leukemia. *J Clin Oncol* 2005;**23**(26):6296–305.

66. Orr MS, Scherf U. Large-scale gene expression analysis in molecular target discovery. *Leukemia* 2002;**16**(4):473–7.

67. Chen Z, Li J, Wei L. A multiple kernel support vector machine scheme for feature selection and rule extraction from gene expression data of cancer tissue. *Artif Intell Med* 2007;**41**(2):161–75.

68. Lee Y, Lee CK. Classification of multiple cancer types by multicategory support vector machines using gene expression data. *Bioinformatics* 2003;**19**(9):1132–9.

69. Andreopoulos B, An A, Wang X, Schroeder M. A roadmap of clustering algorithms: finding a match for a biomedical application. *Brief Bioinform* 2009;**10**(3):297–314.

70. Do JH, Choi DK. Clustering approaches to identifying gene expression patterns from DNA microarray data. *Mol Cells* 2008;**25**(2):279–88.

71. Liu W, Yuan K, Ye D. Reducing microarray data via nonnegative matrix factorization for visualization and clustering analysis. *J Biomed Inform* 2008;**41**(4):602–6.

72. Liu Z, Chen D, Bensmail H, Xu Y. Clustering gene expression data with kernel principal components. *J Bioinform Comput Biol* 2005;**3**(2):303–16.

73. Komura D, Nakamura H, Tsutsumi S, Aburatani H, Ihara S. Multidimensional support vector machines for visualization of gene expression data. *Bioinformatics* 2005;**21**(4):439–44.

74. Bicciato S, Luchini A, Di Bello C. Marker identification and classification of cancer types using gene expression data and SIMCA. *Methods Inf Med* 2004;**43**(1):4–8.

75. Valk PJ, Verhaak RG, Beijen MA *et al.* Prognostically useful gene-expression profiles in acute myeloid leukemia. *New Engl J Med* 2004;**350**(16):1617–28.

76. Baldus CD, Bullinger L. Gene expression with prognostic implications in cytogenetically normal acute myeloid leukemia. *Semin Oncol* 2008;**35**(4):356–64.

77. Sridhar K, Ross DT, Tibshirani R, Butte AJ, Greenberg PL. Relationship of differential gene expression profiles in CD34+ myelodysplastic syndrome marrow cells to disease subtype and progression. *Blood* 2009;**114**(23):4847–58.

6

The integrated approach to the diagnosis of hematological malignancies

Mike A. Scott and Wendy N. Erber

The preceding chapters have illustrated that the analysis of hematological malignancies utilizes a range of cellular and genetic techniques of increasing sophistication and sensitivity. These generate bio-information of greater complexity than ever before, thereby requiring extensive data interpretation and integration. Only when the results of all test parameters are viewed together can the data facilitate an accurate and timely diagnosis, give prognostic indices, and be useful for monitoring treatment and/or disease progression. This approach necessitates a centralized laboratory facility staffed with a multi-skilled medical and scientific workforce focused on hemato-oncology diagnostics. They must be capable of carrying out a wide repertoire of diagnostic investigations and have the ability to interpret the data. This integrated approach to hemato-oncology diagnostics has proven advantages for clinicians and their patients. These comprehensive diagnostic centers are now being established in a number of countries. This chapter describes the structure of and role for integrated hemato-oncology diagnostic services.

What is an integrated hemato-oncology diagnostic service?

An integrated hematological malignancy (or hemato-oncology) diagnostic service is a comprehensive diagnostic facility for the processing and analysis of pathology samples from patients with, or suspected of having, a hematological neoplasm (Figure 6.1). Multiple test modalities are completed on a single sample, the results integrated and interpreted within the clinical context, a single report generated, and the information communicated to the requesting clinician. The concept is of *"one patient, one diagnosis, one report"* and this is only achievable with a multi-disciplinary laboratory

performing all the relevant and up-to-date investigations. Many of these are investigations that would previously have been performed in different departments or disciplines of pathology. The integrated approach places the emphasis on achieving the most accurate diagnosis and because of the range of testing it crosses traditional boundaries between pathology disciplines. A laboratory of this type should provide the highest quality, most cost-effective, modern and efficient diagnostic service for as many patients as possible.

A comprehensive hemato-oncology laboratory should be able to provide as extensive a test repertoire as possible (as detailed below) in order to meet the diagnostic requirements of the WHO classification [1]. A truly integrated diagnostic service should have all testing facilities in one location, i.e. morphology, phenotyping and genetic analyses, and ideally should be co-located within the same laboratory. This facilitates sample triage, determination of testing strategy, discussion and integration of results and clinical interpretation to reach a WHO diagnosis. It also maximizes efficiency by streamlining and prioritizing investigations, avoids unnecessary duplication and minimizes turn-around time. These and other advantages of such a comprehensive integrated environment are listed in Table 6.1.

The laboratory should be staffed by scientific and medical personnel (hematologists, hemato-pathologists and/or histopathologists) with significant knowledge of the biology and genetics of hematological malignancies and extensive experience in diagnostic methodology. They require appropriate expertise, a range of skills and a flexible and readily adaptive approach to scientific advance. They should have a working understanding of the laboratory processes and the need to integrate data in order to reach a diagnosis. The laboratory personnel need to have regular discussions to determine protocols, including which tests to perform,

Diagnostic Techniques in Hematological Malignancies, ed. Wendy N. Erber. Published by Cambridge University Press.
© Cambridge University Press 2010.

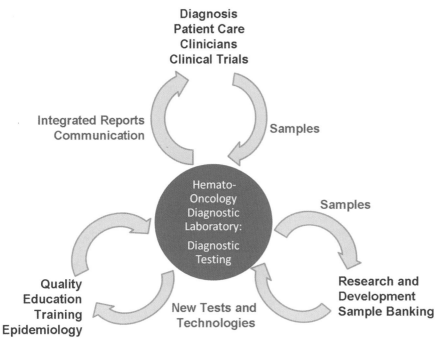

Figure 6.1. Structure of an integrated diagnostic service.

when they should be used and on which samples. Furthermore, they need to be flexible to clinical needs, be able to prioritize urgent samples and to understand that one result may be of greater importance than another in a given situation. They must also be capable of adopting new technologies and, of equal importance, replacing out-dated tests when required.

Why do we need integrated hemato-oncology diagnostic services?

Over the past decade there have been a number of significant clinical and scientific developments in hemato-oncology which have contributed to the need for integrated diagnostic laboratories. These, which will be discussed below, include:

1. Scientific advances.
2. The *WHO Classification of Tumours of Haematopoietic and Lymphoid Tissues.*
3. Modernization of clinical hemato-oncology practice.
4. Guidelines and regulations.

Scientific advances

Until the 1980s, the diagnosis of hematological malignancies relied largely on morphological assessment and cytochemistry. There was limited use of polyclonal antibodies and immunocytochemistry and cytogenetics was in its infancy. The introduction of monoclonal antibodies in the 1980s signaled the birth of a new era in diagnostic hematopathology. Cell immunology using immunocytochemistry and flow cytometry, as described in Chapters 2 and 3 respectively, has subsequently revolutionized many aspects of the diagnosis of hematological malignancies. These technologies have become essential additions to the diagnostic armamentarium. Most recently this has involved the development of highly sensitive multi-parameter flow cytometry that enables simultaneous evaluation of eight or more surface and intra-cellular molecules at the single cell level. This powerful and sophisticated technology is amenable to clinical analysis and residual disease monitoring of neoplastic hematopoietic cells. This requires significant technical expertise, standardization of testing strategies and bioinformatic analysis to enable efficient data interpretation for clinical use [2,3]. Immunocytochemistry has also evolved and has become routine in the analysis of bone marrow biopsies. Standardized methodologies and automation of testing and interpretation are becoming essential as clinical decisions are made on the basis of results generated.

Table 6.1 Advantages and activities of hemato-oncology diagnostic services.

Regional diagnostic center of excellence

Diagnostic standardization

Uniform approaches to disease monitoring

Amalgamation of results of all test parameters

Single integrated report with full interpretation and WHO classification

Improved communication between pathologists and clinicians

Improved clinical care

Potential for personalized medicine and appropriate targeted therapies

Rapid response to scientific and technical developments

Database of cases

Audit of laboratory data

Prioritization of testing, efficient and reduced turn-around-time

Retrospective case review

Epidemiological studies

Sample banking

Participation in research and development

Close ties with multiple clinical service units, and national trials

Center of expertise for teaching and training

Equity of patient access

Supports clinical excellence

There have also been major and perhaps even more significant advances in the field of genetics. New genetic abnormalities of clinical significance have been discovered, some of which are of key importance in defining specific hematological malignancies or in providing prognostic information. For example:

1. Recurrent genetic translocations associated with specific malignancies, e.g. acute myeloid leukemias and some types of lymphoma.
2. Rearrangements within the immunoglobulin and T-cell receptor genes enabling lymphoid cell clonality to be demonstrated at the genetic level [4].
3. Point mutations, e.g. *JAK2*, *MPL* and *TET2* mutations in myeloproliferative neoplasms [5–7]; *FLT3*, *NPM1* and *CEBPA* mutations in some types of acute myeloid leukemia [8].

4. IgV_H mutation status and prognosis in chronic lymphocytic leukemia.

New genetic techniques have also been developed, e.g. FISH, PCR, RT-PCR, aCGH, gene expression analysis, which have been described in detail in Chapters 4 and 5. Many of these are now performed as standard at diagnosis, for prognosis and follow-up of sequential samples in disease monitoring. The provision of these complex and rapidly changing tests is best served by a centralized specialist diagnostic unit, thus enabling the most appropriate tests to be performed and at the correct timing during and following therapy.

With the increasing number of test options available, it is neither technically feasible nor cost-effective for the above-mentioned, clinically important, complicated and expensive analyses to be performed in all routine laboratories. This is one of the main drivers behind the development of integrated hemato-oncology diagnostic services. Comprehensive laboratories are better placed to be able to provide these new technologies for a large patient cohort covering a number of referral institutions within a geographical area.

WHO Classification of Tumours of Haematopoietic and Lymphoid Tissues

The adoption of the WHO classification of hematopoietic neoplasms in 2001, and the subsequent revision in 2008, has had a major effect on diagnostic hemato-oncology practice [1]. The classification has emphasized the importance of a multi-parameter approach incorporating clinical and diagnostic information to define disease entities. The role and validity of the classification has been demonstrated as follows:

1. Use in international studies to standardize diagnostic criteria.
2. Its reproducibility has been shown to enhance the interpretation of clinical studies [9].
3. Introduced the concept of pathologic predictors of therapeutic response and outcome.
4. Demonstrated importance in prognostic prediction.
5. Diagnostic hematologists and hematopathologists, clinical hematologists, physicians and oncologists use the same terminology for hematological malignancies.

Overall the WHO classification has been highly beneficial and resulted in diagnostic services and clinicians communicating using the same "language." However, to be able to use the WHO classification efficiently and achieve its aims, all clinical information and laboratory results (morphology, phenotype and genetics) must be amalgamated; this is best achieved in an integrated testing environment.

Modern clinical hemato-oncology practice

Modern clinical hemato-oncology practice uses intensive therapeutic regimens, targeted therapies and transplantation. These modern treatment strategies place increasing and new demands on diagnostic laboratories. Clinicians require ever more detailed information regarding a disease and its clinical status, e.g. the ability to identify "molecular remission" and early "molecular relapse" for some disorders. To detect these early warnings of impending relapse requires highly sensitive molecular monitoring. This form of disease monitoring provides a sensitive indicator of the need to commence pre-emptive therapy, a strategy adopted for acute promyelocytic leukemia and chronic myeloid leukemia (see Chapters 8 and 13, respectively). This illustrates why diagnostic laboratories require a complete range of highly sensitive tests in their repertoire to support the increasingly sophisticated and patient-oriented therapeutic strategies. Information that clinicians now seek from the diagnostic service includes:

1. A precise diagnosis and WHO classification.
2. Identification of morphologic, phenotypic or genetic markers associated with prognosis.
3. Knowledge of potential therapeutic targets.
4. Regular monitoring for low-level residual disease, including molecular remission, and with increasing sensitivity.
5. Results of diagnostic tests to be generated in a timely fashion.
6. Data interpretation within the clinical context.
7. Single integrated diagnostic report.
8. Communication with clinicians.
9. Participation in clinical meetings.

National guidelines and regulations

Some countries are now supporting, recommending or legislating that diagnostic services for hematological malignancies be centralized [10]. The aims of these national initiatives have included, but are not restricted to:

1. Providing diagnostic excellence to as large a patient population as possible.
2. Rationalizing complex testing.
3. Addressing concerns of inter-observer variability in morphology.
4. Standardization of methodology.
5. Addressing the lack of quality control in diagnostic testing.
6. Ensuring equity of patient access.
7. Improving quality of patient care.

In the UK, regional hemato-oncology diagnostic services have been established in a number of major centers. These serve geographical regions with populations of 3–4 million and between 10 and 20 referring clinical hematology units [10,11]. The guidelines in the UK have stipulated that these services have appropriately qualified medical and scientific staff and apply a range of diagnostic tests to establish accurate and precise diagnoses of hematological malignancies. Results must be integrated and interpreted by experts who work together with the referring clinical hematologists and care teams. Different models have been established in other countries. In Germany, for example, a national 'Acute and Chronic Leukemias' competence network has been developed. The network, which comprises over 300 centers, works towards standardization of diagnostic procedures in leukemia [12]. Initiatives are also in place to further integrate all major regional diagnostic groups to achieve greater standardization of testing and disease monitoring.

How does an integrated hemato-oncology diagnostic service work?

An integrated hemato-oncology diagnostic service has many functions (Figure 6.1). These include:

1. Specimen analysis: from sample reception and testing to a completed report being issued to the referring clinician.
2. Education and training.
3. Research and development.
4. Participation in clinico-pathological conferences.
5. Maintenance of data via dedicated information technology systems.

These roles have grown, and will continue to evolve due primarily to the introduction of new scientific and technological advances which will further advance our understanding of malignant hematological disorders. A description follows of the practical aspects of an integrated service illustrating the concept of *"one patient, one diagnosis, one report."*

Sample receipt, triage and analysis

Specimens received in the laboratory (by courier or post) are initially assessed for:

1. Patient demographics.
2. Clinical information, specifically the provisional diagnosis.
3. Stage of disease (diagnosis or follow-up).
4. Sample type (i.e. blood, bone marrow aspirate, bone marrow trephine, lymph node).
5. Tests requested.

The sample will first be assessed for its integrity and registered in the laboratory computer system. An initial morphology screen ("specimen triage") of an appropriately stained sample should then be performed to give a rapid "working diagnosis," determine the most appropriate diagnostic pathway to follow and define the range of investigations required (Figure 6.2). The sample may need to be aliquoted to provide material for all the necessary tests. Sample information, including the tests being undertaken,

should be entered into the computer; this data entry is crucial for sample tracking.

Testing protocols, or diagnostic pathways, should be developed by the laboratory in collaboration with referring hematologists. These should be based on WHO diagnostic criteria and published literature. These should be adopted as standardized testing strategies. They incorporate multiple test modalities (see below) and will assist in ensuring reproducibility, avoid unnecessary test duplication and be of value for case comparisons and audit. Different pathways may need to be developed for diagnostic and follow-up samples as the information required differs. An illustrative example of a diagnostic pathway for a newly presenting case of acute leukemia is shown in Figure 6.3. This pathway can be used as a template for other malignancies with modifications and exclusions as required. For example, flow cytometry is generally not required in the investigation of myeloproliferative neoplasms.

The diagnostic sample

The first sample received on a patient (the "diagnostic sample") should have as complete a multi-parameter diagnostic work-up as possible. This initial evaluation is to obtain maximal cellular and genetic information about the disease. This gives a "biological baseline" from which clinical, therapeutic and disease monitoring decisions will be made. Thorough primary testing using multiple test modalities is valid:

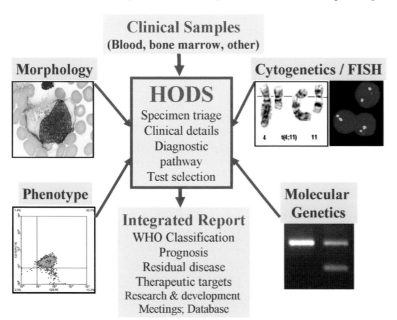

Figure 6.2. Schematic diagram illustrating the functioning of an integrated hemato-oncology diagnostic laboratory. HODS: Hemato-Oncology Diagnostic Service.

115

1. To ensure an accurate diagnosis and classification according to WHO criteria.
2. To identify phenotypic or genotypic markers of prognosis.
3. To identify potential therapeutic targets, e.g. CD20 expression in B-cell malignancies.
4. To identify the most appropriate and sensitive disease-associated marker to use for therapeutic monitoring.
5. Multiple confirmatory tests provide a form of internal quality assurance.

All test types will be reported and a final integrated report should be prepared on completion of all diagnostic testing on this primary sample. The final report includes results of all test modalities and the final WHO diagnosis (see below). This will require incorporating and comparing results of all tests that may detect the same abnormality (e.g. karyotype, FISH and RT-PCR in the diagnosis of chronic myeloid leukemia). Results of prognostic significance should also be incorporated in the report and conveyed to the clinician. The prognostic information may be:

1. A single piece of genetic or phenotypic information, e.g. the presence of a *FLT3* ITD in acute myeloid leukemia; ploidy in B lymphoblastic leukemia/lymphoma.
2. Multiple genetic defects, such as complex karyotypes in myelodysplasia.

3. An amalgamation of phenotypic and genetic results. Table 6.2 gives an example of prognostic indicators available for chronic lymphocytic leukemia (see also Chapter 9).

Table 6.2. Poor prognostic indicators in chronic lymphocytic leukemia.

Clinico-hematologic parameter	Prognostic characteristic
Hematological and biochemical	Anemia and/or thrombocytopenia Lymphocyte doubling time Organomegaly β2-microglobulin Lactate dehydrogenase
Lymphocyte morphology	Atypical morphological features
Bone marrow trephine biopsy histology	Diffuse marrow infiltration
Cell phenotype	CD20 antigen intensity CD38 expression ZAP-70 expression CD49d expression
Genetic abnormalities	*TP53* mutations del17p *ATM* mutations Genetic complexity Clonal evolution Short telomere length
Immunoglobulin analysis	Unmutated IgV$_H$ IgV$_H$3–21 gene usage B-cell receptor stereotype

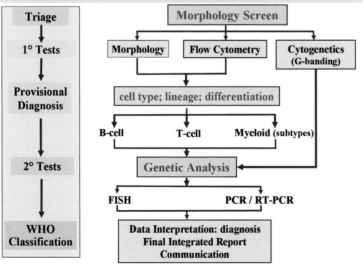

Diagnostic Pathway Testing Strategy: Acute Leukaemia

Triage → 1° Tests → Provisional Diagnosis → 2° Tests → WHO Classification

Morphology Screen → Morphology, Flow Cytometry, Cytogenetics (G-banding)

cell type; lineage; differentiation

B-cell, T-cell, Myeloid (subtypes)

Genetic Analysis

FISH, PCR / RT-PCR

Data Interpretation: diagnosis Final Integrated Report Communication

Figure 6.3. Example of a diagnostic pathway for acute leukemia testing.

Follow-up and disease monitoring

An increasingly important role of the integrated laboratory is disease monitoring on sequential follow-up samples. This is to determine whether there is evidence of:

1. Complete remission, i.e. no evidence of disease by standard criteria, e.g. < 5% morphologically detectable blast cells in acute leukemia.
2. Minimal residual disease, i.e. persistence of small numbers of malignant cells following therapy which are undetectable by conventional methods.

The importance of this has increased due to new therapies which have the potential to cure and because of the instigation of, or changes to, therapy once low-level residual disease is detected. The tests to be performed during and after completion of therapy will be based on the knowledge of the disease as determined at diagnosis, together with knowledge of the sensitivities of each test modality (Table 6.3). This tailored approach minimizes unnecessary testing and maximizes the quality of information available to the clinician. The most appropriate test or tests to perform will therefore be determined by:

1. Sample type, i.e. blood, bone marrow aspirate or bone marrow trephine.
2. Knowledge of the cellular and genetic features of the disease that can be used to distinguish neoplastic cells from normal hematopoietic cells.

3. Required sensitivity of detection; levels of less than 0.01% may be required in some disorders.
4. The clinical urgency.

Figure 6.4 illustrates a case of acute myeloid leukemia showing the difference in sensitivities between morphology, cytogenetics and molecular genetics in monitoring the therapeutic response. This highlights the relative lack of sensitivity of morphology and FISH for the assessment of "complete remission" compared with molecular monitoring using RT-PCR.

Internationally standardized treatment response criteria have been devised for some malignancies. These commonly include clinical, biochemical and radiological parameters together with cellular (morphologic, phenotypic and/or genetic) features. This is illustrated by the disease response criteria for essential thrombocythemia, which are based on clinical, morphological and molecular characteristics (Table 6.4) [13]. Response criteria for plasma cell myeloma are also defined by a combination of features, i.e. morphology ($\leq$ 5% plasma cells), immunophenotyping (absence of clonal plasma cells), paraprotein and serum free light chain levels and disappearance of plasmacytomas [14,15]. As response assessment for many malignancies requires integration of multiple pieces of data together with clinical information, discrepancies can occur and these must be resolved. Discrepant results may be due to sampling differences, different sensitivities of the methods used and/or different interpretations.

Table 6.3. Test sensitivity for disease monitoring.

Test type	Features	Sensitivity
Morphology	Distinct light microscopic cell appearances Disease specific Abnormal topography on bone marrow trephine biopsy	0.1–3%
Immunophenotype Flow cytometry Immunocytochemistry	Cellular antigen expression Disease-associated phenotype Localized antigen-positive cells in the bone marrow trephine	0.01–1%
Karyotype (G-banding)	To detect chromosome structure Labor intensive and poor sensitivity Requires a genetic marker of disease Good specificity	1–5%
Fluorescence *in situ* hybridization	Requires a genetic marker of disease Labor intensive Increased sensitivity when combined with phenotypic cell identification (FICTION)	0.1–3%
PCR, RT-PCR and real-time quantitative PCR	Requires a genetic marker of disease Sensitive	0.0001–0.01%

Table 6.4. International criteria for residual disease and treatment response for essential thrombocythemia [13].

Response definitions	Complete response	Partial response	No response
Clinical/hematologic response	No disease-related symptoms, and Normal spleen size on imaging, and Platelet count ≤ 400 × 10⁹/L, and Leukocyte count ≤ 10 × 10⁹/L	Do not fulfill complete response criteria, platelet count ≤ 600 × 10⁹/L or > 50% decrease from baseline	Any response that does not meet partial response criteria
Molecular response (only applied if the baseline mutant allele burden is > 10%)	Reduction of any molecular abnormality (e.g. *JAK2*; *MPL*) to undetectable levels	1. A ≥ 50% reduction from baseline in patients with < 50% mutant allele burden at baseline, or 2. Reduction of ≥ 25% from baseline in patients with > 50% mutant allele burden at baseline	Any response that does not meet partial response criteria
Bone marrow histological response	Bone marrow histologic remission Absence of megakaryocytic hyperplasia		

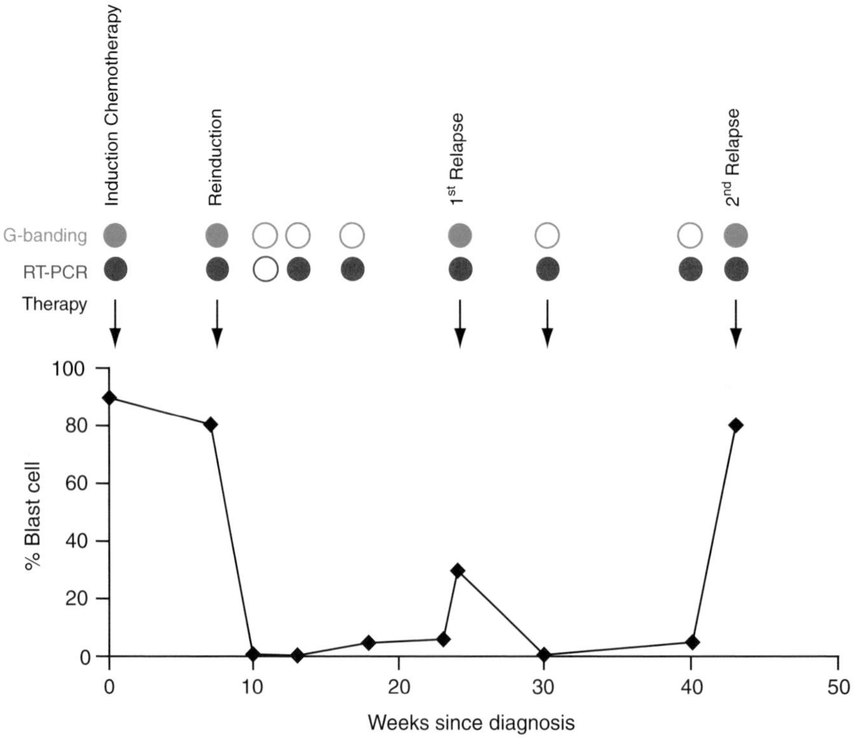

Figure 6.4. A case of acute myeloid leukemia with translocation t(8;16)(p11:p13); *MOZ-CBP*. This demonstrates the difference in sensitivity of morphology, cytogenetics (green) and RT-PCR (red) for disease monitoring (open circles indicate negative and closed circles a positive result).

Resolution will generally require discussion with the treating clinician and may require the "worst" result to be adopted [16]. These issues highlight the importance of clinical input in result interpretation in residual disease analysis. Clinical status of the patient in addition to knowledge of the therapy administered and its timing, as well as biochemical and radiological data are essential [16]. The clinical chapters that follow will describe in detail the optimal methods for monitoring individual diseases.

Requirements for an integrated hemato-oncology diagnostic service

An integrated hemato-oncology laboratory must be able to provide excellence in morphology, together with state-of-the-art immunocytochemistry, flow cytometry, cytogenetic and molecular genetic analyses. Ideally this should be for both primary hematological samples, i.e. blood and bone marrow, and relevant tissue biopsy specimens such as lymph nodes [10]. In practice, it may not always be feasible to include tissue biopsies due to internal arrangements within institutions. The components of an integrated laboratory are described.

Morphology

Morphological assessment of the blood, bone marrow and other diagnostic material (e.g. body fluids, tissue biopsies) remains the cornerstone for the diagnosis of the majority of hematological malignancies. Expertise in the light-microscopic appearances of the range of hematological malignancies is therefore essential. For some malignancies the morphology may be diagnostic and supplementary investigations are confirmatory. For others, the morphological appearances together with the clinical information will be the "screen" to determine the pathway to follow and the range of ancillary tests required to classify the malignancy. Morphology is also used for disease monitoring and may suffice in some situations where:

1. The neoplastic cell has a distinct appearance, or
2. The cell phenotype is not distinct and there is no genetic marker of the disease.

For example, acute myeloid leukemia which has a normal karyotype and no specific leukemia-associated phenotype but the cells have a distinct morphological appearance. The presence of < 5% blast cells would define "morphological complete remission" [17].

Phenotyping

Cellular immunology is a key component in the assessment of hematological malignancies. Flow cytometry, in particular, is one of the most important test modalities of a centralized integrated facility. This is because of its wide applicability to cellular samples and speed resulting in rapid turn-around. Immunocytochemistry, performed on cell smears or tissue biopsy specimens, is also critical. This adds the dimension of

morphological identification of the abnormal cells and simultaneous identification of the cell phenotype in routinely processed material, and especially, bone marrow trephine biopsies (see Chapter 2). A central referral laboratory must therefore be able to offer:

1. Multi-parameter flow cytometry (minimum four-color analysis) (see Chapter 3).
2. Automated immuno-enzyme staining techniques, including double labeling, suitable for smears and fixed tissue biopsies (see Chapter 2).
3. Immunofluorescent microscopy, specifically to detect abnormal PML protein (see Chapter 2).
4. Use of an extensive range of antibodies, sufficient to meet the diagnostic criteria for common and rare diagnoses, and to detect antigens of prognostic importance and targets of immunotherapy.
5. The potential to combine immunofluorescence and fluorescence *in situ* hybridization (FISH) in order to detect relevant genetic abnormalities by FICTION (see Chapters 2 and 4) [17,18].

Flow cytometry and immunocytochemistry can both be useful for disease monitoring if the neoplastic cells have a disease-associated phenotype that enables them to be distinguished from normal cells. Examples include:

1. *T lymphoblastic leukemia/lymphoma*: TdT/ cytoplasmic CD3 dual-positive cells in blood or bone marrow (see Chapter 7).
2. *Hairy cell leukemia*: CD11c/CD103/T-bet-positive light chain-restricted B-cells in blood or bone marrow [19,20] (see Chapter 9).
3. *Angioimmunoblastic T-cell lymphoma*: CD10-positive T-cells (see Chapter 11) [21].
4. *Chronic lymphocytic leukemia*: CD5-positive light chain-restricted B-cells with weak CD22 and CD81 expression [22] (see Chapter 9).

Highly skilled scientific personnel are required with the ability to perform, interpret and understand the limitations of multi-parameter flow cytometry. This is particularly the case for modern flow cytometry, which, with its increasing complexity (> four-color analyses), requires standardization of antibody panels, fluorochromes and data analysis [3]. There is an increasing number of validated antibodies and an ever-expanding repertoire of phenotyping applications, the technology is becoming more sophisticated and data interpretation more complex.

Because of these complexities, uniform flow cytometric strategies are being developed and standardized (e.g. EuroFlow Consortium) should be used [2,23].

Cytogenetics

As discussed in Chapter 4, the detection of chromosomal abnormalities is an essential element in the multimodal assessment of hematological malignancies and should be included in an integrated diagnostic laboratory. For some disorders genetic abnormalities are the key defining feature. For others, genetic alterations may be closely associated with a clinical entity and their detection may prove useful to confirm a diagnosis and for disease monitoring. Decisions about the need for cytogenetic analysis usually follow preliminary morphological assessment. In some situations the optimal genetic analysis (i.e. which test and/or which FISH probes) will also be guided by results of cell phenotyping (specifically knowledge of the cell lineage and stage of differentiation). Scientific expertise is required, particularly for conventional karyotyping of metaphases (the "gold standard") but also for FISH, which is increasingly being utilized to pin-point specific chromosomal abnormalities. Since FISH can be performed both on metaphase spreads and routine hematological specimens (cell smears and paraffin-embedded tissue sections), and takes only 2–3 days to perform, its role is increasing. FISH can be used to target specific genetic lesions, e.g. *PML-RARA* of t(15;17) in acute promyelocytic leukemia or 11q23 abnormalities in *MLL* leukemias, and thereby provides early and rapid diagnostic genetic information. Other examples where the early demonstration of specific genetic abnormalities may be important for instigation of therapy include:

1. Demonstration of t(9;22); *BCR-ABL1* in an unexplained neutrophilia, thereby confirming the diagnosis of chronic myelogenous leukemia.
2. Identification of del(17p) in chronic lymphocytic leukemia and its association with a poor prognosis.

Cytogenetics can also be applied for disease monitoring but with relatively low sensitivity. Conventional karyotyping is generally regarded as being insufficiently sensitive (1–5%), but in some situations may be the only objective measure of disease. FISH, with sensitivities of 0.1–3% neoplastic cells, can be used to target specific known disease-associated genetic aberrations. FICTION, or combined immunophenotyping and FISH, can increase the sensitivity of detection as only cells of known phenotype will be analyzed for the genetic defect [18].

Genetic testing of hematological malignancies is a rapidly evolving field. Regional or centralized services should have the flexibility and skill to integrate new, complex and expensive technologies and applications, such as multicolor FISH, spectral karyotyping, comparative genomic hybridization and array-based whole genome analysis screening into their test repertoire [24].

Molecular genetics

As described in Chapter 5, molecular genetic analysis provides sensitive technology for the detection and quantitation of molecular abnormalities for diagnosis, prognosis and residual disease monitoring over a range of hematological malignancies. Testing for the molecular consequence of acquired genetic change is the most rapidly evolving area of diagnostics in hematopathology. As for cytogenetics, the decisions as to which molecular tests should be performed at diagnosis are based on the results of other investigations, primarily morphology and phenotyping. Molecular tests generally complement and add value to the results obtained by conventional karyotyping and FISH; however, because of their increased sensitivity, they are of particular value in disease monitoring [25,26]. Whether a particular neoplasm can be monitored by molecular techniques will generally have been determined by the baseline molecular genetic work-up at diagnosis. This highlights the importance of a thorough assessment at diagnosis as PCR-based techniques (e.g. PCR, RT-PCR, quantitative RT-PCR) can only be used to detect a subset of molecular abnormalities that occur in hematological malignancies. For this reason it is important to know that a genetic abnormality can be detected in the malignant cells in a specific patient at diagnosis and that the test in question can be used for disease monitoring.

Genetic rearrangements that can currently be detected using PCR include:

1. Fusion genes as a consequence of translocations and occasionally deletions.
2. Over-expression of oncogenes.
3. Point mutations which are cryptic by conventional cytogenetic methods.

Many of these changes carry prognostic significance and may be useful in guiding treatment aimed at controlling specific genetic defects, e.g. all-*trans* retinoic acid in APML and imatinib mesylate in CML, and determination of IgV_H mutational status in chronic lymphocytic leukemia.

The increased sensitivity of PCR and other novel quantitative assays permits detection of low levels of residual disease below the threshold detectable by morphological examination and cytogenetic analysis (Figure 6.4). This allows continued monitoring of patients and the opportunity to institute therapy prior to clinical relapse whilst the tumor burden is still relatively low. The most sensitive techniques in routine use are those that can detect defects at the molecular level. PCR, RT-PCR, quantitative PCR and sequencing can all be used if there is a known detectable abnormality, such as:

1. IG or T-cell receptor gene rearrangements in B- and T-lymphoid neoplasms.
2. Gene translocations, e.g. t(15;17); *PML-RARA*, t(14;18); *BCL2-IgH@*, t(9;22); *BCR-ABL1*.
3. Gene mutations, e.g. *NPM1* or *FLT3*.
4. Unique genetic sequences which can be detected using patient-specific primers, e.g. in B lymphoblastic leukemia/lymphoma.
5. Detection of tumor-specific DNA sequences.

Due to the complexity of the analyses, the range of tests and applications, the rapid changes in technology and the scientific expertise needed, molecular genetics is best served within a specialized centralized service. Standardized approaches to testing, including test selection, timing and utilization of international protocols (e.g. BIOMED-2) should be used [4]. The results of molecular tests must not be interpreted in isolation; they must always be interpreted together with other test modalities. Changes in technology, for example, multiplex PCR, large-scale mutation detection and gene expression profiling, are becoming available for routine diagnostics and will further improve the repertoire of diagnostic and prognostic information available to the clinical teams [27,28].

The integrated report

The integrated final report, an essential output of a hemato-oncology diagnostic service, should be generated on completion of all test modalities. This final report should be generated by the specialist hematologist or hematopathologist and provide the following information:

1. Summary of the results of all tests performed.
2. WHO classification.
3. Prognostic information.
4. Recommendations for further testing, as required.
5. Name of the reporting hematologist or hematopathologist.

Ideally the integrated report should support the inclusion of morphological and other images, e.g. karyotype, FISH, flow cytometry plots or PCR gels (see Figure 6.5 for an example of an integrated report for a case of acute myeloid leukemia). The report should be accessible electronically to referring clinicians via a secure web-based IT system (see below). This has the benefit of significantly enhancing the validity and efficiency of communication and is far superior to paper-based or standard laboratory information systems for dissemination of complex diagnostic information. All integrated reports should also be incorporated into a hemato-oncology database [29]. This is useful, not only for the individual patient (e.g. comparisons between presentation and relapse), but also for audit, epidemiological studies, teaching and research. It is important to remember that individual interim reports must also be issued as different test types take different times to complete. This ensures the clinician is kept up-to-date with all results as they become available.

Information technology

The laboratory must have a quality information technology (IT) system which meets the following requirements:

1. Permits electronic requesting and reporting.
2. Records sample receipt and specimen registration.
3. Allows full tracking of samples and tests.
4. Data and result entry with all diagnostic information incorporated into a single computer file.
5. Capable of generating a final integrated report.
6. Able to incorporate images.
7. Web-based access for referring clinicians to integrated reports on-line in host hospitals.
8. Able to be used to build a comprehensive searchable database or case-file system for follow-up, teaching, presentations, audit and research.

Figure 6.5. Example of an integrated hemato-oncology report.

The report image contains:

HAEMATO-ONCOLOGY DIAGNOSTIC REPORT

Demographics

Patient Name:	Other, Alison	Hospital Number:	10064921
D.O.B:	12.09.1964	Sample ID:	2009:HO21D1
Consultant:	Dr Y Street	Sample Date:	18.12.2009
Ward:	A7	Sample Time:	12:30

Clinical Details
? Acute leukaemia – blast cells present in peripheral blood.
Past history of carcinoma of the breast and chemotherapy.

Morphology
Peripheral Blood:
Hb 135g/L; WBC: 58 x 10^9/L; Platelets 73 x 10^9/L.
Blood film: Blast cells with monocytoid differentiation.

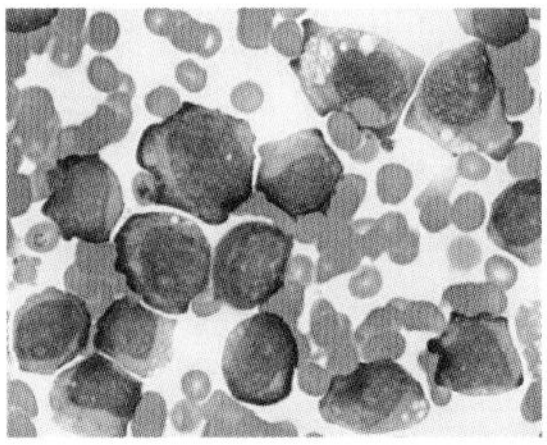

Bone Marrow Aspirate:
Site: Right posterior superior iliac crest.
Cellularity: Markedly hypercellular.
95% blast cells with minimal monocytoid differentiation and show erythrophagocytosis.
Acute monoblastic leukaemia

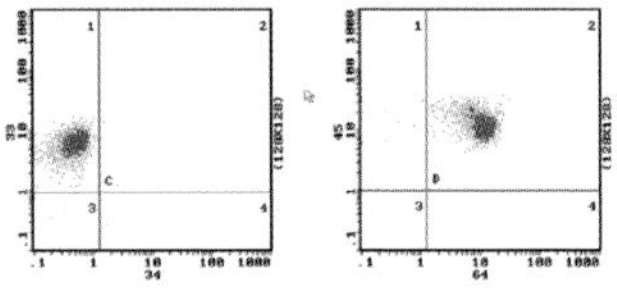

Bone Marrow Trephine:
Hypercellular marrow replaced by blast cells.
Phenotype: CD45, CD33 and lysozyme positive.
Marrow involvement by acute myeloid leukaemia with monocytoid differentiation.

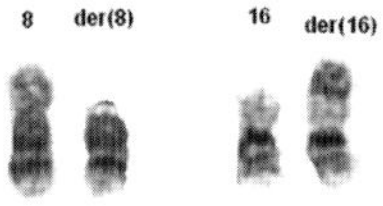

Flow Cytometry:
Positive: CD13, CD14, CD33, CD64.
Negative: CD34, CD117 and MPO.
Phenotype of acute myeloid leukaemia with monocytoid differentiation.

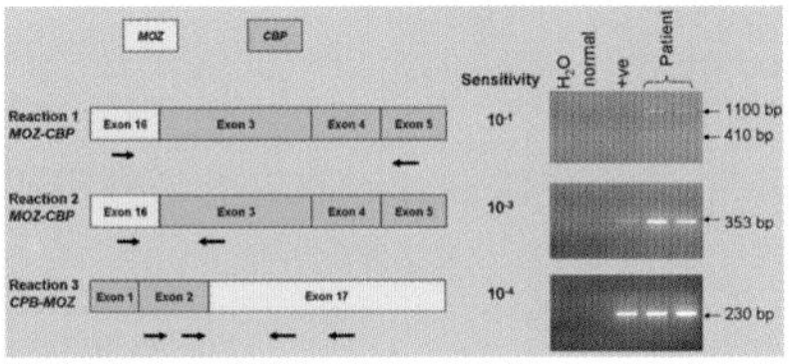

Cytogenetics:
46,XX,t(8;16)(p11.2;p13.3) [20]

Molecular Analysis:
MOZ-CBP and *CBP-MOZ* fusion transcripts detected by RT-PCR.

Summary and WHO Classification
Acute Monoblastic Leukaemia with t(8;16)(p11.2;p13.3)

This type of leukaemia is commonly secondary (therapy-related), associated with blast cells with erythrophagocytosis and has a poor prognosis.
Recommend residual disease monitoring by RT-PCR for *MOZ-CBP*

Authorised by:	Date:
Reported by:	Date:

9. Enable extraction of population-based epidemiological and statistical data.
10. Be secure, enabling access to results to be restricted to the specific referring clinician or institution and the laboratory.
11. Able to monitor workload and be used for service planning.

Communication with clinicians

Communication is critical to the success of this integrated approach. There must be excellent lines of communication between sections within the diagnostic laboratory and between the clinician and the diagnostic service. The diagnostic hematologist and laboratory personnel must be aware of the clinical situation of the patient, i.e. clinical details, stage of disease, clinical protocols and proposed management plan. The clinician also needs to understand the repertoire of tests available, the sample types required, the limitations and sensitivities of the tests. Results must be made available in a timely manner to meet clinical requirements and with appropriate interpretive comments. The diagnosis must be classified according to agreed standardized criteria with internationally accepted criteria being utilized wherever possible. For most entities this is likely to be based on the WHO classification; if another classification scheme is being applied, it must be clear to the referring clinicians which is being used. There should be regular clinico-pathological meetings of clinicians and diagnostic hematologists/hemato-pathologists to discuss and review clinical and diagnostic information (including morphological images, flow cytometry and genetic data). In the UK this is in the form of multidisciplinary team meetings [10]. These forums ensure that results for all patients are discussed in context and are used appropriately in clinical decision-making.

Other activities of a hemato-oncology diagnostic service

Quality assurance, audit and governance

A hemato-oncology diagnostic service, like any other pathology laboratory, must ensure the quality of its results and be able to demonstrate this to its stakeholders (i.e. clinician users, patients, funders). This should be done by regularly reviewing policies and procedures, testing strategies, equipment and laboratory structure to be confident that they are appropriate, up-to-date and in accordance with clinical requirements and national and/or international regulations. Participation in external quality assurance programmes is crucial due to the complexity of many of the analyses. This ensures that the results are accurate, reproducible and there is inter-laboratory comparability [30]. Internal quality also can be demonstrated by showing concordance of results obtained in the laboratory by different methods. For example:

1. *Acute promyelocytic leukemia*: morphology, phenotype, PML protein, FISH, karyotype and RT-PCR results should all be concordant.
2. *B-cell clonality*: results obtained by flow cytometry showing light chain restriction and immunoglobulin gene rearrangement by PCR should be concordant.
3. *Chronic myelogenous leukemia*: results of karyotyping, FISH and RT-PCR should all agree on the presence of t(9;22); *BCR-ABL1*.

Regular audits should be performed to assess the laboratory and its compliance with procedures. It provides a means to assess requesting practices, test utilization, workload and turn-around time. Clinical audit should also be performed to assess the disease

repertoire. Through this process, important new clinical data, such as epidemiological data, identification of rare entities or emergent diseases can be extracted and studied. Stakeholders should be provided with material detailing the range of services, samples required, anticipated turn-around times and any new developments or tests available. Governance issues should be monitored by the laboratory and reported to clinical users. Information that should be made available to stakeholders includes:

1. Number of requests.
2. Range of tests available.
3. Workload data for individual test types.
4. Turn-around-times to ensure clinical needs and guidelines are being adhered to.
5. External quality assurance results.
6. Accreditation status with national bodies (if appropriate).

Feedback from clinical users and other stakeholders to the laboratory is valuable; this can be constructive and help in maintaining quality and for service improvement. Users should therefore be encouraged to comment on the service in the form of complaints, compliments, recommendations for change (including new investigations), and suggested opportunities for service improvements.

Service improvement and technology development

An integrated diagnostic service needs the flexibility to allocate resources and the expertise to be able to modify practice, such as:

1. Responding rapidly to scientific advances.
2. Introducing new tests and new technologies.
3. Providing investigations for new applications.

Being a centralized service, any new tests developed will become available to a large number of patients in a short time period. The advantages of this were demonstrated with the rapid introduction and routine uptake of molecular genetic testing for *JAK2* and *MPL* mutations in the investigation of possible myeloproliferative neoplasms.

Research and development

A centralized hemato-oncology laboratory should be an active participant in research and development. This may be performed in isolation or in collaboration with academic centers or national bodies (e.g. clinical trials, technology development). Research should utilize the strengths of the diagnostic service and the availability of large numbers of clinical samples. Sample banking should be encouraged but is dependent on institutional ethical approval, compliance with national regulations, patient consent and a secure database. Samples that could be banked include purified neoplastic cells, specific cell subpopulations, cellular components, DNA, RNA, protein and plasma from a range of hematological disorders that would be amenable to translational research.

Staff, education and training

The integrated multi-disciplinary hemato-oncology laboratory must have a highly focused well-trained medical and scientific workforce. The staff must understand the benefits of integrated working and the rationale for working across traditional pathology boundaries. Education and staff training are important activities of a hemato-oncology diagnostic service. Integrated diagnostic centers are the ideal location for post-graduate medical and scientific training and sub-specialization. This is because of the highly qualified scientific and medical personnel with expertise in the pathology and investigation of clonal hematological disorders and the number and range of clinical cases available on which to teach and train. Education and training are therefore key functions and should be one of the strengths of the service.

Advantages of the integrated approach to hemato-oncology diagnostics

Regional multi-disciplinary centers for hemato-oncology diagnosis are the ideal model for the full assessment of hematological malignancies and compliance with the WHO classification. There are many advantages for patients and clinicians, primarily in quality (Table 6.1). This approach supports excellence in patient care, teaching and research and is cost-effective, patient-focused and efficient. It provides a critical mass of scientific and medical expertise which is available to a large number of patients, many of whom would not otherwise benefit from such proficiency. A significant benefit is therefore an equitable

Table 6.5. Requirements for a regional hemato-oncology diagnostic service.

Commitment from users and funders to centralize testing and integrate data

Regional cooperation and coordination

Medical and scientific expertise in hemato-oncology diagnosis

Transport systems for specimen delivery

Appropriate equipment and other technical resources

Financial support

Excellent communication with referring centers, including regular team meetings

Information technology systems and support for rapid provision of results

Commitment to education and training

service for patients, irrespective of their geographical location within a region. Inter-regional collaborations are more easily achieved and will support national and international networks. Centralized diagnostic facilities are better able to respond to new demands, be they clinical, scientific (e.g. introduction of new investigations), political or economic, and should be sustainable. However, the major gains are the ability to integrate results of all tests performed, generate a pathology report of clinical relevance and communicate information to clinicians. This is a patient-focused approach from which clinical benefits will inevitably follow.

There are a number of requirements that must be met for integrated services to be a success (Table 6.5). There must be a major commitment from clinician users, scientific staff and funders to centralize testing, and a guarantee that the information technology requirements will be met. Without these the clinical advantages will be difficult to achieve. There are economic implications with initial capital investment, staffing and ongoing running costs. However, this is offset by the clinical advantages, savings in critical mass and equity of access.

The extent of testing and ability to meet all WHO criteria may be dependent on the financial resources and medical and scientific skills available. It may not be possible, for example, to provide a complete test repertoire, specifically in resource-poor countries. It is already acknowledged that molecular techniques are not readily available in some jurisdictions due to restricted facilities, and, in others, advanced scientific technologies may be available without ready access to skilled personnel [31]. International networks and collaborations between large diagnostic facilities should be able to address some of these limitations.

Conclusion

Integrated hemato-oncology diagnostic testing and reporting ensures the most accurate diagnosis is achieved for as large a patient population as possible, in a timely and cost-effective manner. Such multi-disciplinary laboratories have proved their advantages for clinicians and their patients: they are efficient, generate accurate results, are scientifically robust and meet clinical needs and the WHO diagnostic requirements. They also give a platform to provide rapid responses to technological change and for service development. Integrated diagnostic laboratories should be the standard of care for the diagnosis of hematological malignancies.

References

1. Swerdlow SH, Campo E, Harris NL et al. (eds.). *WHO Classification of Tumours of Haematopoietic and Lymphoid Tissues*, 4th edn. Lyon: IARC; 2008.

2. Pedreira CE, Costa ES, Almeida J et al. A probabilistic approach for the evaluation of minimal residual disease by multiparameter flow cytometry in leukemic B-cell chronic lymphoproliferative disorders. *Cytometry A* 2008;**73A**(12):1141–50.

3. Pedreira CE, Costa ES, Barrena S et al. Generation of flow cytometry data files with a potentially infinite number of dimensions. *Cytometry A* 2008;**73** (9):834–46.

4. van Dongen JJ, Langerak AW, Bruggemann M et al. Design and standardization of PCR primers and protocols for detection of clonal immunoglobulin and T-cell receptor gene recombinations in suspect lymphoproliferations: report of the BIOMED-2 Concerted Action BMH4-CT98–3936. *Leukemia* 2003;**17**(12):2257–317.

5. Baxter EJ, Scott LM, Campbell PJ et al. Acquired mutation of the tyrosine kinase JAK2 in human myeloproliferative disorders. *Lancet* 2005;**365** (9464):1054–61.

6. James C, Ugo V, Le Couedic JP et al. A unique clonal JAK2 mutation leading to constitutive signalling causes polycythaemia vera. *Nature* 2005;**434**(7037):1144–8.

7. Delhommeau F, Dupont S, Della Valle V et al. Mutation in TET2 in myeloid cancers. *New Engl J Med* 2009;**360**(22):2289–301.

8. Falini B, Mecucci C, Tiacci E et al. Cytoplasmic nucleophosmin in acute myelogenous leukemia with a normal karyotype. *New Engl J Med* 2005;**352** (3):254–66.

9. Jaffe ES, Harris NL, Stein H, Isaacson PG. Classification of lymphoid neoplasms: the microscope as a tool for disease discovery. *Blood* 2008;**112** (12):4384–99.

10. Jack A. Organisation of neoplastic haematopathology services: a UK perspective. *Pathology* 2005;**37** (6):479–92.

11. Richards SJ, Jack AS. The development of integrated haematopathology laboratories: a new approach to the diagnosis of leukaemia and lymphoma. *Clin Lab Haematol* 2003;**25**(6):337–42.

12. Hehlmann R, Berger U, Aul C et al. The German competence network 'Acute and chronic leukemias'. *Leukemia* 2004;**18**(4):665–9.

13. Barosi G, Birgegard G, Finazzi G et al. Response criteria for essential thrombocythemia and polycythemia vera: result of a European LeukemiaNet consensus conference. *Blood* 2009;**113**(20):4829–33.

14. Durie BG, Harousseau JL, Miguel JS et al. International uniform response criteria for multiple myeloma. *Leukemia* 2006;**20**(9):1467–73.

15. Kyle RA, Rajkumar SV. Criteria for diagnosis, staging, risk stratification and response assessment of multiple myeloma. *Leukemia* 2009;**23**(1):3–9.

16. Dirnhofer S, Went P, Tichelli A. Diagnostic problems in follow-up bone marrow biopsies of patients treated for acute and chronic leukaemias and MDS. *Pathobiology* 2007;**74**:6.

17. de Greef GE, van Putten WL, Boogaerts M et al. Criteria for defining a complete remission in acute myeloid leukaemia revisited. An analysis of patients treated in HOVON-SAKK co-operative group studies. *Br J Haematol* 2005;**128**(2):184–91.

18. Fend F, Tzankov A, Bink K et al. Modern techniques for the diagnostic evaluation of the trephine bone marrow biopsy: methodological aspects and applications. *Prog Histochem Cytochem* 2008; **42**(4):203–52.

19. Johrens K, Stein H, Anagnostopoulos I. T-bet transcription factor detection facilitates the diagnosis of minimal hairy cell leukemia infiltrates in bone marrow trephines. *Am J Surg Pathol* 2007; **31**(8):1181–5.

20. Johrens K, Happerfield LC, Brown JP et al. A novel CD11c monoclonal antibody effective in formalin-fixed

tissue for the diagnosis of hairy cell leukemia. *Pathobiology* 2008;75(4):252–6.

21. Baseggio LBF, Morel D, Delfau-Larue MH *et al.* Identification of circulating CD10 positive T cells in angioimmunoblastic T-cell lymphoma. *Leukaemia* 2006;**20**(2):8.

22. Rawstron AC, Villamor N, Ritgen M *et al.* International standardized approach for flow cytometric residual disease monitoring in chronic lymphocytic leukaemia. *Leukemia* 2007;**21**(5):956s–64.

23. Pedreira CE, Costa ES, Arroyo ME, Almeida J, Orfao A. A multidimensional classification approach for the automated analysis of flow cytometry data. *IEEE Trans Biomed Eng* 2008;**55**(3):1155–62.

24. Maciejewski JP, Tiu RV, O'Keefe C. Application of array-based whole genome scanning technologies as a cytogenetic tool in haematological malignancies. *Br J Haematol* 2009;**146**(5):479–88.

25. Bench AJ, Erber WN, Scott MA. Molecular genetic analysis of haematological malignancies: I. Acute leukaemias and myeloproliferative disorders. *Clin Lab Haematol* 2005;**27**(3):148–71.

26. Bench AJ, Erber WN, Follows GA, Scott MA. Molecular genetic analysis of haematological

malignancies: II. Mature lymphoid neoplasms. *Int J Lab Hematol* 2007;**29**(4):229–60.

27. Kohlmann A, Kipps TJ, Rassenti LZ *et al.* An international standardization programme towards the application of gene expression profiling in routine leukaemia diagnostics: the Microarray Innovations in LEukemia study prephase. *Br J Haematol* 2008;**142**(5):802–7.

28. Mills KI, Kohlmann A, Williams PM *et al.* Microarray-based classifiers and prognosis models identify subgroups with distinct clinical outcomes and high risk of AML transformation of myelodysplastic syndrome. *Blood* 2009;**114**(5):1063–72.

29. Dugas M, Schoch C, Schnittger S *et al.* A comprehensive leukemia database: integration of cytogenetics, molecular genetics and microarray data with clinical information, cytomorphology and immunophenotyping. *Leukemia* 2001;**15**(12):1805–10.

30. Spagnolo DV, Ellis DW, Juneja S *et al.* The role of molecular studies in lymphoma diagnosis: a review. *Pathology* 2004;**36**(1):19–44.

31. Gujral S. Hematolymphoid neoplasms: World Health Organization versus rest of the world. *Leukemia* 2009;**23**(5):978.

7 Acute lymphoblastic leukemia

Elaine Coustan-Smith and Dario Campana

Introduction

Acute lymphoblastic leukemia (ALL), also known as lymphoblastic leukemia/lymphoma in the WHO classification, is a malignant expansion of immature lymphoid cells that results from multi-step genetic changes in a single lymphoid progenitor cell. Its incidence peaks between the ages of 2 and 4 years; rates are lower during later childhood, adolescence and young adulthood but the incidence rises in the sixth decade, reaching a second, smaller peak in the elderly [1]. ALL is the most common malignancy diagnosed in patients younger than 15 years [1]. Childhood ALL appears to have a prenatal origin in many cases [2]. In the case of identical twins, when leukemia occurs in one twin, there are a 20% probability that it will also occur in the other twin due to ALL transfer through the placental circulation. In identical twins with the t(4;11); (q21;q23) *MLL-AFF1*, the chances of ALL becoming clinically overt in the other twin in a short period of time are nearly 100%. The concordance rate in twins is lower in cases of ALL with the *ETV6-RUNX1* fusion or T-cell phenotype, probably because of the requirement for additional genetic events for leukemic transformation [1].

A small proportion of patients (< 5%) have hereditary genetic abnormalities that predispose to the disease, including Down syndrome, ataxia telangiectasia and Bloom's syndrome; children with Down syndrome have a 10- to 30-fold higher risk of developing ALL [1]. It was recently shown that germline single nucleotide polymorphisms in the *ARID5B* and *IKZF1* genes are more frequent in children with hyperdiploid B-lineage ALL, suggesting that these germline variants affect the propensity to develop ALL [3,4].

Acquired genetic changes that are likely to contribute to the development of ALL include the dysregulation of genes encoding transcription factors and signaling molecules, resulting in a subversion of hematopoietic cell homeostasis [1]. Cooperating lesions in genes encoding key regulators of lymphoid-cell differentiation may also play an important role. For example, deletions and translocations involving the *PAX5* gene have been recently described in approximately one-third of cases of childhood and adult B-lineage ALL [5,6], with alterations in other genes involved in B-cell development, i.e. *TCF3*, *EBF*, *LEF1*, *Ikaros* (*IKZF1*) and *Aiolos*, detected in a lower number of cases [5]. Alterations of these genes would be predicted to block or delay normal B-progenitor cell differentiation, thus contributing to leukemogenesis.

General laboratory features at presentation

The clinical and general laboratory features of ALL at presentation usually reflect the degree of bone marrow (BM) replacement and the extent of extramedullary dissemination of leukemic cells. Blood examination typically reveals anemia, neutropenia and thrombocytopenia. Hemoglobin is commonly < 8 g/dL. Initial leukocyte counts may range from 0.1 to 1500×10^9/L. Most patients have circulating leukemic blast cells but in cases with low initial counts (< 2×10^9/L) lymphoblasts may be absent in blood smears. Hypereosinophilia may be present but is rare.

The differential diagnosis of ALL includes other leukemias, as well as viral infections such as infectious mononucleosis. In the latter cases, detection of atypical lymphocytes or elevated viral titers aid in the diagnosis. Patients with pertussis or parapertussis may have marked lymphocytosis, but the affected cells are mature lymphocytes rather than lymphoblasts. Childhood ALL should also be distinguished from pediatric small round cell tumors that involve the bone marrow, including neuroblastoma, rhabdomyosarcoma and retinoblastoma. Generally, in such cases, a primary lesion can be found by routine diagnostic studies, and disseminated tumor cells often form clumps. Besides morphological differences, immunophenotyping is required to conclusively distinguish ALL from activated lymphocytes and solid tumor cells (see below).

Investigations to make the diagnosis and determine prognosis

General principles

Modern diagnosis of leukemia relies on a multidisciplinary approach involving morphology, cytochemistry, immunophenotyping, cytogenetics and molecular genetics. The first step in the laboratory diagnosis of ALL is the morphological analysis of bone marrow smears stained with Wright-Giemsa or May–Grünwald Giemsa stains, and cytochemical stains. If there is significant bone marrow fibrosis (in children, more likely to occur among those with B-lineage hyperdiploid ALL) it may be difficult to obtain an adequate bone marrow aspirate, and a bone marrow trephine biopsy may be required to establish the diagnosis. Although these procedures may be sufficient to distinguish ALL from non-lymphoid leukemias, they do not provide any definitive determination of the cellular and biologic subtype of ALL.

Immunophenotyping not only allows a definitive diagnosis of ALL but can also distinguish leukemias of B- and T-cell origin, establish the stage of maturation of the leukemic cell population, and identify markers that can be used to monitor the presence of minimal residual disease (MRD) during treatment. With current therapies, immunophenotyping provides somewhat limited prognostic information in ALL. Nevertheless, the distinction between B- and T-lineage leukemia is widely used for risk assignment, and the discrimination between B-lineage ALL from B-cell progenitor ALL is used to select between substantially different chemotherapy regimens [1]. More recently, it was shown that patients with early T-cell precursor (ETP) ALL, which can be identified by immunophenotyping, respond extremely poorly to chemotherapy and require alternative treatment strategies [7]. The extent of the immunophenotypic panels to be used at diagnosis depends on the intent

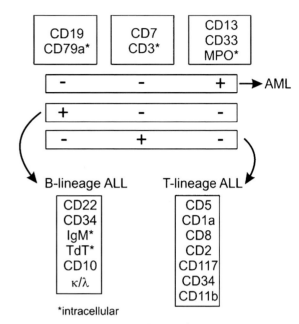

Figure 7.1. Minimum panel of markers for the immunophenotypic classification of ALL. The markers listed in the upper part of the figure discriminate between the main subtypes of acute leukemia in the vast majority of cases. A second set of markers (bottom) can then be tested according to the results of the initial screening. Note that CD79a is weakly expressed in approximately one-third of T-lineage ALL cases, a proportion of ALL cases expresses CD13 and/or CD33, and some AML cases express CD7 and/or CD19. In a small proportion of cases (< 10%) results may be equivocal after the first screening. The second set of markers should elucidate the diagnosis in virtually all of these cases.

of the analysis. If this is simply to establish the diagnosis of ALL and identify the presenting features that are prognostically important with current therapy then a relatively small panel of antibodies, such as those shown in Figure 7.1, is sufficient. A two-step procedure involving screening with the most lineage-specific antibodies, followed by other markers selected according to the results of the first screening, is particularly effective although it might be difficult to fit into the routine schedule of a laboratory that processes many samples daily.

Genetic abnormalities are strongly associated with response to therapy in B-lineage ALL (Table 7.1); their identification is critical for optimal risk-classification. For example, the t(9;22)(q34;q11) translocation and the corresponding *BCR-ABL1* gene fusion are associated with unfavorable treatment response in both children and adults with ALL [1,8]. Conversely, the *ETV6-RUNX1* abnormality and hyperdiploidy (>50 chromosomes) are associated with a favorable treatment response in children with ALL [1,9]. Therefore,

Table 7.1. Main recurrent genetic abnormalities in B-lineage ALL and their relation to immunophenotypic features and prognosis.

Cytogenetics/ FISH abnormality	Molecular abnormality	Prevalence		Characteristic immunophenotype	Prognosis
		Children	Adults		
t(9;22)(q34;q11)	BCR-ABL1	3%	25%	None	Unfavorable
t(4;11)(q21;q23) t(11;19)(q23;q13.3)	MLL-AFF1 MLL-ELL	8%	10%	CD10$^-$, NG2$^+$, CD15$^+$, CD65$^+$	Unfavorable in infants
t(12;21)(p13;q22)	ETV6-RUNX1	22%	2%	Frequently CD13$^+$ and/or CD33$^+$	Favorable
Hyperdiploidy 51–65 chromosomes		25%	7%	CD45 dim	Favorable
Hypodiploidy < 45 chromosomes		1%	2%	None	Unfavorable
t(1;19)(q23;p13.3)	TCF3-PBX1	5%	3%	Cytoplasmic μ+	Favorable
t(X;14)(p22;q32) or t(Y;14)(p11;q32) del(X)(p22.33p22.33) or del(Y)(p11.32p11.32)	IGH-CRLF2 CRLF2 deletions	5%		None	
	IKZF1 deletions or mutations	15%		None	Unfavorable

risk assignment can be considerably refined by determining the presence of these abnormalities. While conventional cytogenetic techniques can detect all major translocations found in ALL as well as determine ploidy status, some abnormalities such as *ETV6-RUNX1* are generally undetectable by conventional cytogenetics and require fluorescence *in situ* hybridization (FISH) or molecular analysis [10].

In principle, it is possible to distinguish genetic subtypes of ALL by their immunophenotype (Table 7.1) [11]. For example, ALL with rearrangements of the *MLL* gene usually have a very distinct marker profile. In general, however, immunophenotypic recognition of genetic subtype is not sufficiently reliable to be used for treatment stratification. DNA index (DI) analysis by flow cytometry, however, can determine changes in ploidy with a high degree of accuracy and this approach is often used instead of cytogenetics to classify high hyperdiploidy (DI ≥1.16) ALL, a feature associated with favorable treatment response. An exciting recent advance is the development of assays that allow the direct detection of fusion transcripts in leukemic cells by using flow cytometry. The assay that is currently commercially available detects BCR-ABL1 and its reliability has been convincingly demonstrated [12]. Assays to detect other abnormalities should be available soon.

Table 7.2. WHO classification of acute lymphoblastic leukemia.

B lymphoblastic leukemia

B lymphoblastic leukemia, NOS

B lymphoblastic leukemia with recurrent genetic abnormalities

B lymphoblastic leukemia with t(9;22)(q34;q11.2); BCR-ABL1

B lymphoblastic leukemia with t(v;11q23); MLL rearranged

B lymphoblastic leukemia with t(12;21)(p13;q22); TEL-AML1 (ETV6-RUNX1)

B lymphoblastic leukemia with hyperdiploidy

B lymphoblastic leukemia with hypodiploidy

B lymphoblastic leukemia with t(5;14)(q31;q32); IL3-IGH

B lymphoblastic leukemia with t(1;19)(q23;p13.3); TCF3-PBX1

T lymphoblastic leukemia

Below is a summary of the major subtypes of ALL that can be distinguished by various techniques and their main features. The classification and nomenclature used for ALL in the 2008 revision of the WHO Classification of Hematopoietic and Lymphoid Tissues is shown in Table 7.2 [13].

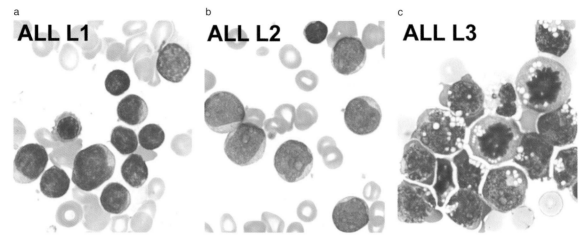

Figure 7.2. Morphological features of ALL cells. Shown are examples according to the FAB classification. Bone marrow smears were stained with Wright–Giemsa (images courtesy of Dr. Mihaela Onciu, St. Jude Children's Research Hospital, Memphis, TN).

Morphology and cytochemistry

The French–American–British (FAB) classification distinguished three morphological subtypes of ALL (L1, L2 and L3) (Figure 7.2). ALL L1 cells are relatively small (they can be as small as a mature lymphocyte), with scanty cytoplasm, a round or slightly indented nucleus, fine or slightly coarse chromatin, and inconspicuous nucleoli. In some cases (ALL L2), the leukemic cell population is morphologically heterogeneous, with smaller blasts admixed with larger lymphoblasts, with prominent nucleoli. Cytoplasmic granules can be seen in some cases and are usually amphophilic (of fuchsia color), in contrast to primary myeloid granules (of deep purple color), corresponding to mitochondria. B ALL blasts are usually distinct from early pre-B ALL and T ALL blasts and are characterized by intensely basophilic cytoplasm, prominent nucleoli and cytoplasmic vacuolation (ALL L3). This terminology for blast cell morphology is no longer applied in the WHO classification.

Analysis of cell morphology is not sufficient to differentiate ALL and acute myeloid leukemia with certainty. Cytochemical stains that can aid this distinction, but are now rarely used, include Sudan black, myeloperoxidase and non-specific esterases (e.g. α-naphthyl butyrate and α-naphthyl acetate esterase); these generally do not stain ALL blasts. The presence of residual normal myeloid precursors may result in a low percentage of myeloperoxidase-positive cells, which should not be confused with ALL cells.

Bone marrow trephine biopsies are only essential when the aspirate yields a "dry tap." However, a trephine is commonly taken in other circumstances. The marrow is diffusely infiltrated by a relatively homogeneous population of blast cells which are of small to intermediate size with a high nuclear:cytoplasmic ratio and fine chromatin (Figure 7.3). Nucleoli are commonly present but may be inconspicuous. Mitotic figures are commonly seen. Immunocytochemistry can be performed on the trephine section for CD3, CD7, CD10, CD34, CD79a and TdT (Figure 7.3). The distinction from acute myeloid leukemia can be made based on the absence of myeloperoxidase.

Central nervous system leukemia

Leukemic blast cells are identified at diagnosis in the cerebrospinal fluid (CSF) of approximately one third of children and 5–10% of adults with ALL, most of whom have no neurological symptoms. Although central nervous system (CNS) leukemia is defined by the presence of at least five leukocytes per μL of CSF and the detection of leukemic blast cells (Figure 7.4), or cranial nerve palsy (Table 7.3), the presence of any leukemic cells in the CSF (even from introduction due to a traumatic lumbar puncture) predicts an increased risk of relapse in children with ALL. In cases with borderline CSF leukocyte counts and/or uncertain morphological findings, additional tests may be necessary. Molecular genetic studies to detect specific gene fusions or antigen receptor gene rearrangements could be helpful but are not routinely

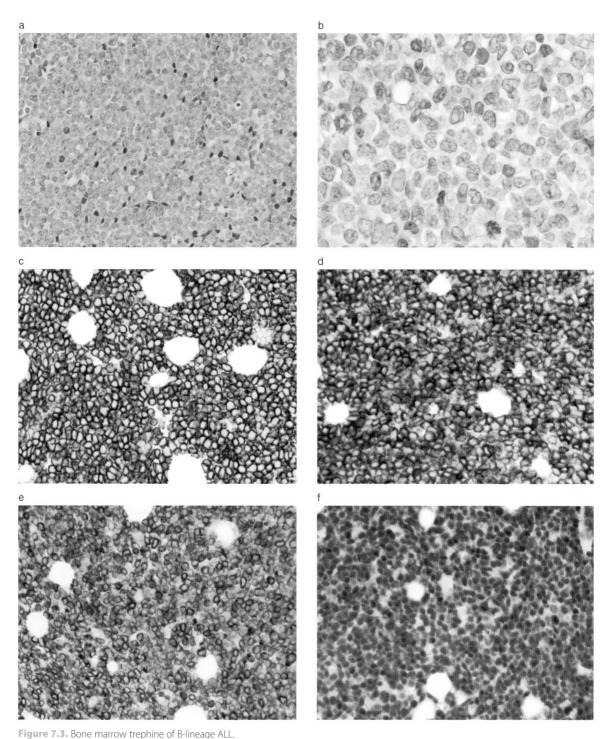

Figure 7.3. Bone marrow trephine of B-lineage ALL.
a. Hematoxylin and eosin (H&E) stained section showing the diffuse infiltrate of monomorphic blast cells.
b. Higher power view showing the cytological details and some pleomorphism of nuclear shape and the indistinct nucleoli.
c. The blast cells are CD34-positive, (d) CD10-positive, (e) CD79a-positive and (f) TdT-positive (immunoperoxidase and DAB substrate).
Images courtesy of Dr. Wendy Erber, Addenbrooke's Hospital, Cambridge, UK.

performed. Flow cytometric analysis can also be informative but requires a substantial number of cells. Staining cytocentrifuge preparations with antibodies to terminal deoxynucleotidyl transferase (TdT) and observation by fluorescence microscopy is probably the most widely applicable method to clarify suspect CSF findings, although the method is tedious and time-consuming (Figure 7.4).

Immunophenotyping

B-lineage ALL

B-lineage ALL cells at any stage of maturation express CD19 antigen and, in almost all cases, have cytoplasmic CD22 and CD79α. CD22 is prominent in the cytoplasm among the most immature cases [11].

Table 7.3. CNS status classification.

Status	Leukocytes (per μL)	Lymphoblasts
CNS1	<5	No
CNS2	<5	Yes
CNS3*	≥5	Yes

*Presence of cranial nerve palsies indicates CNS3 even with <5 leukocytes per L and/or absent lymphoblasts.

Antigen expression can also be used to subtype cases, based on phenotypic differentiation (see Figure 2.1), into early pre-B ALL, pre-B ALL and B-cell ALL.

Early pre-B ALL cases also express CD10 and TdT (approximately 90% of cases), and CD34 (more than 75% of cases). Early pre-B ALL cells lack expression of surface and cytoplasmic immunoglobulins [11]. CD20 is present in one-half of cases and its intensity can increase during treatment [14]. ALL cases with rearrangement of the *MLL* gene typically have an early pre-B ALL phenotype with distinctive phenotypic features such as expression of CD15, CD65 and chondroitin proteoglycan sulfate (NG2), and absence of CD10. Hyperdiploidy (chromosome number > 50) is typically associated with weak or undetectable CD45 expression [11].

Pre-B ALL is defined by the presence of cytoplasmic immunoglobulin μ heavy chains in the lymphoblasts with no detectable surface immunoglobulins; in rare cases leukemic cells express both cytoplasmic and surface immunoglobulin μ heavy chains without κ or λ light chains [11]. Pre-B ALL cells usually express CD10 and TdT, with approximately two-thirds of cases also expressing CD34; CD20 expression is variable. The t(1;19)(q23;p13) or the der(19)t(1;19)(q23;p13) genetic abnormalities are found in 20–25% of pre-B ALL cases.

B-cell ALL is characterized by the expression of surface immunoglobulin μ heavy chains plus either κ or λ light chains [11]. Commonly, cells have L3 morphology

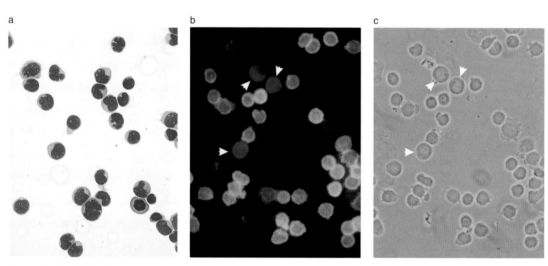

Figure 7.4. CNS leukemia.
a. Cytocentrifuge preparation of cerebrospinal fluid (CSF) from a patient with ALL stained with Wright–Giemsa showing ALL blasts (image courtesy of Dr. Mihaela Onciu, St. Jude Children's Research Hospital, Memphis, TN).
b. Cytocentrifuge preparation of CSF from another patient with ALL stained with anti-TdT (red; tetramethylrhodamine) and anti-CD3 (green; fluorescein isothiocyanate) antibodies. TdT-positive ALL blasts (arrows) are admixed with normal T-cells.
c. The same microscopic field as in **b** viewed by phase contrast microscopy; arrows point to the TdT-positive blasts.

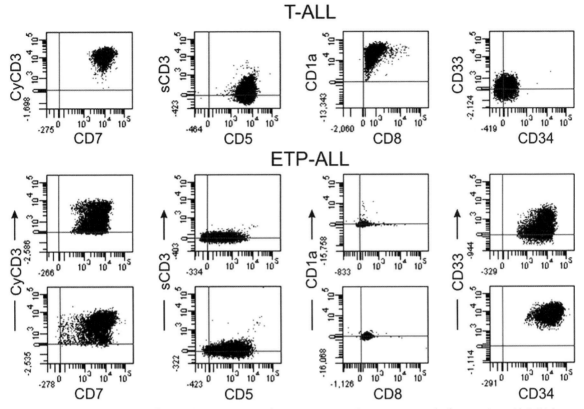

Figure 7.5. Immunophenotypic differences between T-ALL and ETP-ALL. Diagnostic bone marrow samples from a patient with T-ALL (top row) and two patients with ETP-ALL (middle and bottom rows) were analyzed by flow cytometry. Biexponential dot plots are shown.

(according to the FAB classification), express CD20, and frequently CD10; CD34 is negative. An uncommon subtype of B-cell ALL is characterized by blast cells with L1 or L2 morphology, and expression of TdT and/or CD34.

T-lineage ALL

T-lineage ALL cells express CD7 and CD3 antigens, the latter most frequently only in the cytoplasm [11]. Other markers commonly expressed include CD2, CD5 and TdT; CD1a, surface CD3, CD4 and CD8 are detected in approximately 40% of cases. HLA-DR expression is uncommon, and 40–45% of cases are CD10$^+$ and/or CD21$^+$. CD79α is weakly expressed in approximately one third of cases.

T-lineage ALL can be divided into three stages of immunophenotypic differentiation reflecting normal stages of thymic differentiation (see Figure 2.2): early (CD7$^+$, cCD3$^+$, surface CD3$^-$, CD4$^-$ and CD8$^-$), mid or common (cCD3$^+$, surface CD3$^-$, CD4$^+$, CD8$^+$ and CD1a$^+$), and late (surface CD3$^+$, CD1a$^-$ and either CD4$^+$ or CD8$^+$) [11]. However, many cases

have immunophenotypic patterns that do not fit these thymic maturation stages. T-cell receptor (TCR) proteins are heterogeneously expressed in T-lineage ALL. In approximately two-thirds of cases, membrane CD3 and TCR proteins are absent. In half of these cases, however, TCR proteins (TCRβ, TCRα or both) are present within the cytoplasm. Most cases with membrane CD3 and TCR chains express the TCRαβ, whereas a minority express TCRγδ proteins.

A subtype of T-ALL, named ETP-ALL, with the gene expression profile of normal early T-cell precursor cells, has recently been identified [7]. This leukemia is derived from a population of recent immigrants from the bone marrow to the thymus and which retain multi-lineage differentiation potential [7]. These leukemias are CD7- and CD3-positive (mostly only in the cytoplasm), lack CD1a and CD8 expression, have weak or absent CD5 expression and express at least one stem cell or myeloid-associated antigen (e.g. CD34, CD117, CD13, CD33, CD11b) (Figure 7.5). These cases are characterized by a

133

dismal response to therapy and a high rate of relapse [7].

Cytogenetics and molecular genetics

ALL with *BCR-ABL1*

The t(9;22)(q34;q11.2) fuses the 5′ portion of *BCR* to the 3′ portion of *ABL1* [1,10]. In ALL, breaks tend to occur in the minor breakpoint cluster regions, forming a 190 kDa *BCR-ABL1*. This alteration results in a constitutively active ABL tyrosine kinase that induces aberrant signaling and activates multiple cellular pathways. Expression of the BCR-ABL1 chimeric protein results in malignant transformation of hematopoietic cells and causes leukemia in murine experimental systems. Genome-wide analysis of *BCR-ABL1* ALL samples revealed deletions of *Ikaros* (*IKZF1*) in 84% of cases [15]. Deletions of *IKZF1* were not found in chronic phase chronic myelogenous leukemia (CML) samples but appeared to be acquired at the time of transformation into lymphoid blast crisis. *BCR-ABL1* ALL has a poor prognosis with standard chemotherapy [1,8]. The development of the tyrosine kinase inhibitor imatinib mesylate and second-generation inhibitors such as nilotinib and dasatinib has dramatically changed clinical management of *BCR-ABL1* leukemias and substantially improved treatment response [16].

ALL with *MLL* gene rearrangements

Structural alterations involving band 11q23 of chromosome 11 are the most frequent cytogenetic abnormality in infant ALL [1,10]. In most cases, the target is the *MLL* gene (for Mixed-Lineage Leukemia; also known as *HRX*, *ALL-1* and *TRX1*) which encodes a DNA-binding protein that regulates the expression of many genes crucial for hematopoiesis including multiple *HOX* genes [1,10] (Figure 7.6). The most common 11q23 abnormality in ALL is the t(4;11) (q21;q23), which produces a chimeric protein that contains the N-terminal portion of *MLL* linked to the C-terminal portion of *AFF1*. However, *MLL* can also associate with more than 50 other genes in less common translocations [17]. Several genes normally expressed in non-lymphoid hematopoietic lineages are over-expressed in *MLL*-rearranged ALL, including *FLT3*, *LMO2* and HOX genes, such as *HOXA9*, *HOXA5*, *HOXA4* and *HOXC6* [1,10]. Treatment outcome of childhood ALL with an *MLL* gene rearrangement differs by age group with infants having the worst outcome [18].

ALL with *TEL-AML1* (*ETV6-RUNX1*)

The t(12;21)(p13;q22) translocation brings together the 5′ portion of the *TEL* (*ETV6*) gene and the nearly complete *AML1* (*RUNX1*) gene [1,10]. This translocation can usually be detected only by FISH (Figure 7.6b) or reverse-transcriptase polymerase chain reaction (RT-PCR). The non-translocated *ETV6* allele is frequently deleted. The *ETV6* gene belongs to the *Ets* family of transcription factors and appears to have an essential role in hematopoiesis. *RUNX1* encodes a transcription factor that binds DNA as a heterodimer with core binding factor (CBF) β and is essential for the development of definitive hematopoiesis. Experimental evidence suggests that *TEL-AML1* endows preleukemic cells with altered self-renewal and survival properties, which have a higher risk of evolving into leukemia-initiating cells [2]. In most studies, childhood ALL with *TEL-AML1* was associated with excellent response to therapy [9].

Hyperdiploid and hypodiploid ALL

Leukemic lymphoblasts with a chromosome number of 51–65 (Figure 7.6c) have a marked propensity to undergo apoptosis, and accumulate greater quantities of methotrexate and its active polyglutamate metabolites [1]. These features help to explain the relatively low leukemic burden at presentation and the favorable prognosis of this ALL subtype. Among chromosomes that are overrepresented, only the trisomies of chromosome 4, 10 and 17 have been shown to be associated with a favorable prognosis in some studies [19]. There is no association between treatment response and hyperdiploidy with 47–50 chromosomes or near-triploidy (69–81 chromosomes), which frequently also have the *ETV6-RUNX1* abnormality [1]. Cases with near-tetraploidy (82–94 chromosomes) are more frequently of T-cell immunophenotype. Hypodiploidy (< 45 chromosomes) occurs in < 2% of ALL cases and is associated with a poor outcome, which is worse in cases with < 44 chromosomes [20].

ALL with *E2A-PBX1* (*TCF3-PBX1*)

The t(1;19)(q23;p13) translocation juxtaposes the *E2A* (*TCF3*) gene on chromosome 19 and the *PBX1* gene on chromosome 1 (Figure 7.6d). The resulting E2A-PBX1 fusion protein contains the transcriptional activation domains of E2A linked to the DNA-binding domain of PBX1 and the encoded protein inappropriately activates the transcription of

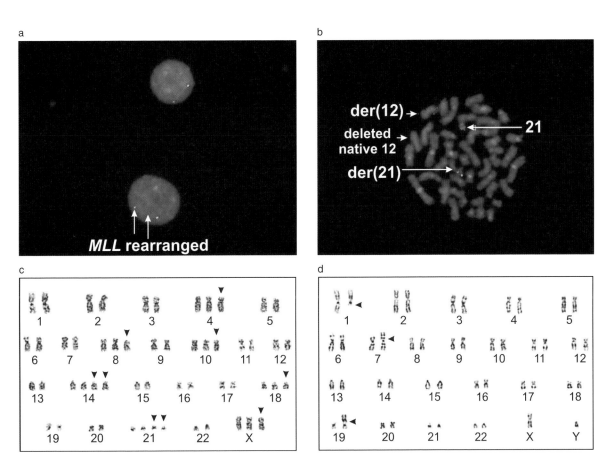

Figure 7.6. Cytogenetic abnormalities in ALL.
a. Interphase FISH showing the rearrangement of the *MLL* gene using a breakapart probe (Abbott/Vysis); the top nucleus is normal and has two *MLL* signals, the bottom nucleus is abnormal and the arrows show the split signals.
b. Metaphase FISH showing the t(12;21)(p13;q22) using the *ETV6-RUNX1* extra-signal probe (Abbot/Vysis); the *ETV6* native signal is deleted.
c. Hyperdiploid 51+ ALL; arrows point to trisomy of chromosomes 4, 8, 10, 18 and X, and tetrasomy of chromosomes 14 and 21.
d. t(1;19)(q23;p13.3) translocation with arrows showing the derivative chromosomes 1 and 19, and isochromosome 7q.
Illustrations courtesy of Dr. Susana C. Raimondi, St Jude Children's Research Hospital, Memphis, TN.

genes normally regulated by PBX1 [1,10]. Another *E2A* fusion gene is created by the t(17;19)(q22;q13), in which *E2A* is fused to the gene that encodes the transcription factor hepatic leukemia factor (*HLF*). The t(1;19)(q23;p13) abnormality was previously reported to be associated with unfavorable outcome in studies; however, with current therapy this leukemia subtype has an excellent treatment response although they still have increased risk of CNS relapses [21].

Novel subtypes of B-lineage ALL identified by genome-wide screens

Microarray methods for measuring gene expression can identify profiles that distinguish cases with the abovementioned genetic abnormalities as well as other novel subtypes. To this end, a subset of ALL, identified by hierarchical cluster analysis of gene expression data, comprised many cases that clustered with *BCR-ABL1*-positive cases and had an unfavorable outcome [22]. The majority of cases with *BCR-ABL1*-like disease also had deletions in genes involved in B-cell development such as *PAX5* and *IKZF1*. Another study using single nucleotide polymorphism arrays showed that *IKZF1* deletions and mutations were associated with a *BCR-ABL1*-like gene expression profile and strongly predicted poor response to chemotherapy and relapse [23]. Genomic re-sequencing of *JAK1* and *JAK2* in 187 cases of B-lineage ALL classified as "high-risk" by clinical criteria and lack of favorable genetic abnormalities, identified 19 with heterozygous, somatic mutations which resulted in constitutive activation of the JAK-STAT signaling pathway; most of these cases also had *IKZF1* alterations [24].

Genetic subtypes of T-lineage ALL

Several genes in T-ALL, such as *SCL* (*TAL-1*), *LMO1* (*TTG-1*), *LMO2* (*TTG-2*), *HOX11* (*TLX1*) and *HOX11L2* (*TLX3*), are dysregulated by translocation to the TCR locus resulting in overexpression [1,10]. *LMO1* is inserted into the *TCRαδ* locus in the t(11;14)(p15;q11), while *LMO2* is inserted into this locus in the t(11;14)(p13;q11). In a small fraction of cases, the *SCL* gene (involved in early hematopoiesis and located on chromosome 1) is inserted into the *TCRδ* locus on chromosome 14. More frequent (approximately 25% of cases) is the internal deletion in the $5'$ untranslated region of *SCL*, which juxtaposes a locus called *SIL* with the *SCL* coding region, resulting in the expression of a fused *SIL-SCL* transcript that encodes a normal SCL protein. An additional alteration found in more than 50% of T-cell ALL cases is the deletion from chromosome 9p21of the *INK4b-ARF-INK4a* locus, which encode the p16^{INK4a}, p15^{INK4b} and p19^{ARF}, regulators of cell cycle and apoptosis.

Levels of *HOX11*, *TAL1* and *LYL1* mRNA expression have been used to recognize distinct subtypes of T-ALL [25,26]. Activating mutations of *NOTCH1* are frequently found in T-ALL and have been implicated in its pathogenesis [27]. Although there has been some discussion on their prognostic significance, most studies showed either a favorable or no prognostic impact [28]. Adult patients whose cells have low *ERG* and *BAALC* gene expression reportedly have a better outcome [29]. Among childhood cases, those bearing the gene expression profile of ETP have a dismal outcome [7]. The prevalence of this subset in adults is unclear.

Studies at diagnosis to identify markers for disease monitoring

Immunophenotyping

ALL cells express immunophenotypic features that distinguish them from normal hematopoietic cells, including hematogones [30]. The most widely applicable leukemia-associated immunophenotypes are constituted by markers expressed during normal lympho-hematopoiesis but found in abnormal combinations in leukemic cells; these phenotypes have been termed "aberrant" or "asynchronous." In cases of T-lineage ALL, residual disease can be monitored by tracking cells expressing markers, such as nuclear TdT in combination with T-cell antigens; this combination is only expressed by normal thymocytes and not peripheral blood or bone marrow cells. Finally, expression of fusion proteins derived from chromosomal breakpoints, such as *BCR-ABL1*, *ETV6-RUNX1* or *TCF3-PBX1*, and ectopic expression of proteins promoted by gene translocations, such as expression of PBX1 in lymphoblasts (PBX1 is normally confined to non-lymphoid cells), could potentially be used to identify residual ALL cells. However this approach has not been extensively explored due to the lack of suitable antibodies for reliable flow cytometric analysis.

Leukemia-associated markers for MRD studies can be identified at diagnosis in virtually all patients with ALL (Table 7.4) [30]. Immunophenotypes sufficiently dissimilar from those of normal cells are expressed by the majority of cells in approximately 95% of cases. This therefore allows a sensitivity of 0.01% for MRD detection. Obviously, the identification of such markers requires the testing of large panels of antibodies, well beyond those required for initial classification of the leukemia for diagnostic purposes. We therefore use a two-stage approach to establish the immunophenotypic signature that will be used for MRD studies in follow-up samples in B-lineage ALL. The first stage involves screening markers potentially over- and under-expressed by combining the individual antibodies with CD19. After the aberrantly expressed markers have been identified, the second stage consists of re-staining cells with the selected markers in 4–8 color combinations; this includes markers such as CD19, CD10, CD34 and TdT to produce a cell profile characteristic of the leukemic clone. This cell profile will then be used to identify leukemic cells during treatment.

To be reliable the immunophenotypes used to distinguish leukemic cells from normal cells must be truly leukemia-specific. While some immunophenotypes are apparently restricted to leukemic cells when compared with results obtained in bone marrow samples from healthy adult donors, it is evident that they are not when one examines bone marrow samples proliferating after chemotherapy.

Table 7.4. Marker combinations used to monitor minimal residual disease (MRD) at St Jude Children's Research Hospital.

ALL subtype	Marker combinations	Frequency (%)*
T-lineage ALL	anti-TdT / CD5 / CD3	90
	CD34 / CD5 / CD3	30
B-lineage ALL		
CD10+ cases	CD19 / CD34 / CD10 / CD58	37
	CD19 / CD34 / CD10 / CD38	54
	CD19 / CD34 / CD10 / CD45	30
	CD19 / CD34 / CD10 / anti-TdT	21
	CD19 / CD34 / CD10 / CD13	5
	CD19 / CD34 / CD10 / CD66c	15
	CD19 / CD34 / CD10 / CD33	3
CD10− cases	CD19 / CD34 / CD10 / CD15	48
	CD19 / CD34 / CD133 / CD10	33
	CD19 / CD34 / NG-2 / CD10	35

* Percentage of cases within a leukemia subtype in which the marker combination indicated was used to monitor MRD with a sensitivity of 10^{-4}. Data are from a group of 470 pediatric patients with newly diagnosed ALL (T-lineage ALL, 56; B-lineage ALL CD10+, 391; B-lineage ALL CD10−, 23).

Molecular genetics

Molecular markers to track ALL cells during treatment can be identified at diagnosis in the majority of cases. Gene fusions, such as *BCR-ABL1*, *MLL-AFF1*, *TCF3-PBX1* and *ETV6-RUNX1*, resulting in the expression of aberrant mRNA transcripts, are convenient markers for this purpose [31]. Recurrent abnormalities suitable for routine studies in clinical samples are present in approximately 40% of children and 50% of adults with ALL. It is likely that additional genetic targets will become available with the discovery of new genetic abnormalities afforded by the application of whole-genome screening technologies.

The second group of PCR targets for MRD studies in ALL is represented by the clonal rearrangement of immunoglobulin (*IG*) and T-cell receptor (*TCR*) genes whose junctional regions are unique to the leukemic clone [32]. The presence of clonal *IG* and/or *TCR* gene rearrangements at diagnosis is screened by using PCR primers matched to the V and J regions of various *IG* and *TCR* genes. If an apparently clonal rearrangement is found, one must ensure that it is derived from ALL cells and not from normal cells by analyzing the PCR product for their clonal origin, e.g. by heteroduplex

analysis (Figure 7.7a). The ALL-derived PCR products are then used for direct sequencing of the junctional regions of the *IG/TCR* gene rearrangements which, in turn, is used to design junctional region-specific oligonucleotides, also called allele-specific oligonucleotides. Clonal *IG/TCR* gene rearrangements can also be detected with high-resolution electrophoresis systems, such as radioactive fingerprinting or fluorescent gene scanning, without the need for patient-specific oligonucleotides, but this approach has a considerably lower sensitivity, usually not better than 0.1% [32].

The majority (>95%) of B-lineage ALL cases have *IG* gene rearrangements. Cross-lineage *TCR* gene rearrangements also occur in up to 90% of cases of B-lineage ALL. *TCR* genes are rearranged in most cases of T-lineage ALL with cross-lineage *IG* gene rearrangements occurring in approximately 20% of T-ALL. Of note, infant *MLL-AFF1* ALL has a high prevalence of immature, non-productive and/or oligoclonal antigen-receptor gene rearrangements [32].

Monitoring treatment response and disease progression

General principles

Examination of bone marrow smears is performed periodically during treatment to determine the degree of treatment response and detect leukemia relapse. However, the sensitivity and accuracy of this test is limited because the morphology of ALL cells can be virtually indistinguishable from that of lymphoid precursors (hematogones) and activated mature lymphocytes. The distinction between leukemic and normal cells becomes particularly challenging when bone marrow lympho-hematopoiesis is recovering after chemotherapy or transplantation, with hematogones representing 5% or more of the total cellular population.

Precision in determining the degree of early treatment response is important to predict the risk of relapse and therefore inform therapeutic decisions [30]. Efforts to develop assays for detecting MRD, i.e. leukemia undetectable by morphology, evolved from the identification of unique features of ALL cells and development of robust detection methods, to the determination of the clinical significance of MRD. This has culminated in the incorporation of MRD testing in clinical trials. MRD reflects the influence of multiple variables on treatment response,

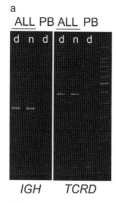

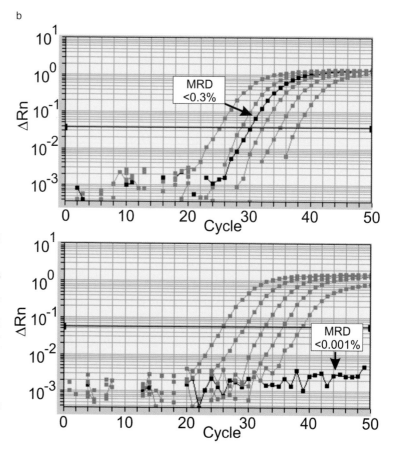

Figure 7.7. Antigen receptor gene rearrangement studies.
a. Heteroduplex analysis of *IGH* (FR2B-JHU) and *TCRD* (Vdelta2-N-Ddelta3) gene rearrangements in bone marrow mononuclear cells of B-lineage ALL. DNA was analyzed under denaturing (d) or non-denaturing conditions (n) and DNA from the peripheral blood of four healthy donors (PB) was used as control. In the ALL samples clonal bands are visible irrespective of denaturation.
b. MRD monitoring in two patients with B-lineage ALL using real-time quantitative PCR and *IGH* genes as targets. Gray lines correspond to signals obtained with serial dilutions of diagnostic DNA in DNA from peripheral blood of healthy donors. The black lines correspond to the signal obtained in the follow-up sample. MRD-positive (0.3%; top) and MRD-negative (< 0.001%; bottom) are shown; in both cases, the primers were a patient-specific primer combined with a JH4 primer.

including clinical features, pharmacogenomic and pharmacokinetic variables, and cellular and genetic leukemia characteristics. Not surprisingly, treatment response measured by MRD assays is currently the strongest prognostic factor for patients with ALL.

Practical considerations for minimal residual disease studies

The main features of currently available MRD assays are summarized in Table 7.5.

Flow cytometry

Minimal residual disease detection by flow cytometry is becoming increasingly used for risk assignment in patients with ALL. It must be stressed, however, that simple availability of a flow cytometer and experience in leukemia immunophenotyping is not sufficient to perform MRD studies proficiently. This is because

MRD testing requires a solid knowledge of the immunophenotype of bone marrow cells under different conditions, including suppression during chemotherapy, and regeneration after cessation of chemotherapy or post-transplant. Chemotherapy might decrease the expression of some markers, and the recovery phase may dramatically increase the percentage of immature lymphoid cells. Bone marrow samples collected in these circumstances may appear very different from that of healthy adult donors and the differences could mask the presence of residual leukemia, or be confused with residual leukemia.

The sensitivity of flow cytometry depends on the robustness of the set of leukemia-associated immunophenotypes and on the number of cells acquired. As explained above, the best leukemia-associated immunophenotypes should be selected at diagnosis. During MRD testing, it is important to acquire sufficient cells to achieve a high sensitivity of detection [30].

Table 7.5. Methods for monitoring minimal residual disease (MRD) in acute lymphoblastic leukemia (ALL).

Method	Percent of cases with marker	Routine sensitivity	Main advantages	Main disadvantages
Flow cytometric detection of abnormal phenotypes	98%	0.01%	Rapid Precise Allows overview of normal hematopoiesis	Requires solid knowledge of the immunophenotype of normal cells for correct interpretation
PCR amplification of *IG* or *TCR* genes	90%	0.01–0.001%	Highly sensitive	Preparation of patient-tailored assay is laborious
RT-PCR amplification fusion transcripts	<50%	0.1–0.001%	Stable targets Detection of pre-leukemic clones	MRD estimates can be imprecise

Thus, if a sensitivity of 1 leukemic cell in 10 000 is desired, one must acquire at least 100 000 mononuclear cells so that at least 10 leukemic "events" are present. Currently, reliable leukemia-associated immunophenotypes that afford a sensitivity of 1 in 10 000 can be identified in > 95% of patients with ALL [30]. Specific advantages of flow cytometry include:

1. The capacity to analyze the status of normal hematopoietic cells while searching for MRD.
2. The identification of markers that can be used to sort leukemic cells for biological and genetic studies.
3. The ability (afforded by modern 8-plus color flow cytometers) to analyze multiple biological features of ALL cells while detecting MRD.

In our laboratory, we typically require 2 mL of bone marrow for MRD studies and prepare mononuclear cell preparations. These generate cleaner flow cytometry plots which facilitate analysis. The mononuclear cell preparations can also be used for PCR studies. Other investigators, however, have reported informative results by flow cytometry after red cell lysis separation.

Molecular genetics

A strong suit of PCR amplification of fusion transcripts is the stable association between the molecular abnormality and the leukemic clone, irrespective of changes caused by therapy or clonal selection [31]. In addition, positive MRD-findings may indicate the presence of pre-leukemic or "stem" cells, which could be undetectable by other methods. However, an important disadvantage of PCR monitoring is that the estimate of the percentage of leukemic cells present may be imprecise. This is because the amount of

transcripts per leukemic cell may vary from patient to patient with the same genetic subtype of ALL, and can be affected by chemotherapy and sample integrity [31].

PCR amplification of antigen-receptor genes is a very reliable and accurate method for monitoring MRD and can be used in the majority of cases of childhood and adult ALL [32]. Because rearranged *IG* and *TCR* genes are present in one copy per cell, a precise quantitation of MRD can be achieved particularly by using limiting-dilution methods or real-time PCR (Figure 7.7b). *IG* and *TCR* genes in ALL might undergo continuing or secondary rearrangements, resulting in oligoclonality, i.e. the presence of sub-clones having distinct clonal *IG/TCR* gene rearrangements [32]. Minor clones, undetected at diagnosis, may become predominant during the course of the disease, leading to the recommendation of targeting two or more different rearrangements. Indeed, multiple targets are identifiable in the majority of ALL cases; however multiple targets that allow detection of MRD with a high sensitivity (e.g. 0.01%) are not identifiable in approximately 30% of cases [33]. Nevertheless, it is unclear to what extent clonal evolution impacts the reliability of MRD detection, particularly at early stages of treatment.

Flow cytometry versus molecular genetics: which test to perform?

When applied in parallel to study MRD in the same samples, flow cytometry and PCR amplification of *IG/TCR* genes yield remarkably similar measurements, if MRD is present at a ≥ 0.01% level [30]. Flow cytometry results can be obtained within a few hours of sample collection. The development of a patient-specific PCR assay is time-consuming but, once the assay is developed, MRD estimates can also be obtained quite rapidly. Because of the time required to develop a patient-specific PCR assay, flow cytometry may be preferable for studies at very early time points during therapy while PCR may be preferable for studies at the end of therapy or post-transplant because of higher sensitivity. Our current strategy is to use flow cytometry to monitor MRD during remission induction therapy, and develop a PCR assay for IG/TCR genes only if a suitable immunophenotype is not identified at diagnosis.

Blood versus bone marrow: which sample to use?

In patients with B-lineage ALL, MRD is usually present at higher levels in bone marrow than in peripheral blood. In T-lineage ALL, however, MRD levels in peripheral blood are similar to those in bone marrow [34]. Therefore, with T-lineage ALL it is our current practice to use blood (5–10 mL are requested) rather than marrow to monitor MRD post-remission induction.

Prognostic significance of minimal residual disease in childhood ALL

The prognostic value of MRD detected during the first 2–3 months of therapy in childhood ALL has been demonstrated in numerous studies [30]. MRD can also help identify

1. Patients with a higher risk of relapse among those with specific ALL subtypes as well as among patients with first-relapse ALL who achieve a second remission.
2. Patients with "isolated" extramedullary relapse.
3. Patients undergoing allogeneic stem cell transplantation [30].

A cut-off level of 0.01%, the typical limit of detection for routine flow cytometric and molecular assays, has been shown to discriminate patients with different risks of relapse. For example, patients with MRD $\geq 0.01\%$ in bone marrow at any treatment interval had a significantly higher risk of relapse in earlier St Jude studies [35], and MRD $\geq 0.01\%$ on day 29 was the strongest prognostic indicator in studies of the Children's Oncology Group [36]. Other investigators (i.e. from the EORTC group, the Austrian BFM group, and the Dana-Farber Cancer Institute ALL Consortium) found that a cut-off level of 0.1% at the end of remission induction and at subsequent time points was particularly informative [37–39].

By MRD testing during the early phases of treatment it is possible to identify patients with a very high risk of relapse and are candidates for allogeneic hematopoietic stem cell transplantation. For example, MRD $\geq 1\%$ at the end of remission induction therapy was associated with an extremely high rate of relapse in St Jude studies [35]. Investigators of the I-BFM Study Group reported that patients whose bone marrow had MRD $\geq 0.1\%$ on both day 33 and day 78 of treatment had a relapse rate of 75% [33]. At the other end of the spectrum, a group of patients show remarkably good responses to remission induction therapy, resulting in undetectable (<0.01%) MRD after only 2–3 weeks of therapy [40]. We found that 183 of 402 patients (45.5%) with B-lineage ALL were MRD <0.01% after 19 days of treatment and had an excellent prognosis overall. A simple and economical test was devised to detect this subgroup of patients [41] who may be considered for reduction in treatment intensity.

Genetic abnormalities in childhood ALL are associated with a different prevalence of MRD during remission induction therapy. In B-lineage ALL, MRD on days 19 and 43 of treatment is much more prevalent in those with BCR-ABL1 ALL, and less prevalent in patients with ETV6-RUNX1, hyperdiploid (>50 chromosomes) and TCF3-PBX1 ALL [42]. In addition, patients with B-lineage ALL and mutations or deletions of IKZF1 are more likely to have MRD detected during remission induction therapy than those without this abnormality [43]. Finally, among patients with T-lineage ALL, those with ETP-ALL have strikingly higher levels of MRD during remission induction therapy [7].

Prognostic significance of minimal residual disease in adult ALL

Presence of MRD by PCR amplification of antigen-receptor genes post-remission induction therapy correlated with a poorer outcome in adult patients with Philadelphia chromosome-negative B-lineage ALL enrolled in or treated according to the UKALL XII protocol [44]. PCR amplification of antigen-receptor genes could recognize three risk-groups among standard-risk patients enrolled in GMALL trials from 1997 to 2002: low-risk (10%) with <0.01% MRD on day 11 and day 24, high-risk (23%) with MRD $\geq 0.01\%$ until week 16, and intermediate-risk (67%) with intermediate levels of MRD; the risk of relapse for the three groups was 0%, 94% and 47% respectively [45]. Conversion to MRD positivity post-consolidation was an adverse prognostic indicator [46]. Studies using fusion transcripts and/or *IG/TCR* gene rearrangements as targets indicated that MRD at the end of consolidation was the most significant risk factor for relapse in patients treated according to the NILG-ALL 09/00 protocol [47]. Studies by flow cytometry indicated that in patients with Philadelphia-negative ALL, MRD ≥ 0.1% after remission induction therapy was an independent predictor for relapse in the Polish Adult Leukemia Group ALL 4–2002 study [48]. MRD measurements prior to allogeneic hematopoietic stem cell transplant have also been shown to predict treatment outcome [47,49].

Feasibility of minimal residual disease testing for routine risk classification

It is feasible to routinely test MRD for risk classification in the majority of patients, even in multi-center studies. For example, among 2086 patients (97.3%) with B-lineage ALL enrolled on the Children's Oncology Group 9900 protocols, a flow cytometry MRD test with a 0.01% sensitivity could be performed on day 29 in 92% of patients [36]. Of the 3341 diagnostic samples examined in the AIEOP-BFM 2000 trial, only 305 (9.1%) lacked a suitable gene rearrangement target for PCR analysis or had a target not sufficient to reach a sensitivity of 0.01%; 2365 (70.8%) patients had at least two sensitive targets for MRD analysis [33]. In the St Jude Total XV trial flow cytometry and/or PCR amplification of antigen-receptor genes were used to monitor MRD in pediatric ALL. Flow cytometry was applied in patients with B-lineage ALL and T-ALL. In B-lineage ALL both flow cytometry (482 of 492 patients [98%]) and PCR (403 of 492 [82%]) were performed; the two methods, in combination, could be applied to study 491 of 492 (99.8%) patients [50]. The single patient with no available immunophenotypic MRD marker or antigen-receptor gene rearrangements had a MLL-MLLT3 fusion transcript and was monitored by RQ-PCR using that marker.

The AIEOP-BFM group currently uses MRD by PCR amplification of antigen-receptor genes to classify patients into three risk groups:

1. Standard risk (MRD negative on days 33 and 78).
2. Intermediate risk (any MRD positivity on days 33 and 78 but < 0.1% on day 78).
3. High risk (MRD ≥ 0.1% on day 78) [33].

St Jude Children's Research Hospital uses MRD levels by flow cytometry or PCR on day 15 and day 42 for treatment assignment. Patients with MRD of ≥1% on day 15 receive intensified remission induction therapy; further intensification is reserved for patients with ≥5% leukemic cells. By contrast, patients with MRD <0.01% on day 15 receive a slightly less intensive reinduction therapy and lower cumulative doses of anthracycline. Patients with standard-risk ALL who have MRD of ≥0.01% on day 42 are reclassified as high-risk; patients with MRD ≥ 1% are eligible for transplant in first remission. MRD monitoring is stopped in patients with B-lineage ALL who are MRD negative on day 42.

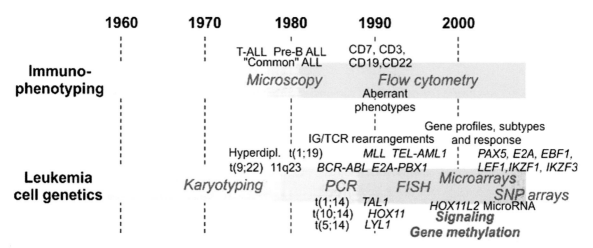

Figure 7.8. Schematic representation of the progress in understanding the biology of ALL during the last 50 years. The advent of new technologies (in red) and related discoveries is shown in approximate chronological order.

Table 7.6. Summary of tests for the diagnosis and follow-up of acute lymphoblastic leukemia (ALL).

Test	Application	
	Diagnosis	**Follow-up**
Morphology (+/− cytochemistry)		
Bone marrow aspirate	Assessment of bone marrow cellularity Determine diagnosis/differential diagnosis	Assessment of treatment response Assessment of hematopoietic recovery Detection of impending relapse Low sensitivity for detecting residual disease (~5%)
Bone marrow trephine	May be required in cases with significant bone marrow fibrosis and difficult marrow aspirate	To estimate the decrease in bone marrow cellularity during early phases of therapy To assess bone marrow recovery with prolonged cytopenias (preferable to the aspirate)
CSF	Determination of CNS involvement TdT staining may be required	Determination of CNS involvement TdT staining may be required
Flow cytometry	Definitive diagnosis of ALL Identification of stage of cell maturation. Detect prognostic features (DI ≥1.16, ETP-ALL) Identify markers for MRD monitoring	Monitoring MRD
Cytogenetics		
Karyotype, ploidy	Corroboration of ALL diagnosis Identification of genetic abnormalities with prognostic significance, e.g. *BCR-ABL1*; *MLL* rearrangements; hyperdiploidy (> 50 chromosomes); hypodiploidy (< 45 chromosomes)	Assessment of treatment response Detection of impending relapse Low sensitivity for detecting residual disease (~5%)
FISH	Corroboration of ALL diagnosis Identification of genetic abnormalities with prognostic significance e.g. *ETV6-RUNX1*	Assessment of treatment response Detection of impending relapse Low sensitivity for detecting residual disease (~5%)
Molecular genetics		
Gene fusions	Corroboration of ALL diagnosis Identification of genetic abnormalities with prognostic significance, e.g. *BCR-ABL1*; *MLL* rearrangements; *ETV6-RUNX1* Identify abnormalities for MRD	Monitoring MRD
IG and *TCR* gene rearrangements	Corroboration of ALL diagnosis (rare) Identification of markers for MRD	Monitoring MRD

Sequential MRD monitoring continues in patients with B-lineage ALL who are MRD positive and in any patient with T-lineage ALL.

Our team also uses MRD to guide treatment for patients with first-relapse ALL who achieve a second remission. Those with persistent MRD are candidates for transplant whereas those who achieve MRD negativity (in the context of other favorable clinical features) are eligible for continuing chemotherapy. For patients who undergo transplant, additional courses of chemotherapy may be administered in efforts to reduce MRD levels before transplant.

Concluding comments

There has been phenomenal progress in the understanding of the biology of ALL over the last three decades (Figure 7.8). With current methods and the wealth of expertise accumulated over the years, the diagnosis of ALL can be performed quickly and accurately (Table 7.6). Gaining additional information beyond diagnosis, such as the identification of biological and genetic features with prognostic importance and the selection of targets for MRD studies, requires more specialized tests. Although these tests add significantly to the initial laboratory costs, they could improve the quality of treatment and should ultimately pay for themselves.

Recently developed methodologies, such as arrays to screen genome-wide expression of mRNA and microRNA, as well as gene methylation status, genomic gains and losses and single nucleotide polymorphisms are likely to find their way in the diagnostic procedures in the future. Some of these methods have already been proven to identify subtypes of ALL that cannot be discriminated with the routine methods currently used. Their application appears to be particularly promising to identify ALL subtypes with prognostic significance and provide clues about pathways that could be targeted by molecular therapies. Conceivably, a single gene expression test by microarray could provide a classification as robust as that provided by immunophenotypic and genetic studies combined.

It is unquestionable that MRD tests allow leukemia "remission" to be defined in a way that is much more accurate and rigorous than the one afforded by conventional morphological techniques. Incorporating MRD to guide treatment decisions promises to result in significantly higher cure rates and lower treatment toxicities.

Acknowledgments

We thank Drs. Mihaela Onciu, Susana Raimondi, Jeffrey Jacobsen and Wendy Erber for providing images for the figures and helpful discussions, and Pat Stow for antigen receptor gene rearrangement studies.

References

1. Pui CH, Robison LL, Look AT. Acute lymphoblastic leukaemia. *Lancet* 2008;**371**:1030–43.

2. Hong D, Gupta R, Ancliff P *et al.* Initiating and cancer-propagating cells in *TEL-AML1*-associated childhood leukemia. *Science* 2008;**319**:336–9.

3. Trevino LR, Yang W, French D *et al.* Germline genomic variants associated with childhood acute lymphoblastic leukemia. *Nat Genet* 2009;**41**:1001–5.

4. Papaemmanuil E, Hosking FJ, Vijayakrishnan J *et al.* Loci on 7p12.2, 10q21.2 and 14q11.2 are associated with risk of childhood acute lymphoblastic leukemia. *Nat Genet* 2009;**41**:1006–10.

5. Mullighan CG, Goorha S, Radtke I *et al.* Genome-wide analysis of genetic alterations in acute lymphoblastic leukaemia. *Nature* 2007;**446**:758–64.

6. Familiades J, Bousquet M, Lafage-Pochitaloff M *et al.* PAX5 mutations occur frequently in adult B-cell progenitor acute lymphoblastic leukaemia and PAX5 haploinsufficiency is associated with *BCR-ABL1* and *TCF3-PBX1* fusion genes: a GRAALL study. *Leukemia* 2009;**23**:1989–1998.

7. Coustan-Smith E, Mullighan CG, Onciu M *et al.* Early T-cell precursor leukaemia: a subtype of very high-risk acute lymphoblastic leukaemia. *Lancet Oncol* 2009;**10**:147–56.

8. Rowe JM. Optimal management of adults with ALL. *Br J Haematol* 2009;**144**:468–83.

9. Rubnitz JE, Wichlan D, Devidas M *et al.* Prospective analysis of TEL gene rearrangements in childhood acute lymphoblastic leukaemia: a Children's Oncology Group study. *J Clin Oncol* 2008;**26**:2186–91.

10. Harrison CJ. Cytogenetics of paediatric and adolescent acute lymphoblastic leukaemia. *Br J Haematol* 2009;**144**:147–56.

11. Campana D, Behm FG. Immunophenotyping of leukemia. *J Immunol Methods* 2000;**243**:59–75.

12. Weerkamp F, Dekking E, Ng YY *et al.* Flow cytometric immunobead assay for the detection of BCR-ABL fusion proteins in leukemia patients. *Leukemia* 2009;**23**:1106–17.

13. Vardiman JW, Thiele J, Arber DA *et al.* The 2008 revision of the World Health Organization (WHO) classification of myeloid neoplasms and acute leukemia: rationale and important changes. *Blood* 2009;**114**:937–51.

14. Dworzak MN, Schumich A, Printz D *et al.* CD20 up-regulation in pediatric B-cell precursor acute lymphoblastic leukemia during induction treatment: setting the stage for anti-CD20 directed immunotherapy. *Blood* 2008;**112**:3982–8.

15. Mullighan CG, Miller CB, Radtke I *et al.* BCR-ABL1 lymphoblastic leukaemia is characterized by the deletion of *Ikaros*. *Nature* 2008;**453**:110–14.

16. Ottmann OG, Pfeifer H. First-line treatment of Philadelphia chromosome-positive acute lymphoblastic leukaemia in adults. *Curr Opin Oncol* 2009;**21** Suppl 1:S43–6.

17. Meyer C, Kowarz E, Hofmann J *et al.* New insights to the MLL recombinome of acute leukemias. *Leukemia* 2009;**23**:1490–9.

18. Pui CH, Chessells JM, Camitta B *et al.* Clinical heterogeneity in childhood acute lymphoblastic leukemia with 11q23 rearrangements. *Leukemia* 2003;**17**:700–6.

19. Sutcliffe MJ, Shuster JJ, Sather HN *et al.* High concordance from independent studies by the

Children's Cancer Group (CCG) and Pediatric Oncology Group (POG) associating favorable prognosis with combined trisomies 4, 10, and 17 in children with NCI Standard-Risk B-precursor Acute Lymphoblastic Leukemia: a Children's Oncology Group (COG) initiative. *Leukemia* 2005;**19**:734–40.

20. Nachman JB, Heerema NA, Sather H *et al.* Outcome of treatment in children with hypodiploid acute lymphoblastic leukemia. *Blood* 2007;**110**:1112–15.

21. Jeha S, Pei D, Raimondi SC *et al.* Increased risk for CNS relapse in pre-B cell leukemia with the t(1;19)/ *TCF3-PBX1*. *Leukemia* 2009;**23**:1406–9.

22. den Boer ML, van Slegtenhorst M, de Menezes RX *et al.* A subtype of childhood acute lymphoblastic leukaemia with poor treatment outcome: a genome-wide classification study. *Lancet Oncol* 2009;**10**:125–34.

23. Mullighan CG, Su X, Zhang J *et al.* Deletion of *IKZF1* and prognosis in acute lymphoblastic leukemia. *New Engl J Med* 2009;**360**:470–80.

24. Mullighan CG, Zhang J, Harvey RC *et al.* *JAK* mutations in high-risk childhood acute lymphoblastic leukemia. *Proc Natl Acad Sci USA* 2009;**106**:9414–18.

25. Ferrando AA, Neuberg DS, Staunton J *et al.* Gene expression signatures define novel oncogenic pathways in T cell acute lymphoblastic leukemia. *Cancer Cell* 2002;**1**:75–87.

26. Ferrando AA, Neuberg DS, Dodge RK *et al.* Prognostic importance of *TLX1* (*HOX11*) oncogene expression in adults with T-cell acute lymphoblastic leukaemia. *Lancet* 2004;**363**:535–6.

27. Weng AP, Ferrando AA, Lee W *et al.* Activating mutations of *NOTCH1* in human T cell acute lymphoblastic leukemia. *Science* 2004;**306**:269–71.

28. Larson GA, Chen Q, Kugel DS *et al.* The impact of *NOTCH1*, *FBW7* and *PTEN* mutations on prognosis and downstream signaling in pediatric T-cell acute lymphoblastic leukemia: a report from the Children's Oncology Group. *Leukemia* 2009;**23**:1417–25.

29. Baldus CD, Martus P, Burmeister T *et al.* Low *ERG* and *BAALC* expression identifies a new subgroup of adult acute T-lymphoblastic leukemia with a highly favorable outcome. *J Clin Oncol* 2007;**25**:3739–45.

30. Campana D. Status of minimal residual disease testing in childhood haematological malignancies. *Br J Haematol* 2008;**143**:481–9.

31. Gabert J, Beillard E, van der Velden V *et al.* Standardization and quality control studies of 'real-time' quantitative reverse transcriptase polymerase chain reaction of fusion gene transcripts for residual disease detection in leukemia – a Europe Against Cancer program. *Leukemia* 2003;**17**:2318–57.

32. van der Velden VH, van Dongen JJ. MRD detection in acute lymphoblastic leukemia patients using *Ig/TCR* gene rearrangements as targets for real-time quantitative PCR. *Methods Mol Biol* 2009;**538**:115–50.

33. Flohr T, Schrauder A, Cazzaniga G *et al.* Minimal residual disease-directed risk stratification using real-time quantitative PCR analysis of immunoglobulin and T-cell receptor gene rearrangements in the international multicenter trial AIEOP-BFM ALL 2000 for childhood acute lymphoblastic leukemia. *Leukemia* 2008;**22**:771–82.

34. Coustan-Smith E, Sancho J, Hancock ML *et al.* Use of peripheral blood instead of bone marrow to monitor residual disease in children with acute lymphoblastic leukemia. *Blood* 2002;**100**:2399–402.

35. Coustan-Smith E, Sancho J, Hancock ML *et al.* Clinical importance of minimal residual disease in childhood acute lymphoblastic leukemia. *Blood* 2000;**96**:2691–6.

36. Borowitz MJ, Devidas M, Hunger SP *et al.* Clinical significance of minimal residual disease in childhood acute lymphoblastic leukemia and its relationship to other prognostic factors. a Children's Oncology Group study. *Blood* 2008;**111**:5477–85.

37. Cave H, van der Werff ten Bosch J, Suciu S *et al.* Clinical significance of minimal residual disease in childhood acute lymphoblastic leukemia. European Organization for Research and Treatment of Cancer – Childhood Leukemia Cooperative Group. *New Engl J Med* 1998;**339**:591–8.

38. Dworzak MN, Froschl G, Printz D *et al.* Prognostic significance and modalities of flow cytometric minimal residual disease detection in childhood acute lymphoblastic leukemia. *Blood* 2002;**99**:1952–8.

39. Zhou J, Goldwasser MA, Li A *et al.* Quantitative analysis of minimal residual disease predicts relapse in children with B-lineage acute lymphoblastic leukemia in DFCI ALL Consortium Protocol 95–01. *Blood* 2007;**110**:1607–11.

40. Coustan-Smith E, Sancho J, Behm FG *et al.* Prognostic importance of measuring early clearance of leukemic cells by flow cytometry in childhood acute lymphoblastic leukemia. *Blood* 2002;**100**:52–8.

41. Coustan-Smith E, Ribeiro RC, Stow P *et al.* A simplified flow cytometric assay identifies children with acute lymphoblastic leukemia who have a superior clinical outcome. *Blood* 2006;**108**:97–102.

42. Campana D. Molecular determinants of treatment response in acute lymphoblastic leukemia. *Hematology Am Soc Hematol Educ Program* 2008;366–73.

43. Mullighan CG, Su X, Zhang J *et al.* Deletion of IKZF1 and prognosis in acute lymphoblastic leukemia. *New Engl J Med* 2009;**360**:470–80.

44. Mortuza FY, Papaioannou M, Moreira IM *et al.* Minimal residual disease tests provide an independent predictor of clinical outcome in adult acute lymphoblastic leukemia. *J Clin Oncol* 2002;**20**:1094–104.

45. Bruggemann M, Raff T, Flohr T *et al.* Clinical significance of minimal residual disease quantification in adult patients with standard-risk acute lymphoblastic leukemia. *Blood* 2006;**107**:1116–23.

46. Raff T, Gokbuget N, Luschen S *et al.* Molecular relapse in adult standard-risk ALL patients detected by prospective MRD monitoring during and after maintenance treatment: data from the GMALL 06/99 and 07/03 trials. *Blood* 2007;**109**:910–15.

47. Bassan R, Spinelli O, Oldani E *et al.* Improved risk classification for risk-specific therapy based on the molecular study of MRD in adult ALL. *Blood* 2009;**113**:4153–62.

48. Holowiecki J, Krawczyk-Kulis M, Giebel S *et al.* Status of minimal residual disease after induction predicts outcome in both standard and high-risk Ph-negative adult acute lymphoblastic leukaemia. The Polish Adult Leukemia Group ALL 4–2002 MRD Study. *Br J Haematol* 2008;**142**:227–37.

49. Wassmann B, Pfeifer H, Stadler M *et al.* Early molecular response to posttransplantation imatinib determines outcome in MRD+ Philadelphia-positive acute lymphoblastic leukemia (Ph+ ALL). *Blood* 2005;**106**:458–63.

50. Pui CH, Campana D, Pei D *et al.* Treating childhood acute lymphoblastic leukemia without cranial irradiation. *New Engl J Med* 2009;**360**:2730–41.

8 Acute myeloid leukemia

David Grimwade

Introduction

Acute myeloid leukemia (AML) encompasses a highly heterogeneous group of clonal disorders arising in hematopoietic progenitors that are characterized by a block in differentiation and outgrowth of myeloid blasts giving rise to bone marrow failure. Although AML is not particularly common, affecting approximately 3 individuals per 100 000 population per year in Western countries (i.e. ~2000 new cases per year in the UK), it is challenging and expensive to treat, representing a significant burden on healthcare systems. Given that AML is predominantly a disease of the elderly, with markedly higher incidence in individuals over 60 years of age, this disease is set to become an increasing problem as the population ages.

Molecular basis of AML

The last three decades have witnessed major advances in deciphering the cytogenetic and molecular lesions underlying the pathogenesis of AML. These have not only afforded significant insights into disease biology, but also proved helpful in providing prognostic information and underpinned the development of molecularly targeted and risk-stratified treatment approaches. A further benefit of improved understanding of the molecular basis of AML coupled with the development of sensitive quantitative polymerase chain techniques has been the possibility to assess treatment response at the submicroscopic level (i.e. detection of minimal residual disease, MRD), thereby affording the opportunity to tailor therapy more precisely to the needs of the individual patient.

Chromosomal abnormalities in AML

Approximately 60% of AML exhibit an abnormal karyotype, with the pattern of changes differing according to the age of presentation (reviewed in [1]). In children and younger adults, balanced chromosomal translocations are relatively common, while in older patients AML is more frequently associated with chromosomal losses and gains, often in the context of a complex karyotype. To date, over a hundred recurring balanced chromosomal rearrangements associated with AML have been characterized at the molecular level [2]. Such rearrangements typically lead to the formation of chimeric fusion proteins, which play a key role in mediating the leukemic phenotype. A significant proportion of chromosomal rearrangements disrupt genes encoding transcription factors which are involved in the regulation of normal hematopoiesis (reviewed in [3]). Notable examples include genes encoding the α and β subunits of the heterodimeric core binding factor (CBF) complex disrupted by the t(8;21)(q22;q22) and the inv(16)(p13q22)/t(16;16)(p13;q22) rearrangements, respectively, and which between them, occur in ~13% of AML cases arising in younger adults (Figure 8.1). These chromosomal abnormalities lead to formation of the *AML1* (*CBFα2/RUNX1*)-*ETO* (*RUNX1T1*) and *CBFβ-MYH11* fusions (Figure 8.1) and predict a relatively favorable prognosis (Figure 8.2). Another hematopoietic transcription factor gene targeted in AML is *RARA* (retinoic acid receptor alpha) resulting from rearrangements of 17q21 in acute promyelocytic leukemia (APL). Seven fusion partners of *RARA* have been identified to date [4], with the vast majority (>95%) involving the *PML* gene as a result of the t(15;17)(q22;q12–21), which accounts for ~10% of AML arising in children and younger adults (Figure 8.1). Chromosomal rearrangements involving 3q26, such as inv(3)(q21q26)/t(3;3)(q21;q26) are associated with up-regulation of the transcription factor EVI1, occur in ~2% of AML and predict a dismal prognosis [5] (Figure 8.2).

Diagnostic Techniques in Hematological Malignancies, ed. Wendy N. Erber. Published by Cambridge University Press.
© Cambridge University Press 2010.

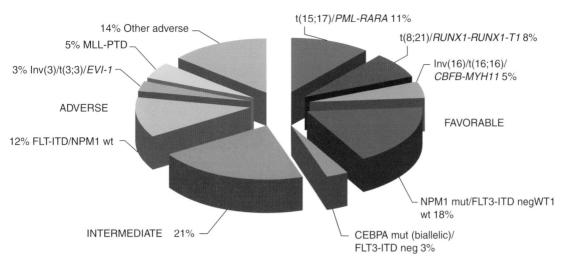

Figure 8.1. Frequency of prognostically relevant molecular and cytogenetic subgroups of AML arising in younger adults.
Frequencies of the various entities specified in Table 8.5 are based on a synthesis of published data [14,21,23,25,28–31] and analysis of adults with
AML entered into the MRC AML10 and 12 trials [32].
Reproduced courtesy of the American Society of Hematology (Grimwade D, Hills RK. Independent prognostic factors for AML outcome.
Hematology Am Soc Hematol Educ Program 2009; 385–95) with permission.

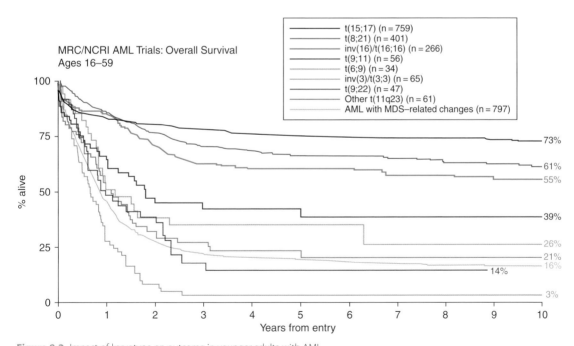

Figure 8.2. Impact of karyotype on outcome in younger adults with AML.
Overall survival is shown for adults with AML (median age 43 years, range 16–59) treated in successive Medical Research Council/National Cancer
Research Institute trials (MRC AML10, AML12, AML15) according to cytogenetic entities specified in the 2008 WHO classification [36]. All
patients with t(15;17) received an extended course of ATRA in addition to anthracycline-based chemotherapy.
Reproduced courtesy of the American Society of Hematology (Grimwade D, Hills RK. Independent prognostic factors for AML outcome.
Hematology Am Soc Hematol Educ Program 2009; 385 95) with permission.

Retention of dimerization and/or DNA-binding domains within the chimeric fusion proteins generated by AML-associated balanced chromosomal rearrangements can deregulate downstream target genes and impact on the pathways in which the respective translocation partners normally function. A growing family of oncogenic fusion proteins, which include those involving *TEL* (*ETV6*) as a result of 12p translocations (present in ~1% of AML), *RUNX1* and *RARA* have been shown to recruit nuclear co-repressor complexes including histone deacetylase. This leads to transcriptional repression of genes implicated in normal hematopoietic differentiation (reviewed in [6]). Involvement of genes that encode proteins with a direct influence on chromatin remodeling, or with transcriptional regulatory properties, provides another recurring theme in the development of AML. Amongst this group are rearrangements disrupting genes encoding *MOZ*, *TIF2*, p300 and *CBP*, as well as translocations involving 11q23 leading to rearrangements of the mixed lineage leukemia (*MLL*) gene [7]. Over 50 *MLL* fusion gene partners have been characterized to date, with the most common in AML (occurring in ~3% of cases) being *MLLT3* (*AF9*), *MLLT1* (*ENL*), *MLLT10* (*AF10*), *MLLT4* (*AF6*) and *ELL*, as a result of translocations involving 9p22, 19p13.3, 10p11~13, 6q27 and 19p13.1, respectively [8]. Deregulation of class I homeobox (*HOX*) genes, which encode transcription factors that play a key role in pattern formation and organogenesis during embryonic development, as well as contributing to the organization and regulation of hematopoiesis, is a common feature in AML pathogenesis. AML-associated translocations also involve genes encoding components of the nuclear pore complex, which plays a role in transport between nucleus and cytoplasm, i.e. *NUP98* and *CAN* (*NUP214*) disrupted respectively by translocations involving 11p15 and by 9q34 rearrangements, notably the t(6;9)(p23;q34) giving rise to the *DEK-NUP214* fusion, present in ~1% of AML [9].

Molecular mechanisms in AML cases with unbalanced chromosomal abnormalities remain poorly understood. Leukemias with particular trisomies have been found to be enriched for specific mutations, for example presence of partial tandem duplications of the *MLL* gene in the context of +11 [10]. Approximately 15% of AML cases that lack balanced chromosomal abnormalities have a complex karyotype, often associated with partial or complete loss of chromosomes 5 and/or 7 [1]. Defining the genes implicated in the development of myelodysplasia (MDS) and AML characterized by deletions of the long arms of chromosome 5 and 7 has been the subject of intense research interest for many years. Haplosufficiency of a number of genes appears likely to play an important role in disease pathogenesis, with recent studies implicating α-catenin and *RPS14* in MDS/AML with 5q deletions [11–13]. Complex karyotype predicts a very poor prognosis in AML and abnormalities of p53 are particularly common in this group.

Molecular genetics of AML

A substantial proportion of AML cases (~40%) have a normal karyotype. In recent years there have been significant advances in defining genomic variations of pathogenic and independent prognostic relevance in this group of patients, with mutation status of the genes encoding Fms-like tyrosine kinase 3 (*FLT3*), nucleophosmin (*NPM1*) and CCAAT/enhancer binding protein alpha (*CEBPA*) shown to be of major importance (reviewed [14]).

FLT3 is a receptor tyrosine kinase expressed on hematopoietic progenitors, which is mutated in approximately a third of AML, including those with normal karyotype (reviewed [15]). The majority of mutations are internal tandem duplications (ITDs) that lead to in-frame insertions within the juxta-membrane region of the receptor. Less frequent are mutations involving the region encoding the activation loop (tyrosine kinase domain, TKD), which most commonly affect codons aspartate 835 and isoleucine 836 (D835/I836), found in approximately 7% of patients with AML [15]. Both classes of mutation lead to constitutive activation of the receptor and are associated with higher presenting white blood cell counts (WBC) [15,16]. While there are conflicting data concerning the prognostic implications of the TKD mutations [16–18], studies have consistently found that presence of FLT3-ITD provides a major independent adverse prognostic indicator, associated with an increased risk of relapse and poorer overall survival [14,15]. Worse outcomes are observed in those patients with high FLT3-ITD allelic ratios [19–21] indicative of homozygous mutations generated by acquired uniparental disomy (UPD) [22].

The discovery by Falini and colleagues in 2005 that one-third of AML cases, including approximately 50% with normal karyotype, harbor heterozygous mutations in the carboxy-terminus of the nucleolar phosphoprotein, nucleophosmin (*NPM1*) [23] provided a major step forward in understanding the molecular genetics of this disease. Over 40 mutations have been described. These lead to gain of a nuclear export signal combined with loss of at least one of the tryptophan residues at positions 288 and 290 that are involved in nucleolar targeting. These act in concert to delocalize the protein to the cytoplasm (designated NPMc+ AML) [24]. The majority of cases exhibit the Type A mutation (70–80%), with Types B and D accounting for a further 10% and 5% each. There is increasing evidence that *NPM1* mutations represent primary lesions in leukemogenesis, being mutually exclusive of balanced translocations [25]. Interestingly, *NPM1* mutation and FLT3-ITD commonly co-exist in normal karyotype AML, suggesting that they may cooperate in generating the leukemic phenotype. Presence of an *NPM1* mutation is associated with monocytic blast cell morphology and higher presenting WBC, even allowing for *FLT3* mutation status [24].

CEBPA, a transcription factor involved in normal myelopoiesis, is mutated in approximately 10% of AML, and particularly cases with a normal karyotype [3]. Mutations commonly involve the amino-terminal region of CEBPA, leading to expression of a truncated protein, or the carboxy-terminus, disrupting regions required for dimerization and/or DNA binding. In a significant proportion of AML cases with *CEBPA* mutations, both alleles are involved. These may be homozygous mutations resulting from acquired UPD involving the *CEPBA* locus on chromosome 19 [22] or biallelic compound heterozygous mutations involving amino- and carboxy-terminal regions. Interestingly, it has emerged that some patients harbour a germline mutation in *CEBPA*, with acquisition of a second mutation involved in progression to AML [26]. In a proportion of AML cases, the *CEBPA* locus has been shown to be inactivated by an alternative mechanism involving epigenetic silencing [27]. A number of studies have reported that *CEBPA* mutations predict a relatively favorable outcome in AML [14,28,29]. More recent reports, which have considered larger patient cohorts, suggest this effect relates to the group with biallelic mutations, who tend to have a normal karyotype and lack FLT3-ITD mutations [30,31].

A number of other recurring mutations have been identified in AML patients. *RAS* mutations are relatively common, occurring in ~15% of cases, with evidence to date suggesting that they are prognostically neutral (reviewed in [14]). Whereas, partial tandem duplications in the *MLL* gene and mutations in the Wilms' Tumor (*WT1*) gene, each found in ~10% of normal karyotype AML, have been associated with a poor prognosis (reviewed in [32]). Mutations in the *TET2* gene have recently been identified in ~10% of AML [33], including a quarter with secondary disease [34], and may also confer a poor prognosis [33]. Other recurrent mutation targets in AML include *PTPN11*, *RUNX1*, *CBL*, IDH1 and IDH2. Although mutations in the *KIT* gene are relatively uncommon in AML as a whole, they occur in ~25% of CBF leukemia and have been associated with a significantly poorer prognosis (reviewed in [35]).

Factors predisposing to AML

In the vast majority of AML patients, the disease arises spontaneously, with no known predisposing factors. However, a number of genetic abnormalities are now recognized to confer a significant risk for the development of AML (Table 8.1). The most common of these is Down syndrome with trisomy 21, which in conjunction with acquired mutation in the *GATA1* gene predisposes to the development of a myeloproliferative disorder during early childhood. This can resolve spontaneously (transient abnormal myelopoiesis) or progress to acute megakaryoblastic leukemia [36]. Familial AML is extremely rare and has been associated with mutations in genes encoding the hematopoietic transcription factors CEBPA and RUNX1, with the latter being associated with Familial Platelet Disorder (reviewed in [37]). Various bone marrow failure syndromes predispose to AML, including Shwachman–Diamond, associated with a ribosomal protein gene defect, dyskeratosis congenita and Fanconi anemia (reviewed in [38]). Mutations in the *FANCA* gene account for ~65% of Fanconi anemia, associated with a 35–50% risk of progression to AML by 40 years of age [39]. Defects in genes encoding other proteins involved in DNA damage and repair responses also predispose to AML, which include *BLM* and *TP53* in Bloom's and Li Fraumeni syndromes, respectively [37].

Approximately 25–35% of AML cases evolve from a prior hematological condition, particularly MDS and myeloproliferative neoplasms [36,40]. A further 10–15% of AML arise following exposure to DNA-damaging agents [41]. Therapy-related leukemias are emerging as an increasing healthcare problem as more patients survive their primary cancers following treatment with chemotherapy and/or radiotherapy. The disease characteristics of therapy-related leukemias

Table 8.1. Factors predisposing to the development of secondary acute myeloid leukemia (AML).

Genetic predisposition
  Down syndrome
  Fanconi anemia

Other inherited bone marrow failure syndromes:
  Shwachman–Diamond
  Diamond–Blackfan
  Kostmann's
  Familial platelet disorder
  Dyskeratosis congenita

DNA repair defects e.g. Bloom's syndrome

Other tumor predisposition syndromes e.g. Li–Fraumeni

Prior hematologic disorder
  Chronic myeloid leukemia
  Other myeloproliferative disorders
  Myelodysplastic syndrome
  Paroxysmal nocturnal hemoglobinuria

Exposure to environmental or therapeutic agents
  Chronic exposure to benzene and derivatives
  Ionizing radiation
  Chemotherapeutic agents
    Alkylating agents
    Topoisomerase II targeting drugs

tend to differ according to the causative agent. Exposure to alkylating agents is associated with development of MDS/AML characterized by loss of chromosome 5 and/or 7 material after a latency period of several years. Whereas, secondary leukemias arising following treatment with agents targeting topoisomerase II, including epipodophyllotoxins (e.g. etoposide), anthracyclines (e.g. epirubicin) and anthracenediones (e.g. mitoxantrone) exhibit a shorter latency period (typically 1–4 years) and are characterized by balanced translocations, particularly involving *MLL* at 11q23, *NUP98* at 11p15, *RUNX1* at 21q22 and *RARA* at 17q21 [36,41]. However, a significant proportion of patients developing t-MDS/AML have been exposed to multiple chemotherapy drugs as well as radiotherapy, making it difficult to identify the causative agent with any certainty. There is considerable interest in investigating whether particular individuals might be at risk of developing therapy-related leukemias. A number of studies have suggested that various polymorphisms that affect drug metabolism and detoxification may affect susceptibility (reviewed in [41]).

Classification of AML

The first classification systems for AML were developed by the French, American and British (FAB)

collaborative group over 30 years ago, defining eight subtypes (designated AML FAB M0-M7) based upon morphological features, apparent maturity of leukemic blasts and lineage involvement [42]. However, with improved understanding of the biology of AML, the FAB system has been superseded by the classification schemes developed by the World Health Organization (WHO) [36,43]. The 2001 WHO classification for the first time defined subsets of AML according to the underlying cytogenetic/molecular lesion, i.e. APL with t(15;17);*PML-RARA* and its molecular variants, CBF leukemia with t(8;21); *RUNX1-RUNX1T1 (AML1-ETO)* or inv(16)/t(16;16); *CBFB-MYH11* and AML with 11q23/*MLL* translocations were specifically recognized as disease entities. AML with MDS-related features and therapy-related leukemias arising following exposure to alkylating agents/radiotherapy or drugs targeting topoisomerase II were also defined [43]. A morphological classification was retained to categorize cases not falling into one of these "specific" clinical, morphological or cytogenetic groups. These morphological groups were based on the FAB categories M0, M1, M2, M4, M5, M6 and M7. Three new categories were added, namely acute basophilic leukemia, acute panmyelosis with marrow fibrosis and myeloid sarcoma. A major difference between the FAB and WHO classifications lies in the minimum bone marrow blast percentage used as a "cut-off" to separate MDS from AML, with the WHO system dropping the FAB threshold of blast cells from 30% to 20%. Indeed for cases with clonal abnormalities in the form of t(15;17)(q22;q12–21), inv (16) or t(8;21), a diagnosis of AML can be made irrespective of blast percentage according to the WHO system.

The WHO classification system was updated in 2008 (Table 8.2) [36]. In this the list of cytogenetic abnormalities defining "AML with recurrent genetic abnormalities" was expanded to include t(3;3)(q21; q26)/inv(3)(q21q26);*RPN1-EVI1* and t(6;9)(p23; q34);*DEK-NUP214*, both of which occur in 1–2% of AML and have characteristic morphological features. AML with t(1;22)(p13;q13);*RBM15-MKL1* was also included; this is a very rare entity associated with acute megakaryoblastic leukemia in infancy. In addition AML t(9;11)(p22;q23) with *MLLT3-MLL* fusion, which occurs in ~1% of AML, was distinguished from cases with other 11q23 abnormalities. The new WHO classification also lists a number of cytogenetic abnormalities which can be used to define AML

Table 8.2. WHO classification (2008) of acute myeloid leukemia (AML) and related precursor neoplasms and acute leukemias of ambiguous lineage (adapted from references [36,46]).

Acute myeloid leukemia (AML) with recurrent genetic abnormalities
 AML with t(8;21)(q22;q22); *RUNX1-RUNX1T1*
 AML with inv(16)(p13.1q22) or t(16;16)(p13.1;q22); *CBFB-MYH11*
 Acute promyelocytic leukemia (APL) with t(15;17)(q22;q12); *PML-RARA*[a]
 AML with t(9;11)(p22;q23); *MLLT3-MLL*[b]
 AML with t(6;9)(p23;q34); *DEK-NUP214*
 AML with inv(3)(q21q26.2) or t(3;3)(q21;q26.2); *RPN1-EVI1*
 AML (megakaryoblastic) with t(1;22)(p13;q13); *RBM15-MKL1*
 Provisional entity: AML with mutated NPM1
 Provisional entity: AML with mutated CEBPA

AML with myelodysplasia-related changes[c]

Therapy-related myeloid neoplasms[d]

AML, not otherwise specified (NOS)
 AML with minimal differentiation
 AML without maturation
 AML with maturation
 Acute myelomonocytic leukemia
 Acute monoblastic/monocytic leukemia
 Acute erythroid leukemia
  Pure erythroid leukemia
  Erythroleukemia, erythroid/myeloid
 Acute megakaryoblastic leukemia
 Acute basophilic leukemia
 Acute panmyelosis with myelofibrosis (acute myelofibrosis; acute myelosclerosis)

Myeloid sarcoma (extramedullary myeloid tumor; granulocytic sarcoma; chloroma)

Myeloid proliferations related to Down syndrome
 Transient abnormal myelopoiesis (transient myeloproliferative disorder)
 Myeloid leukemia associated with Down syndrome

Blastic plasmacytoid dendritic cell neoplasm

Acute leukemias of ambiguous lineage
 Acute undifferentiated leukemia
 Mixed phenotype acute leukemia with t(9;22)(q34;q11.2); *BCR-ABL1*[e]
 Mixed phenotype acute leukemia with t(v;11q23); *MLL* rearranged
 Mixed phenotype acute leukemia, B/myeloid, NOS
 Mixed phenotype acute leukemia, T/myeloid, NOS
 Provisional entity: Natural-killer (NK) cell lymphoblastic leukemia/lymphoma

For a diagnosis of AML, a marrow blast count of ≥ 20% is required, except for AML with the recurrent genetic abnormalities t(15;17), t(8;21), inv (16) or t(16;16) and some cases of erythroleukemia.
[a] Other recurring translocations involving *RARA* should be reported accordingly: i.e. APL with t(11;17)(q23;q12)/*ZBTB16-RARA*, with t(11;17)(q13; q12)/*NUMA1-RARA*, t(5;17)(5q35;q12)/*NPM1-RARA*, t(4;17)(q12;q21)/*FIP1L1-RARA*, *STAT5B-RARA* and *PRKAR1A-RARA* (fusion partners located on 17q).
[b] Other translocations involving *MLL* should be reported accordingly: e.g. AML with t(6;11)(q27;q23); *MLLT4-MLL*; AML with t(11;19)(q23;p13.3); *MLL-MLLT1*; AML with t(11;19)(q23;p13.1); *MLL-ELL*; AML with t(10;11)(p12;q23); *MLLT10-MLL*.
[c] >20% blood or marrow blasts *and* any of the following: previous history of myelodysplastic syndrome (MDS), or myelodysplastic/ myeloproliferative neoplasm (MDS/MPN); myelodysplasia-related cytogenetic abnormality (see below); multi-lineage dysplasia; *and* absence of both prior cytotoxic therapy for unrelated disease and aforementioned recurring genetic abnormalities; cytogenetic abnormalities sufficient to diagnose AML with myelodysplasia-related changes are:
– complex karyotype (defined as three or more chromosomal abnormalities
– unbalanced changes: −7 or del(7q); −5 or del(5q); i(17q) or t(17p); −13 or del(13q); del(11q); del(12p) or t(12p); del(9q); idic(X)(q13);
– balanced changes: t(11;16)(q23;p13.3); t(3;21)(q26.2;q22.1); t(1;3)(p36.3;q21.1); t(2;11)(p21;q23); t(5;12)(q33;p12); t(5;7)(q33;q11.2); t(5;17)(q33; p13); t(5;10)(q33;q21); t(3;5)(q25;q34).
[d] Cytotoxic agents implicated in therapy-related hematologic neoplasms: alkylating agents; ionizing radiation therapy; agents targeting topoisomerase II; others.
[e] *BCR-ABL1*-positive leukemia may present as mixed phenotype acute leukemia, but should be treated as *BCR-ABL1*-positive acute lymphoblastic leukemia.

cases as "MDS-related" even in the absence of dysplastic features (see legend to Table 8.2). Two molecular genetic abnormalities, i.e. mutation of the *NPM1* and *CEBPA* genes, were introduced into the classification as provisional disease entities (Table 8.2). Criteria used to define therapy-related leukemias were altered, with no distinction between cases arising following alkylating agents, radiotherapy or drugs targeting topoisomerase II, recognizing that patients are often exposed to combination therapy. Myeloid proliferations arising in patients with Down syndrome were also considered as separate entities.

Investigations to diagnose AML

Morphological assessment of peripheral blood and bone marrow

A range of tests is required to establish the diagnosis and classify cases of AML according to the WHO classification (Table 8.3). Figures 8.3–8.6 illustrate diagnostic morphological, phenotypic and genetic features of a range of AML subtypes. Morphological analysis of peripheral blood (PB) and bone marrow (BM) smears stained with Wright Giemsa or May–Grünwald Giemsa is clearly the first step in investigating a patient with suspected AML. Bone marrow aspirates should be examined for morphological classification and identification of multi-lineage dysplasia. Cytochemistry using myeloperoxidase (MPO) or Sudan black B stain, and a combined esterase stain to confirm myeloid lineage involvement and subclassification may be performed, but are not essential and now rarely required. This is particularly so if flow cytometry is performed for cytoplasmic MPO. However, a toluidine blue stain is necessary to establish a suspected diagnosis of acute basophilic leukemia [44]. In cases of suspected APL, immunocytochemical staining of BM smears (or PB smears for cases with circulating leukemic cells) using monoclonal or polyclonal antibodies to PML protein is particularly valuable as a rapid diagnostic test for presence of the PML-RARA fusion (evidenced by microspeckled nuclear staining pattern); this indicates those patients who are likely to benefit from molecularly targeted therapies i.e. all-*trans* retinoic acid (ATRA) and arsenic trioxide (ATO) (Figure 8.3d).

A bone marrow trephine is indicated in patients in whom bone marrow aspiration yields a "dry tap." A trephine biopsy is essential to detect marrow fibrosis and may facilitate identification of presence of multi-lineage dysplasia (defined as ≥50% dysplastic cells in two of erythroid, megakaryocytic and granulocytic/monocytic lineages) in conjunction with the aspirate. A diagnosis of acute panmyelosis with marrow fibrosis can only be made with a trephine, requiring immunocytochemistry with antibodies identifying CD34, MPO, glycophorin and megakaryocyte antigens (CD61 or Factor VIII) to identify and quantify the blast percentage and multi-lineage involvement [44]. Bone marrow trephines should be avoided in patients with suspected APL due to the associated coagulopathy and risk of hemorrhagic complications [45].

Immunophenotyping

Immunophenotyping should utilize a minimum of three-color flow cytometry and is essential for establishing a diagnosis of AML in cases that are negative for cytochemical MPO, e.g. AML with minimal differentiation and acute megakaryoblastic leukemia [44]. Both surface and intracellular antigens should be studied. Standard panels have been published which can be applied in the diagnosis of AML and acute leukemias with mixed phenotype, such as those detailed in the European LeukemiaNet guidelines and in Chapter 3 [46] (Table 8.4). It is important to be aware that cross-lineage expression of lymphoid markers in AML is relatively common (reviewed in [46]). Indeed, expression of B-lineage-affiliated antigens CD19 and CD79a in AML with t(8;21)(q22; q22);*RUNX1-RUNX1T1* is well recognized, while the T-lineage-associated antigen CD2 has been reported in inv(16)(p13.1;q22);*CBFB-MYH11*-associated AML and in APL, particularly the hypogranular variant form. Cross-lineage antigen expression is one of the features used to define leukemia-associated aberrant immunophenotypes (LAIPs) used for detection of minimal residual disease (MRD) (reviewed in [47]). Identification of LAIPs requires diagnostic material to be analyzed in specialist reference laboratories with more extensive antibody panels based on at least 4-color technology. Panels are being amended as 6–10 color technology becomes more widely available, which should enhance the reliability of flow cytometry-based approaches to MRD detection.

Table 8.3. Test/procedures to establish baseline status of acute myeloid leukemia (AML).

Test/Procedure	General practice	Clinical trial
Tests to establish the diagnosis		
Full blood count and differential, blood film	Yes	Yes
Bone marrow aspirate	Yes	Yes
Bone marrow trephine biopsy	Optional[a]	Optional[a]
Immunophenotyping	Yes	Yes
Cytogenetics	Yes	Yes
RUNX1-RUNX1T1, *CBFB-MYH11*, or other gene fusion screening	Optional[b]	Yes[b]
PML-RARA RT-PCR, PML immunofluorescence test	Yes[c]	Yes[c]
Additional tests/procedures at diagnosis		
Demographics and medical history[d]	Yes	Yes
Performance status (ECOG/WHO score)	Yes	Yes
Analysis of co-morbidities	Yes	Yes
Biochemistry, coagulation tests, urine analysis[e]	Yes	Yes
Serum pregnancy test[f]	Yes	Yes
Information on oocyte and sperm cryopreservation	Optional[g]	Optional[g]
HLA-typing, CMV testing	Optional[h]	Optional[h]
Hepatitis A, B, C; HIV-1 testing	Yes	Yes
Chest X-ray, 12-lead ECG; echocardiography (on indication)	Yes	Yes
Lumbar puncture[i]	No	No
Biobanking[j]	Optional[j]	Yes
Prognostic marker assessment		
NPM1, *CEBPA*, *FLT3* gene mutation	Optional[k]	Yes
WT1, *RUNX1*, *MLL*, *TET2*, *KIT*, *RAS*, *TP53*, IDH1, IDH2 gene mutation	No	Investigational
ERG, *MN1*, *EVI1*, *BAALC* gene expression	No	Investigational
Identification of markers for MRD detection	No	Investigational

Adapted from European LeukemiaNet AML Guidelines [46].

[a] Recommended in patients with a dry tap, but not recommended in patients with suspected acute promyelocytic leukemia (APL).

[b] Should be performed if chromosome morphology is of poor quality, if there is typical morphology but the suspected cytogenetic abnormality is not present and if patient is eligible for intensive therapy including allogeneic transplantation.

[c] Recommended in patients with suspected APL. In the presence of the PML-RARA fusion, PML immunofluorescence test shows a characteristic microspeckled staining pattern in leukemic blasts (see Figure 8.3d).

[d] Including age, occupation, race or ethnicity, family history, previous exposure to toxic agents, history of hematologic disorder or malignancy, therapy for prior malignancy, information on smoking.

[e] *Biochemistry*: glucose, sodium, potassium, calcium, creatinine, aspartate amino transferase (AST), alanine amino transferase (ALT), alkaline phosphatase, lactate dehydrogenase, bilirubin, urea, total protein, uric acid, total cholesterol, total triglycerides, creatinine phosphokinase (CPK). *Coagulation tests*: prothrombin time (PTT), international normalized ratio (INR) where indicated, activated partial thromboplastin time (aPTT), thrombin time. *Urine analysis*: pH, glucose, erythrocytes, leukocytes, protein, nitrite.

[f] In women with childbearing potential.

[g] Cryopreservation to be undertaken in accordance with the wish of the patient.

[h] HLA typing and CMV testing should be performed in those patients eligible for allogeneic stem cell transplantation.

[i] Required in patients with clinical symptoms suspicious of central nervous system involvement; patient should be evaluated by imaging study for intracranial bleeding, leptomeningeal disease, and mass lesion; lumbar puncture considered optional in other settings (e.g. high WBC count).

[j] Pretreatment leukemic bone marrow and blood sample and constitutional DNA. Biobanking should also be performed in general practice if at all possible.

[k] Strongly encouraged in AML with normal karyotype.

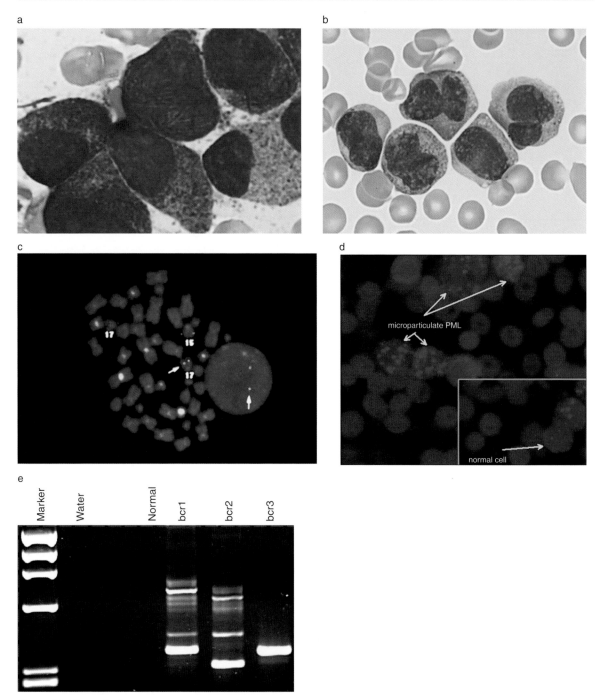

Figure 8.3. Diagnosis of acute promyelocytic leukemia.

a. Blasts of classical (hypergranular) acute promyelocytic leukemia (FAB type M3). A "faggot cell" with bundles of Auer rods can be seen.

b. Hypogranular variant (M3v) form of acute promyelocytic leukemia.

c. Detection of *PML-RARA* fusion gene by fluorescence *in situ* hybridization (FISH) using locus-specific cosmid probes in an APL case where fusion was the result of an interstitial insertion of chromosome 15-derived material including *PML* (green) within the *RARA* locus (red) on chromosome 17, leading to a fusion signal (arrow) and "split" *RARA* signal. (FISH analysis performed by Patricia Gorman, Cancer Research UK, London.)

d. Detection of presence of PML-RARA by PML immunofluorescence test, revealed by microspeckled nuclear staining pattern of PML antibody (PG-M3) as compared to discrete pattern of nuclear dots in cells lacking PML-RARA fusion (inset panel). (Figure provided by Dr. Sylvie Freeman, University of Birmingham.)

e. Detection of *PML-RARA* by RT-PCR. Multiplex PCR using breakpoint specific primers identifies the three main types of fusion transcript.

a

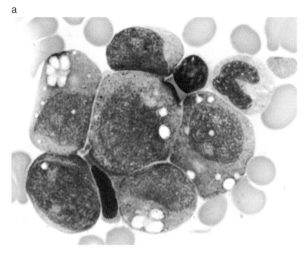

b

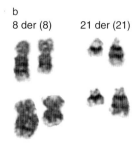

8 der (8)   21 der (21)

Figure 8.4. AML with t(8;21)(q22;q22); *RUNX1-RUNX1T1* (*AML1-ETO*). a. Bone marrow morphology showing myeloblasts with maturation to promyelocytes and myelocytes. b. G-banding partial karyotype of t(8;21)(q22;q22) showing the normal (left) and derivative rearranged (right) chromosomes 8 and 21.

Cytogenetic analysis

As discussed previously, conventional cytogenetics has a critical role in the analysis of AML; for technical details the reader is referred to Chapter 4. Cytogenetics serves to:

1. Identify a number of chromosomal abnormalities that confirm a clinical diagnosis of AML irrespective of the BM blast percentage (see Table 8.2).
2. Distinguish subgroups of patients who may benefit from molecularly targeted therapies (i.e. ATRA and ATO in APL with t(15;17);*PML-RARA* and imatinib in Ph-positive leukemias).
3. Provides key independent prognostic information (reviewed in [1]).

Therefore cytogenetics is a *mandatory* component of the routine diagnostic work-up for AML [46]. Cytogenetic analysis is best conducted using pre-treatment BM aspirate samples, although abnormal karyotypes can be established from PB specimens where the former are unevaluable. Analysis of at least 20 evaluable metaphases is required for the diagnosis of normal karyotype AML and examination of a comparable number of metaphases is recommended to define an abnormal karyotype [46].

Fluorescence *in situ* hybridization (FISH) can detect a number of AML-associated genetic abnormalities, including *PML-RARA*, *RUNX1-RUNX1T1*, *CBFB-MYH11*, *MLL* fusions, *BCR-ABL*, *EVI-1*, complex karyotypes and loss of *TP53*. It can be used to:

1. Identify abnormalities which may establish the diagnosis of AML.
2. Help inform treatment approach.
3. Predict clinical outcome.

It can either be performed as a primary diagnostic test or reserved for when karyotyping fails. The latter approach necessitates fixed cell pellets being stored routinely for subsequent analysis. The most appropriate FISH tests to be conducted (i.e. which probes to use) in any given patient may be influenced by:

1. The presence of suggestive morphological features indicative of a particular disease entity (e.g. M4Eo morphology predicting presence of *CBFB-MYH11* fusion).
2. Clinical characteristics of the patient (e.g. marked coagulopathy in APL with *PML-RARA* fusion).
3. Other known mutations.

Extensive laboratory tests are not indicated in patients with confirmed AML and poor performance status in whom curative therapy is not planned. There is also little value in performing FISH analyses in patients already shown to have AML with mutations in *NPM1* or *CEBPA*, as these do not occur with any frequency in AML with balanced chromosomal rearrangements or a complex karyotype. In patients with a relevant family history and/or suggestive clinical features detected on physical examination (e.g. café au lait spots, skeletal abnormalities) additional cytogenetic

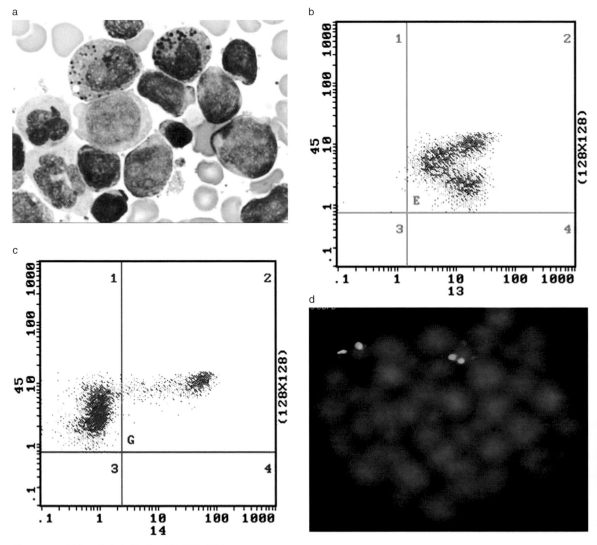

Figure 8.5. AML with inv(16)(p13.1q22); *CBFB-MYH11*.
a. Bone marrow morphology showing myeloblasts, a monoblast, granulocytic differentiation and abnormal baso-eosinophil precursors.
b. Flow cytometry showing three sub-populations of blast cells based on varying intensity of CD13 and CD45 antigen expression.
c. Flow cytometry showing the subpopulation of blast cells with strongest CD45 positivity to express CD14 monocyte-associated antigen (monoblasts).
d. Metaphase FISH for *CBFB* using a breakapart probe showing the normal red/green fusion signal and a rearranged *CBFB* (separated red and green signals) on the abnormal chromosome 16.

tests should be performed, looking for evidence of chromosomal instability (diepoxybutane/mitomycin-c stress test) [48].

Routine molecular diagnostics

Molecular diagnostic assays are best performed on nucleic acid extracted from BM samples. When marrow is not available, fusion genes and mutations can generally be reliably identified using blood (particularly if blasts predominate). Ideally DNA and RNA should be extracted and viable cells stored; however, where cell numbers are limiting RNA extraction should be prioritized, as this is suitable for molecular screening for fusion genes and leukemia-associated mutations. Ideally diagnostic material should be stored for future research, along with constitutional DNA extracted from buccal swabs or other non-leukemic tissue, subject to appropriate ethical approval and informed patient consent.

Molecular screening for chimeric fusion genes

PML-RARA fusion gene: When APL is suspected molecular analysis for the *PML-RARA* fusion gene should be performed. This should be done irrespective of patient age to identify those likely to benefit from molecularly targeted therapies (ATRA and ATO) and to establish the *PML* breakpoint location necessary for subsequent MRD detection [45].

RUNX1-RUNX1T1 and CBFB-MYH11 fusion genes: Molecular screening for presence of these fusion genes is also relevant in younger non-APL patients who are suitable for intensive treatment approaches including allogeneic transplantation. This is important as the overt cytogenetic lesion is not detected in ~10% of cases with CBF leukemia due to cryptic, simple variant or more complex rearrangements or cytogenetic failures (reviewed in [1]). Cases that are molecularly positive in the absence of the associated cytogenetic lesion should be subject to confirmation by reverse transcriptase polymerase chain reaction (RT-PCR) performed

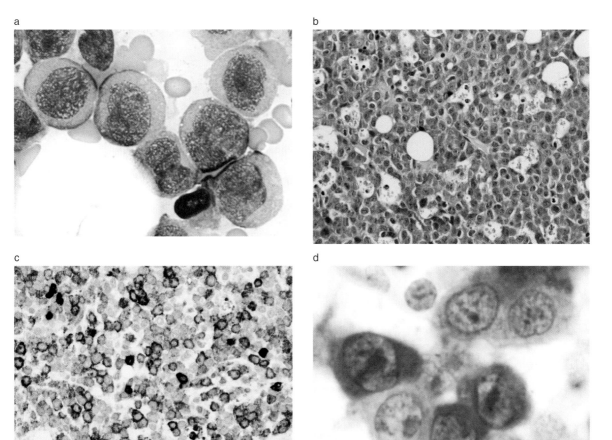

Figure 8.6. Acute monoblastic leukemia with *NPM1* exon 12 mutation.
a. Bone marrow aspirate morphology showing monoblasts.
b. Bone marrow trephine showing a monomorphic blast cell infiltrate of intermediate sized cells (hematoxylin and eosin (H&E)).
c. CD15 positivity of the myeloblasts in the bone marrow trephine (immunoperoxidase stain).
d. Cytoplasmic localization of NPM (immuno-alkaline phosphatase staining) of the bone marrow trephine biopsy.
e. Melt curve analysis for *NPM1* exon 12 mutations showing normal wildtype single peaks (red). Three AML samples with *NPM1* mutations (other colors) have different melt profiles corresponding to the presence of mutant and wildtype alleles.
f. High resolution capillary gel electrophoresis for *NPM1* exon 12 mutations. PCR amplification of DNA containing the *NPM1* exon 12 mutation yields a PCR product (*) that is four base pairs longer than the wildtype allele. (Red peaks are size markers).

e

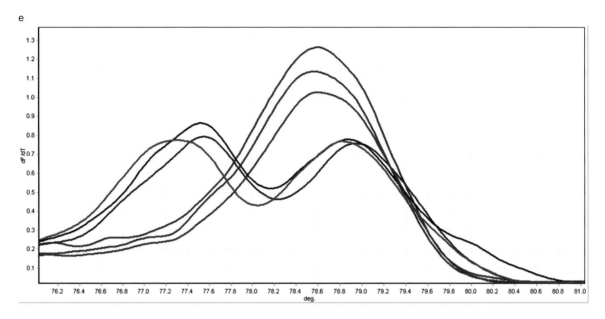

f

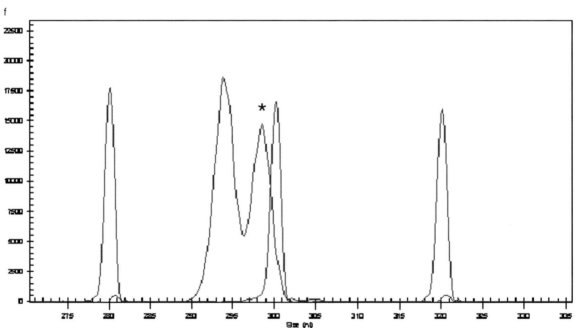

Figure 8.6. (cont.)

in an independent laboratory and FISH. These analyses respectively serve to exclude the possibility that the result was spurious due to PCR contamination or was unlikely to be of clinical relevance, should the fusion gene have arisen in a minor clone. However, it is important to appreciate that small insertion events can potentially be missed by FISH when using large probes, hence molecular screening for CBF leukemia is best undertaken by RT-PCR, for which standardized optimized protocols have been published by the BIOMED-1 group [49]. Patients with CBF leukemia identified on molecular screening are assumed to be biologically similar to those with the overt cytogenetic lesion. Recognition of such cases is clinically relevant,

Table 8.4. Immunophenotyping panel for the diagnosis of acute myeloid leukemia (AML) and mixed phenotype acute leukemia.

Diagnosis of AML[a]

Precursor stage	CD34, CD38, CD117, CD133, HLA-DR
Granulocytic markers	CD13, CD15, CD16, CD33, CD65, cytoplasmic myeloperoxidase (cMPO)
Monocytic markers	Non-specific esterase (NSE), CD11c, CD14, CD64, lysozyme, CD4, CD11b, CD36, NG2 homologue[b]
Megakaryocytic markers	CD41 (glycoprotein IIb/IIIa), CD61 (glycoprotein IIIa), CD42 (glycoprotein 1b)
Erythroid marker	CD235a (glycophorin A)

Diagnosis of mixed phenotype acute leukemia[c]

Myeloid lineage	MPO *or* evidence of monocytic differentiation (at least two of the following: NSE, CD11c, CD14, CD64, lysozyme)
B-lineage	CD19 (strong) with at least one of the following: CD79a, cCD22, CD10, *or* CD19 (weak) with at least two of the following: CD79a, cCD22, CD10
T-lineage	cCD3, or surface CD3

Adapted from European LeukemiaNet AML Guidelines [46].
[a] For the diagnosis of AML, the table provides a list of selected markers rather than a mandatory marker panel.
[b] Most cases with 11q23 abnormalities express the NG2 homolog (encoded by *CSPG4*) reacting with the monoclonal antibody 7.1.
[c] Requirements for assigning more than one lineage to a single blast population adopted from the WHO classification (see Table 8.2). Note that the requirement for assigning myeloid lineage in mixed phenotype acute leukemia is more stringent than for establishing a diagnosis of AML. Note also that mixed phenotype acute leukemia can be diagnosed if there are separate populations of lymphoid and myeloid blasts.

since they represent a group of patients who may be spared routine use of allogeneic transplant in first remission and can benefit from MRD monitoring by real-time quantitative polymerase chain reaction (RQ-PCR). Routine provision of samples for molecular diagnostics in the CBF leukemias is important to establish breakpoint location (variable for *CBFB-MYH11*) and to provide a baseline fusion transcript level for subsequent MRD assessment.

BCR-ABL1 fusion: Although rare in AML (~1%), molecular screening for the *BCR-ABL1* fusion may also be worth including in the diagnostic panel. This will identify those patients with a very poor prognosis, who could potentially benefit from molecularly targeted therapy with imatinib and other tyrosine kinase inhibitors.

FIP1L1-PDGFRA fusion: In AML with a marked eosinophilic component and negative for *CBFB-MYH11* there may be merit in screening for the *FIP1L1-PDGFRA* fusion using PCR or FISH-based approaches, given the sensitivity of this disease entity to imatinib [50].

Other fusion genes: Beyond identifying patients who can potentially be subject to MRD monitoring by RQ-PCR, more extensive screening for a wider range of AML fusion genes is of limited clinical utility and is currently not recommended [46].

Mutation screening

The diagnostic work-up for AML patients lacking APL or CBF leukemia subtypes and who are candidates for intensive treatment, should be routinely screened for mutations that may impact upon management and clinical outcome. A number of studies have highlighted the complex interplay of mutations affecting *NPM1*, *CEBPA* and *FLT3* on clinical outcome. Such information is increasingly being used to direct use of allogeneic transplantation in first remission (reviewed in [32]).

FLT3 mutations: For detection of *FLT3*-ITD mutations it is important to use a methodology that allows quantification of the mutant allele (e.g. Genescan) [20], since higher mutant ratios have been associated with poorer prognosis [19–21]. The prognostic significance of TKD mutations remains uncertain and based

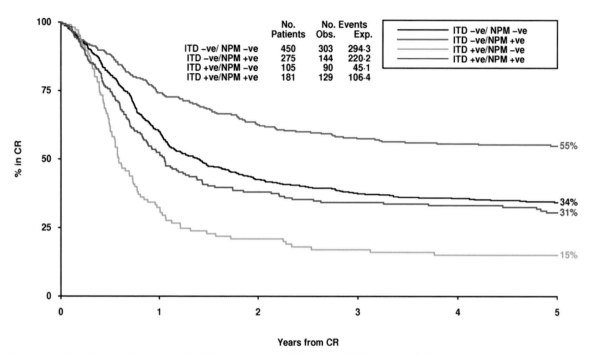

Figure 8.7. Impact of *NPM1* and *FLT3*-ITD mutations in younger adults treated in the UK NCRI AML trials. Adapted from [21] with permission.

on current evidence there appears to be little merit in screening for this mutation outside clinical trials evaluating FLT3 inhibitor therapy.

NPM1 exon 12 mutations: Molecular screening for *NPM1* exon 12 mutations is most appropriately restricted to AML cases lacking any of the balanced chromosomal abnormalities recognized in the WHO classification. A number of methods are available to detect mutations in the *NPM1* gene [51]. Presence of an *NPM1* mutation to some extent ameliorates the adverse prognosis associated with *FLT3*-ITD, while *NPM1*-positive/*FLT3*-ITD-negative AML has a particularly favorable prognosis (Figure 8.7). *NPM1* mutations have been shown to provide highly sensitive and reliable targets for MRD detection [47,52]. There is preliminary evidence to suggest, albeit based on analysis of small sample sizes, that patients with mutant *NPM1* may benefit from ATRA therapy [53].

CEBPA mutations: Protocols have been established for mutation screening of *CEBPA* [26,29–31]. However, this is more challenging than analysis of *FLT3* and

NPM1, given that mutations are widely distributed and the gene is highly GC-rich. Routine screening strategy may be influenced by the observation that favorable disease outcome correlates with presence of biallelic *CEBPA* mutations in the absence of *FLT3*-ITD [30–32]. Accordingly, *CEBPA* mutation screening could reasonably be restricted to cases that are:

1. *FLT3*-ITD-negative.
2. *NPM1* mutation-negative.
3. Do not have balanced cytogenetic abnormalities.
4. Do not have adverse risk cytogenetics (defined below).

Other mutations: In situations in which clinical features suggest that AML has arisen on the background of a predisposing genetic disorder (e.g. Down syndrome, Fanconi anemia), input should be sought from specialist laboratories for additional molecular characterization to help inform patient management.

Establishing baseline disease status

Having established a diagnosis of AML, apart from the cytogenetic and molecular genetic characteristics of the leukemic clone, a number of factors need to be taken into account that are highly relevant to patient management. These include consideration of the patient's age and performance status, ascertaining the presence and nature of any co-morbidities (e.g. impaired cardiac, renal, pulmonary or hepatic function, history of previous cancer), establishing whether the leukemia has arisen *de novo* or secondary to an antecedent hematologic disorder or previous chemotherapy/radiotherapy exposure, the presenting WBC, presence of extramedullary disease and the patient's wishes with respect to therapy in the context of the predicted prognosis. Pregnancy status of women of childbearing age should be established prior to treatment. Steps to preserve fertility should be considered where possible. Therefore, a considerable number of baseline factors need to be taken into account at diagnosis of AML that are relevant for patient management (Table 8.3).

Investigations for risk stratification, determining prognosis and treatment approach

Routine investigations

A critical first step in assessing any patient with suspected AML is rapid scrutiny of the PB and BM morphology to determine whether the patient is likely to have APL, or another disease subtype. APL should be considered as a medical emergency requiring immediate treatment with ATRA and supportive care measures to reduce the risk of death due to the associated coagulopathy [45]. In patients with suspected APL, BM samples should be analyzed by PML immunofluorescence, cytogenetics and molecular diagnostics using RT-PCR to establish the presence of the *PML-RARA* fusion [45]. For patients with documented *PML-RARA* positivity, ATRA and reduced intensity anthracycline-based treatment protocols have become a standard of care [45]. In recent years, regimens based entirely on molecularly targeted therapies (i.e. ATRA, ATO +/− gemtuzmab ozogamicin) have been developed. The place of these chemotherapy-free treatment approaches is being evaluated in randomized clinical trials; however, they are increasingly being applied in patients with *PML-RARA+* APL who are considered unfit for standard anthracycline-based therapy [45]. Given the high risk of death in untreated APL, treatment should not be delayed until results of laboratory investigations

are available [45]. Any patients with suspected APL in whom routine investigations do not identify a *PML-RARA* fusion should be discussed with a reference laboratory considering the possibility of an alternative fusion partner, which has an important bearing upon ATRA sensitivity. For example, APL with t(11;17)(q23; q21) giving rise to the *PLZF(ZBTB16)-RARA* fusion is resistant to ATRA, whereas t(5;17)(q35;q21);*NPM1-RARA*, t(4;17)(q12;q21);*FIP1L1-RARA* and t(11;17)(q13;q21);*NuMA-RARA* are ATRA-sensitive [45]. The use of ATO should be restricted to *PML-RARA+* APL, since this agent is ineffective in *PLZF-RARA+* APL and untested in other molecular subtypes.

For patients with AML other than APL, pre-treatment cytogenetic analysis is fundamental to determine treatment approach and predicting outcome. Indeed, in multivariable analyses taking into account age, type of AML (*de novo*/secondary) and presenting WBC, diagnostic karyotype emerges as the most significant prognostic factor [32]. Patients with CBF leukemia i.e. with t(8;21)(q22;q22) or inv(16)(p13q22)/t(16;16)(p13;q22) treated with intensive chemotherapy involving cytarabine at a range of doses typically have a relatively favorable prognosis (Figure 8.2, Table 8.5). In this favorable risk group, relapse rates are too low and salvage rates too high for there to be any survival benefit for allogeneic transplantation in first remission [32]. Conversely, adults presenting with AML with the following cytogenetic abnormalities with other changes or complex karyotype (more than three unrelated abnormalities) have a very poor prognosis with conventional chemotherapy:

1. abn(3q) [excluding t(3;5)(q21~25;q31~35)/*NPM1-MLF1*].
2. inv(3)(q21q26)/t(3;3)(q21;q26).
3. add(5q), del(5q) or −5.
4. add(7q), del(7q) or −7.
5. t(6;11)(q27;q23).
6. t(10;11)(p11~13;q23).
7. other t(11q23) [excluding t(9;11)(p21~22;q23) and t(11;19)(q23;p13)]
8. t(9;22)(q34;q11).
9. −17 and abn(17p).

Patients with these abnormalities are considered candidates for allogeneic transplant and experimental treatment approaches [32]. These adverse risk cytogenetic abnormalities are present in a quarter of AML cases in patients >60 years and predict a dismal prognosis (<5% survival at 5 years) [32]. Therefore there may be a

Table 8.5. Pre-treatment cytogenetic and molecular entities shown to predict disease outcome in multivariable analysis studies conducted in younger adults [32,65].

	Cytogenetic/molecular abnormality	Comments
Favorable	t(15;17)(q22;q12~21);*PML-RARA* t(8;21)(q22;q22);*RUNX1-RUNX1T1* inv(16)(p13q22)/t(16;16)(p13;q22);*CBFB-MYH11* *NPM1* mutant/*FLT3*-ITD neg, *WT1* wild type *CEBPA* mutant (biallelic, *FLT3*-ITD negative)	Irrespective of additional cytogenetic abnormalities
Intermediate	Entities not classified as favorable or adverse	
Adverse	abn(3q) [excluding t(3;5)(q21~25;q31~35)], inv(3)(q21q26)/t(3;3)(q21;q26);*EVI-1* expression add(5q), del(5q), −5 −7, add(7q), del(7q) t(6;11)(q27;q23), t(10;11)(p11~13;q23), other t(11q23) [excluding t(9;11)(p21~22;q23) and t(11;19)(q23;p13)] t(9;22)(q34;q11), −17, abn(17p) with other changes Complex (>3 unrelated abnormalities)	Excluding cases with favorable karyotype
	FLT3-ITD	In absence of favorable karyotype. Particularly poor prognosis with high level *FLT3*-ITD mutant ratio or if *FLT3*-ITD accompanied by *WT1* mutation
	MLL-PTD *RUNX1* mutation	

rationale for performing rapid cytogenetic analysis to inform treatment approach for older AML patients in whom APL is not suspected and outside a clinical trial. This group of patients may be candidates for experimental treatment approaches or supportive care, depending upon patient wishes. In pediatric patients, outcomes for the standard and adverse risk groups are generally better than in adults, such that relatively few children are considered candidates for transplant in first complete remission.

There are several limitations in the use of karyotype as the sole risk stratification tool to determine treatment approach. These include failed cytogenetic analyses, presence of cryptic chromosomal rearrangements, and notably because of the substantial proportion of AML cases with normal karyotype, now known to be highly heterogeneous at the molecular level [32]. Therefore, as detailed above, in patients entered into clinical trials and those who are eligible for allogeneic transplantation, cytogenetics is increasingly being complemented by targeted molecular screening to predict outcome and inform treatment strategy (Table 8.3).

Having excluded a diagnosis of APL or CBF leukemia, molecular screening for *NPM1* and *FLT3*-ITD mutations can identify patients with favorable (NPMc positive/*FLT3*-ITD negative) and very poor (*NPM1* wild type/*FLT3*-ITD positive) prognoses, similar to those observed in patients with CBF leukemia and adverse karyotype, respectively (Figure 8.7). In the absence of *FLT3*-ITD, presence of *CEBPA* mutation (particularly affecting both alleles) also predicts a favorable outcome similar to that of CBF leukemia [32]. These observations have led to suggestions that AML patients with unmutated *FLT3* in the presence of *NPM1* or biallelic *CEBPA* mutations (which between them account for 23% of younger adults with AML) may represent a further group of patients who may not benefit from routine use of allogeneic transplant in first complete remission [28,32]. Conversely, in non-APL, non-CBF AML patients with *FLT3*-ITD and wildtype *NPM1* and *CEBPA*, a number of groups advocate the use of allogeneic transplant in first remission given their poor prognosis with conventional therapy (reviewed in [32]).

Investigational assays

The ever-increasing number of molecular markers identified in AML presents an ongoing challenge to determine which provide information of therapeutic and independent prognostic relevance, once other well-established pre-treatment factors are taken into account. Mutations in the *N-* and *K-RAS* genes are common in AML but do not impact upon prognosis and are not helpful in predicting response to the farnesyl transferase inhibitor tipifarnib (reviewed in [1,14]). Mutation of the *RUNX1* gene occurs in ~3% of AML and is particularly associated with trisomy 13, trisomy 21 and cases with minimal differentiation [1]. *PTPN11* (encoding SHP-2) is mutated in ~4% and associated with monocytic leukemia and monosomy 7 [1]. Studies are in progress to assess the value of molecular screening for mutations in the *IDH1* and *IDH2* genes. Mutations in *cKIT* are present in ~3% of AML and are associated with trisomy 4 and CBF leukemia; in the latter group they have been associated with a poor prognosis and are therapeutically relevant, leading to the evaluation of tyrosine kinase inhibitors within the context of clinical trials [35]. Partial tandem duplications of *MLL* (*MLL*-PTD) predict a poor outcome and may become relevant for molecularly targeted therapies in the future [14]. Adverse outcome has also been associated with over-expression of a number of genes including *BAALC*, *EVI1*, *MN1* and *ERG* (reviewed in [14,32]). While over-expression of *EVI1* can be associated with cytogenetically cryptic 3q26 abnormalities [5], the molecular basis of upregulation of other genes which have been associated with poorer prognosis remains poorly understood. Since the level of expression of these markers appears to be a continuum in AML, "up-regulation" has been defined variously on the basis of expression levels falling within the upper quartile or above the median. As such, cases with very similar levels of expression and comparable outcomes could just straddle the cut-point and end up being assigned to different risk groups. Given this limitation, establishing the clinical utility of such markers as tools to achieve greater individualization of patient care will necessitate:

1. Setting of robust validated expression thresholds relative to standard housekeeping genes (e.g. *ABL*), and
2. Evidence that these defined thresholds refine outcome prediction after allowing for cytogenetics and the mutation status of *NPM1*, *FLT3*-ITD and *CEBPA*.

It is possible that the relative expression of some of these markers reflect differences in the nature of the hematopoietic progenitors subject to leukemic transformation, and/or the characteristics and relative size of the leukemic stem cell compartment.

Immunophenotypic profiles of the leukemic population may provide similar prognostic information. Previous studies have shown that BCL2/BAX ratio and drug resistance protein expression are predictive of treatment response and risk of relapse [32]. Similarly, poor outcomes have been observed in AML with a relatively large early progenitor population defined by a CD34+/CD38– phenotype [54]. These parameters may become increasingly relevant as newer agents that modulate drug resistance or target the leukemic stem cell pool become available. Expression of factors that may relate to interactions of leukemic cells with the bone marrow microenvironment (e.g. VEGF, CXCR4, reviewed in [55]) or gene variants that influence drug handling have also been found to impact on outcome. However, their relationship to other well-established prognostic factors is poorly defined and hence their clinical utility remains to be established.

A number of studies have highlighted the potential of microarrays to evaluate expression of mRNA transcripts or microRNAs as a tool to distinguish subgroups of patients with differing prognosis (reviewed in [56]). These platforms have shown their capacity to identify well-recognized cytogenetically or molecularly defined subsets of leukemia, such as those with t(15;17);*PML-RARA* [56]. A key question is whether these approaches will realize their promise to identify targets or discrete constellations of novel markers that distinguish patients at differing risk of relapse and which are:

1. Independent of well-established prognostic factors.
2. Can be accurately measured in a robust fashion.
3. Validated in independent data sets.

Given the considerable challenges relating to the performance of microarrays and conduct of the downstream bioinformatic analyses in a standardized fashion, these technologies appear unlikely to shape the way individual AML patients will be treated in the very near future. Similarly, in the absence of clinically available drug resistance modulators, assays evaluating p-glycoprotein activity and other resistance pathways remain investigational.

Disease monitoring: detection of minimal residual disease

Response to induction therapy has long been recognized as a major independent prognostic factor in AML, predicting risk of relapse and overall survival, leading to the development of standardized response criteria [57]. While the percentage of residual leukemic blasts following induction has been used to refine risk stratification, morphological appearances can be difficult to interpret. To provide a more objective and sensitive approach to assess treatment response to induction therapy numerous studies have applied flow cytometry or real-time quantitative PCR (RQ-PCR) to detect minimal residual disease (MRD). The former depends upon the characterization of an aberrant "leukemia-associated immunophenotype" (LAIP) of the blast population at diagnosis, which can be defined in over 90% of AML cases (reviewed in [47]). LAIPs have traditionally been classified into three groups, although there is overlap between the last two. These are:

1. Cross-lineage expression of lymphoid antigens on myeloid cells.
2. Asynchronous expression of antigens, e.g. blast cells express antigens that are normally present on mature myeloid cells.
3. Under- or over-expression of antigens.

Defined LAIPs differ in their specificity and thus sensitivity; cross-lineage expression of lymphoid antigens usually provides the highest specificity. Typically flow cytometry can detect ~1 AML cell in 1000–10 000 normal bone marrow cells. The sensitivity depends on the upper level of frequency of rare cells of identical phenotype in normal and regenerating marrow.

The RQ-PCR approach relies on the detection of:

1. Leukemia-specific targets, including:
   a. Fusion genes, e.g. *PML-RARA*, *RUNX1-RUNX1T1* and *CBFB-MYH11*.
   b. Mutations, e.g. mutant *NPM1*.
2. Transcripts that are commonly upregulated in AML, particularly *WT1* [47].

Standardized RQ-PCR assays for these various AML targets have been developed by laboratories participating in the Europe Against Cancer (EAC) and European LeukemiaNet programs [58–60]. The EAC

group also undertook a systematic evaluation of housekeeping genes to allow reliable normalization of MRD results, with *ABL* emerging as the preferred reference gene [59]. For RQ-PCR assays detecting *NPM1* mutations or fusion gene transcripts, maximal sensitivities range between 1 in 10^3–10^6 depending upon the relative level of expression (as compared with the housekeeping gene) that may vary between molecular subtypes of AML and cases with the same target (reviewed in [47]). The establishment of a standardized *WT1* assay [60] is relevant to assess responses to novel WT1-targeted therapies that are now entering early phase clinical trials. MRD monitoring strategies using *WT1* need to take into account that transcripts can be detected in normal marrow and to a lesser extent peripheral blood. This suggests that RQ-PCR assays using this target may be most informatively deployed to measure early treatment responses, rather than providing a sensitive "universal marker" for MRD detection, as had originally been hoped [47,60].

Retrospective studies using RQ-PCR detection of *WT1* transcripts (evaluable in ~45% of AML patients) or flow cytometry to assess reduction in leukemic burden following induction and consolidation therapy have shown that both approaches can distinguish patients at differing risk of relapse within cytogenetic risk groups (Figure 8.8a); they retain their prognostic significance when other factors such as age and type of AML (*de novo*/secondary) are taken into account [47,60,61]. Studies using RQ-PCR have also consistently shown that response kinetics are predictive of risk of subsequent relapse in CBF leukemias, although the relationship to other prognostic factors such as presenting leukocyte count and *KIT* mutation status remains unclear (reviewed in [47]).

In addition to investigating the potential of MRD detection to provide a risk stratification tool, longitudinal monitoring may provide early warning of impending relapse, allowing the opportunity for pre-emptive therapy (Figure 8.8b). This approach has been most extensively studied in APL in which molecular monitoring for residual disease has now been introduced into routine clinical practice. Notably, the International Working Group for development of standardized response criteria in AML included recognition of achievement of molecular remission as a critical therapeutic goal in the management of APL [57]. Indeed, in the Medical Research Council (MRC) AML15 trial sequential monitoring using the standardized EAC *PML-RARA* RQ-PCR assay was shown to

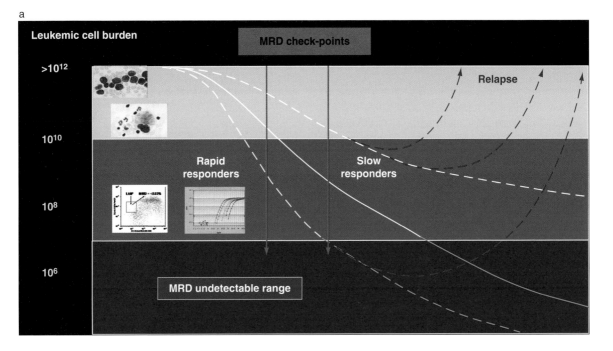

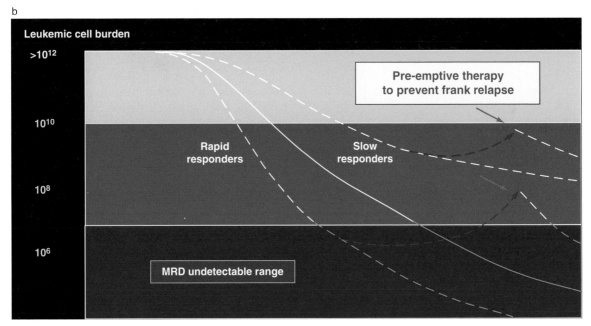

Figure 8.8. Strategies for use of minimal residual disease detection to direct treatment of AML.
a. Application of MRD assessment at early time-points during treatment to provide a risk stratification tool. Patients with slow kinetics of disease response as determined by flow cytometry [61] or RQ-PCR (detecting *WT1* transcripts [60]) exhibit an increased rate of subsequent relapse.
b. RQ-PCR may also be applied for sequential MRD monitoring, identifying patients with persistent PCR positivity or molecular relapse, allowing pre-emptive therapy to prevent clinical relapse. This strategy has been successfully used in the management of APL [62].

provide the strongest predictor of relapse, far superior in multivariable analyses to presenting leukocyte count [62], which has traditionally been used to provide the framework for risk-stratified treatment approaches in this subtype of AML [45]. Evidence to date suggests that sequential MRD monitoring to direct pre-emptive therapy can reduce rates of frank relapse and improve survival in APL [45,62]. Analysis of paired blood and marrow samples using the standardized EAC RQ-PCR assay has shown that the latter sample source affords approximately 1.5 log greater sensitivity for detection of MRD than blood [62]; therefore use of blood for MRD assessment is not recommended [45]. Taking into account that the EAC *PML-RARA* assay usually affords a sensitivity of 1 in 10^4 when applied to patient marrow samples, and considering that fusion transcripts typically rise by ~1 log per month in relapsing patients, to predict relapse and have sufficient time to deliver pre-emptive therapy to prevent relapse, marrow samples should be taken at the end of consolidation and at 3-month intervals for ~36 months. Timing of the next MRD assessment should be brought forward if the previous sample was sub-optimal (i.e. failed to afford a sensitivity of at least 1 in 10^4), or yielded equivocal results [45,62]. If PCR positivity is detected, a bone marrow aspirate should be repeated within 2 weeks and samples sent to two laboratories (to be tested by RQ-PCR and FISH) [44,45]. Should PCR positivity be detected in the repeat samples with a stable or rising *PML-RARA* level and confirmed in an independent laboratory, the patient is deemed to be in "molecular relapse" and immediate therapeutic intervention (e.g. with ATO) is indicated to prevent relapse [45].

While MRD monitoring has been widely applied in APL and is assuming greater importance as de-intensified molecularly targeted approaches are being investigated, the clinical utility of MRD monitoring in other subsets of AML remains to be firmly established. A recent large German study has shown that RQ-PCR detection of *NPM1* mutations provides a powerful independent predictor of disease relapse [52]. Clinical trials are in progress to assess the use of sequential MRD monitoring by RQ-PCR assay in CBF leukemia to direct additional therapy, such as KIT inhibitors and allogeneic transplantation. A major challenge for large-scale clinical trials is to establish optimal MRD monitoring schedules and determine predictive thresholds of MRD at particular time-points. This is fundamental to addressing the key question as to whether MRD assessment can identify in a more reliable fashion those patients most (and least) likely to benefit from allogeneic transplantation as compared to traditional prognostic factors and whether MRD-directed therapy can lead to meaningful improvements in clinical outcome.

Laboratory assessment of relapsed disease and in patients undergoing stem cell transplantation

In patients with recurrence of AML and who are fit for salvage therapy, laboratory assessment is valuable to:

1. Distinguish true relapse with recurrence of the original leukemic clone from secondary MDS/AML induced by first-line anti-leukemic therapy.
2. Help inform therapy.
3. Predict outcome.

Laboratory assessment should include cytogenetic analysis, flow cytometry and banking of material for molecular analysis. Cytogenetic findings at relapse, the timing of relapse following first-line therapy, patient age and performance status all have a critical bearing on disease outcome (reviewed in [63]).

In patients who are candidates for transplantation, MRD detection is increasingly being applied to guide treatment, with studies in *PML-RARA*+ APL again providing proof of principle. In patients with relapsed APL, achievement of further molecular remission is critical for any chance of cure of the disease. Autologous transplantation can provide an effective approach to consolidation in APL patients achieving molecular remission and in whom a satisfactory PCR-negative harvest can be obtained [45]. For patients who fail to achieve molecular remission with salvage therapy, allogeneic transplantation is the preferred treatment approach [45]. In APL patients, sequential MRD monitoring following transplant can be helpful in guiding the need for further treatment intervention, for example with ATRA and ATO. In allografted patients with any subtype of AML, there is also scope to treat residual or recurrent disease with relaxation of immune suppression and donor leukocyte infusion. Based upon the experience in chronic myelogenous leukemia, this approach is most likely to be effective when applied in the context of minimal residual disease rather than in clinical relapse. Preliminary data using a range of MRD targets are very encouraging (reviewed in [64]) and with the development of more sensitive chimerism assays it may become increasingly possible to refine immunotherapy according to the needs of the individual patient and reduce risk of disease relapse.

Concluding remarks

In addition to the expansion of the repertoire of assays used to evaluate newly diagnosed patients with AML, the next few years are likely to see more widespread use of MRD assessment to determine treatment approach [66,67]. For patients with fusion gene transcripts, RQ-PCR provides the most reliable methodology and international efforts are underway to establish optimal time-points for MRD sampling and thresholds of fusion gene expression that are predictive of long-term outcome. A key challenge is to determine the most appropriate way to monitor patients who lack a suitable fusion gene marker, whether by RQ-PCR detection of genes which are typically over-expressed in AML or by use of flow cytometry. It is clear that the leukemia laboratory is set to play an ever-increasingly important role in optimizing and individualizing the management of patients with AML.

Acknowledgments

The author gratefully acknowledges Leukaemia and Lymphoma Research of Great Britain and the National Institute for health Research (NIHR) for support of minimal residual disease studies in the UK National Cancer Research Institute AML trials. Support of the Minimal Residual Disease Workpackage (WP12) of the European LeukemiaNet is also gratefully acknowledged. The author wishes to thank Dr. Robert Hills for helpful discussions and preparation of the figures.

References

1. Grimwade D. Impact of cytogenetics on clinical outcome in AML. In Karp, JE (ed.), *Acute Myelogenous Leukemia*. Totowa, NJ: Humana Press; 2007: 177–92.

2. Mitelman Database of Chromosome Aberrations in Cancer (2009). Mitelman F, Johansson B, Mertens F (eds.), http://cgap.nci.nih.gov/Chromosomes/ Mitelman

3. Rosenbauer F, Tenen DG. Transcription factors in myeloid development: balancing differentiation with transformation. *Nat Rev Immunol* 2007;**7**:105–17.

4. Grimwade D, Mistry AR, Solomon E, Guidez F. Acute promyelocytic leukemia: A paradigm for differentiation therapy. *Cancer Treat Res*, 2009;**145**: 219–35

5. Lugthart S, van Drunen E, van Norden Y *et al*. High EVI1 levels predict adverse outcome in acute myeloid leukemia: prevalence of EVI1 overexpression and chromosome 3q26 abnormalities underestimated. *Blood* 2008;**111**:4329–37.

6. Guidez F, Zelent A. Role of nuclear receptor corepressors in leukemogenesis. *Curr Top Microbiol Immunol* 2001;**254**:165–85.

7. Plass C, Oakes C, Blum W, Marcucci G. Epigenetics in acute myeloid leukemia. *Semin Oncol* 2008;**35**: 378–87.

8. Harper DP, Aplan PD. Chromosomal rearrangements leading to *MLL* gene fusions: clinical and biological aspects. *Cancer Res* 2008;**68**:10024–7.

9. Moore MA, Chung KY, Plasilova M *et al*. NUP98 dysregulation in myeloid leukemogenesis. *Ann N Y Acad Sci* 2007;**1106**:114–42.

10. Caligiuri MA, Strout MP, Oberkircher AR *et al*. The partial tandem duplication of ALL1 in acute myeloid leukemia with normal cytogenetics or trisomy 11 is restricted to one chromosome. *Proc Natl Acad Sci USA* 1997;**94**:3899–902.

11. Liu TX, Becker MW, Jelinek J *et al*. Chromosome 5q deletion and epigenetic suppression of the gene encoding alpha-catenin (CTNNA1) in myeloid cell transformation. *Nat Med* 2007;**13**:78–83.

12. Ebert BL, Pretz J, Bosco J *et al*. Identification of RPS14 as a 5q- syndrome gene by RNA interference screen. *Nature* 2008;**451**:335–9.

13. Ebert BL. Deletion 5q in myelodysplastic syndrome: a paradigm for the study of hemizygous deletions in cancer. *Leukemia* 2009;**23**:1252–6.

14. Mrózek K, Marcucci G, Paschka P, Whitman SP, Bloomfield CD. Clinical relevance of mutations and gene-expression changes in adult acute myeloid leukemia with normal cytogenetics: are we ready for a prognostically prioritized molecular classification? *Blood* 2007;**109**:431–48.

15. Scholl C, Gilliland DG, Fröhling S. Deregulation of signaling pathways in acute myeloid leukemia. *Semin Oncol* 2008;**35**:336–45.

16. Mead AJ, Linch DC, Hills RK *et al*. FLT3 tyrosine kinase domain mutations are biologically distinct from and have a significantly more favorable prognosis than FLT3 internal tandem duplications in patients with acute myeloid leukemia. *Blood* 2007;**110**:1262–70.

17. Bacher U, Haferlach C, Kern W *et al.* Prognostic relevance of FLT3-TKD mutations in AML: the combination matters – an analysis of 3082 patients. *Blood* 2008;**111**:2527–37.

18. Whitman SP, Ruppert AS, Radmacher MD *et al.* FLT3 D835/I836 mutations are associated with poor disease-free survival and a distinct gene-expression signature among younger adults with de novo cytogenetically normal acute myeloid leukemia lacking FLT3 internal tandem duplications. *Blood* 2008;**111**:1552–9.

19. Whitman SP, Archer KJ, Feng L *et al.* Absence of the wild-type allele predicts poor prognosis in adult de novo acute myeloid leukemia with normal cytogenetics and the internal tandem duplication of FLT3: a Cancer and Leukemia Group B study. *Cancer Res* 2001;**61**:7233–9.

20. Thiede C, Steudel C, Mohr B *et al.* Analysis of FLT3-activating mutations in 979 patients with acute myelogenous leukemia: association with FAB subtypes and identification of subgroups with poor prognosis. *Blood* 2002;**99**:4326–35.

21. Gale RE, Green C, Allen C *et al.* The impact of FLT3 internal tandem duplication mutant level, number, size, and interaction with NPM1 mutations in a large cohort of young adult patients with acute myeloid leukemia. *Blood* 2008;**111**:2776–84.

22. Fitzgibbon J, Smith LL, Raghavan M *et al.* Association between acquired uniparental disomy and homozygous gene mutation in acute myeloid leukemias. *Cancer Res* 2005;**65**:9152–4.

23. Falini B, Mecucci C, Tiacci E *et al.* Cytoplasmic nucleophosmin in acute myelogenous leukemia with a normal karyotype. *New Engl J Med* 2005;**352**:254–66.

24. Falini B, Nicoletti I, Martelli MF, Mecucci C. Acute myeloid leukemia carrying cytoplasmic/mutated nucleophosmin (NPMc+ AML): biologic and clinical features. *Blood* 2007;**109**:874–85.

25. Haferlach C, Mecucci C, Schnittger S *et al.* AML with mutated *NPM1* carrying a normal or aberrant karyotype show overlapping biological, pathological, immunophenotypic, and prognostic features. *Blood* 2009;**114**:3024–32.

26. Pabst T, Eyholzer M, Haefliger S *et al.* Somatic CEBPA mutations are a frequent second event in families with germline CEBPA mutations and familial acute myeloid leukemia. *J Clin Oncol* 2008;**26**:5088–93.

27. Figueroa ME, Wouters BJ, Skrabanek L *et al.* Genome-wide epigenetic analysis delineates a biologically distinct immature acute leukemia with myeloid/T-lymphoid features. *Blood* 2009;**113**:2795–804.

28. Schlenk RF, Döhner K, Krauter J *et al.* Mutations and treatment outcome in cytogenetically normal acute myeloid leukemia. *New Engl J Med* 2008;**358**:1909–18.

29. Marcucci G, Maharry K, Radmacher MD *et al.* Prognostic significance of, and gene and microRNA expression signatures associated with, *CEBPA* mutations in cytogenetically normal acute myeloid leukemia with high-risk molecular features: a Cancer and Leukemia Group B Study. *J Clin Oncol* 2008;**26**:5078–87.

30. Wouters BJ, Löwenberg B, Erpelinck-Verschueren CA *et al.* Double *CEBPA* mutations, but not single *CEBPA* mutations, define a subgroup of acute myeloid leukemia with a distinctive gene expression profile that is uniquely associated with a favorable outcome. *Blood* 2009;**113**:3088–91.

31. Green CL, Koo KK, Hills RK *et al.* Prognostic significance of *CEBPA* mutations in a large cohort of younger adult patients with acute myeloid leukemia. Impact of double *CEBPA* mutations and the interaction with FLT3 and *NPM1* mutations. *J Clin Oncol* 2010;**28**:2739–47.

32. Grimwade D, Hills RK. Independent prognostic factors for AML outcome. *Hematology Am Soc Hematol Educ Program* 2009; 385–95.

33. Abdel-Wahab O, Mullally A, Hedvat C *et al.* Genetic characterization of TET1, TET2, and TET3 alterations in myeloid malignancies. *Blood* 2009;**114**:144–7.

34. Delhommeau F, Dupont S, Della Valle V *et al.* Mutation in *TET2* in myeloid cancers. *New Engl J Med* 2009;**360**:2289–301.

35. Mrózek K, Marcucci G, Paschka P, Bloomfield CD. Advances in molecular genetics and treatment of core-binding factor acute myeloid leukemia. *Curr Opin Oncol* 2008;**20**:711–18.

36. Swerdlow SH, Campo E, Harris NL *et al.* (eds.). *World Health Organization Classification of Tumours of Haematopoietic and Lymphoid Tissues*, 4th edn. Lyon: IARC Press; 2008.

37. Owen C, Barnett M, Fitzgibbon J. Familial myelodysplasia and acute myeloid leukaemia – a review. *Br J Haematol* 2008;**140**:123–32.

38. Dokal I, Vulliamy T. Inherited aplastic anaemias/bone marrow failure syndromes. *Blood Rev* 2008;**22**:141–53.

39. de Winter JP, Joenje H. The genetic and molecular basis of Fanconi anemia. *Mutat Res* 2009;**668**:11–19.

40. Estey E, Döhner H. Acute myeloid leukaemia. *Lancet* 2006;**368**:1894–907.

41. Godley LA, Larson RA. Therapy-related myeloid leukemia. *Semin Oncol* 2008;**35**:418–29.

42. Bennett JM, Catovsky D, Daniel MT *et al.* Proposed revised criteria for the classification of acute myeloid

leukemia. A report of the French-American-British Cooperative Group. *Ann Intern Med* 1985;**103**:620–5.

43. Jaffe ES, Harris NL, Stein H, Vardiman JW (eds.). *World Health Organization Classification of Tumours: Pathology and Genetics of Tumours of Haematopoietic and Lymphoid Tissues*. Lyon: IARC Press; 2001.

44. Milligan DW, Grimwade D, Cullis JO *et al.* Guidelines on the management of acute myeloid leukaemia in adults. *Br J Haematol* 2006;**135**:450–74.

45. Sanz MA, Grimwade D, Tallman MS *et al.* Management of acute promyelocytic leukemia: recommendations from an expert panel on behalf of the European LeukemiaNet. *Blood* 2009;**113**:1875–91.

46. Döhner H, Estey EH, Amadori S *et al.* Diagnosis and management of acute myeloid leukemia in adults: recommendations from an international expert panel, on behalf of the European LeukemiaNet. *Blood* 2010;**115**:453–74.

47. Freeman SD, Jovanovic JV, Grimwade D. Development of minimal residual disease directed therapy in acute myeloid leukemia. *Semin Oncol* 2008;**35**:388–400.

48. Pinto FO, Leblanc T, Chamousset D *et al.* Diagnosis of Fanconi anemia in patients with bone marrow failure. *Haematologica* 2009;**94**:487–95.

49. van Dongen JJM, Macintyre EA, Gabert JA *et al.* Standardized RT-PCR analysis of fusion gene transcripts from chromosome aberrations in acute leukemia for detection of minimal residual disease. *Leukemia* 1999;**13**:1901–28.

50. Metzgeroth G, Walz C, Score J *et al.* Recurrent finding of the *FIP1L1-PDGFRA* fusion gene in eosinophilia-associated acute myeloid leukemia and lymphoblastic T-cell lymphoma. *Leukemia* 2007;**21**:1183–8.

51. Gulley ML, Shea TC, Fedoriw Y. Genetic tests to evaluate prognosis and predict therapeutic response in acute myeloid leukemia. *J Mol Diagn* 2010;**12**:3–16.

52. Schnittger S, Kern W, Tschulik C *et al.* Minimal residual disease levels assessed by *NPM1* mutation specific RQ-PCR provide important prognostic information in AML. *Blood* 2009;**114**:2220–31.

53. Schlenk RF, Döhner K, Kneba M *et al.* Gene mutations and response to treatment with all-trans retinoic acid in elderly patients with acute myeloid leukemia. Results from the AMLSG Trial AML HD98B. *Haematologica* 2009;**94**:54–60.

54. van Rhenen A, Feller N, Kelder A *et al.* High stem cell frequency in acute myeloid leukemia at diagnosis predicts high minimal residual disease and poor survival. *Clin Cancer Res* 2005;**11**:6520–7.

55. Lane SW, Scadden DT, Gilliland DG. The leukemic stem cell niche – current concepts and therapeutic opportunities. *Blood* 2009;**114**:1150–7.

56. Wouters BJ, Löwenberg B, Delwel R. A decade of genome-wide gene expression profiling in acute myeloid leukemia: flashback and prospects. *Blood* 2009;**113**:291–8.

57. Cheson BD, Bennett JM, Kopecky KJ *et al.* Revised recommendations of the International Working Group for Diagnosis, Standardization of Response Criteria, Treatment Outcomes, and Reporting Standards for Therapeutic Trials in Acute Myeloid Leukemia. *J Clin Oncol* 2003;**21**:4642–9.

58. Gabert JA, Beillard E, van der Velden VHJ *et al.* Standardization and quality control studies of 'real-time' quantitative reverse transcriptase polymerase chain reaction of fusion gene transcripts for residual disease detection in leukemia – a Europe Against Cancer program. *Leukemia* 2003;**17**:2318–57.

59. Beillard E, Pallisgaard N, van der Velden VHJ *et al.* Evaluation of candidate control genes for diagnosis and residual disease detection in leukemic patients using 'real-time' quantitative reverse-transcriptase polymerase chain reaction (RQ-PCR) – a Europe Against Cancer program. *Leukemia* 2003;**17**:2474–86.

60. Cilloni D, Renneville A, Hermitte F *et al.* Real-time quantitative PCR detection of minimal residual disease by standardized WT1 assay to enhance risk stratification in acute myeloid leukemia: A European LeukemiaNet study. *J Clin Oncol* 2009;**27**:5195–201.

61. Maurillo L, Buccisano F, Del Principe MI *et al.* Toward optimization of postremission therapy for residual disease-positive patients with acute myeloid leukemia. *J Clin Oncol* 2008;**26**:4944–51.

62. Grimwade D, Jovanovic JV, Hills RK *et al.* Prospective minimal residual disease monitoring to predict relapse of acute promyelocytic leukemia and to direct pre-emptive arsenic trioxide therapy. *J Clin Oncol* 2009;**27**:3650–8.

63. Craddock C, Tauro S, Moss P, Grimwade D. Biology and management of relapsed acute myeloid leukaemia. *Br J Haematol* 2005;**129**:18–34.

64. Bacher U, Zander AR, Haferlach T *et al.* Minimal residual disease diagnostics in myeloid malignancies in the post transplant period. *Bone Marrow Transplant* 2008;**42**:145–57.

65. Grimwade D, Hills RK, Moorman AV *et al.* Refinement of cytogenetic classification in acute myeloid leukemia: determination of prognostic significance of rare recurring chromosomal abnormalities among 5876 younger adult patients treated in the United Kingdom Medical Research Council trials. *Blood* 2010;**116**:354–65.

66. Rubnitz JE, Inaba H, Dhal G *et al*. Minimal residual dieases-directed theropy for childhood acute myeloid leukemia: results of the AML02 multicentre trial. *Lancet Oncol* 2010;**11**:543–52.

67. Corbacioglu A, Scholl C, Schlenk RF *et al*. Prognostic impact of minimal residual dieases in CBFB-MYH11-positive acute myeloid leukemia. *J Clin Oncol* 2010 Jul 12 [Epub ahead of print].

9 Mature B-cell leukemias

Constantine S. Tam and Michael J. Keating

Introduction

The mature B-cell leukemias are a pathologically diverse group of diseases that share commonalities in clinical presentation and behavior. Early stage patients are often diagnosed incidentally on a routine complete blood count and blood film, whereas advanced stage patients present with lymphadenopathy, organomegaly, bone marrow infiltration and cytopenias. All of these leukemias are considered "indolent" in that they tend to progress relatively slowly (over months to years), and all are currently incurable with conventional therapy but are often exquisitely sensitive to the graft-versus-leukemia effect of allogeneic stem cell transplantation.

Precise classification of mature B-cell leukemias is important as each entity confers a different prognosis and requires individual treatment approaches. Most mature B-cell lymphomas can be defined using morphological and immunophenotypic markers. More recently, with the discovery of recurrent cytogenetic and molecular genetic rearrangements in individual leukemia subtypes, it has become possible to fine-tune the classification of mature B-cell leukemias using genetic features. The majority of this chapter will be devoted to the discussion of chronic lymphocytic leukemia (CLL), the most common mature B-cell leukemia (Figure 9.1), which serves as the prototypical disease in this category.

Chronic lymphocytic leukemia

Clinical example

A 56-year-old man presented for a routine physical examination. A full blood examination was requested

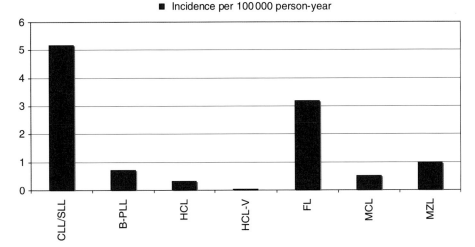

Figure 9.1. Incidence of mature B-cell leukemias in Western populations. Note that the incidence given for follicular lymphoma (FL), mantle cell lymphoma (MCL) and marginal zone lymphoma (MZL) include both nodal and leukemic presentations (modified from Morton *et al.* [1]). CLL/SLL, chronic lymphocytic leukemia/small lymphocytic lymphoma (the tissue variant of CLL); B-PLL, B-Cell prolymphocytic leukemia; HCL, hairy cell leukemia; HCL-V, HCL variant.

Diagnostic Techniques in Hematological Malignancies, ed. Wendy N. Erber. Published by Cambridge University Press.
© Cambridge University Press 2010.

and showed a lymphocytosis of $18 \times 10^9/L$. A repeat test four weeks later showed the lymphocytosis to persist. How should this patient be evaluated?

Chronic lymphocytic leukemia is the most common adult leukemia in the Western world, with an annual incidence of approximately 5 per 100 000 persons in the USA, being similar between white Americans and African–Americans [1]. Curiously, CLL is rare in oriental populations, accounting for less than 5% of adult leukemias in China [2]. The mean age of presentation is 65 years, and there is a male predominance with a male : female ratio of approximately 1.5–2.0.

Establishing the diagnosis

Morphology: Morphologically, CLL cells are typically bland, small lymphocytes with clumped chromatin and scanty cytoplasm (Figure 9.2a). "Smudge," "smear" or "basket" cells are often present and may be prognostically important [3]. Increased numbers of prolymphocytes (Figure 2b) has been historically associated with aggressive disease: patients with >55% prolymphocytes are considered B-cell prolymphocytic leukemia (see below), whereas "typical CLL" is associated with <10% prolymphocytes [4]. Patients with 10–55% prolymphocytes have intermediate disease features and are traditionally classified as "CLL/PLL"; within the context of clinical trials and modern treatment algorithms these patients are generally managed as if they have typical CLL.

Atypical morphology in CLL is not uncommon and may include larger forms with less condensed chromatin and nuclear irregularities; these findings may be particularly common in patients with trisomy 12. Because of this variation in disease morphology, in modern practice, CLL is most commonly defined by its characteristic immunophenotype.

The bone marrow infiltrate in CLL may be interstitial, nodular or diffuse ("packed"). The cytological features of the neoplastic cells are comparable to that seen in the blood or bone marrow aspirate, i.e. small cells with a high nuclear : cytoplasmic ratio and condensed nuclear chromatin. Larger cells may be present and these are the proliferation centers of the CLL (Figure 9.3). Immunocytochemistry can be performed on the bone marrow biopsy to demonstrate the CLL phenotype (see below).

Immunophenotype: Flow cytometry of the peripheral blood is the most common method for confirming a diagnosis of CLL. The typical immunophenotypic profile for CLL is that of a mature B-cell (CD19-and CD79a-positive) with aberrant CD5 expression, CD23 positivity and dim expression of CD20 and surface immunoglobulin [5] (Figure 9.4). CD43 is usually positive. CD79b and FMC7 are absent or weakly expressed. CD23 expression is of importance as the major differential diagnosis of a CD5-positive mature B-cell leukemia is mantle cell lymphoma in leukemic phase (see below), which is typically CD23 negative.

Matutes *et al.* proposed the use of a scoring system to differentiate CLL from other mature B-cell leukemias [6]. This system initially used five markers for features typical of CLL:

1. CD5 positivity.
2. CD23 positivity.
3. FMC7 negativity.
4. Weak expression of surface immunoglobulin.
5. Weak or absent expression of CD22.

In a large cohort of cases with a variety of circulating B-leukemia or B-lymphoma cells, 87% of patients with CLL were found to have scores of 4 or 5, whereas 89% and 72% of other B-leukemias and B-lymphomas had scores of 0 or 1, respectively [6]. A later refinement of this scoring system replaced CD22 with CD79b (typically absent in CLL), and broadened the criteria for defining CLL to 3–5 points [7]. This refinement improved diagnostic accuracy from 91.8–96.8% [7].

In CLL in transition to B-PLL (CLL/PLL), there may be two distinct populations on flow cytometry, with the B-PLL population being larger and showing brighter expression of CD20 and surface immunoglobulin. In contrast to *de novo* B-PLL, which is usually CD5-negative, transformed prolymphocytes in CLL/PLL often retain CD5 expression [5]. "Atypical" CLL (as defined by the "Matutes score") may be CD23-negative or show increased expression of surface immunoglobulin, FMC7 and/or CD20; these cases may be associated with the trisomy 12 cytogenetic abnormality [8].

The typical flow cytometry panel for CLL will include a tube assessing the co-expression of CD19 and CD38, an important prognostic indicator (see below).

Cytogenetic and molecular genetic features: Cytogenetic studies in CLL have traditionally been hampered by the low mitotic activity of the tumor cells *in vitro*. In a large study of peripheral blood mononuclear cell karyotyping in 433 patients with

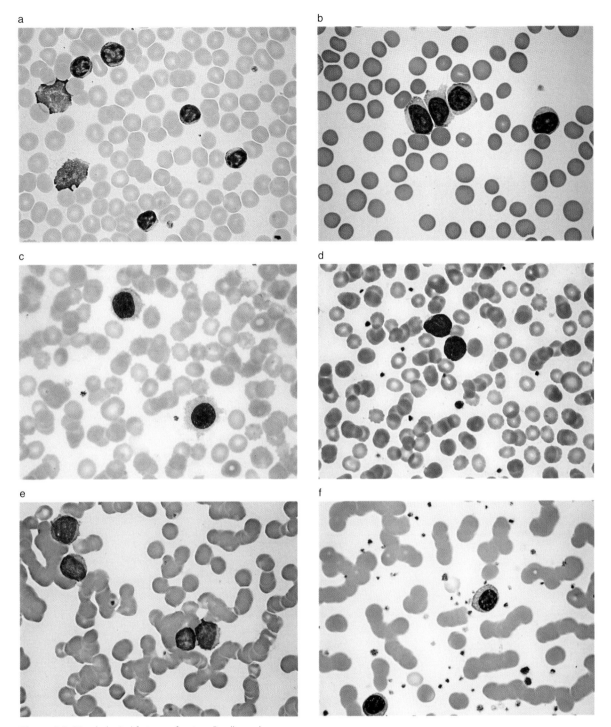

Figure 9.2. Morphological features of mature B-cell neoplasms.

a. CLL: Tumor cells are small lymphocytes with clumped chromatin and scanty cytoplasm. Note the presence of "smudge" cells.

b. B-PLL: Prolymphocytes are twice the size of mature lymphocytes, with condensed chromatin and a single prominent nucleolus.

c. HCL: Hairy cells can be scanty in the blood, but have a distinctive appearance with abundant, weakly basophilic or gray cytoplasm with circumferential "hairy" projections and an oval or bean-shaped nucleus displaying homogeneous, moderately clumped chromatin.

d. Follicular lymphoma: Lymphoma cells are small cells, with a high nuclear : cytoplasmic ratio, condensed homogeneous chromatin and a characteristic fine nuclear cleft.

e. Mantle cell lymphoma. The lymphoma cells are pleomorphic with both small- and medium-sized forms present, and a variety of nuclear morphology.

f. Lymphoplasmacytic lymphoma. Circulating lymphoplasmacytoid cells and background rouleaux due to paraprotein.

   Photographs courtesy of Dr. A George, St Vincent's Pathology, Melbourne, Victoria, Australia.

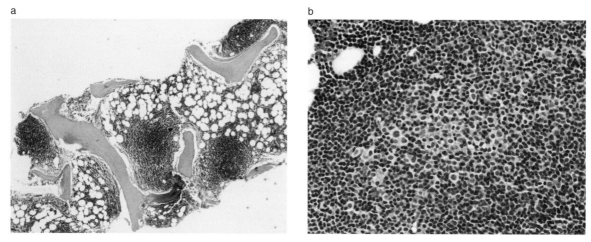

Figure 9.3. Chronic lymphocytic leukemia in a bone marrow trephine (H & E stain).
a. Low power view showing an interstitial nodular pattern of infiltration by CLL.
b. Higher power of a CLL nodule showing nucleolated larger cells in the center and peripherally located small mature CLL lymphocytes.

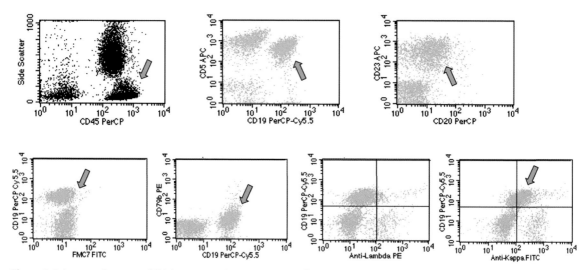

Figure 9.4. Immunophenotype of CLL (green arrows). Note expression of CD5, CD19, CD23; dim expression of CD20; and negative expression of FMC7 and CD79b. Surface immunoglobulin expression is weak and shows kappa light chain restriction.
Figure courtesy of Ms. I Cutter, St Vincent's Pathology, Melbourne, Victoria, Australia.

CLL, clonal abnormalities were identified in only 50% [9]. Thus, the field of CLL genetics was slow to progress until the widespread availability of fluorescent *in situ* hybridization (FISH) probes for common cytogenetic aberrations [10]; this showed that approximately 80% of CLL samples harbor one or more karyotypic aberration. This high aberration rate has since been confirmed by modern cultivation techniques (using an immuno-stimulatory

CpG-oligonucleotide and IL-2) capable of generating metaphases from > 98% of tested samples [11].

Cytogenetic features are most useful in prognostication of CLL, and not in classification. One possible exception is isolated trisomy 12, which is common in CLL and uncommon in other mature B-cell leukemias [9]. The other "recurrent" CLL abnormalities (deletion of 11q22.3, deletion of 13q14 and deletion of 17p13) are non-specific and may be found in disparate tumors such as mantle cell lymphoma and prolymphocytic leukemia.

Monoclonal B-cell lymphocytosis

With increasing use of flow cytometry to investigate minimal (and often transient) elevations in peripheral lymphocyte count, there is an increasing number of otherwise healthy subjects who are identified to have clonal B-cell populations of uncertain significance. These populations often display a classic CLL immunophenotype, and are present in approximately 5% of normal populations over 65 years of age [12]. In first-degree relatives of patients with CLL, small clonal B-cell populations are detectable in 13.5% [13]. In order to differentiate subjects with small B-cell clones of uncertain significance from patients with CLL, the International Workshop on Chronic Lymphocytic Leukemia (IWCLL) working group has arbitrarily defined CLL as requiring persistent elevation of circulating B-lymphocytes to $\geq 5 \times 10^9$/L [14]. Subjects displaying lower levels of clonal B-cell populations have "monoclonal B-lymphocytosis" (MBL), a state analogous to that of monoclonal gammopathy of uncertain significance (MGUS). Recent studies have shown that similar cytogenetic aberrations occur in subjects with MBL and in patients with CLL [15], that MBL precedes CLL in the majority of patients [15], and that the risk of conversion from MBL to CLL requiring treatment occurs at a rate of approximately 1% per year [16].

Currently, there is no agreed consensus as to when patients with an unexplained lymphocytosis should be further investigated by flow cytometry in order to diagnose MBL or CLL. The authors' practice is to perform flow cytometry if the lymphocytosis is persistent for more than 8 weeks at a borderline level ($<10 \times 10^9$/L), or for more than 4 weeks at a more moderate level ($\geq 10 \times 10^9$/L).

Staging and prognostication

Clinical example

The patient presented above (page 175) was confirmed to have CLL by morphology and flow cytometry ("Matutes score" = 5). What diagnostic tests are useful in staging and prognostication?

Clinical staging: CLL is staged based on clinical examination and peripheral blood findings. The two most commonly used systems are the Rai system (mainly

Table 9.1. Clinical staging systems in chronic lymphocytic leukemia (CLL).
(A) Clinical stage according to Binet [50]

	Number of involved lymph node areas[a]	Hemoglobin (g/L)	Platelets $\times 10^9$/L
Binet A	0–2	> 100	> 100
Binet B	> 2	> 100	> 100
Binet C	any	< 100 or	< 100

(B) Clinical stage according to Rai [51]

0	Blood and bone marrow involvement only
I	Lymphadenopathy
II	Splenomegaly/hepatomegaly
III	Hemoglobin < 110 g/L
IV	Platelet count $< 100 \times 10^9$/L

[a] Each of the following five regions counts as one area: palpable nodes in the neck, axillae and groins, clinically enlarged spleen and liver.

used in the USA) and the Binet system (mainly used in Europe) (Table 9.1). Although the exact cut-offs are slightly different, the major message is the same between the two systems: patients with features of bone marrow failure (low hemoglobin and/or platelets) fare the worst, followed by patients with widespread lymphadenopathy and/or organomegaly, and patients with either low-volume nodal disease or peripheral blood lymphocytosis only (Rai stage 0) fare the best.

A simple indicator of the proliferative capacity, or "pace," of the disease is the lymphocyte doubling time. Many patients present for initial assessment with a record of past blood counts, prior to the realization that they have CLL. Patients with short doubling times progress more rapidly to clinical symptoms requiring therapy, and experience inferior survival [17]. The assessment is simple and objective, and is one of the most important parameters with which to prospectively monitor disease progress. In clinical practice, patients without symptoms of progressive leukemia can be monitored with 3-monthly blood counts for one year, followed by 6-monthly blood counts if the disease remains non-progressive.

Although clinical staging and lymphocyte doubling time have stood the test of time and proven to be predictive of outcomes in both observation and therapeutic studies, they are intrinsically retrospective in nature and do not allow accurate prognostication of patients presenting in early stage disease, which now accounts for > 80% of patients at CLL diagnosis. Thus, there is substantial impetus to the development of novel prognostic markers to help prognosticate and guide decision-making at the time of initial disease diagnosis.

Morphology – prolymphocytes and smudge/smear cells: As discussed above, an increased proportion of prolymphocytes in the peripheral blood was associated with inferior outcomes in early studies [4]. Additionally, data from the Mayo group suggested that greater than 30% smudge cells on the routine blood smear may be a favorable factor in patients with newly diagnosed CLL [3].

Flow cytometry – CD38 and ZAP-70: The two most important markers of prognosis as determined by flow cytometry are CD38 and ZAP-70 expression. Whereas CD38 is regularly included in the diagnostic antibody panel for CLL in most laboratories, the status of ZAP-70 is controversial and it is not yet regarded as a routine test (see discussion later).

CD38 is a trans-membrane glycoprotein first characterized in 1980 as a T-cell differentiation antigen. It came to light as a prognostic marker in CLL when it was found to be strongly correlated with the immunoglobulin V_H gene (IgV_H) somatic mutation status, a key prognostic factor in CLL. Specifically, patients with unmutated IgV_H were more likely to have $\geq 30\%$ CD19/38 co-expression in the peripheral blood, and such patients were less likely to respond to chemotherapy and had reduced survival [18]. As IgV_H sequencing and mutation status determination was not routinely available in many diagnostic laboratories, it was proposed that CD38 percentage be used as a surrogate marker of IgV_H mutation status [18].

Subsequent studies have shown that CD38 is unreliable as a surrogate marker of IgV_H mutation status, but that CD38 positivity in itself confers an adverse prognostic significance. However, there remains considerable controversy regarding levels for defining CD38 positivity, with various studies suggesting 30%, 20% and even 7% as the ideal cut-off [18–20]. Another study suggested that it is the presence of *any* CD38 positive population, rather than a cut-off level, that is prognostic [21]. Finally, there is emerging evidence

that CD38 expression on CLL cells may be dynamic and may differ between blood, tissue and marrow compartments [21]. In practice, since most patients are confirmed to have CLL by flow cytometry of the peripheral blood, it is most pragmatic to define CD38 positivity by either the 20% or 30% threshold in peripheral blood samples.

ZAP-70 (zeta-associated protein 70) is a tyrosine kinase normally expressed in T- and NK-cells, where it plays a critical role in T-cell signaling [22]. It was identified in CLL in microarray experiments comparing patients with unmutated and mutated IgV_H genes, where it was shown that ZAP-70 was aberrantly and differentially expressed in patients with unmutated IgV_H. Therefore, ZAP-70 was developed initially as a surrogate marker for IgV_H mutation status [22], where it showed concordance of 77–95% [22–24]. Subsequent studies have shown that ZAP-70 may be more predictive of aggressive disease features than IgV_H mutation status, with patients discordantly positive for ZAP-70 and mutated IgV_H behaving similarly to unmutated, ZAP-70 positive patients [24]. Patients with usage of the V_H3–21 chain, which is an aggressive subset within the mutated IgV_H population, often show discordant positivity for ZAP-70 [25]. Therefore, there is little controversy regarding the importance of ZAP-70 as a prognostic factor.

The major controversy surrounding ZAP-70 lies with its measurement. It is most commonly measured by flow cytometry, where the major limitation is its relatively weak expression on CLL cells, and strong expression in T- and NK-cells. Therefore, a reliable flow cytometry strategy must take steps to separate ZAP-70 expression on malignant CLL cells, from that of background T- and NK-cell populations. Three major flow cytometry strategies have been published [22–24] (Table 9.2). Subsequent to their publication, many groups have attempted to optimize the flow cytometry assay, and it is clear that a number of factors including sample integrity, permeabilization procedure, antibody clone and fluorochrome choice and local factors all impact on the performance of the test. At present, no standard method for ZAP-70 assessment exists, and groups (including our center) have shown that measurement of ZAP-70 by other methods such as RT-PCR and immunocytochemistry may be similarly prognostic [26].

Cytogenetic and molecular genetic features: The landmark study be by Döhner *et al.*, showed FISH aberrations to be organized in a hierarchical model.

Table 9.2. Published methods for the assessment of ZAP-70 by flow cytometry.

Method [Ref.]	Sample	Antibody clone + fluorochrome	ZAP-70 negative cutoff	Counting ZAP-70 positive CLL cells
Crespo [22]	PB mononuclear cells or whole blood	2F3.2 (Upstate) FITC	Defined by expression in endogenous T/NK population (as identified by CD3+ or CD56+ staining). At least 1000 T/NK-cells analyzed	Proportion of CD5/19-positive population expressing ZAP-70 above cut-off
Orchard [23]	PB mononuclear cells	2F3.2 (Upstate) FITC	Defined by isotype control	T/NK-cell recognized either as distinct "bright" population or by CD2 or CD3 staining, and subtracted from total ZAP-70-positive population
Rassenti [24]	PB mononuclear cells	1E7.2 Alexa-488	Defined by threshold gates set on a normal donor (such that 0.1% of lymphocytes are CD19- and ZAP-70-positive)	Proportion of cells in the right upper quadrant (CD19 and ZAP-70 co-expressing) as defined by normal donor cut-off

Deletions of 17p13 are associated with the most aggressive disease features and shortest median survival (32 months), followed by deletions of 11q22–23 (79 months), trisomy 12q13 (114 months), "negative" FISH panel (111 months) and deletions of 13q14 (133 months) (Figure 9.5) [10]. Note that in this model the most adverse aberration confers the prognostic implication (i.e. a patient with both deletions of 13q14 and 17p13 would be regarded as being in the most adverse category of 17p13 deletion). Currently available commercial FISH probe "panels" target the four most important genetic aberrations listed above, with individual laboratories sometimes employing additional probes directed against 6q21, 8q24 and 14q32. An example of a FISH test is shown in Figure 9.6.

Based on these data, FISH is now regarded as one of the most important prognostic markers in CLL. In particular, CLL with deletion of 17p13 is said to be associated with relentlessly aggressive disease, poor response to chemotherapy and short survival, with several groups advocating early allogeneic transplantation for all such patients. Indeed, the experience with frontline chemotherapy trials in both Germany and UK supported this view, with median survivals of 16 and 11 months after fludarabine-based chemotherapy, respectively [27,28]. The UK data suggested that there may be a "threshold" effect of 17p13 deletion, with

patients displaying < 20% deletion behaving similarly to patients without 17p13 deletion [27]. This "threshold" has not been confirmed in the German studies [28]. However, 17p13 deletion is uncommon in early stage CLL, being found in only 5–7% of patients at the time of diagnosis, compared with a much higher prevalence (30–40%) in heavily pre-treated patients. Therefore, much of the poor prognosis associated with 17p13 deletion may simply be due to its prevalence in patients with advanced, multiply relapsed disease.

In order to better define the significance of 17p13 deletion in early stage CLL, our group analyzed the outcome of 99 patients found to have deletion of 17p13 prior to commencement of therapy [29]. In this study, only half of patients with early stage, asymptomatic 17p13 deletion progressed to requiring chemotherapy over 3 years, with patients remaining in stable non-progressive disease for up to 70 months (the limit of the current follow-up). Therefore, in our view, the finding of 17p13 deletion in patients with early stage CLL should not prompt therapeutic intervention outside of current guidelines for genetically unselected patients.

Recent data have also suggested that advances in rituximab-containing chemotherapy regimens may have modified the prognostic significance of deletions of 11q22–23, such that it may no longer be a marker

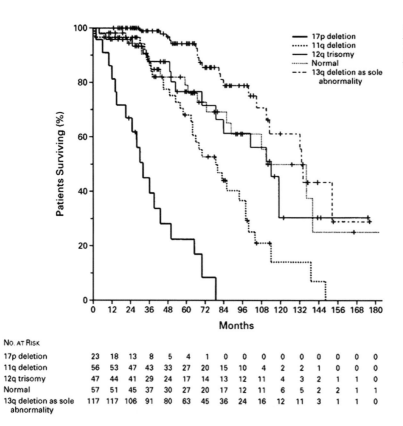

Figure 9.5. Survival in patients with CLL from date of diagnosis, as influenced by FISH findings. Reprinted with permission from Döhner [10].

No. AT RISK

17p deletion	23	18	13	8	5	4	1	0	0	0	0	0	0	0	0
11q deletion	56	53	47	43	33	27	20	15	10	4	2	2	1	0	0	0
12q trisomy	47	44	41	29	24	17	14	13	12	11	4	3	2	1	1	0
Normal	57	51	45	37	30	27	20	17	12	11	6	5	2	2	1	1
13q deletion as sole abnormality	117	117	106	91	80	63	45	36	24	16	12	11	3	1	1	0

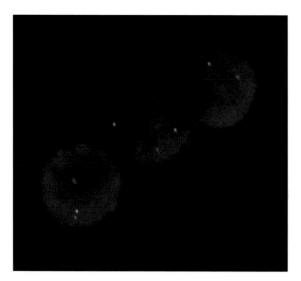

Figure 9.6. Interphase FISH testing in CLL. The red signal is the *ATM* gene (11q22.3) and the green signal is the *TP53* gene (17p13.1). The probe used is the p53/*ATM* dual color probe from Kreatech Diagnostics. Three cells are present: one with normal signal pattern (two green and two red signals), and two showing loss of one *ATM* signal. Photograph courtesy of A/Prof L Campbell, Victorian Cancer Cytogenetics Service, Melbourne, Victoria, Australia.

of inferior treatment outcome [30]. In addition, patients with trisomy 12 CLL may have increased expression of CD20, making these cells particularly susceptible to rituximab therapy [8]. Further clarification of the significance of FISH aberrations in the context of modern combination chemotherapy is ongoing.

A major pitfall of FISH testing is that it only identifies aberrations specifically probed for, in comparison to the genome-wide information available with conventional karyotyping. Current efforts to overcome the poor cytogenetic yield of CLL include improved culture techniques capable of producing an abnormality rate comparable to FISH, and genome-wide "array" platforms [11]. Preliminary data from these new platforms suggest that the complexity of cytogenetic changes is a predictor of aggressive disease and poor outcome. Further studies to define the exact prognostic significance of novel karyotypic aberrations are ongoing.

IgV_H mutation status: Somatic mutation of the IgV_H gene is a marker of B-cell maturation in the follicular germinal center, and IgV_H mutation status was one of the first novel markers shown to be prognostically important in CLL. Approximately 50% of patients with CLL have an unmutated IgV_H, and these patients experience more rapid disease progression, and have inferior survival, compared with their mutated IgV_H counterparts [18,31]. When IgV_H mutation status was first described, sequencing was poorly available in clinical laboratories, sparking the search for surrogate markers such as CD38 and ZAP-70. With increasing availability of high-throughput sequencing services and on-line immunoglobulin gene databases, IgV_H mutation status is now routinely available at selected clinical centers.

Although various studies have suggested differing optimal cut-offs for dividing mutated and unmutated IgV_H mutation status, the 2.0% cut-off as proposed by the original studies is now commonly accepted. Hence, CLL samples showing 2.0% or more sequence deviation from germline are defined as being IgV_H-mutated. It is also increasingly recognized that there are specific subsets of patients with mutated IgV_H who have aggressive disease features, similar to those of patients with unmutated IgV_H. The best recognized subset is mutated IgV_H patients that utilize the V_H3-21 family of genes. In a German study comparing FISH parameters, IgV_H mutation status and ZAP-70 expression in patients with B-CLL, the V_H3-21 cases were mostly discordantly Ig V_H-mutated and ZAP-70 positive [25]. The existence of these poor prognostic subsets in the IgV_H-mutated group may explain why ZAP-70 may be more effective at predicting aggressive disease than IgV_H mutation status.

Other tests: There are a large number of emerging prognostic markers for CLL, many of which have yet to transition from the research to the clinical domain. Of special mention are simple biochemical markers available in most clinical laboratories, in particular beta-2-microglobulin (β2m) and lactate dehydrogenase (LDH). β2m is the invariable light chain of the class I HLA

molecule. In our institutional experience, β2m is consistently one of the most important independent determinants of outcome, predicting for early requirement for initial therapy, poor response to both chemotherapy and chemo-immunotherapy regimens, and inferior survival across virtually all therapeutic trials [32]. It is likely to be a summation marker of disease bulk and proliferative activity, and the patient's renal function. LDH is a proliferative marker which is usually elevated in patients with histologic (Richter) transformation.

Are bone marrow aspirate and trephines still necessary in patients with CLL?: Most of the diagnostic and prognostic tests in CLL can be performed in the peripheral blood. Indeed, for certain tests such as FISH panels, peripheral blood may be preferable to the marrow due to a greater proportion of cells being malignant CLL cells. The only prognostic tests requiring bone marrow aspirate are conventional cytogenetic testing and bone marrow histology. A diffuse pattern of marrow infiltration is associated with reduced survival in the alkylator era [33], however this probably represents the effects of a heavy tumor burden. Many CLL physicians choose not to perform bone marrow aspirate and trephine at the time of initial diagnosis. In such cases, bone marrow examination is recommended prior to the initiation of chemotherapy, in order to document the extent and pattern of involvement, and to obtain samples for conventional cytogenetic testing. The latter test is not only important for assessment of the CLL karyotype, but also in documenting baseline cytogenetic status in patients who may later develop therapy-related myelodysplasia [34].

Summary of prognostic markers: All patients should be evaluated and staged clinically (Table 9.1), and peripheral blood examined for presence of smudge/smear cells and prolymphocytes. Serial blood counts, where available, provide a useful retrospective guide to the pace of disease progression and doubling time. Serum markers, particularly β2m and LDH, continue to be useful and widely available surrogates of disease burden and activity. With regards the "novel" markers, current evidence supports the characterization of CD38 status, FISH aberrations, IgV_H mutation status and sub-family usage (where available) in patients with newly diagnosed CLL. ZAP-70, although a powerful and independent marker, is hampered by difficulties in testing and may be employed if demonstrated to be reliably measured and validated against clinical endpoints by the testing laboratory.

International response criteria

Clinical example

Prognostic testing of this patient identified him to have unfavorable risk factors including an unmutated IgV$_H$ gene and deletion of 11q22–23 by FISH. After 18 months of observation, the patient developed tiredness, progressive splenomegaly and anemia. He received six cycles of chemotherapy in combination with rituximab and had a good response with no clinical (clinical examination and blood count) evidence of disease at the end of treatment. How should he be staged for response?

The response criteria for patients with CLL following therapy are standardized and are summarized in Table 9.3 [14]. At present, patients are staged by clinical history, physical examination and a blood count. Of relevance is the importance of bone marrow aspirate and trephine in establishing complete response or "nodular partial response." The identification of residual lymphoid nodules in the bone marrow is important as this is the last site of morphological disease to be cleared. Longitudinal studies have shown that patients with residual marrow nodules (nodular partial response) have inferior remission durations than patients in complete response (Figure 9.7). With the advent of immunocytochemistry, it is possible to determine whether the residual nodules in the marrow are predominantly B-cells (i.e. presumed residual CLL), or predominantly T-cell nodules (i.e. presumed reactive nodules). However, the ability of immunocytochemistry to predict remission durations has not been confirmed in prospective studies and this technique is likely to be superseded by more sensitive minimal residual disease testing methodologies, as detailed below.

Table 9.3. IWCLL response categories in chronic lymphocytic leukemia. Adapted from [14].

IWCLL response	Clinical assessment (Examination + blood tests)	Bone marrow assessment (2 months after last treatment)
Complete response	Peripheral blood lymphocytes < 4.0 × 10^9/L Lymph nodes ≤ 1.5cm[a] No hepatosplenomegaly[a] No constitutional symptoms Hemoglobin > 11 g/dL Neutrophils > 1.5 × 10^9/L Platelets > 100 × 10^9/L	Less than 30% lymphocytes in marrow aspirate Absence of lymphoid nodules on marrow trephine
Complete response with incomplete marrow recovery (provisional entity)	Same as complete response, except blood recovery parameters (hemoglobin, neutrophils and/or platelets) not met	Same as complete response
Nodular partial response	Same as complete response	Less than 30% lymphocytes in marrow aspirate Residual lymphoid nodules on marrow trephine Immunocytochemistry may be helpful
Partial response	Peripheral blood lymphocytes decrease ≥ 50% Reduction in lymph node size ≥ 50%[a] Reduction in hepatomegaly Reduction in splenomegaly ≥ 50%[a] **and** improvement in one blood count lineage: hemoglobin > 11 g/dL, neutrophils > 1.5 × 10^9/L, platelets > 100 × 10^9/L or improvement of ≥ 50% over baseline	Reduction in marrow infiltrate ≥ 50% (marrow re-evaluation generally not indicated outside of clinical trial)

All responses should be maintained for at least 2 months

[a] Assessment of lymph nodes, hepatomegaly and splenomegaly is by physical examination outside the context of a clinical trial; in a clinical trial, CT assessment of abdominal nodes is recommended before and after treatment.

Time to Disease Progression By Chemotherapy Response

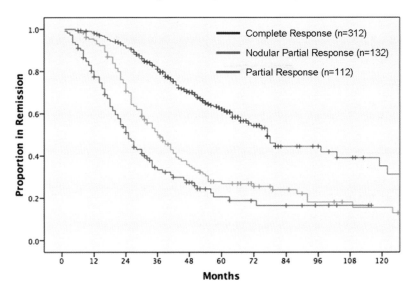

Figure 9.7. Time to progression for patients in various IWCLL response categories, from completed MD Anderson Cancer Center studies. Patients in complete response consistently enjoy superior remission durations than those in nodular partial response or partial response (p<0.001).

Minimal residual disease

The definition of complete remission requires <30% marrow lymphocytes without regard to the nature of these lymphocytes. This morphological definition is insensitive to small amounts of disease, and as highly effective chemo-immunotherapy treatment regimens evolve, there is an increasing need for tests to quantify minimal residual disease (MRD) at a submicroscopic level. The easiest way to accomplish this is with flow cytometry. We have previously shown that standard flow cytometry (capable of detecting approximately one CLL cell in 100 lymphocytes) is meaningful in predicting remission duration, and that the use of an even more sensitive molecular technique (ligase chain reaction) further refined the ability to identify those patients with the best clinical outcomes (Figure 9.8). Subsequently standardized methods of MRD assessment have emerged.

The two standard techniques of MRD assessment are allele-specific oligonucleotide polymerase chain reaction (ASO-PCR) [35] and four-color flow cytometry (Figure 9.9) [36]. The principles of these techniques are outlined in Table 9.4. Both techniques are capable of detecting MRD at a level of 1 in 10^4 cells. In the recent German CLL Study Group study of frontline chemo-immunotherapy, MRD proved to be one of the strongest determinants of remission duration [37], confirming that the goal of modern CLL therapy should be to eliminate all detectable MRD.

B-cell prolymphocytic leukemia

Clinical example

A 66-year-old man presents with poor energy, involuntary loss of weight and abdominal discomfort due to splenomegaly. A blood count shows lymphocytosis of $121 \times 10^9/L$ with numerous prolymphocytes. How should this patient be investigated?

B-cell prolymphocytic leukemia (B-PLL) is a rare leukemia, occurring in fewer than 1 per 100 000 person-years in Western populations (Figure 9.1b). Most patients are over 60 years old, with a balanced male:female distribution [4]. It is an aggressive disease with a median survival of approximately 3 years [4,38].

Establishing the diagnosis

Morphology: Morphologically, patients with B-PLL have a peripheral lymphocytosis with >55% (often close to 100%) prolymphocytes. Prolymphocytes are twice the size of a mature lymphocyte, with a round nucleus, condensed chromatin pattern and a single prominent nucleolus (Figure 9.2b). Although there are some significant morphological differences, it is

181

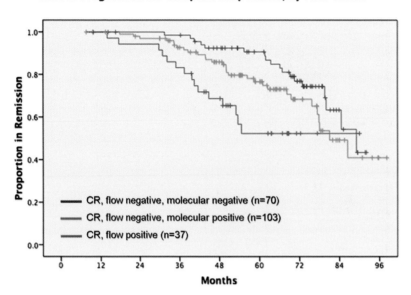

Time to Progression for Complete Responders, by MRD Status

Figure 9.8. Minimal residual disease (MRD) studies are valuable in patients in morphological complete remission (CR) (p=0.007). Data from the MD Anderson Cancer Center Phase II Study of Fludarabine, Cyclophosphamide and Rituximab.

not always possible to differentiate between B-PLL and T-PLL morphologically.

Immunophenotype: The immunophenotype of B-PLL is that of a B-cell (CD19- and CD79a-positive) with brighter expression of surface immunoglobulin, CD20, CD22, CD79b and FMC-7 than CLL. CD5, CD10 and CD23 are typically negative [5].

Cytogenetic and molecular genetic features: Early case series of B-PLL included cases with the t(11;14)(q13;q32) translocation. Such cases are now considered mantle cell lymphoma in leukemic phase (see below). The diagnosis of B-PLL under the 2008 World Health Organization classification requires exclusion of t(11;14)(q13;q32) by FISH and/or molecular studies. There are no karyotypic aberrations specific to B-PLL.

Staging and prognostication

No staging system exists for B-PLL. The majority of patients present with systemic symptoms, splenomegaly, marked lymphocytosis and anemia [4]. Due to the rarity of the condition, prognostic markers in B-PLL have not been defined. One published study evaluated IgV$_H$ mutation status, ZAP-70 and FISH in 19 cases of *de novo* B-PLL. In this study, the distribution of unmutated IgV$_H$ gene usage (53%) and ZAP-70 positivity

(57%) in B-PLL was similar to that reported for CLL populations, but unlike the situation in CLL, there was no relationship between an unmutated IgV$_H$ gene and ZAP-70 positivity [38]. IgV$_H$ mutation status and ZAP-70 expression had no impact on survival. FISH deletion of 17p13.1 was common, occurring in 53% of cases, and was found mainly in patients with an unmutated IgV$_H$. Patients with 17p13.1 deletion had a reduced median survival of 12 months (versus 40 months for 17p13.1 non-deleted, $p = 0.24$) [38].

Hairy cell leukemia

Clinical example

A 56-year-old man presented with tiredness and was found to be pancytopenic with absolute monocytopenia. Splenomegaly was evident on clinical examination. He underwent an attempted bone marrow aspirate which yielded a "dry tap." How should he be investigated?

Hairy cell leukemia (HCL) is a rare leukemia, with an incidence of less than 1 per 100 000 person-years (Figure 9.1). The median age at presentation is 55 years, with a striking (5:1) male predominance [39]. With the advent of purine analog-based chemotherapy, long-lasting remissions are now achievable in the majority of patients [39]. This unique sensitivity to

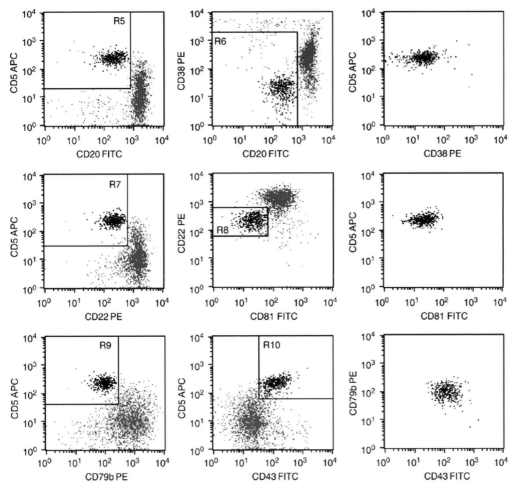

Figure 9.9. Standardized 4-color flow cytometry MRD assessment in CLL. CLL cells can be identified as CD5+ events that express CD20, CD22 (R7), CD81(R8) and CD79b(R9) weakly, and CD43(R10) strongly.
Reprinted with permission from [36].

purine analog makes HCL an important diagnosis to consider in patients presenting with bone marrow failure, despite the rarity of the condition.

Establishing the diagnosis

Morphology: Hairy cell lymphocytes have a distinctive appearance, being small- to medium-sized cells displaying abundant, weakly basophilic or light gray cytoplasm with numerous circumferential "hairy" or irregular projections (Figure 9.2c). The nucleus is usually oval or bean-shaped with homogeneous, moderately clumped chromatin. Nucleoli are typically absent. These cells are often infrequent in the peripheral blood and can be inconspicuous. A common peripheral blood "clue" to

the presence of HCL is marked monocytopenia (the mechanism of which remains undefined).

Due to the fibrotic nature of the disorder, bone marrow aspirates are often "dry taps" yielding poor quality specimens for diagnostic work-up. When sufficient HCL cells are present, a classic cytochemical finding is tartrate-resistant acid phosphatase (TRAP) stain positivity. Bone marrow trephine histology typically shows a widely spaced infiltrate with a classic "fried egg" appearance due to the abundant cytoplasm (Figure 9.10). Immunocytochemistry can be performed on sections of the bone marrow biopsy to demonstrate the neoplastic cells are of B-cell origin (CD20, CD79a, PAX5 positive) and express CD11c antigen (Figure 9.10c). Reticulin fibrosis is usually

Table 9.4. Minimal residual disease (MRD) assessment in CLL. Current studies indicate that MRD detection is more sensitive in marrow aspirate than peripheral blood. Adapted from [35,36].

MRD assessment methodology	Principle of test	Advantages	Disadvantages
Allele-Specific Oligonucleotide Polymerase Chain Reaction (ASO-PCR)	The unique IgH complementary determining region III (CDRIII) of CLL cells provides a specific clonal marker for PCR testing Patient-specific primers are generated by amplifying CLL cell CDRIII using consensus primers, and sequencing the clonal PCR product. Cloning may be required in some patients These primers are then used to detect minimal residual disease (by PCR amplification) following treatment	Considered gold standard for MRD detection (sensitive to 1 in 10^4 cells or better) Samples for MRD testing can be stably stored, for transportation and testing at a later date. Suitable for batch-testing	Sequencing of CDRIII may not be successful in all patients, even when cloning techniques are employed Requires availability of pre-treatment material Sequencing and generation of patient-specific primers is labor intensive Turn-around time for PCR testing of MRD is slower than flow cytometry
Multi-color flow cytometry	CLL has a unique flow cytometry signature, allowing its separation from normal B-cells and hematogones Samples are analyzed using 3 standard antibody combinations (CD5/CD19 with CD20/CD38, CD81/CD22 and CD79b/CD43). A target of ≥ 500 000 events is acquired and MRD is present if greater than 50 CLL cells are detected in ≥ 2 of 3 tubes Relative to normal B-cells, CLL cells can be identified as CD5+ events that express CD20, CD22, CD81 and CD79b weakly, and CD43 strongly	Similar sensitivity to ASO-PCR (sensitive to 1 in 10^4 cells) Does not require pre-treatment sample to be available, or patient-specific material to be generated Fast turn-around time compared with ASO-PCR.	Variation in interpretation is required for patients with atypical CLL phenotypes (e.g. strong CD20 expression, weak CD43 expression). Knowledge of baseline phenotype is desirable. May not be possible to acquire sufficient events in poor quality specimens Requires fresh blood or marrow samples, not suitable for batch-testing

present and mesh-like in appearance. When there is low-volume and patchy marrow infiltration, this subtle involvement by HCL can be missed by an inexperienced morphologist.

Immunophenotype: The classic immunophenotype of HCL is a B-cell with bright surface immunoglobulin, CD20, FMC-7 and CD22 expression, and co-expression of one or more HCL-associated markers (i.e. CD11c, CD25 and/or CD103) (Figure 9.11). CD5, CD10 and CD23 are usually negative [5]. CD11c may also be weakly expressed by CLL, B-PLL and marginal zone lymphomas, and some cases of CLL can be CD25-positive. Therefore, there is significant interest in identifying new markers specific for HCL.

Of these new markers, the ones most commonly used in clinical practice are DBA44 and annexin A1 [40,41]. Both markers are effective immunocytochemical stains when performed on bone marrow trephine biopsies. DBA44 has the advantage of being restricted to areas of lymphoid infiltration, but is less specific for

HCL than annexin A1. Annexin A1, on the other hand, is positive in background marrow myeloid and T-cells and should be interpreted using a concurrent CD20 immunostain to highlight areas of B-cell infiltration. Other promising new markers for HCL include CD123, T-bet and monoclonal antibodies which identify TRAP.

Cytogenetic and molecular genetic features: No cytogenetic abnormality is specific for HCL. The majority of cases are IgV$_H$-mutated, consistent with a post-germinal center cell of origin [42].

Staging and prognostication

Hairy cell leukemia is unique in that results following purine analog therapy are exceptionally favorable, such that no important prognostic markers currently exist. With current chemotherapy, approximately 80–90% of patients achieve complete remission lasting five or more years, and those who relapse are often successfully re-treated [39,43]. In a large cohort of 349 patients treated

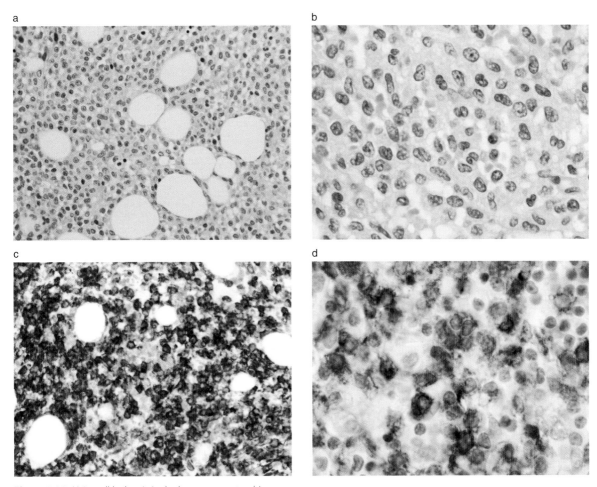

Figure 9.10. Hairy cell leukemia in the bone marrow trephine.
a. Diffuse bone marrow infiltrate and a virtual absence of normal hematopoiesis.
b. Cytological detail of hairy cells. The cells are well spaced due to abundant cytoplasm and the nuclei are pleomorphic.
c. CD11c positivity of the hairy cells (immunoperoxidase stain).
d. CD20 positivity of hairy cells (×1000; immunoperoxidase stain) showing persistent disease following therapy.

with cladribine therapy, the only independent associates of inferior survival were baseline white cell count > 15 × 10^9/L and age > 50 years [39].

Hairy cell leukemia variant

The term "hairy cell leukemia variant" was used to describe cases with atypical clinical, morphological, cytochemical or phenotypic features. The atypical morphological features include high white cell count, lack of monocytopenia and cells with prominent nucleoli. The atypical cytochemical and immunophenotypic features are negativity for TRAP, CD25 and annexin-A1. They may be positive for CD11c, CD103 and DBA44, and may show a widely spaced, diffuse pattern of infiltration on

bone marrow trephine biopsy. These cases are said to have a less favorable response to purine analog chemotherapy. In the 2008 World Health Organization classification of hematopoietic and lymphoid neoplasms, these cases are no longer considered biologically related to HCL. Hairy cell leukemia ariants are regarded as splenic lymphomas and, as such, are listed under the heading of "splenic B-cell lymphoma/leukemia, unclassifiable".

Leukemic phase of mature B-cell lymphomas

A discussion follows of lymphomas that are typically based primarily either in lymph nodes or extranodal lymphoid tissues, and which may spill over into the

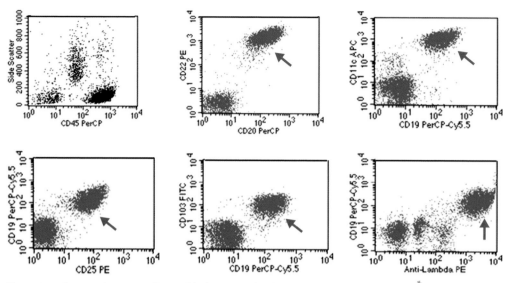

Figure 9.11. Immunophenotype of hairy cell leukemia. Note bright expression of CD20 and CD22, expression of CD11c, CD25 and CD103, and lambda light chain restriction (arrows). Figure courtesy of Ms. I Cutter, St Vincent's Pathology, Melbourne, Victoria, Australia.

peripheral blood as a consequence of heavy systemic involvement. In uncommon cases, these lymphomas can present predominantly as circulating disease without significant clinical lymphadenopathy, thus mimicking the primary low-grade B-cell leukemias such as CLL. These lymphomas will not be discussed in detail, but rather the peripheral blood morphological and immunophenotypic features are focused on as these may assist in making the correct diagnosis. Chapter 11 gives a more detailed account of lymphomas and the laboratory techniques used for disease staging.

Follicular lymphoma

Follicular lymphoma is the second most common type of non-Hodgkin lymphoma [44]. The bone marrow is involved in 40–70% of cases, and circulating lymphoma cells are present in a significant minority of patients. Circulating follicular lymphoma cells are typically small, with a high nuclear : cytoplasmic ratio, condensed chromatin and a characteristic fine nuclear cleft (Figures 9.2d). The immunophenotype is that of a B-cell (moderate to strong expression of CD19, CD20, CD22, CD79a and surface immunoglobulin), with expression of the follicle center cell markers CD10 and BCL-6 [5]. CD5, CD23 and CD43 are negative. Most patients with circulating cells have the diagnosis confirmed by lymph node and/or bone marrow biopsy. The classical cytogenetic/molecular aberration of follicular

lymphoma is over-expression of the BCL-2 protein due to a translocation with the IgH gene, and evidence of t(14;18)(q32;q21). The genetic translocation can be detected by karyotyping, FISH and/or RT-PCR. BCL-2 over-expression can be assessed by immunocytochemistry and will be present in 80–90% of cases.

Mantle cell lymphoma

Mantle cell lymphoma is a non-Hodgkin lymphoma with a relatively aggressive clinical course. Circulating lymphoma cells are seen at some stage in the illness in up to 77% of patients [45]. A diagnostic clue in the peripheral blood is the marked pleomorphism of the cells, which can range from small (CLL-like) forms to medium (or occasionally large) cells with irregular, angular or cleft nuclei and multiple nucleoli (Figure 9.2e). Patients with the blastoid variant have increased proportions of the larger cells and an open chromatin pattern similar to that of lymphoblasts [46]. There is also a small cell variant that resembles CLL morphologically. The immunophenotype is moderate expression of CD19, CD20, CD22, CD79a and surface immunoglobulin with co-expression of CD5 and CD43 antigens. Therefore, the major differential diagnosis by flow cytometry is CLL. However, mantle cell lymphoma is CD23-negative and usually expresses CD20, FMC-7 and surface immunoglobulin at a brighter intensity than CLL.

The classical cytogenetic/molecular aberration of mantle cell lymphoma is over-expression of cyclin D1 (also known as BCL-1) protein due to a translocation with the *IgH* gene, and evidence of t(11;14)(q13;q32). The genetic translocation is best tested by FISH, but is also evaluable by karyotyping and RT-PCR. Evidence of cyclin D1 over-expression is tested by immunocytochemistry and will be present in almost all cases. The existence of "cyclin D1-negative" mantle cell lymphomas, where the tumor displays classical morphology and immunophenotype but is negative for the t(11;14)(q13;q32) translocation by FISH and cyclin D1 is not over-expressed by immunocytochemistry, has been controversial until recently. Gene expression array studies now confirm that such cases do exist and that dysregulation of cyclin D2 or cyclin D3 account for their pathophysiology [47].

Marginal zone lymphoma

There are four subtypes of marginal zone lymphoma (MZL): extranodal, splenic, nodal and leukemic. Extranodal, splenic and nodal MZL are genetically distinct disorders grouped together because of a common immunophenotype and presumed cell of origin (i.e. post-germinal center, marginal zone B-cell). Leukemic MZL, in contrast, is a controversial entity that may represent a separate disease, or alternatively early forms of one of the other subtypes of MZL [48].

Immunophenotypically all subtypes of MZL are monoclonal B-cells (expression of CD19, CD20, CD79a and light chain restricted surface immunoglobulin) that express the marginal zone cell associated antigens CD21 and CD35. CD11c may be positive (particularly in splenic MZL) but is typically less bright than in hairy cell leukemia. Cases of MZL are otherwise negative for CD5, CD10, CD23, CD43, CD103 and cyclin D1 antigens. Morphologically MZL lymphoma cells tend to be either bland, small lymphocytes, or alternatively (in the case of splenic MZL) lymphocytes with short, polar villous projections. The main differentiating feature is that they do not express antigens typical of other B-cell neoplasms, i.e. CLL (CD5 and CD23), follicular lymphoma (CD10), mantle cell lymphoma (CD5 and cyclin D1) or hairy cell leukemia (CD103 and annexin A1) [5]. Hence MZL is primarily an immunophenotypic diagnosis of exclusion.

The discovery of this diagnosis on peripheral blood should prompt careful physical examination and investigation of the gastrointestinal tract (for extranodal MZL), evaluation for lymphadenopathy by computerized tomography (for nodal MZL), and radiological measurement of spleen size (for splenic MZL). Patients without any identifiable foci of disease following these above-mentioned investigations may be considered "leukemic MZL" [48]. The investigation for additional sites of disease is important as the subtypes differ greatly in treatment strategies (e.g. *Helicobacter pylori* eradication for gastric extranodal MZL, compared with splenectomy for splenic MZL) and prognosis. There is also an association between splenic MZL and hepatitis C infection.

Lymphoplasmacytic lymphoma

Lymphoplasmacytic lymphoma (LPL) is characterized by a spectrum of neoplastic cells ranging from small bland B-lymphocytes to plasmacytoid lymphocytes and plasma cells (Figure 9.2f). It includes Waldenström macroglobulinemia, defined as a subset of LPL cases with bone marrow infiltration and an IgM paraprotein of any concentration [49].

In the 2008 World Health Organization classification, this label can only be applied if the diagnostic criteria for another B-cell neoplasm (many of which can have lymphoplasmacytoid variants) are not met. This is particularly problematic in the case of MZL, which can display prominent lymphoplasmacytoid morphology and which has no distinguishing immunophenotypic features. In practice, the clinical picture dominates the diagnostic decision-making process. For example, a patient with a small paraprotein and prominent spleen is best classified as splenic MZL, whereas a patient with circulating lymphoplasmacytoid cells, high IgM paraprotein, hyperviscosity and heavy marrow infiltrate is best classified as LPL/Waldenström macroglobulinemia.

Conclusions

Currently, accurate diagnosis of a circulating B-cell lymphoproliferative disorder relies mostly on immunophenotypic features (as assessed by flow cytometry), supplemented by clinical and morphological findings. Increasingly, individual diseases are defined by distinct cytogenetic and molecular features, with the salient example being the requirement for t(11;14)(q13;q32) [or equivalent] in mantle cell lymphoma, and reclassification of cases formerly considered to be B-PLL based on this cytogenetic finding. There is increasing appreciation that CLL is not a single disease, but rather a heterogeneous collection of related disorders, and further subclassification of this diagnosis is likely to occur in future studies. Already, patients with 17p13 deletion CLL are recognized to have an inferior prognosis compared with other subtypes of CLL, and specific treatment strategies targeting this particular group of patients are being trialed. Finally, new tools such as gene arrays will be increasingly used in the clinical setting, particularly in cases where the diagnosis is difficult to establish, such as in cases of cyclin D1-negative mantle cell lymphoma.

References

1. Morton LM, Wang SS, Devesa SS *et al*. Lymphoma incidence patterns by WHO subtype in the United States, 1992–2001. *Blood* 2006;**107**:265–76.

2. Tam CS. The rare entity of chronic lymphocytic leukemia in Chinese patients: is it the same disease as in Western patients? *Leuk Lymphoma* 2008;**49**:1841–2.

3. Nowakowski GS, Hoyer JD, Shanafelt TD *et al*. Percentage of smudge cells on routine blood smear predicts survival in chronic lymphocytic leukemia. *J Clin Oncol* 2009;**27**:1844–9.

4. Melo JV, Catovsky D, Gregory WM, Galton DA. The relationship between chronic lymphocytic leukaemia and prolymphocytic leukaemia. IV. Analysis of survival and prognostic features. *Br J Haematol* 1987;**65**:23–9.

5. Weisberger J, Wu CD, Liu Z *et al*. Differential diagnosis of malignant lymphomas and related disorders by specific pattern of expression of immunophenotypic markers revealed by multiparameter flow cytometry. *Int J Oncol* 2000;**17**:1165–77.

6. Matutes E, Owusu-Ankomah K, Morilla R *et al*. The immunological profile of B-cell disorders and proposal of a scoring system for the diagnosis of CLL. *Leukemia* 1994;**8**:1640–5.

7. Moreau EJ, Matutes E, A'Hern RP *et al*. Improvement of the chronic lymphocytic leukemia scoring system with the monoclonal antibody SN8 (CD79b). *Am J Clin Pathol* 1997;**108**:378–82.

8. Tam CS, Otero-Palacios J, Abruzzo LV *et al*. Chronic lymphocytic leukaemia CD20 expression is dependent on the genetic subtype: a study of quantitative flow cytometry and fluorescent in-situ hybridization in 510 patients. *Br J Haematol* 2008;**141**:36–40.

9. Juliusson G, Oscier DG, Fitchett M *et al*. Prognostic subgroups in B-cell chronic lymphocytic leukemia defined by specific chromosomal abnormalities. *New Engl J Med* 1990;**323**:720–4.

10. Dohner H, Stilgenbauer S, Benner A *et al*. Genomic aberrations and survival in chronic lymphocytic leukemia. *New Engl J Med* 2000;**343**:1910–16.

11. Dicker F, Schnittger S, Haferlach T, Kern W, Schoch C. Immunostimulatory oligonucleotide-induced metaphase cytogenetics detect chromosomal aberrations in 80% of CLL patients: A study of 132 CLL cases with correlation to FISH, IgVH status, and CD38 expression. *Blood* 2006;**108**:3152–3160.

12. Ghia P, Prato G, Scielzo C *et al*. Monoclonal CD5+ and CD5- B-lymphocyte expansions are frequent in the peripheral blood of the elderly. *Blood* 2004;**103**:2337–42.

13. Rawstron AC, Yuille MR, Fuller J *et al*. Inherited predisposition to CLL is detectable as subclinical monoclonal B-lymphocyte expansion. *Blood* 2002;**100**:2289–90.

14. Hallek M, Cheson BD, Catovsky D *et al*. Guidelines for the diagnosis and treatment of chronic lymphocytic leukemia: a report from the International Workshop on Chronic Lymphocytic Leukemia (IWCLL) updating the National Cancer Institute-Working Group (NCI-WG)1996 guidelines. *Blood* 2008;**111**:5446–56.

15. Rawstron AC, Bennett FL, O'Connor SJ *et al*. Monoclonal B-cell lymphocytosis and chronic lymphocytic leukemia. *New Engl J Med* 2008;**359**:575–83.

16. Landgren O, Albitar M, Ma W *et al*. B-cell clones as early markers for chronic lymphocytic leukemia. *New Engl J Med* 2009;**360**:659–67.

17. Montserrat E, Sanchez-Bisono J, Vinolas N, Rozman C. Lymphocyte doubling time in chronic lymphocytic leukaemia: analysis of its prognostic significance. *Br J Haematol* 1986;**62**:567–75.

18. Damle RN, Wasil T, Fais F *et al*. Ig V gene mutation status and CD38 expression as novel prognostic indicators in chronic lymphocytic leukemia. *Blood* 1999;**94**:1840–7.

19. Ibrahim S, Keating M, Do KA *et al*. CD38 expression as an important prognostic factor in B-cell chronic lymphocytic leukemia. *Blood* 2001;**98**:181–6.

20. Krober A, Seiler T, Benner A *et al*. V(H) mutation status, CD38 expression level, genomic aberrations, and survival in chronic lymphocytic leukemia. *Blood* 2002;**100**:1410–16.

21. Ghia P, Guida G, Stella S *et al*. The pattern of CD38 expression defines a distinct subset of chronic lymphocytic leukemia (CLL) patients at risk of disease progression. *Blood* 2003;**101**:1262–9.

22. Crespo M, Bosch F, Villamor N *et al*. ZAP-70 expression as a surrogate for immunoglobulin-variable-region mutations in chronic lymphocytic leukemia. *New Engl J Med* 2003;**348**:1764–75.

23. Orchard JA, Ibbotson RE, Davis Z *et al*. ZAP-70 expression and prognosis in chronic lymphocytic leukaemia. *Lancet* 2004;**363**:105–11.

24. Rassenti LZ, Huynh L, Toy TL *et al*. ZAP-70 compared with immunoglobulin heavy-chain gene mutation status as a predictor of disease progression in chronic lymphocytic leukemia. *New Engl J Med* 2004;**351**:893–901.

25. Krober A, Bloehdorn J, Hafner S *et al*. Additional genetic high-risk features such as 11q deletion, 17p deletion, and V3–21 usage characterize discordance of ZAP-70 and VH mutation status in chronic lymphocytic leukemia. *J Clin Oncol* 2006;**24**:969–75.

26. Schlette E, Admirand J, Wierda W *et al*. p53 expression by immunohistochemistry is an important determinant of survival in chronic lymphocytic leukemia patients receiving frontline chemoimmunotherapy. *Leukemia Lymphoma* 2009;**50**:1597–605.

27. Catovsky D, Richards S, Matutes E *et al*. Assessment of fludarabine plus cyclophosphamide for patients with chronic lymphocytic leukaemia (the LRF CLL4 Trial): a randomised controlled trial. *Lancet* 2007;**370**:230–9.

28. Stilgenbauer S, Krober A, Busch R *et al*. 17p deletion predicts for inferior overall survival after fludarabine-based first line therapy in chronic lymphocytic leukemia: first analysis of genetics in the CLL4 trial of the GCLLSG. *ASH Annual Meeting Abstracts* 2005;**106**:715.

29. Tam CS, Shanafelt TD, Wierda WG *et al*. De novo deletion 17p13.1 chronic lymphocytic leukemia shows significant clinical heterogeneity: the M. D. Anderson and Mayo Clinic experience. *Blood* 2009;**114**:957–64.

30. Tsimberidou AM, Tam CS, Wierda WG *et al*. The prognostic significance of 11q deletion detected by fluorescence in situ hybridization (FISH) in untreated chronic lymphocytic leukemia (CLL): the MDACC experience. *ASH Annual Meeting Abstracts* 2007;**110**:2078.

31. Hamblin TJ, Davis Z, Gardiner A, Oscier DG, Stevenson FK. Unmutated Ig V(H) genes are associated with a more aggressive form of chronic lymphocytic leukemia. *Blood* 1999;**94**:1848–54.

32. Tam CS, O'Brien S, Wierda W *et al*. Long-term results of the fludarabine, cyclophosphamide, and rituximab regimen as initial therapy of chronic lymphocytic leukemia. *Blood* 2008;**112**:975–80.

33. Rozman C, Montserrat E, Rodriguez-Fernandez JM *et al*. Bone marrow histologic pattern – the best single prognostic parameter in chronic lymphocytic leukemia: a multivariate survival analysis of 329 cases. *Blood* 1984;**64**:642–8.

34. Tam CS, Seymour JF, Prince HM *et al*. Treatment-related myelodysplasia following fludarabine combination chemotherapy. *Haematologica* 2006;**91**:1546–50.

35. Provan D, Bartlett-Pandite L, Zwicky C *et al*. Eradication of polymerase chain reaction-detectable chronic lymphocytic leukemia cells is associated with improved outcome after bone marrow transplantation. *Blood* 1996;**88**:2228–35.

36. Rawstron AC, Villamor N, Ritgen M *et al*. International standardized approach for flow cytometric residual disease monitoring in chronic lymphocytic leukaemia. *Leukemia* 2007;**21**:956–64.

37. Boettcher S, Fischer K, Stilgenbauer S *et al*. Quantitative MRD assessments predict progression free survival in CLL patients treated with fludarabine and cyclophosphamide with or without rituximab – a prospective analysis in 471 patients from the randomized GCLLSG CLL8 Trial. *ASH Annual Meeting Abstracts ASH Annual Meeting Abstracts* 2008;**112**:326.

38. Del Giudice I, Davis Z, Matutes E *et al*. IgVH genes mutation and usage, ZAP-70 and CD38 expression provide new insights on B-cell prolymphocytic leukemia (B-PLL). *Leukemia* 2006;**20**:1231–7.

39. Saven A, Burian C, Koziol JA, Piro LD. Long-term follow-up of patients with hairy cell leukemia after cladribine treatment. *Blood* 1998;**92**:1918–26.

40. Hounieu H, Chittal SM, al Saati T *et al*. Hairy cell leukemia. Diagnosis of bone marrow involvement in paraffin-embedded sections with monoclonal antibody DBA.44. *Am J Clin Pathol* 1992;**98**:26–33.

41. Falini B, Tiacci E, Liso A *et al*. Simple diagnostic assay for hairy cell leukaemia by immunocytochemical detection of annexin A1 (ANXA1). *Lancet* 2004;**363**:1869–70.

42. Arons E, Sunshine J, Suntum T, Kreitman RJ. Somatic hypermutation and VH gene usage in hairy cell leukaemia. *Br J Haematol* 2006;**133**:504–12.

43. Else M, Ruchlemer R, Osuji N *et al*. Long remissions in hairy cell leukemia with purine analogs: a report of 219 patients with a median follow-up of 12.5 years. *Cancer* 2005;**104**:2442–8.

44. Armitage JO, Weisenburger DD. New approach to classifying non-Hodgkin's lymphomas: clinical features of the major histologic subtypes. Non-Hodgkin's Lymphoma Classification Project. *J Clin Oncol* 1998;**16**:2780–95.

45. Cohen PL, Kurtin PJ, Donovan KA, Hanson CA. Bone marrow and peripheral blood involvement in mantle cell lymphoma. *Br J Haematol* 1998;**101**:302–10.

46. Singleton TP, Anderson MM, Ross CW, Schnitzer B. Leukemic phase of mantle cell lymphoma, blastoid variant. *Am J Clin Pathol* 1999;**111**:495–500.

47. Fu K, Weisenburger DD, Greiner TC *et al*. Cyclin D1-negative mantle cell lymphoma: a clinicopathologic study based on gene expression profiling. *Blood* 2005;**106**:4315–21.

48. Tam CS, Prince HM, Westerman D, Seymour JF, Juneja S. Leukaemic subtype of marginal zone lymphoma: a presentation of three cases and literature review. *Leukemia Lymphoma* 2004;**45**:705–10.

49. Owen RG, Treon SP, Al Katib A *et al*. Clinicopathological definition of Waldenstrom's macroglobulinemia: consensus panel recommendations from the Second International Workshop on Waldenstrom's Macroglobulinemia. *Semin Oncol* 2003;**30**:110–15.

50. Binet JL, Auquier A, Dighiero G *et al*. A new prognostic classification of chronic lymphocytic leukemia derived from a multivariate survival analysis. *Cancer* 1981;**48**:198–206.

51. Rai KR, Sawitsky A, Cronkite EP *et al*. Clinical staging of chronic lymphocytic leukemia. *Blood* 1975;**6**:219–34.

10 Mature T-cell and natural-killer cell leukemias

Kaaren K. Reichard and Kathryn Foucar

Introduction

Mature T-cell and natural-killer cell (NK-cell) leuke-mias consist of T-cell prolymphocytic leukemia (T-PLL), T-cell large granular lymphocytic leukemia (T-LGL), chronic lymphoproliferative disorder of NK-cells (NK-CLPN), adult T-cell leukemia/lym-phoma (ATLL) and Sézary syndrome (SS). These dis-orders comprise a relatively uncommon group of neoplasms which, with the exception of T-PLL, lack a recurrent cytogenetic "marker." Consequently, the successful diagnosis of a mature T/NK-cell leukemia requires the integration of a variety of parameters.

The evaluation of a patient for a possible T/NK-cell chronic lymphoproliferative disorder is generally triggered by a symptom. Some of these symptoms are non-specific such as fatigue, secondary infection and bleeding, all of which are linked to underlying hematopoietic compromise. Other symptoms are somewhat more disease-specific including skin man-ifestations in SS, and less often in ATLL (> 50%) and T-PLL (20%). Some patients with mature T/NK-cell leukemias are severely symptomatic (especially patients with T-PLL and ATLL), while other patients may be entirely asymptomatic (NK-CLPN and T-LGL). In these asymptomatic patients, the work-up is generally triggered by an abnormal blood count.

The blood count is typically the starting point for a more "refined" diagnostic work-up. The blood count parameters, including morphological review and dif-ferential cell count, highlight an absolute lymphocyto-sis in patients with T/NK leukemias, or at least an increase in the absolute number of large granular lymphocytes (LGLs) in patients with either T-LGL or NK-CLPN. The white blood cell count (WBC) is typ-ically markedly elevated in patients with T-PLL and at least moderately elevated in patients with ATLL and SS. The WBC is much more variable in patients with T-LGL or NK-CLPN, but there is an absolute increase in LGLs even in cases in which the absolute lympho-cyte count is within the normal range.

In addition to the WBC and absolute lymphocyte count determination, assessment of other hemato-logical parameters is also essential. The evaluation of red blood cell parameters, absolute neutrophil count and platelet counts generally provide information pre-dicting the degree of bone marrow effacement by the neoplasm, although other mechanisms for cytopenias are operative in T-LGL.

The morphological features of the abnormal lym-phocyte population are critical in guiding differential diagnostic considerations and evaluating for response to therapy and relapse. By definition, the nuclear fea-tures are "mature" in that the nuclear chromatin is at least moderately condensed. Other nuclear features such as nuclear contours (round, clefted, cerebriform or lobulated) are useful in ranking differential diag-nostic considerations. Assessment of the cytoplasm of the abnormal lymphoid population is essential in doc-umenting the distinctive, sparse cytoplasmic granules in T-LGL and NK-CLPN; cytoplasmic features are not generally contributory in the other mature T-cell leukemias.

Comprehensive multi-color flow cytometric immunophenotyping is the "gold standard" technique for determining lineage and stage of maturation of T-cell disorders (Table 10.1) [1–5]. Mature T-cell leukemias *lack* the classic profile of immature T-cells (T lymphoblasts) such as weak CD45, CD34, TdT, CD1a and weak to negative surface CD3 expression. Instead, mature T-cell leukemias express bright CD45, strong surface CD3, and usually either CD4 or CD8, although some mature T-cell leukemias can

---

Table 10.1. Stage of maturation of T-cell disorders [1–5].

Stage of maturation	Immunophenotype	Neoplasms/comments
T-lymphoblast	CD34, TdT, cCD3, CD7	T-lymphoblastic leukemia/lymphoma
Cortical thymocyte	cCD3, CD1a, CD7, TdT, TCR, CD4, CD8	T-lymphoblastic leukemia/lymphoma
Mature helper T cell	CD3, CD7, TCR, CD4, CD5	T-cell prolymphocytic leukemia (25% aberrantly co-express CD4 and CD8) Sézary syndrome (CD7–) Adult T-cell leukemia/lymphoma (CD25+, CD7–)
Mature cytotoxic/suppressor T cell	CD3, CD7, TCR, CD8, CD5	T-cell large granular lymphocytic leukemia (CD57+) Rare adult T-cell leukemia (CD7–, CD25+)

c = cytoplasmic. TCR = T-cell receptor alpha/beta.

aberrantly co-express both CD4 and CD8 antigens, a feature of T-PLL. In addition, other patterns of *aberrant* antigen expression are critical in the subclassification of mature T-cell leukemias and these will be discussed in detail in this chapter. The immunophenotypic profile of NK-cells is somewhat more problematic, although typical features of NK-cells include cytoplasmic but *not* surface CD3 expression, as well as CD56 expression.

In addition to establishing lineage and stage of maturation of T/NK-cell disorders, immunophenotyping can also be used to distinguish naïve T-cells (CD45RA positive) from memory T-cells (CD45RO-positive). Furthermore, assessment of antigens linked to function status (e.g. CD25) and various adhesion antigens (CD56 and CD57) are also commonly used in the immunophenotypic assessment of T/NK-cell neoplasms [3,6].

For many mature T- and NK-cell leukemias, the integration of clinical, hematological, morphological and immunophenotypic information is the diagnostic "end point," and a definitive diagnosis of T-PLL, ATLL or SS can be rendered. This is especially true if the absolute lymphocyte count is significantly elevated and morphological features are consistent with an overt neoplastic process. Even though inv(14)(q11q32) is characteristic of T-PLL, documentation of this cytogenetic abnormality is not a diagnostic requirement [1,6]. However, molecular confirmation of T-cell clonality is often necessary in T-LGL, because the absolute lymphocyte count is often not impressive in these patients, and because many non-neoplastic disorders are linked to an increase in cytotoxic/suppressor T-cells.

The confirmation of an overt NK-CLPN is even more challenging, since there are neither confirmatory cytogenetic nor molecular tests available to exclude non-neoplastic causes of an absolute NK-cell lymphocytosis. Specialized flow cytometric immunophenotypic testing for families of surface killer activating or inhibitory receptors has been suggested as a modality to distinguish neoplastic NK-cells (restricted surface-killer inhibitory receptor profile) from reactive NK-cells (polytypic surface killer inhibitory receptor profile) [7].

This chapter will guide the diagnostician in terms of a logical, cost-effective case assessment, provide information about the fairly limited number of potential therapeutic targets, and provide recommendations for assessing response to therapy and disease relapse for mature T- and NK-cell leukemias.

T-cell prolymphocytic leukemia (T-PLL)

Diagnostic aspects

The diagnosis of T-PLL is made using a combination of clinical and laboratory findings (Table 10.2) [8,10]. A complete history and physical examination (lymphadenopathy, splenomegaly, skin rash), complete blood count with differential, peripheral blood smear review and immunophenotyping should be performed. Cytogenetic studies are not required but may be useful in diagnostically difficult cases to reveal a characteristic abnormality [e.g. inv(14)(q11q32) or t(X;14)(q28;q11)]. A bone marrow biopsy is generally not necessary.

Table 10.2. Laboratory evaluation of T-cell prolymphocytic leukemia [8–10].

Test/Procedure	Frequency and comments
Blood count with differential count (blood)	At diagnosis Marked absolute lymphocytosis with distinctive morphology; prominent nucleolus and scant, agranular cytoplasm with blebbing (75%) Ongoing regular monitoring for response to therapy
Flow cytometric immunophenotyping (blood)	At diagnosis Confirm mature T-cell phenotype; CD3+, CD4+ (65% of cases) Unique CD4 and CD8 dual positivity (25% of cases) Assess presence of CD52 for targeted therapy Other T-cell markers (CD2, CD5 and CD7) generally present Surface CD3 may be weak Subsequent monitoring may be performed to assess disease resistance and/or protocol requirements
Bone marrow (BM) examination	Not necessary unless protocol requirement Diffuse BM effacement
Assessment for potential targeted therapy (blood)	Determine if CD52 expressed for alemtuzumab therapy
Cytogenetics (blood)	Generally not necessary unless protocol requirement May be helpful in a diagnostically challenging case to assess for characteristic inv(14)(q11q32) (70% of cases) Complex karyotype typical
Molecular assessment for clonality (blood)	Not usually required for diagnosis T-cell receptor clonality expected
Minimal residual disease detection	As needed or per protocol T-cell receptor clonality (expected sensitivity of $1/10^4$ to $1/10^5$ cells) If aberrant T-cell phenotype (e.g. dual CD4/CD8 positive) sensitivity $1/10^4$ cells
Pre-transplant assessment	Blood count Flow cytometric immunophenotyping and/or T-cell receptor clonality studies Transplant considered at initial response to therapy

Blood count: The WBC in T-PLL is most often markedly elevated (> 100×10^9/L). Concomitant anemia and thrombocytopenia are common and serum studies for HTLV-1 are negative.

Morphology: T-PLL cells are predominantly small to medium with round or irregular nuclear contours, mature chromatin, a prominent nucleolus, and scant, agranular cytoplasm with blebbing (Figure 10.1). In approximately one fourth of cases, the cells are small with indistinct nucleoli (so-called small cell variant). Rarely, cells show marked nuclear irregularity, similar to the cytological features seen in Sézary syndrome or adult T-cell leukemia/lymphoma. The bone marrow is diffusely infiltrated by T-PLL.

Immunophenotype: Flow cytometry demonstrates that T-PLL cells are of post-thymic derivation and express surface CD2, CD3 (may be weak), CD5 and CD7 and lack expression of immature markers (TdT, CD1a, CD34). In contrast to other mature T-cell leukemia mimics, CD7 is usually strongly expressed. In ~65% of cases, the tumor cells are CD4+, while ~25% cases show a relatively unique dual CD4 and CD8 positivity. The majority of cases are T-cell receptor alpha/beta positive. TIA-1 and natural-killer associated markers (CD16, CD56) are negative. Immunohistochemistry for TCL-1 is highly specific and sensitive for T-PLL amongst mature T-cell lymphoproliferative disorders [11]. Assessment for the high expression of CD52 for potential targeted therapy (e.g. alemtuzumab) may be done.

Cytogenetics: Cytogenetics is generally not essential for diagnosis. However, in cases difficult to distinguish from Sézary syndrome, chromosomal studies may be useful. T-PLL is characterized by a complex karyotype and recurrent abnormalities most often involve chromosomes 8, 11, 14 and X [12]. Inversion (14)(q11q32) is distinctive in T-PLL and seen in > 70% of cases. This inversion, or more rarely the translocation t(14;14)(q11;q32), results in the juxtaposition of the T-cell receptor alpha *TRA@* (14q11) and *TCL1A* (14q32) genes with subsequent constitutive activation of TCL-1. Translocation t(X;14)(q28;q11) is less common but results in the juxtaposition of *TRA@* (14q11) and *MTCP1* (Xq28). Abnormalities of chromosome 8 including iso8q are frequent. Mutations in the *ATM* gene (11q22) are often detected by molecular

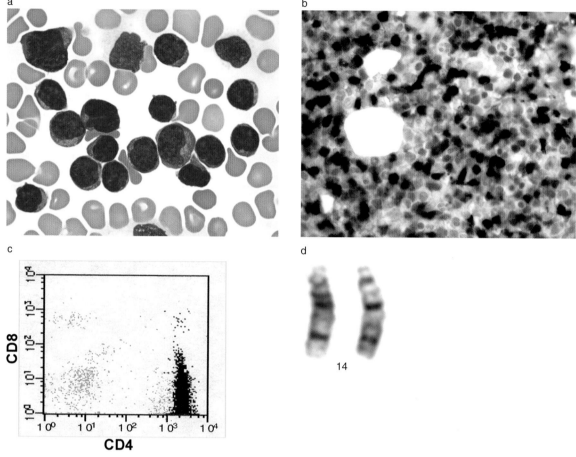

Figure 10.1. T-cell prolymphocytic leukemia.
a. Cytological features of T-PLL in peripheral blood. Note the cytoplasmicprotrusions from some cells
b. A bone marrow core biopsy section stained for TCL-1 by immunohistochemistry.
c. Flow cytometric immunophenotyping showing the T-cells to be CD4+, CD8–.
d. Conventional karyotyping showing inv(14) (q11q32)

and FISH studies. Confirmation of T-cell receptor gamma clonality is generally not necessary in the presence of otherwise typical clinical, laboratory, morphological and immunophenotypic features.

Clinical aspects

Given that T-PLL is an aggressive disease with less than one year median survival, most patients are treated if possible. Although outcome in T-PLL has improved with alemtuzumab (CD52 monoclonal antibody), the responses remain transient and disease progression is unavoidable. Thus, for patients showing an initial response to therapy, consideration should be given to autologous or allogeneic hematopoietic stem cell transplantation [13].

Disease monitoring

Therapeutic response may be assessed by evaluating for improvements in clinical and hematological findings (e.g. decreased hepatosplenomegaly, lymphadenopathy, skin rash, normalization of peripheral blood cell counts). Evaluation for minimal residual disease may be achieved with flow cytometric immunophenotyping if an aberrant T-cell expression pattern is present or with T-cell receptor gamma gene rearrangement studies.

T-cell large granular lymphocytic leukemia (T-LGL)

Diagnostic aspects

T-cell large granular lymphocytic (T-LGL) leukemia is diagnosed using a combination of clinical and laboratory findings (Table 10.3 and Figure 10.2) [14–17]. A blood count with differential, peripheral blood smear review, immunophenotyping and T-cell receptor clonality studies should be performed. A bone marrow biopsy is generally not necessary unless there is clinical suspicion for an additional accompanying disorder (e.g. myelodysplasia) or if the absolute lymphocyte count is <0.5 × 10^9/L. The bone marrow core biopsy often shows subtle interstitial and sinusoidal infiltrates.

Morphology: The blood cell count will reveal, in addition to variable cytopenias, an absolute lymphocytosis (>1.0–2.0 × 10^9/L) with typical large granular lymphocyte (LGL) morphology. However, up to one-third of newly diagnosed patients show an absolute lymphocyte count <0.5 × 10^9/L.

Immunophenotype: T-LGL leukemia exhibits a mature cytotoxic T-cell phenotype (CD3+, CD8+, CD57+) and is nearly always of alpha/beta T-cell receptor type. Rare cases are CD4+ and/or of gamma/delta T-cell receptor type Immunophenotypic clues to clonality are gained by aberrant expression of other T-cell markers (CD5, CD7 most commonly), as well as Vβ restriction or monotypic killer cell immunoglobulin-like receptor (KIR) expression (CD157b, CD158a, CD158e). Given

Table 10.3. Laboratory evaluation of T-cell large granular lymphocytic leukemia [14–17].

Test/Procedure	Frequency and comments
Blood count with differential count	At diagnosis Variable degree of absolute lymphocytosis (usually >1.0–2.0 × 10^9/L) Typical LGL morphology (inconspicuous nucleoli and abundant pale blue cytoplasm containing variable numbers and sizes of azurophilic granules)
Flow cytometric immunophenotyping	At diagnosis Confirm mature T-cell phenotype; CD3+, CD8+, CD57+; nearly all cases alpha/beta subtype Aberrant expression of CD2, CD3, CD5 and/or CD7 Vβ restriction or monotypic killer cell immunoglobulin-like receptor (KIR) expression (CD157b, CD158a, CD158e) may help distinguish from reactive process Subsequent monitoring may be performed to assess disease resistance and/or for protocol requirements
Bone marrow (BM) examination	Generally not necessary unless protocol requirement, suspicion for a second BM disorder and/or absolute lymphocytosis < 0.5 × 10^9/L Infiltrate predominantly interstitial and intra-sinusoidal Infiltrate may be difficult to identify on morphological review alone Immunohistochemistry for CD3/CD8 reveals pattern and extent
Assessment for potential targeted therapy	Determine if CD2 present for potential siplizumab therapy Determine if CD52 present for potential alemtuzumab therapy Determine if CD122 present for potential miK-beta-1 therapy
Cytogenetics	Generally not necessary unless protocol requirement No specific recurrent abnormalities
Molecular assessment for clonality (blood)	Generally required at diagnosis to distinguish from non-neoplastic LGL proliferation T-cell receptor clonality expected
Minimal residual disease detection	Flow cytometric or molecular tests not needed as clinical and hematological improvements do not correlate with a reduction in LGL burden Blood count with differential will document persistent or improved cytopenia(s)
Pre-transplant assessment	CBC will reveal progressive disease Bone marrow biopsy could be considered to assess for marrow percent involvement or evidence of another, concurrent disease process

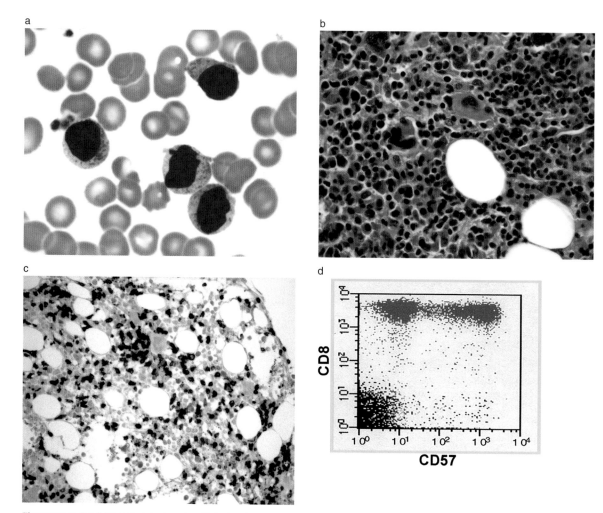

Figure 10.2. T-cell large granular lymphocytic leukemia.
a. Peripheral blood showing numerous large granular lymphocytes.
b. Bone marrow biopsy where the infiltrate is relatively inconspicuous by hematoxylin and eosin staining (H&E).
c. Immunoperoxidase staining for CD3 highlights the infiltration of the bone marrow core biopsy by T-LGL.
d. Flow cytometric immunophenotyping shows a significant population of CD8+ CD57+ cytotoxic, suppressor T-cells.

the availability of certain targeted therapies, confirmation of the presence of CD2, CD52 and/or CD122 may be helpful. A more aggressive form of T-LGL leukemia often exhibits immunophenotypic differences including expression of CD26 and CD56 and lack of CD57.

Molecular genetics: Confirmation of T-cell receptor gamma clonality is a key component in the establishment of the diagnosis of T-LGL leukemia. Chronic and transient elevations of T-LGLs are well-known and require distinction from true T-LGL leukemia. Non-neoplastic LGL conditions show oligoclonal or polyclonal T-cell receptor patterns.

Clinical aspects

The indications for treatment in T-LGL leukemia include recurrent infections, symptomatic thrombocytopenia or anemia, symptomatic splenomegaly, severe neutropenia and severe B symptoms. For the 30% of patients who are asymptomatic and lack severe cytopenia(s) a "watch and wait" approach is advocated. Such individuals are managed conservatively and indications for subsequent testing (e.g. blood count) should be driven by development of symptomatology.

Patients requiring therapy are identified based on the above-mentioned indications with immunosuppression playing the major role in treatment regimens. It has been recommended that such patients be enrolled in a clinical trial or treated with methotrexate, cyclophosphamide or cyclosporin A with or without corticosteroids. In general, patients will require lifelong therapy to maintain a durable response. Hematopoietic growth factors (granulocyte colony stimulating factor) may also be used in patients with severe neutropenia and/or recurrent infections. Antibiotics are often also utilized in this setting. Splenectomy is not routinely performed although may show success in rare individuals. If there is no response to the initial therapy, based on clinical, physical and/or blood count factors, reassignment to a clinical trial, treatment with second-line therapy (e.g. alemtuzumab) or hematopoietic stem cell transplantation are considered.

In addition to the general principle of immunosuppressive therapy for T-LGL leukemia, specific therapeutic targets are also being investigated, predominantly in Phase I and Phase II clinical trials. These include therapies against CD2, CD52, CD122 and others (Table 10.3).

Disease monitoring

In the majority of patients, there is no need to perform follow-up flow cytometric or molecular tests as clinical and hematologic improvements do not correlate with a reduction in LGL burden [18]. A routine blood count with differential may document the persistent or improved cytopenia(s). Clinical findings and physical examination are adequate to assess the response to treatment based on the resolution of recurrent infections and improvement in B symptoms and splenomegaly. Currently it is recommended that one wait to assess response until after 4 months of therapy as it may take 6–8 weeks to see any initial improvement. The lack of a significant response to therapy after four months or evidence of worsening disease will be evident from these monitoring modalities. In progressive disease, hematopoietic stem cell transplantation may be a treatment option. No additional testing is necessary per se for the T-LGL leukemia itself, as increasing tumor burden is likely evident from the ongoing tests; clinical findings, physical exam and blood count. Bone marrow biopsy could be considered to assess for marrow percent involvement or evidence of another, concurrent disease process such as myelodysplasia.

Chronic lymphoproliferative disorders of NK-cells (NK-CLPN)

The diagnostic approach in a case of possible NK-CLPN requires that four initial requirements be met:

1. Documentation of increased circulating large granular lymphocytes (LGLs) ($\geq 2 \times 10^9$/L) (blood count and differential cell count).
2. Documentation that LGLs are NK cells (*not* cytotoxic/suppressor T-cells) (flow cytometric immunophenotyping).
3. Documentation that the increased circulating NK large granular lymphocytosis is sustained for over six months (repeat blood count and leukocyte differential cell counts).
4. Exclusion of reactive causes of NK-cell lymphocytosis (clinical and laboratory evaluations to *exclude* infection, underlying neoplasm, vasculitis, neuropathy and autoimmune disorders) [7].

Once these four initial requirements have been met, the final diagnosis of the WHO 2008 provisional category of NK-CLPN may require sophisticated flow cytometric immunophenotyping for killer inhibitory receptor profile, possible bone marrow examination, and tests to exclude an Epstein–Barr-related lesion (Table 10.4) (Figure 10.3) [2,7,19–25]. The extent of testing performed is highly patient-specific. For example, asymptomatic patients with intact hematopoietic lineage cell counts may require only infrequent blood counts and differential cell counts with even less frequent monitoring by flow cytometric immunophenotyping of blood. In contrast, either symptomatic patients or patients in whom the diagnosis is not clear-cut, may require additional testing including bone marrow examination and possible molecular assessment, especially if T-cell disorders are to be excluded. Intrasinusoidal localization is a somewhat distinctive feature of NK-CLPN in bone marrow and, in general, immunohistochemical assessment is necessary to delineate the pattern and extent of bone marrow infiltration (Figure 10.3).

Prototypic morphological and immunophenotypic features of NK-CLPN are illustrated in Figure 10.3. Since most patients are asymptomatic, no therapy may be needed; the clinical course is indolent in these patients and spontaneous remissions may occur [7,21,26].

Table 10.4. Laboratory evaluation of chronic lymphoproliferative disorders of NK-cells [2,7,19,20,22–25].

Test/Procedure	Frequency and comments
Blood count with differential count (blood)	At diagnosis Documentation of sustained LGL for at least six months Infrequent follow-up blood counts if patient asymptomatic Monitor for development of cytopenia(s), especially if patient develops symptoms Monitor for response to therapy (if given for cytopenias or for NK-CLPN)
Flow cytometric immunophenotyping (blood)	Establish NK-cell lineage at diagnosis Assess for aberrant loss of CD2, CD7, CD57 Diminished expression of CD2, CD7 or CD56 may be useful in distinguishing from reactive NK cell proliferation Assess for aberrant expression of CD5 Assess for KIR isoform expression profile on NK-cells (specialized laboratory test) Assess for response to therapy
Bone marrow examination (at diagnosis)	May not be necessary in asymptomatic patients Assess for pattern and extent of NK-CLPN infiltration on clot or core biopsy sections utilizing immunohistochemical staining for CD3 (cytoplasmic), CD56 (usually positive), TIA-1 (highlights cytoplasmic granules) Diminished expression of CD2, CD7 or CD56 may be useful in distinguishing from reactive NK-cell proliferation Typical NK-CLPN infiltrates in bone marrow are intra-sinusoidal and interstitial
Repeat bone marrow examination	May not be necessary Performance and frequency are patient-specific Can be used to assess response to therapy May be useful for evaluation of new onset cytopenias
Cytogenetics (bone marrow preferred)	Karyotype usually normal Not recommended as routine test for diagnosis
Molecular assessment for clonality (blood)	Normal Not recommended unless T-LGL is under consideration Gene expression profiling may distinguish neoplastic from reactive NK-cell proliferations (not routine test) PCR-based assessment of KIR genotypes may be helpful in distinguishing NK-CLPN from benign conditions (not routine test)
Assessment for EBV in NK cells (tissue, cell block section)	EBER *in situ* hybridization staining on tissue sections Should be negative NK-CLPN *not* EBV-related neoplasm Positive result should prompt consideration of aggressive NK-cell leukemia

KIR = Killer Ig-like inhibitory receptors, EBER = EBV RNA.

Adult T-cell leukemia/lymphoma

Adult T-cell leukemia/lymphoma (ATLL) is unique among the mature T-cell leukemias in that a viral etiology (human T-cell leukemia virus-1) has been confirmed in conjunction with a specific geographic disease distribution in southwestern Japan, the Caribbean basin, West Africa, Brazil and northern Iran [4,27]. Likewise, as predicted by a viral pathogenesis, there is a broad spectrum of clinical manifestations including smoldering, chronic, lymphomatous and acute forms [4,27–29]. Evolution from carrier state to overt leukemia takes decades and only a small proportion of carriers experience this aggressive transformation [4]. Only the acute form of ATLL with distinctive leukemic manifestations (acute ATL) will be discussed in this chapter.

Despite the long latency of human T-cell leukemia virus-1 (HTLV-1) infection, patients with acute ATL typically manifest with the fairly abrupt onset of symptomatology. These disease manifestations are often systemic and include lymphadenopathy, hepatosplenomegaly, skin lesions and hypercalcemia as well as a leukemic blood and bone marrow picture [4,27–29]. Hypercalcemia is the result of the

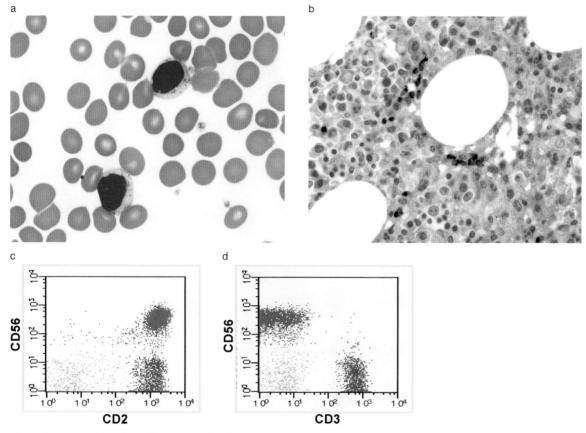

Figure 10.3. Chronic lymphoproliferative disorder of NK-cells.
a. Circulating large granular lymphocytes in the blood.
b. In the bone marrow there is a predilection for sinusoidal infiltration highlighted by TIA-1 immunoperoxidase staining.
c. Flow cytometric immunophenotyping shows a distinct population of CD56+, CD2+ cells.
d. Flow cytometry showing the cells to be CD3–.

constitutive production of parathyroid hormone-related protein by the leukemic cells [30].

Diagnostic aspects

A diagnosis of acute ATL is contingent upon the integration of blood count data, lymphocyte morphology, flow cytometric immunophenotyping and serologic studies for HTLV-1 (Table 10.5 and Figure 10.4) [4,27–29].

Morphology: Although a morphological spectrum of lymphocyte morphology has been described, the prototypic circulating leukemic acute ATL cells exhibit mature nuclear chromatin condensation with marked nuclear lobation including clover leaf nuclei (flower cells) which are readily apparent at low magnification (Figure 10.4) [4,6,29,31,32].

Immunophenotype: Flow cytometric immunophenotyping confirms a mature T-cell phenotype with several distinctive and diagnostically useful aberrations. The clear-cut majority of cases of ATL derive from helper (CD4+) T-cells; only very rare cases of either CD8+ ATL or double CD4+ CD8+ cases have been described [4]. In addition, CD7 expression is typically absent, while CD25 is strongly expressed [4,29]. Similarly aberrantly reduced expression of CD3 has been described also in ATL [27].

Clinical aspects

Definitive diagnosis is contingent upon documentation of underlying HTLV-1 infection which can be assessed serologically, although confirmation of clonal integration of HTLV-1 provirus in the host genome

Table 10.5. Laboratory evaluation of adult T-Cell leukemia/lymphoma [4,27–29,31,32].

Test/Procedure	Frequency and comments
Blood count with differential cell count (blood)	At diagnosis Marked absolute lymphocytosis with unique morphology Ongoing regular monitoring for response to therapy
Flow cytometric immunophenotyping (blood)	At diagnosis Confirm mature T-cell phenotype, CD4+, CD7–, CD25+ (Rare CD8+ cases) Reduced CD3 expression common feature Frequency of repeat monitoring may be linked to blood count response or protocol requirements
HTLV viral assessment (serum)	At diagnosis Confirm association with HTLV-1 infection Consider other differential diagnoses if negative
Cytogenetics	Not usually required No recurrent abnormality but clonal abnormalities almost always detected
Molecular (clonality)	Not usually required unless non-neoplastic disorders under consideration Clonal T-cell receptor gene rearrangement expected finding Monoclonal integration of HTLV-1 proviral genome can be assessed (not routine test)
Assessment for potential targeted therapy	Determine if CD52 expressed for potential alemtuzumab therapy Reassess if patient becomes resistant to alemtuzumab
Bone marrow examination	Variable extent of bone marrow effacement Immunohistochemical assessment (CD3, CD4, CD7, CD25) useful in delineating pattern (usually diffuse) and extent of infiltration Repeat bone marrow examination may be useful for monitoring treatment response or if protocol requirement

Alemtuzumab = Campath-1H = humanized IgG CD52 antibody [10].

confirms causality [33]. Unlike chronic ATL, acute ATL is biologically aggressive with median survival times barely exceeding one year [34]. Most cases of acute ATL are resistant to conventional chemotherapy prompting evaluations of alternative therapies [34]. Because most cases of acute ATL express CD52, alemtuzumab may prove to be clinically effective [10]. Recent investigators have tried zidovudine plus alpha-interferon with or without arsenic trioxide for chronic ATL with the goal of inducing remissions of the chronic less biologically aggressive form of ATL, thus preventing subsequent acute transformation [34].

Leukemic cutaneous T-cell lymphoma (Sézary syndrome)

Sézary syndrome (SS) is defined by the presence of erythroderma, generalized lymphadenopathy and circulating Sézary cells [5]. Sézary syndrome can occur *de novo* or in the setting of long-standing mycosis fungoides.

Diagnostic aspects

Sézary syndrome is diagnosed by clinical and laboratory findings (Table 10.6 and Figure 10.5). Integral to the diagnosis is a blood count with absolute Sézary count, flow cytometric analysis and often, T-cell receptor clonality studies. Demonstration of an absolute Sézary count $\geq 1.0 \times 10^9$/L, and/or CD4:CD8 ratio ≥ 10 or an expanded CD4+ T-cell population with aberrant T-cell antigen expression is required [5].

The analysis of and quantification of blood for Sézary cells is integral to the current staging work-up of cutaneous T-cell lymphomas [35,36]. The extent of blood involvement by Sézary cells is used to categorize the "blood" stage of the patient into B0, B1 and B2 (Table 10.7). Flow cytometric analysis and often T-cell receptor clonality studies are needed.

Morphology: The circulating neoplastic cells in primary and secondary SS exhibit characteristic cerebriform nuclear outlines best detected on high magnification (Figure 10.5). The nuclei of Sézary cells are often more hyperchromatic than normal

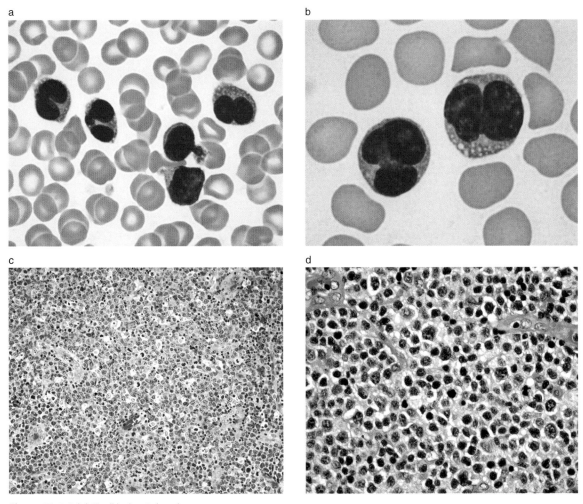

Figure 10.4. Adult T-cell leukemia/lymphoma.
a. Cytological features of ATL cells in the blood.
b. At higher magnification note striking nuclear lobulation of ATL cells in the peripheral blood.
c. Morphological features of acute ATL in a tissue biopsy.
d. Bone marrow biopsy showing extensive diffuse effacement of the marrow.

lymphoid cells and may show a range in cell size. Morphological distinction of small Sézary cells from normal lymphocytes may be challenging. Cells with cytological features of Sézary cells can be present in the blood of healthy control subjects and patients with non-neoplastic cutaneous disorders. Judicious use of ancillary tests such as flow cytometry to discriminate neoplastic cells from non-neoplastic is often necessary. In the bone marrow, the infiltrates are remarkably subtle and scant and often require immunohistochemical stains for identification.

Immunophenotype: Flow cytometric analysis reveals a mature T-cell population most often CD4+ T-helper phenotype. Although by no means specific, compared with other T-cell leukemia disorders, SS exhibits a fairly classic loss or weak expression of CD7 and CD26. CD2, CD3 and CD5 may show aberrant weak or bright expression. The CD4: CD8 ratio typically exceeds 10. Recently the presence of CD158k has been reported as being highly specific and sensitive for Sézary cells [37], and may be particularly useful for minimal residual disease detection.

Caution should be used when interpreting flow cytometric findings as clear-cut evidence of Sézary cells, given that a certain percent of circulating T-cells in healthy individuals and in persons with non-neoplastic cutaneous conditions may show a

Table 10.6. Laboratory evaluation of Sézary syndrome [5,6,36,37,39].

Test/Procedure	Frequency and comments
Skin biopsy	At diagnosis (unless previously diagnosed mycosis fungoides) Dermatopathologist review Immunohistochemistry as needed
Blood tests	Comprehensive metabolic panel Lactate dehydrogenase
Blood count with differential count (blood)	At diagnosis Variable degree of absolute lymphocytosis (usually > 1.0–2.0 × 10^9/L) Typical Sézary morphology (intermediate to large with hyperchromasia and cerebriform nuclei) Absolute Sézary count should be determined for staging (see Table 10.7)
Flow cytometric immunophenotyping (blood)	At diagnosis Confirm mature T-cell phenotype; CD3+, CD4+, CD7–, CD26– All cases alpha/beta subtype Assess for expanded CD4+ population with CD4:CD8 ratio ≥ 10 or evidence of aberrant T-cell antigen expression (other than CD7) CD4+/CD7– ≥ 40% or CD4+/CD26– ≥ 30% of lymphocytes in conjunction with positive T-cell receptor gene rearrangement CD4+/CD7– cells may comprise up to 38% of total lymphocytes in some non-neoplastic conditions The presence of CD158k is highly specific for Sézary cells Subsequent monitoring may be related to assess disease resistance/response and/or protocol requirements
Bone marrow examination	Generally not necessary unless protocol requirement BM often spared or with minimal interstitial involvement irrespective of degree of peripheral blood involvement
Molecular assessment for clonality (blood)	Generally performed at diagnosis T-cell receptor clonality expected; positive clone should be interpreted with caution as may be seen occasionally in non-neoplastic conditions Establishment of the baseline TCR clonal fingerprint may be useful for comparison in follow-up studies for minimal residual disease
Cytogenetics	Generally not necessary unless protocol requirement No specific recurrent abnormalities
Assessment for potential targeted therapy	Assess for CD52 for potential alemtuzumab therapy CD4 positivity for potential zanolimumab therapy
Minimal residual disease detection	Assess for disease response as indicated or per protocol Flow cytometry (CD158k) or clonal T-cell receptor studies

CD3+, CD4+/CD7– immunophenotype. Reference ranges for CD4+/CD7– subsets are as follows. As a percentage of total lymphocytes CD3+/CD4+/CD7– T-cells have been reported as:

- Normal controls: 3–13%.
- Benign dermatoses: 2–38%.

As a percentage of all CD4+ T-cells, those with loss of CD7 have been reported as:

- Normal controls: 3.6–16.5%.
- Reactive dermatoses: 2.1–21%.
- Sézary syndrome: 4.7–96.7% [38].

Therefore, in many cases the flow cytometric results in patients with Sézary syndrome and benign dermatoses may be overlapping. Clinical correlation (including potential therapy) and possible molecular analysis is required to confirm a diagnosis of Sézary syndrome.

Molecular genetics: Molecular analysis for a clonal T-cell receptor (*TCR*) gene rearrangement of blood may be necessary in some cases at presentation to confirm the diagnosis of blood involvement. Establishment of the baseline *TCR* clonal fingerprint may be useful for comparison in follow-up studies of blood for minimal

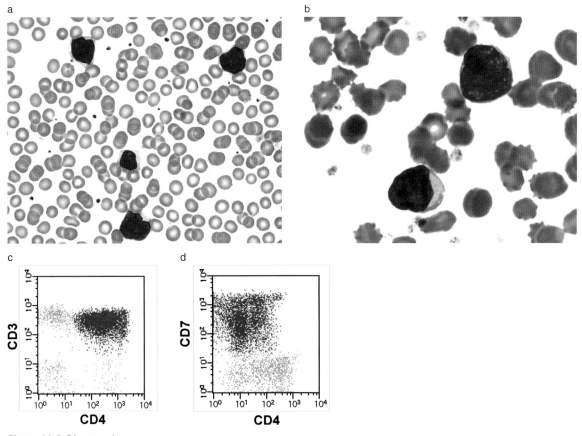

Figure 10.5. Sézary syndrome.
a. Circulating Sézary cells showing prominent variation in size.
b. Blood film at high magnification demonstrating the subtle nuclear convolutions of the Sézary cells.
c. Flow cytometric immunophenotyping showing the cells to be CD3+, CD4+ (red events).
d. There is variable intensity of CD7 expression (red events).

residual disease. T-cell receptor clonality may however be identified in some patients with autoimmune disease and in some healthy adults, and thus should be interpreted in conjunction with the entire clinical context [39].

Clinical aspects

Therapies specifically targeting CD4 and CD52 on Sézary cells (zanolimumab and alemtuzumab) have been utilized, mainly in refractory cutaneous T-cell lymphoma (CTCL) cases. Zanolimumab has been shown to be efficacious [40]. Alemtuzumab is active against Sézary syndrome but is associated with a high risk of opportunistic infections [41]. Consequently, this agent most effective in lower doses as a palliative treatment. Allogeneic and autologous stem cell transplants have been performed in some cases of refractory, progressive CTCL. Although the number of cases is small, allogeneic transplants have seen more durable responses than autologous.

Summary

Mature T-cell and NK-cell lymphoproliferative disorders comprise a fairly rare and limited set of chronic leukemias. Although characteristic hematological and/ or morphological features exist for some of the disorders (e.g. high WBC count in T-PLL, "flower-like" nuclei in ATLL), integration of morphological findings with immunophenotypic and occasionally cytogenetic/molecular studies is required for a definite diagnosis.

Multi-parameter flow cytometric analysis is a necessary and practical upfront approach to these disorders to:

Table 10.7. Categories of blood involvement by Sézary cells in the staging of cutaneous T-cell lymphoma [36].

Category	Definition
B0	Absence of significant blood involvement; < 5% of PB lymphocytes are Sézary cells
B1	Low degree of blood involvement; > 5% of PB lymphocytes are Sézary cells but not B2
B2	High degree of blood involvement; > 1.0×10^9/L Sézary cells

1. Establish lineage (T-cell vs. NK-cell vs. other).
2. Exclude an immature neoplasm (lack of CD34, TdT, CD1a).
3. Provide clues to the diagnosis based on a characteristic antigen profile.
4. Reveal a marker(s) to follow for minimal residual disease (e.g. T-cell aberrancy).

Cytogenetics is generally not helpful in establishing a diagnosis except for the characteristic inversion 14 or t(X;14) seen in T-PLL. Molecular T-cell receptor studies are generally clonal in the T-cell disorders and may be used to follow the patient for disease response/pre-transplantation monitoring. Targeted therapies remain fairly limited for mature T-cell and NK-cell lymphoproliferative disorders. However, progress has been, and continues to be made, particularly with monoclonal antibodies. For example, alemtuzumab, (CD52) is useful in the treatment of T-PLL and refractory cutaneous T-cell lymphoma/Sézary syndrome.

Upfront hematological, morphological, immuno-phenotypic and, as indicated, molecular testing are integral to the diagnosis and subsequent monitoring of T-cell/NK-cell mature leukemias. The generous use of specialized testing techniques at diagnosis allows for the identification of key features/aberrancies that serve as a genetic fingerprint of the disease. These features may then be used for subsequent disease monitoring as needed.

References

1. Catovsky D, Ralfkiaer E. T-cell prolymphocytic leukaemia. In Swerdlow SH, Campo E, Harris N *et al.* (eds.). *WHO Classification of Tumours of Haematopoietic and Lymphoid Tissues*, 4th edn. Lyon: IARC Press; 2008, 270–1.

2. Chan J, Ralfkiaer E, Ko Y-H. Aggressive NK-cell leukaemia. In Swerdlow SH, Campo E, Harris NL *et al.* (eds.), *WHO Classification of Tumours of Haematopoietic and Lymphoid Tissues*, 4th edn. Lyon: IARC Press; 2008, 276–77.

3. Jaffe E, Stein H, Campo E, Pileri S, Swerdlow S. Introduction and overview of the classification of the lymphoid neoplasms. In Swerdlow SH, Campo E, Harris NL *et al.* (eds.), *WHO Classification of Tumours of Haematopoietic and Lymphoid Tissues*, 4th edn. Lyon: IARC Press; 2008, 158–66.

4. Ohshima A, Jaffe ES, Kikuchi M. Adult T-cell leukaemia/lymphoma. In Swerdlow SH, Campo E, Harris NL *et al.* (eds.), *WHO Classification of Tumours of Haematopoietic and Lymphoid Tissues*, 4th edn. Lyon: IARC Press; 2008, 281.

5. Ralfkiaer E. Sézary syndrome. In Swerdlow SH, Campo E, Harris NL *et al.* (eds.), *WHO Classification of Tumours of Haematopoietic and Lymphoid Tissues*, 4th edn. Lyon: IARC Press; 2008, 299.

6. Foucar K. Mature T-cell leukemias including T-prolymphocytic leukemia, adult T-cell leukemia/lymphoma, and Sezary syndrome. *Am J Clin Pathol* 2007;**127**(4):496–510.

7. Villamor N, Chan W, Foucar K. Chronic lymphoproliferative disorders of NK cells. In Swerdlow S, Campo E, Harris N *et al.* (eds.), *WHO Classification of Tumours of Haematopoietic and Lymphoid Tissues*, 4th edn. Lyon: IARC Press; 2008, 274–75.

8. Dearden CE, Matutes E, Cazin B *et al.* High remission rate in T-cell prolymphocytic leukemia with CAMPATH-1H. *Blood* 2001;**98**(6):1721–6.

9. Dungarwalla M, Matutes E, Dearden CE. Prolymphocytic leukaemia of B- and T-cell subtype: a state-of-the-art paper. *Eur J Haematol* 2008;**80**(6):469–76.

10. Jiang L, Yuan CM, Hubacheck J *et al.* Variable CD52 expression in mature T cell and NK cell malignancies: implications for alemtuzumab therapy. *Br J Haematol* 2009;**145**(2):173–9.

11. Herling M, Khoury JD, Washington LT *et al.* A systematic approach to diagnosis of mature T-cell leukemias reveals heterogeneity among WHO categories. *Blood* 2004;**104**(2):328–35.

12. Maljaei SH, Brito-Babapulle V, Hiorns LR, Catovsky D. Abnormalities of chromosomes 8, 11, 14, and X in T-prolymphocytic leukemia studied by fluorescence in situ hybridization. *Cancer Genet Cytogenet* 1998;**103**(2):110–16.

13. Khot A, Dearden C. T-cell prolymphocytic leukemia. *Expert Rev Anticancer Ther* 2009;**9**(3):365–71.

14. Alekshun TJ, Sokol L. Diseases of large granular lymphocytes. *Cancer Control* 2007;**14**(2):141–50.

15. Burks EJ, Loughran TP Jr. Perspectives in the treatment of LGL leukemia. *Leuk Res* 2005;**29** (2):123–5.

16. Mohan SR, Maciejewski JP. Diagnosis and therapy of neutropenia in large granular lymphocyte leukemia. *Curr Opin Hematol* 2009;**16**(1):27–34.

17. Zhang R, Shah MV, Yang J et al. Network model of survival signaling in large granular lymphocyte leukemia. *Proc Natl Acad Sci USA* 2008;**105** (42):16308–13.

18. Sokol L, Loughran TP Jr. Large granular lymphocyte leukemia. *Oncologist* 2006;**11**(3):263–73.

19. Choi YL, Makishima H, Ohashi J et al. DNA microarray analysis of natural killer cell-type lymphoproliferative disease of granular lymphocytes with purified CD3–CD56+ fractions. *Leukemia* 2004;**18**(3):556–65.

20. Epling-Burnette PK, Painter JS, Chaurasia P et al. Dysregulated NK receptor expression in patients with lymphoproliferative disease of granular lymphocytes. *Blood* 2004;**103**(9):3431–9.

21. Foucar K, Matutes E, Dearden C, Catovsky D. Chronic T-cell and natural killer cell leukemias. In Armitage JCB, Dalla-Favera R, Harris NL, Mauch P (eds.), *Non-Hodgkin Lymphoma*. Lippincott Williams & Wilkins; 2009.

22. Lima M, Almeida J, Montero AG et al. Clinicobiological, immunophenotypic, and molecular characteristics of monoclonal CD56–/+dim chronic natural killer cell large granular lymphocytosis. *Am J Pathol* 2004;**165**(4):1117–27.

23. Scquizzato E, Teramo A, Miorin M et al. Genotypic evaluation of killer immunoglobulin-like receptors in NK-type lymphoproliferative disease of granular lymphocytes. *Leukemia* 2007;**21**(5):1060–9.

24. Verheyden S, Bernier M, Demanet C. Identification of natural killer cell receptor phenotypes associated with leukemia. *Leukemia* 2004;**18**(12):2002–7.

25. Zambello R, Falco M, Della Chiesa M et al. Expression and function of KIR and natural cytotoxicity receptors in NK-type lymphoproliferative diseases of granular lymphocytes. *Blood* 2003;**102**(5):1797–805.

26. Rabbani GR, Phyliky RL, Tefferi A. A long-term study of patients with chronic natural killer cell lymphocytosis. *Br J Haematol* 1999;**106**(4):960–6.

27. Yokote T, Akioka T, Oka S et al. Flow cytometric immunophenotyping of adult T-cell leukemia/lymphoma using CD3 gating. *Am J Clin Pathol* 2005;**124**(2):199–204.

28. Liu TY, Chen CY, Tien HF, Lin CW. Loss of CD7, independent of galectin-3 expression, implies a worse prognosis in adult T-cell leukaemia/lymphoma. *Histopathology* 2009;**54**(2):214–20.

29. Nicot C. Current views in HTLV-I-associated adult T-cell leukemia/lymphoma. *Am J Hematol* 2005;**78** (3):232–9.

30. Nadella MV, Dirksen WP, Nadella KS et al. Transcriptional regulation of parathyroid hormone-related protein promoter P2 by NF-kappaB in adult T-cell leukemia/lymphoma. *Leukemia* 2007;**21** (8):1752–62.

31. Uchiyama T. Adult T-cell leukemia. *Blood Rev* 1988;**2** (4):232–8.

32. Uchiyama T, Yodoi J, Sagawa K, Takatsuki K, Uchino H. Adult T-cell leukemia: clinical and hematologic features of 16 cases. *Blood* 1977;**50**(3):481–92.

33. Kamihira S, Sugahara K, Tsuruda K et al. Proviral status of HTLV-1 integrated into the host genomic DNA of adult T-cell leukemia cells. *Clin Lab Haematol* 2005;**27**(4):235–41.

34. Kchour G, Tarhini M, Kooshyar MM et al. Phase 2 study of the efficacy and safety of the combination of arsenic trioxide, interferon alpha, and zidovudine in newly diagnosed chronic adult T-cell leukemia/lymphoma (ATL). *Blood* 2009;**113**(26):6528–32.

35. http://www.nccn.org/professionals/physician_gls/PDF/nhl.pdfMysocisFungoids/Sezary Syndrome(MFSS-1).

36. Olsen E, Vonderheid E, Pimpinelli N et al. Revisions to the staging and classification of mycosis fungoides and Sezary syndrome: a proposal of the International Society for Cutaneous Lymphomas (ISCL) and the cutaneous lymphoma task force of the European Organization of Research and Treatment of Cancer (EORTC). *Blood* 2007;**110**(6):1713–22.

37. Bahler DW, Hartung L, Hill S, Bowen GM, Vonderheid EC. CD158k/KIR3DL2 is a useful marker for identifying neoplastic T-cells in Sezary syndrome by flow cytometry. *Cytometry B Clin Cytom* 2008;**74** (3):156–62.

38. Morice WG, Katzmann JA, Pittelkow MR et al. A comparison of morphologic features, flow cytometry, TCR-Vbeta analysis, and TCR-PCR in qualitative and quantitative assessment of peripheral blood involvement by Sezary syndrome. *Am J Clin Pathol* 2006;**125**(3):364–74.

39. Vonderheid EC, Bernengo MG, Burg G et al. Update on erythrodermic cutaneous T-cell lymphoma: report of the International Society for Cutaneous Lymphomas. *J Am Acad Dermatol* 2002;**46**(1):95–106.

40. Kim YH, Duvic M, Obitz E et al. Clinical efficacy of zanolimumab (HuMax-CD4): two phase 2 studies in refractory cutaneous T-cell lymphoma. *Blood* 2007;**109** (11):4655–62.

41. Ure UB, Ar MC, Salihoglu A et al. Alemtuzumab in Sezary syndrome: efficient but not innocent. *Eur J Dermatol* 2007;**17**(6):525–9.

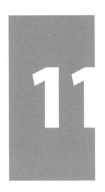

11 Lymphoma

Jennifer Herrick and Ahmet Dogan

Introduction

The cornerstone of the diagnosis of lymphoma is the architectural pattern and cytology of the lesion in the affected tissue and this is supplemented by immunophenotypic, molecular and cytogenetic characteristics. These features together define our modern classification scheme of lymphoma. These same investigations are utilized in the assessment of bone marrow involvement by lymphoma, but with some variations and limitations. The role of bone marrow examination varies according to the subtype of lymphoma. This chapter will provide the general principles and practical guidelines of the most useful diagnostic techniques for the detection of bone marrow involvement by malignant lymphomas. It will detail the typical features and roles of morphology, immunohistochemistry, flow cytometric immunophenotyping, cytogenetic and molecular testing in different types of lymphoma. The existence of significant variations from the classical description will be identified by "caveats." Disease monitoring and pre-transplant assessment will be discussed where applicable. Acronyms used for the various entities are listed in Table 11.1.

General principles of bone marrow evaluation in lymphoma

Bone marrow examination is routinely performed for lymphoma staging. A bone marrow may also be performed as an ad hoc diagnostic procedure in patients suspected of having a neoplasm lymphoma but who are not deemed suitable for a surgical biopsy of the implicated tissue lesion (e.g. thrombocytopenia, anticoagulation, unsuitable for general anesthesia). In many specimens malignancy (hematopoietic or non-hematopoietic) and cell lineage can be established. However, accurate sub-typing may require correlation with a tissue biopsy. In addition, the grade of the tumor in the marrow may not reflect the extramedullary process.

As a practicing clinician or pathologist, it is useful to be aware of the frequency with which the bone marrow is involved by lymphoma as this varies by subtype (Table 11.1) [1]. The extent of ancillary testing should be guided by the indication for the bone marrow examination, i.e. whether it is the primary diagnostic test material thereby necessitating a full work-up, or marrow staging of a previously characterized process. Prudent, cost-effective use of ancillary testing in bone marrow staging or primary diagnosis of lymphoma is recommended but this may not be straightforward. This is because immediate decisions must be made regarding the need for supplementary tests on fresh tissue samples (e.g. flow cytometry, karyotype), versus the limitations posed by bone marrow fixation, decalcification and processing. Table 11.2 lists the samples which are both suitable and unsuitable for the most commonly used ancillary tests in the assessment of lymphoma involving the bone marrow.

It cannot be overemphasized that care must be taken in interpreting the results of ancillary tests in the absence of morphological evidence of lymphoma. Discrepancies can occur due to:

1. Sampling and sensitivity issues giving a positive ancillary test (e.g. flow cytometry) in a morphologically negative sample.
2. Small clonal populations detectable in a small number of patients without evidence of pathological disease.

Diagnostic Techniques in Hematological Malignancies, ed. Wendy N. Erber. Published by Cambridge University Press.
© Cambridge University Press 2010.

Table 11.1. Bone marrow involvement in non-Hodgkin and Hodgkin lymphomas [1,2,14].

Lymphoma subtype	Incidence of bone marrow involvement
Follicular lymphoma (FL), all grades	40–70%
FL, grade 1	30–60%
FL, grade 2	7–46%
FL, grade 3	2–15%
Mantle cell lymphoma (MCL)	50–80%
Splenic marginal zone lymphoma (SMZL)	near 100%
Extranodal marginal zone lymphoma (EMZL)	3–20%
Nodal marginal zone lymphoma (NMZL)	30–40%
Diffuse large B-cell lymphoma (DLBCL)	10–30%
T-cell rich B-cell lymphoma (TCRBCL)	15–60%
Burkitt lymphoma (BL)	15–35%
Classical Hodgkin lymphoma (CHL), all subtypes	4–10%
Nodular sclerosis (NSCHL)	3%
Mixed cellularity (MCCHL)	10%
Lymphocyte rich (LRCHL)	Rare
Lymphocyte depleted (LDCHL)	>50%
NLP Hodgkin lymphoma (NLPHL)	<1%
Anaplastic large cell lymphoma (ALCL)	15–25%
Angioimmunoblastic T-cell lymphoma (AITL)	>50%

3. Highly sensitive techniques may give results that may not carry well-established clinical significance in the absence of morphological correlation.

Due to the importance placed on morphological assessment, it is recommended that bilateral bone marrow trephine (core) biopsies be performed routinely for bone marrow staging of lymphoma; this increases the sensitivity of morphological detection

in both classical Hodgkin lymphoma and non-Hodgkin lymphomas [2]. A general overview of the standard components for evaluating the bone marrow follows.

Primary diagnosis or initial staging bone marrow

Morphology: Both bone marrow aspirate and trephine biopsy samples are both routinely assessed in the staging of lymphoma (see Chapter 1). The aspirate can be used for cytological detail as well as providing samples for flow cytometry, cytogenetics and molecular genetics investigations. A bone marrow "squash" preparation is more sensitive than smears for the detection of bone marrow infiltration; overall the aspirate is less sensitive than the trephine biopsy for the following reasons:

1. Marrow involvement by lymphoma is commonly patchy and paratrabecular and neoplastic cells may not be in the sample, giving a false negative result.
2. Neoplastic infiltrates are commonly enmeshed in a fibrotic framework precluding aspiration, giving a false negative result.
3. The cytology of the lymphoid cells can be used to distinguish between normal and neoplastic, in most instances, but can be difficult for lymphoma subclassification. This requires the use of ancillary test modalities.

The trephine biopsy has a number of advantages over the aspirate because the cells are *in situ*. This enables the topographic distribution of any infiltrate to be assessed in relation to the bone and other cellular elements. The morphological features that are most useful in describing and categorizing lymphomas in the bone marrow are:

1. Distribution pattern i.e. paratrabecular, interstitial, nodular, sinusoidal, diffuse, mixed.
2. Cell size, i.e. smaller, equal or larger than a macrophage or endothelial cell nucleus.
3. Cell type i.e. cleaved, round, monocytoid/plasmacytoid, RS/Hodgkin cells).
4. Associated or accompanying features e.g. plasma cell, amyloid, inflammatory cell, histiocytic or granulomatous collections.

These collective features may be considered diagnostic of a subtype or helpful to considerably narrow a diagnosis. Table 11.3 lists common patterns of lymphomas involving the bone marrow.

Table 11.2. Appropriate samples for bone marrow ancillary testing for lymphoma.

Sample selection for ancillary testing of bone marrow material

	Suitable samples	Unsuitable samples
Immunohistochemistry (IHC)	Core biopsy Aspirate clot/particle preparation	Aspirate smears Touch preparation
in situ Hybridization (ISH)	Core biopsy Aspirate clot/particle preparation	Aspirate smears Touch preparation
Flow cytometry[a]	Liquid aspirate Fresh core biopsy (limited results)	Aspirate smears Aspirate clot section/particle preparation Fixed core biopsy
Karyotyping[b]	Liquid aspirate	Core biopsy Aspirate smears Aspirate clot/part preparation
Fluorescence in situ Hybridization (FISH)	Aspirate smears Liquid aspirate Touch preparations Clot section/part preparation (limited)	Core biopsy
Polymerase chain reaction (PCR)	Liquid aspirate Clot section/particle preparation Aspirate smears (scrape slides)	B5-fixed clot section/particle preparation Core biopsy
Southern blot	Liquid aspirate Frozen tissue Aspirate smears	Aspirate clot section/particle preparation Core biopsy

Ancillary testing possibilities for each component of the bone marrow study

	Acceptable for:	Unacceptable for:
Dried aspirate or peripheral blood smears	Morphology FISH	Flow cytometry IHC PCR
Liquid aspirate or peripheral blood	Flow cytometry[a] PCR (RNA or DNA based) Southern blot FISH Conventional karyotype[b]	Morphology IHC
Clot or particle section Formalin-fixed	Morphology IHC FISH PCR (DNA based only)	Flow cytometry Conventional karyotyping Southern blot
Clot or particle section Mercuric based fixative (B5)	Morphology IHC	Flow cytometry Conventional karyotyping Southern blot PCR FISH
Core biopsy (decalcified) (paraffin embedded)	Morphology IHC	Flow cytometry FISH PCR Southern blot Conventional karyotyping

[a] Flow cytometry acceptable mediums: RPMI, EDTA, ACD, heparin.
[b] Karyotyping acceptable mediums: Prefer heparin, EDTA acceptable.

Table 11.3. Morphological patterns of non-Hodgkin lymphomas in bone marrow core biopsies, differential diagnoses (DDx) and useful IHC panels.

Pattern	Differential Diagnosis
Predominantly paratrabecular	FL, rituximab-induced reactive aggregates
Mixed paratrabecular/interstitial	LPL, EMZL, NMZL, SMZL, MCL
Nodular	MCL, CLL, SMZL, EMZL, NMZL, reactive, AILT
Interstitial	MCL, CLL, DLBCL, ALCL, LPL, HCL, SMZL, NMZL, EMZL, T-PLL
Diffuse	MCL, CLL, DLBCL, ALCL, LPL, HCL, SMZL, NMZL
Sinusoidal	SMZL, EMZL, ALCL, intravascular DLBCL
Singular cells	ALCL, rare DLBCL
Lymphohistiocytic lesions	CHL, TCRBCL, PTCL, ALCL, infection, sarcoid, lipogranulomas, foreign body

Paratrabecular aggregates:

FL, MCL, LPL, MZLs, rituximab-induced reactive aggregates

CD3, CD20, CD5, CD10, BCL-6, cyclin D1, CD138, kappa/lambda

Interstitial infiltrate:

MCL, CLL, DLBCL, ALCL, LPL, HCL, SMZL, NMZL, EMZL, T-PLL

Small cell infiltrate: CD3, CD20, CD5, CD23, cyclin D1, CD138, kappa/lambda, add as needed

Large cell infiltrate: CD3, CD20, CD30, MUM-1, add as needed

Nodular infiltrate:

MCL, CLL, SMZL, EMZL, NMZL, AITL, reactive lymphoid aggregates

CD3, CD20, CD5, CD23, cyclin D1, CD138, kappa/lambda

Lymphohistiocytic aggregates:

DDx: CHL, TCRBCL, PTCL, ALCL (rare), sarcoid, infection, lipogranulomas, foreign body granuloma

CD3, CD20, CD30, CD15, PAX-5, LCA, organism stains as needed

Small/intermediate and/or large cells with irregular nuclear contours:

DDx: PTCL, AITL, ALCL, DLBCL, blastoid MCL

CD3, CD20, CD4, CD8, CD30, ALK, cyclin D1, CD138, add as needed

Note: If the patient has been treated with an anti CD20 monoclonal antibody, an additional pan-B cell marker should be added (i.e. CD19, CD79a, PAX-5). Particular attention should be paid to the correct staining pattern of the antibody (i.e. cytoplasmic, membranous or nuclear) as incorrect staining patterns represent non-specific testing artefact and should not be interpreted as positive.

Caveat: Care should be taken in assigning a paratrabecular pattern to crushed biopsies as non-paratrabecular aggregates can be artefactually juxtaposed to bone trabeculae. The true paratrabecular aggregate should wrap around the bone, not just be located adjacent to it. Paratrabecular aggregates are usually somewhat fibrotic with a linear streaming quality hugging the bone.

Immunohistochemistry: General guidelines for immunohistochemistry (IHC) are outlined in Table 11.3 and described in Chapter 2. The initial immunohistochemical panel used to diagnose lymphoma in the bone marrow should be based on the morphological features (see also Chapter 2). It is important that positive and negative controls are assessed; normal cells that express or lack the relevant antigen should be used as internal positive and negative controls, respectively.

Caveats:

1. Particular attention should be paid to the correct staining pattern for all antibodies (i.e. cytoplasmic, membranous, nuclear). Incorrect staining patterns represent non-specific reactivity and should not be interpreted as positive.
2. Background cell populations which may also express a particular antigen must not be over-interpreted as positive staining. Be sure to correctly assign staining characteristics to the cell population of interest.
3. If the patient has been treated with a therapeutic monoclonal antibody (e.g. CD20 immunotherapy), another lineage-associated marker should be used to assess the presence or absence of the cell line of interest. The antibody effect should be present for approximately five half-lives of the antibody (approximately 15 weeks).

In situ hybridization: *In situ* hybridization (ISH) can be performed on paraffin-embedded tissue and is a useful adjunct to immunohistochemistry. The most commonly used probes in lymphomas are to EBV-encoded RNA (EBER or EBV-ISH) and kappa and lambda light chains of immunoglobulin. Probe binding is detected with chromogenic markers and visualized by standard light microscopy. The ISH-stained slides, unlike FISH, can be stored for historical reassessment (much like immunohistochemical stains).

Flow cytometric immunophenotyping: Flow cytometry immunophenotyping (FCI) is a powerful technique for cell identification in a liquid bone marrow aspirate sample based on antigen expression (see Chapter 3 for details). However, it is only useful if there are adequate cells in the sample and the aspirate is involved by the lymphomatous process; otherwise the results will reflect normal uninvolved marrow or peripheral blood. In mature B-cell neoplasms FCI can identify a disease-associated phenotype and show light chain restriction. For mature T-cell lymphomas FCI can identify aberrant loss of an antigen or an unusually homogeneous immunophenotype.

However, there are some significant limitations to FCI in lymphoma analysis. For example, larger cells such as Reed–Sternberg (RS) cells, lymphocyte predominant "popcorn cells," ALCL and DLBCL are not well represented in the marrow and many T-cell lymphomas do not have an aberrant phenotype. FCI can therefore not be used in isolation to establish the presence or absence of marrow involvement by these lymphoma types. Lymphomas which adhere to the bone marrow and where there is significant fibrosis and are not easily aspirated are also commonly undetectable on FCI, e.g. follicular lymphoma. Therefore, a negative result on flow cytometry does not exclude marrow involvement by lymphoma.

Caveat: Flow cytometry may give false negative results due to sampling issues such as focal disease, fibrosis or adherence to the marrow stroma. Flow cytometry may not accurately quantify neoplastic cells in the marrow due to blood contamination or processing artefact.

Cytogenetics

Conventional karyotyping: Conventional karyotyping has a limited role in the diagnosis or staging of lymphomas in the bone marrow. In most situations a normal karyotype is obtained as the mitotically active background normal hematopoietic cells "swamp" the more slowly dividing lymphoma cells. If a cytogenetically abnormal population is detected, it frequently does not add critical information to the diagnosis; questions about specific chromosomal abnormalities can be more efficiently and rapidly addressed by fluorescence *in situ* hybridization (FISH) studies. Chromosome studies are useful if there is a question of a secondary myeloid process, e.g. therapy-related myelodysplasia following chemotherapy.

FISH: Fluorescence *in situ* hybridization (FISH) studies are very useful for lymphomas that require the presence of a specific genetic anomaly for diagnosis. For others FISH detectable chromosomal abnormalities may be helpful but other quicker and less expensive methods for the same aberrancy may suffice, such as immunohistochemistry. Positive FISH results are rarely entirely disease-specific and must be correlated with other diagnostic modalities to reach a final accurate diagnosis. Also, low percentage positive results

Table 11.4. FISH probes available for lymphoma diagnosis (adapted from [9]).

Chromosome abnormality	FISH probes	Lymphoma type
t(8;14)(q24;q32)	*MYC-IGH; MYC*	BL; DLBCL; FL; MCL; PLL
t(2;8)(p11;q24)	*MYC* breakapart	BL, DLBCL; FL
t(8;22)(q24;q11)	*MYC* breakapart	BL, DLBCL; FL
t(14;18)(q32;q21)	*IGH-BCL2*	FL; DLCL; CLL (rare)
t(3;v)(q27;v)	*BCL6* breakapart	DLBCL; FL
t(11;18)(q21;q21)	*API2-MALT1; MALT1*	EMZL (MALT)
t(14;18)(q32;q21)	*MALT1* breakapart	EMZL (MALT)
t(11;14)(q13;q32)	*CCND1-IGH*	MCL
t(2;v)(p23;v)	*ALK* breakapart	ALCL
del (11)(q22)	*ATM*	CLL
del(13)(q14)	*D13S319*	CLL
del(17)(p13)	*TP53*	CLL
trisomies	Centromere probes	Many subtypes

should be interpreted with caution as some low-level translocations can be seen in normal individuals. FISH probes that are useful in the assessment of lymphoma are listed in Table 11.4.

Molecular genetics

PCR: PCR-based studies for clonal gene rearrangements or specific translocations can be applied to bone marrow and most successfully on liquid aspirate samples. Processing of the bone marrow trephine limits its suitability (see Table 11.2). PCR assays for clonal B-cell gene rearrangements (*IG* PCR) use Ig light and heavy chain primer sets (such as in the BIOMED-2 protocols) and are highly sensitive [3]. When this assay is used neoplasms historically negative for a clone can be shown to have monoclonal rearrangements (i.e. classical Hodgkin lymphoma, nodular LP Hodgkin and many follicular lymphomas). PCR for clonal T-cell gene rearrangements (*TCR*) is generally performed using probes detecting the gamma (*TCRG*) or beta (*TCRB*) region. A combined *TCRG* and *TCRB* PCR approach increases the sensitivity of detecting clonal T-cell populations. All lymphoid cell clonality PCR assays should be interpreted in the context of morphological and immunophenotypic data. This is because

equivocal and positive results can be seen in autoimmune disorders or with restricted T-cell repertoires (e.g. aging) with the potential of false positives.

Caveat: Up to 10% of B-cell lymphomas can have a clonal *TCR* as well as *IG* gene rearrangement and 10% of T-cell lymphomas can have a clonal *IG* rearrangement. Up to 90% of B lymphoblastic leukemia/lymphoma (see Chapter 7) can have a clonal *TCR*, especially in pediatric patients; these should be in the setting of a double positive result for both *IG* and *TCR* rearrangements.

Southern blotting: Southern blotting has been used to establish clonality within DNA segments associated within B, T and EBV genetic material. It has a diagnostic sensitivity of 5% and hence may give false negative results. However, an unequivocally positive band is a solid indicator of a clonal population and very strong evidence for a neoplasm. Southern blotting is labor intensive and has now been replaced by faster, less expensive and more flexible PCR-based tests.

Assessment of residual bone marrow disease and therapeutic monitoring

The crux of remission status surveillance relies on clinical assessment including physical examination, blood counts, imaging/PET scans and monitoring metabolites (i.e. LDH). If the lymphoma involves the blood or was present in the marrow at diagnosis, marrow examination is indicated. Flow cytometric immunophenotyping may be useful for disease monitoring of the peripheral blood or bone marrow aspirate. Because many B-cell neoplasms are treated with a CD20 monoclonal antibody, an additional B-cell marker (as well as CD20) must be included in a panel to allow for the detection of residual neoplastic B-cells. Similarly, expression of additional therapeutic targets (e.g. CD52 and CD25) can be assessed for therapeutic dosing efficacy.

Pre-transplant bone marrow assessment

Not all lymphoma subtypes are treated with stem cell transplant. However, many aggressive or refractory neoplasms are associated with an increased survival with a transplant. Autologous stem cells are commonly used because the mortality and morbidity rates are much more favorable. However this poses the risk of tumor cell contamination and reinfusion due to the high incidence of peripheral blood and/or bone marrow involvement. Pre-transplant tumor cell detection by flow cytometry of the blood and/or bone marrow prior to collection is recommended. *In vivo* or *in vitro* purging of neoplastic cells has been investigated with some reports of a longer relapse-free survival time; however, longer survival studies are needed [4]. Monoclonal immunotherapy in combination with chemotherapy is often used to prepare patients for transplant. If a specimen shows involvement by morphological, flow cytometric, immunocytochemical or clonal molecular gene rearrangement analyses, additional treatment with monoclonal antibody immunotherapy may be used for purging the remaining tumor before transplant. Post harvest *in vitro* purging of the infusion product can also be performed and offers another method of purification.

This overview has discussed the general principles and methods for bone marrow assessment in respect to solid tissue lymphoma. Specific lymphoma types and their features in the bone marrow are addressed in the following section.

Follicular lymphoma

Follicular lymphoma (FL) is a common lymphoma of germinal center B-cell origin which commonly involves the bone marrow (Table 11.1). Ninety percent of cases are associated with the t(14;18)(q32,q21); *IGH-BCL2*. Rearrangements of *BCL6* located on chromosome 3q27 are present in a subset of the remaining cases. Rare t(8;14)(q24;q32); *MYC-IGH* have been reported in FL; however, a more aggressive process such as Burkitt lymphoma should be excluded if this is detected. The incidence of BM involvement in FL is inversely related to the grade of lymphoma. The reported ranges for marrow involvement for grades 1, 2 and 3 are 30–60%, 7–46% and 2–15% respectively; the peripheral blood is involved in approximately 18% of cases [5]. Diagnostic tests for FL include immunohistochemistry, flow cytometry, FISH for t(14;18)(q32, q21); *BCL2-IGH* and PCR. However, these techniques rarely add value as the neoplastic cells do not aspirate reliably and false negative results can be seen [6,7]. Bone marrow trephine morphology alone is usually sufficient in bone marrow staging FL. When there is marrow involvement there may be a difference in the grade of the lymphoma between the bone marrow and the primary tissue; this is termed discordant lymphoma and is important to note. The majority of these are discordant grades of FL or FL and DLBCL in different sites, implying the association of a lower grade process to a more aggressive process within a single clone [5].

Primary diagnosis or initial staging bone marrow

Morphology: The neoplastic cells seldom involve the peripheral blood and are not readily aspirated due to increased fibrosis in the bed of the lymphoid aggregates. If the peripheral blood or bone marrow aspirate are involved, the cells are typically small to medium-sized with distinctly clefted nuclei. The bone marrow trephine (core) biopsy is the mainstay of the bone marrow study. The biopsy typically contains lymphocyte aggregates in a predominantly paratrabecular location forming fibrotic linear networks of small cells with intermixed small cleaved cells (centrocytes) and few larger non-cleaved cells with peripherally localized chromatin (centroblasts). It is because of the patchy and paratrabecular nature of the marrow infiltrate that the aspirate may be normal, even when there is extensive marrow involvement (Figure 11.1).

It is important to note that paratrabecular lymphoid infiltrates are not diagnostic of FL as they can also be seen in MCL, marginal zone lymphomas (MZL) and LPL. However, in these other lymphoma types they usually have a mixed picture with nodular/interstitial infiltrates as well as the paratrabecular lesions. Isolated paratrabecular lesions favor FL. Other distinguishing features are:

1. MCL can have clefted cytology similar to FL; however, cyclin D1 immunostaining or FISH for t(11;14)(q13;q32); *CCND1-IGH* can exclude this possibility, if needed.
2. LPL and MZL usually have round nuclear contours with more moderately abundant cytoplasm and evidence of plasmacytic differentiation.

Ancillary tests in follicular lymphoma

Typical immunophenotype:
    Positive: CD10, CD20, PAX-5, BCL-6, BCL-2, CD23.
    Negative: CD3, CD43, CD5, cyclin D1.
Immunohistochemistry panel: CD3, CD10, CD20, BCL-6, BCL-2, cyclin D1.
Genetics: t(14;18)(q32;q21); *IGH-BCL2*.

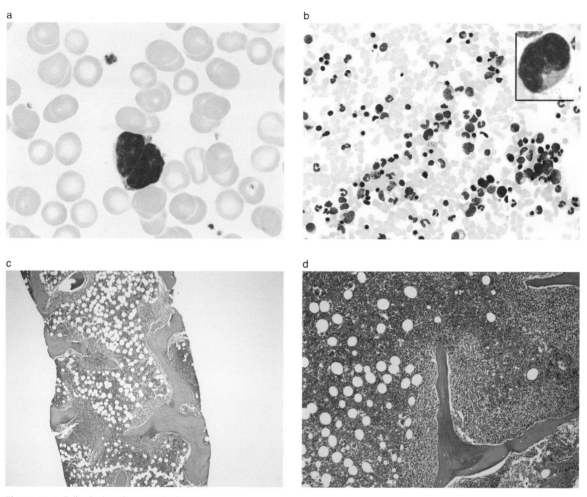

Figure 11.1. Follicular lymphoma in the bone marrow.

a. Peripheral blood: approximately 20% of cases contain cleaved cells in the blood.

b. Wright–Giemsa aspirate smear may not show many neoplastic cells even in extensively involved marrows. Malignant cells are variably sized with clefted nuclear contours (inset).

c. The core biopsy typically contains paratrabecular lymphoid aggregates with intercellular fibrotic bands creating a streaming appearance. Low grade pattern at 40×.

d. 100×.

Immunohistochemistry: If the typical morphological features are present on the H&E stained core biopsy this will suffice for marrow staging. Immunohistochemistry shows the lymphoid aggregates to be comprised of B-cells with significant numbers of admixed small reactive T-cells. The neoplastic B-cells have a germinal center phenotype (BCL-6 or CD10 positive), which is supportive evidence for FL. BCL-2 will be positive on the FL B-cells, reactive T-cells and mantle cells.

Caveats: CD10 and BCL-6 can be negative in FL. Normal T-cells and normal mantle cells express BCL-2.

Flow cytometry: Flow cytometry has limited use in assessing FL involving the bone marrow. If the neoplastic population is detectable by FCI, it expresses B-cell antigens (CD19, CD20), is CD10-positive and frequently has dim to negative surface light chain immunoglobulin expression. Permeabilizing the cells to detect cytoplasmic immunoglobulin will generally show light chain restriction confirming the presence of FL cells. A CD10-positive B-cell population is not specific for FL as this can also be seen in DLBCL, Burkitt lymphoma or an unusual maturing B-ALL. A light chain immunoglobulin-negative, CD19 and CD10-positive population can represent

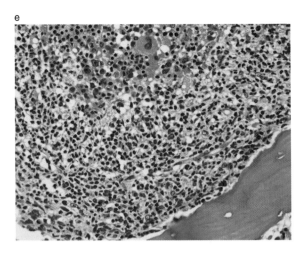

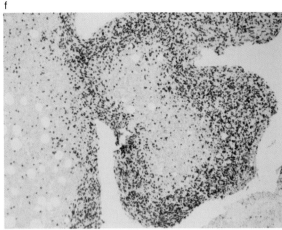

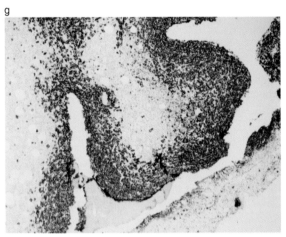

Figure 11.1. (cont.) Follicular lymphoma in the bone marrow.
e. Paratrabecular lymphoid infiltrate in the bone marrow core biopsy (H&E stain) ×100.
f. IHC for CD3 (×400) showing many intermixed reactive T-cells. The presence of these T-cells can make interpretation of small foci difficult.
g. IHC for CD20 (×100) showing a similar pattern to CD3.

hematogones, B-ALL, FL, DLBCL or reactive lymphoid hyperplasia. Sometimes FL cells will be negative for CD10 by FC but show positive expression by IHC. It is not uncommon for FC to be negative on the aspirate even when there is morphological evidence of marrow involvement on the core biopsy [6,7]. This is because of the failure to aspirate the paratrabecular neoplastic cells.

Cytogenetics studies

Karyotyping: Karyotyping the bone marrow is generally not of any use in assessing FL. This is due to the infrequent presence of the population of interest in the aspirate and the low probability of capturing the slowly dividing neoplastic cell karyotype among the rapidly dividing background hematopoiesis. If a t(14;18)(q32;q21) is detected, conventional karyotyping cannot distinguish between *IGH-BCL2* and *IGH-*

MALT1 seen in extranodal marginal zone lymphomas of mucosa-associated tissue (EMZL) [8]. Additional chromosomal anomalies, including gains and losses of chromosomes, are frequently reported in nodal FL which may mirror increasing histological grade.

FISH: FISH studies require the cells of interest to be present in the aspirate smear, touch preparation or clot section/particle preparation. FISH studies for t(14;18)(q32;q21); *IGH-BCL2* can be useful in rare circumstances where the morphology is not classic and to distinguish FL from other small B-cell neoplasms. It is not routinely used to determine whether a lymphoid aggregate is neoplastic or benign. Testing should not be undertaken as a screening procedure without morphological support due to the presence of a low level of the translocation in the normal population, especially in smokers [9].

Molecular diagnostics/PCR: PCR can be used to detect the *BCL2-IGH* fusion in FL. Approximately 75% of cases possess a breakpoint within the MBR region of the *BCL2* gene and in approximately 15% of cases, the breakpoint is within the 5' mcr or mcr region. The location of the *BCL2* breakpoint does not offer prognostic information although patients with a mcr *BCL2* breakpoint tend to present with a higher grade of disease and more frequent extra-nodal involvement. The breakpoint within the *IGH* locus usually lies close to one of the six JH domains. PCR primers are able to detect the *BCL2-IGH* rearrangement in approximately 90% of cases with a t(14;18). This utilizes a multiplex PCR amplification system incorporating a consensus JH primer and a number of different primers specific for each of the breakpoint cluster regions. The identification of the specific *BCL2* breakpoint region by PCR allows the development and use of patient-specific primers for disease monitoring, if required. The small number of t(14;18) cases in which the *BCL2-IGH* rearrangement is not detectable by PCR are likely to possess breakpoints between the MBR and mcr regions or, more rarely, 5' of the *BCL2* locus.

Although PCR for *BCL2-IGH* fusions is available and can be applied to blood and bone marrow aspirate samples, it is not used routinely for marrow staging. FISH is more commonly utilized as it is more sensitive for all possible splicing variants and complex cytogenetic abnormalities involving the *IGH* or *BCL2* genes [8,9,10]. PCR for *IG* gene rearrangements is also not routinely used as this may be falsely negative due to somatic hypermutation. Some cases may however require *IG* PCR to confirm clonality and differentiate from a reactive lymphoid process; a positive result does not help to subtype the neoplasm.

Residual bone marrow disease and therapeutic monitoring

Bone marrow morphology is widely used to assess disease response to treatment or progression/transformation to a more aggressive form of lymphoma. CD20 expression on B-cells assists in the monitoring of rituximab dosing; however, care must be taken interpreting immunostaining following CD20 immunotherapy. This is because the therapeutic antibody interferes with or blocks CD20 receptors and may give a false negative IHC result. Alternate B-cell-associated antibodies (e.g. PAX-5 or CD19) must be used to assess B-cell numbers in the marrow. It is also important to differentiate reactive paratrabecular T-cell aggregates that are commonly associated with rituximab treatment from residual involvement by FL as these have similar morphological appearances. The reactive aggregates will be T-cells (CD3-positive) and not contain many PAX-5 or CD19-positive B-cells. More sophisticated methods of monitoring minimal residual disease are not routinely performed and investigators have found no correlation between numbers of circulating t(14;18)-positive cells and ultimate response to treatment [11]; however, the use of log reductions in quantitative PCR may predict a favorable clinical response or relapse in patients with advanced stage FL [12]. These techniques are not at present used in routine standard disease monitoring.

> *Caveat*: Low levels of t(14;18)(q32;q21); *IGH-BCL2* are detected in normal individuals, especially smokers, which obscures the clinical significance of single data point minimal residual disease testing.

Pre-transplant bone marrow assessment

Imaging/PET scans and other clinical laboratory features are the mainstay of pre-transplant evaluation to assess residual tumor burden. Flow cytometric immunophenotyping or PCR for *IG* or *BCL2* can be performed to assess the presence of tumor cells in the blood or marrow prior to collection of autologous cells for transplantation. If present, *in vivo* purging with cytotoxics and immunotherapy has been reported to be associated with an increased remission rate [13]. The BM biopsy assessment is similar to that performed on the initial evaluation with aforementioned post-treatment caveats in mind.

Mantle cell lymphoma

Mantle cell lymphoma (MCL) is a mature B-cell neoplasm that typically has a more aggressive clinical course than the other small B-cell neoplasms. A subset of MCLs with blood involvement but without demonstrable nodal disease has been shown to have a better prognosis [14,15]. The cell of origin is the naïve B-cell in primary follicles that are pushed to the periphery of the follicle. Following antigen stimulation these cells form the mantle zone surrounding the germinal center. The typical immunophenotype of MCL is a CD5-positive B-cell that is cyclin D1- and CD23-negative. Almost all cases are associated with t(11;14)(q13;q32); *CCND1-IGH*, with very rare cyclin D1-negative cases reported. MCL commonly involves the marrow and can be detected morphologically on aspirate smears, touch preparations and clot sections as well as the core biopsy (Table 11.1). It is readily detectable by flow cytometry and confirmed by FISH or cyclin D1 IHC. Some cases have peripheral blood involvement which can be used for diagnosis.

Primary diagnosis or initial staging bone marrow

Morphology: MCL typically has mature small cell morphology with round to slightly angular or cleaved nuclei. In the bone marrow trephine biopsy, MCL can have a paratrabecular, nodular or interstitial pattern of involvement and have small or large blastoid cells. Because of this topographical heterogeneity it is included in many differential diagnoses. A diagnostic clue is the higher mitotic rate than seen with other small B-cell neoplasms. There are many morphological variants: blastoid and pleomorphic variants contain large cells with finer chromatin or pleomorphic cells with pale cytoplasm and both have very high mitotic rates. Small cell and monocytoid variants mimic CLL and MZL morphologically but there are no proliferation centers (collections of paraimmunoblasts) as seen in CLL/SLL. Mantle cell lymphoma can be detected in aspirate samples but the sensitivity is lower than the trephine biopsy.

Ancillary tests in mantle cell lymphoma

Typical immunophenotype:
   Positive: CD19, CD20 (bright), CD5, CD43, CD45
       (bright), cyclin D1, surface Ig (bright).
   Negative: CD23-negative.
Caveat: can be CD5-negative or CD10-positive.
Immunohistochemistry panel: CD3, CD5, CD10, CD20,
       CD23, CD138, cyclin D1, Ki67, PAX-5, kappa
   and lambda light chains.
Other tests: can also use flow phenotype and cyclin
       D1 or FISH for confirmation.
Genetics: t(11;14)(q13;q32); *CCND1-IGH*.

Immunohistochemistry: Confirmation of the phenotype is usually performed with CD20, CD5 and cyclin D1; however, additional stains may be needed as discussed below (Table 11.5). CD5-negative and CD10-positive cases are well established. Ki67 is recommended to be used as a prognostic indicator in MCL, with >40% positive neoplastic cells being an adverse prognostic sign [10]. Cyclin D1 is not pathognomonic of MCL as other neoplasms are also positive (Table 11.5):

- *Plasma cell neoplasms*: A subset of plasma cell neoplasms are CD20- and cyclin D1-positive by IHC and have t(11;14)(q13;q32); *CCND1-IGH* and lymphocyte-like morphology. Low level cyclin D1 positivity can also be seen in myeloma with trisomy 11. CD43 is positive in both MCL and plasma cells. Plasma cell neoplasms are CD138- and MUM-1-positive whereas MCL is negative, and plasma cells are negative for CD5.
- *Hairy cell leukemia*: Cyclin D1 can be over-expressed in HCL but this is not associated with the *CCND1-IGH* translocation [16]. In rare cases, both MCL and HCL can express CD10. HCL will be associated with an interstitial pattern of marrow infiltration and have distinctive cytology, immunophenotypic and clinical history findings without significant lymphadenopathy.
- *Chronic lymphocytic leukemia*: proliferation centers may sometimes show cyclin D1 staining.

If there is no confirmed diagnosis of MCL from a tissue site, it is prudent to exclude these differential diagnoses when a cyclin D1, CD20-positive cell population is detected in the bone marrow. Very rare cyclin D1-negative MCLs have been reported and have been confirmed to have gene expression profiles similar to that of cyclin D1-positive MCLs. These cases show cyclin D2 and cyclin D3 expression (available in paraffin IHC) and may behave similarly or more indolently than classic MCL cases [17].

Flow cytometry: Flow cytometry is very useful for the diagnosis of MCL as the typical immunophenotype i.e. CD20 (bright), CD5, CD45 (bright)-positive with light chain restriction and CD23, CD103-negative, prompts confirmation of the genetic translocation by FISH or cyclin D1 IHC (Figure 11.2). FCI with CD11c, CD103, CD38 and CD138 can also be used to distinguish cyclin D1-positive HCL and plasma cell neoplasms. See Table 11.5 for a comparison of these entities.

Table 11.5. Comparative immunophenotypes of mantle cell lymphoma (MCL), plasma cell myeloma (PCM), hairy cell leukemia (HCL) and splenic marginal zone lymphoma (SMZL).

	MCL	PCM	HCL	SMZL
CD20	++	−/+	+++	+++
CD19	+	−/+	+++	+++
CD5	+/−	−	−/+	−/+
CD23	−	−	−	−
CD25	−	−	+	−
CD138	−	+	−	−
Annexin-A1	−	−	+	−
TRAP	−	−	+	−/+
CD10	−/+	−/+	−/+	−
CD43	+	+	−	−
CD56	−	+	+	−
CD123	−	−	+	−
MUM1/IRF4	−	+	−	−/+
CD103	−	−	+	−/+
Light chain	surface (++)	cytoplasm	surface (+++)	surface (+++)
Cyclin D1	+	+/−	+/−	−
FISH CCND1-IGH	+	+	−	−

Cytogenetics

Karyotyping: Karyotyping is not routinely used in MCL involving the bone marrow due to the relatively long test result time and the low probability of capturing the neoplastic cell karyotype among the rapidly dividing background hematopoiesis. However, if the translocation is detected, it provides supportive evidence for a definitive diagnosis if morphological and immunophenotypic criteria are met.

FISH: The detection of t(11;14)(q13;q32); *CCND1-IGH* by FISH is a useful way to establish a diagnosis of MCL. If the MCL is limited to the blood and/or bone marrow than FISH for t(11;14)(q13;q32); *CCND1-IGH* is indicated. In general there is no need to perform FISH on the bone marrow if the diagnosis of MCL is already established from solid tissue.

Molecular diagnostics/PCR: PCR for *CCND1-IGH*, the molecular consequence of t(11;14)(q13;q32) is not routinely used in the initial diagnosis or staging of MCL due to its low sensitivity. The genomic breakpoint on chromosome 11 can lie up to 120 kb upstream of the *CCND1* gene. In up to 40% of cases the breakpoint lies within an 85 bp region termed MTC but the remainder are spread throughout a large genomic region upstream of *CCND1*. PCR techniques are only able to identify the cases with breakpoints within the MTC cluster (i.e. 40%) by using a specific primer that anneals just adjacent to the cluster along with a consensus JH-specific primer. Although *IG* PCR can be used to detect B-cell clonality, in general FISH is the genetic test of choice.

Residual bone marrow disease and therapeutic monitoring

Morphology and immunophenotyping are used to monitor residual disease. CD20 immunohistochemistry

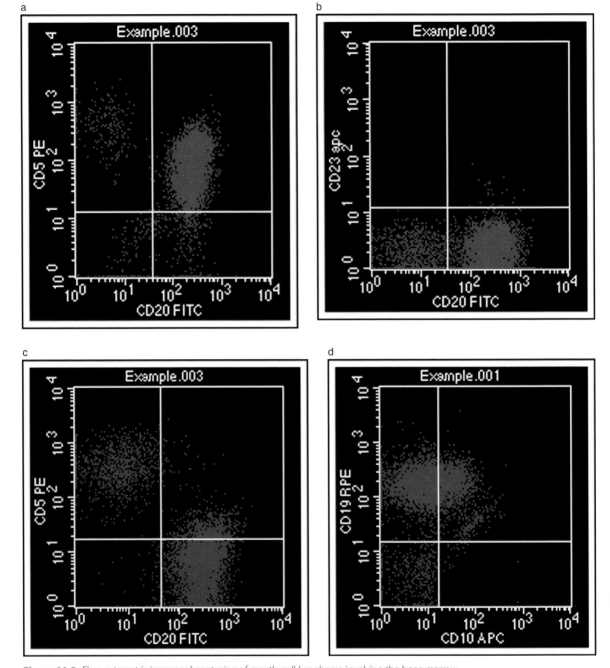

Figure 11.2. Flow cytometric immunophenotyping of mantle cell lymphoma involving the bone marrow.
a. CD20 is moderately bright and the B-cells express CD5.
b. The CD20-positive B-cells are CD23-negative.
c. A subset of MCLs are negative for CD5.
d. CD19-positive with some weak CD10 positivity.

can be used as an indicator of rituximab efficacy. Detection of *CCND1-IGH* by sensitive PCR methods is only applicable for those cases in which the translocation was detectable at diagnosis. PCR for clonal *IG* gene rearrangements can be employed for the remaining 60% of cases to monitor minimal residual disease status [18].

Pre-transplant bone marrow assessment

Pre-transplant evaluation relies on the assessment of tumor burden using imaging/PET scans and other clinical laboratory features. Flow cytometric immunophenotyping or *IG* PCR can be used to assess the presence of tumor cells in the blood or marrow prior to collection of cells for autologous transplantation. If present, *in vivo* purging with immunotherapy may be performed. The BM biopsy assessment is similar to that performed at initial staging evaluation; the aforementioned post-treatment caveats must be taken into consideration (e.g. loss of CD20 expression).

Splenic marginal zone lymphoma

Splenic marginal zone lymphoma (SMZL), a neoplasm of small mature B-cells, invariably involves the spleen and bone marrow but with no significant tissue involvement outside the splenic lymph node region. The putative cell of origin is the post-germinal center marginal zone B-cell of the spleen. The neoplastic B-cells are typically CD5- and CD10-negative although some cases do express CD5 antigen. No recurrent cytogenetic anomalies have been described. The bone marrow and peripheral blood are the usual primary diagnostic samples. Frequently the morphological features in the BM are not sufficient to accurately diagnose SMZL. The major differential diagnosis is HCL due to the overlapping immunophenotype, cytological features and clinical presentations. This distinction is of clinical importance due to the differences in treatment strategies. The current WHO classification acknowledges this diagnostic dilemma with a category of "splenic B-cell lymphoma, unclassified"; this entity encompasses those cases with overlapping or unusual features for SMZL or HCL and hairy cell leukemia variant (HCL-v) [14]. HCL-v typically does not respond to purine analog treatment regimens and should not be classified with HCL – see Chapter 9.

Primary diagnosis or initial staging bone marrow

Morphology: SMZL has a nodular and/or sinusoidal pattern of bone marrow infiltration by predominantly small cells with moderately abundant cytoplasm occasionally with admixed larger immunoblasts. However, SMZL can have an interstitial pattern that mimics HCL. Cytological features in the blood or bone marrow aspirate smears are of small to medium-sized cells with scant to moderately abundant cytoplasm which can have polar villi. Although the cytological features can be similar to HCL, the marrow pattern can be used to distinguish SMZL from HCL [19,20] (Figure 11.3). Splenic diffuse red pulp small B-cell lymphoma (SDRPSBCL) is a described variant with a diffuse red pulp pattern of splenic involvement.

Ancillary tests in splenic marginal zone lymphoma

Typical immunophenotype:
  Positive: CD19, CD20, CD22, CD79a, CD11c, DBA.44,
    BCL-2, IgM, IgD.
  Negative: CD10, CD23, CD25, CD43, BCL-6, cyclin D1,
    CD123, annexin-A1.
  Variable: CD5, CD103. TRAP is negative to weak.
Immunohistochemistry panel: CD3, CD20, CD5, CD10,
    CD25, CD123, BCL-6, annexin A1, cyclin D1.

Immunohistochemistry: IHC on the bone marrow biopsy can be challenging as the primary method for diagnosis of SMZL and to differentiate from HCL. Annexin A1 and TRAP IHC can be very useful as they are negative in SMZL and positive in HCL (see Table 11.5).

Caveat: Annexin-1 is positive in background myeloid and T-cells and can be difficult to interpret if only minimally involved.

Flow cytometry: The classic immunophenotypic profile of SMZL is bright expression of pan-B-cell antigens CD19, CD20, CD22 and surface Ig, and CD11c, and lack of CD10 and CD103 expression (Figure 11.3). CD5 is variably expressed; CD25 and CD123 are

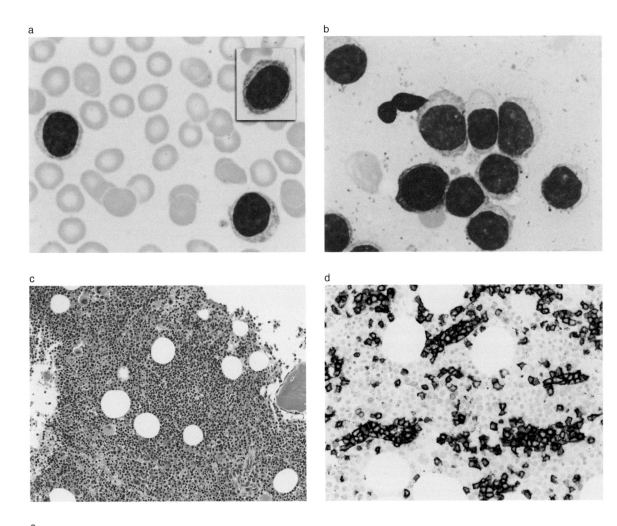

Figure 11.3. Splenic marginal zone lymphoma in the bone marrow.
a. The peripheral blood contains cells with moderately abundant light blue cytoplasm with or without fine cytoplasmic projections (inset).
b. Bone marrow aspirate showing small cells with scant to moderately abundant cytoplasm.
c. The core biopsy pattern is commonly nodular (hematoxylin and eosin (H&E)) 200× and there may be an associated sinusoidal pattern.
d. IHC for CD20 (200×) highlights the lymphoma cells.
e. CD20 (400×).

f1 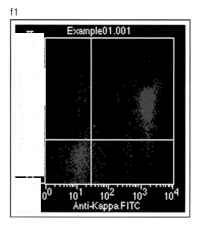 f2 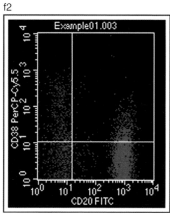 f3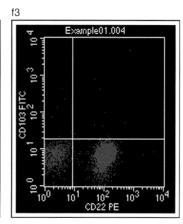

g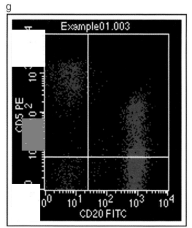

Figure 11.3. (cont.) Splenic marginal zone lymphoma.
f. (f1, f2, f3) Typical flow cytometry plots showing bright surface kappa (f1), CD20 (f2) and CD22, but CD103-negative (f3).
g. An example of partial CD5 expression.

negative in SMZL but positive in HCL. Occasional cases of SMZL are CD103-positive and TRAP, annexin A1, CD25 and CD123 can be used to distinguish these cases from HCL [21] (Table 11.5). The provisional WHO classification category "splenic diffuse red pulp B-cell lymphoma" is associated with intra-sinusoidal bone marrow infiltration and has the following immunophenotype: CD20-, IgG-positive and annexin A1-, CD25-, CD103-, CD123-, CD11c-negative. Occasional cases can be CD103-, CD11c- or CD123-positive [14].

Cytogenetics/FISH: Cytogenetics and FISH do not have a routine role in the diagnosis of SMZL due to the variable and non-specific chromosomal anomalies associated with the entity. A 7q31–32 deletion is present in 40% of cases. Of note, t(14;18)(q32;q21); *IGH-BCL2*, t(11;14)(q13;q32); *CCND1-IGH* and the extranodal MALT translocation, t(11;18)(q21;q21); *AP12-MALT1* are not associated with SMZL [14].

Molecular diagnostics: Molecular testing is rarely used in SMZL. In cases where there is a question as to whether the infiltrate is reactive or neoplastic *IG* PCR for B-cell clonality may be helpful. Other more specific tests for qualitative diagnosis confirmation are not routinely applied.

Residual bone marrow disease and therapeutic monitoring

The mainstays of disease monitoring are flow cytometry to detect a monotypic surface Ig B-cell population, and morphology of the bone marrow core biopsy.

Pre-transplant bone marrow assessment

Transplantation is not a standard treatment choice for SMZL.

Table 11.6. Chromosomal abnormalities (% of cases) according to site in EMZL (MALT) lymphomas (adapted from [14]).

Site	t(11;18)	t(14;18)	t(3;14)	t(1;14)	+3	+18
Stomach	6–26	1–5	0	0	11	6
Intestine	12–56	0	0	0–13	75	25
Ocular/orbit	0–10	0–25	0–20	0	38	13
Salivary glands	0–5	0–16	0	0–2	55	19
Lung	31–53	6–10	0	2–7	20	7
Skin	0–8	0–14	0–10	0	20	4
Thyroid	0–17	0	0–50	0	17	0

Extranodal marginal zone lymphoma of mucosa-associated lymphoid tissue

Extranodal marginal zone lymphoma of mucosa-associated lymphoid tissue (EMZL or MALT) is a neoplasm arising from post-germinal center small mature B-cells. These cells classically have a CD5, CD10-negative phenotype and may have an associated monotypic plasma cell component. The translocations t(11;18)(q21;q21);*API2-MALT1*, t(14;18)(q32;q21); *IGH-MALT1*, t(1;14)(p22;q32);*BCL10-IGH* vary in prevalence in EMZL/MALT lymphomas according to the location of primary involvement [14,22] (Table 11.6).

MALT lymphomas are usually indolent in spite of multifocal organ involvement. Classic staging paradigms used for other types of lymphoma may therefore not be accurate for assessing prognosis. Relatively few EMZL lymphomas involve the bone marrow (overall 3–20%) and the frequency depends on primary disease site. For example, primary gastric cases show infrequent involvement whereas lung and conjunctival/ocular cases more commonly have bone marrow disease [14].

Primary diagnosis or initial staging bone marrow

Morphology: The cells may be very difficult to visualize on peripheral blood or aspirate smears but typically are small to medium sized and have small round nuclei with moderately abundant cytoplasm. The bone marrow trephine biopsy, when involved, shows nodular non-paratrabecular lymphoid aggregates and occasional paratrabecular aggregates [14,19,20], or lymphoma cells surrounding reactive lymphoid aggregates or germinal centers. Scattered large cells (immunoblasts) can be present and be quite prevalent; these should not be over-interpreted as transformation to a more aggressive neoplasm without additional supportive evidence (e.g. necrosis, space-occupying sheets of large cells).

Ancillary tests in extranodal marginal zone (or MALT) lymphoma

Typical immunophenotype:
  Positive: CD19, CD20, CD22, CD79a, CD11c, FMC-7.
  Negative: CD10, CD23, CD25, BCL-6, cyclin D1, CD123, annexin-A1.
  Immunohistochemistry panel: CD3, CD5, CD10, CD20, CD43, BCL-2, CD138, kappa, lambda.

Immunohistochemistry: The immunohistochemical features of EMZL are indistinguishable from nodular MZL and SMZL. The cells express pan B-cell antigens (CD19, CD20, CD22, CD79a) and monotypic kappa or lambda surface immunoglobulin. The majority of cases express BCL-2, 50% CD43 and most cases express IgM. CD10, BCL-6, cyclin D1 and CD23 are negative whilst CD5 and IgD are usually negative but can be expressed in a small number of cases. Annexin A1 and TRAP are negative. Assessment of kappa and lambda light chain expression by IHC or ISH may be useful to detect associated plasma cells with monotypia.

Flow cytometry: FCI is helpful in all marginal zone lymphomas due to the frequent morphological overlap with reactive lymphoid infiltrates. A light chain-restricted CD19, CD20-positive B-cell population lacking CD5 and CD10 with associated monotypic plasma cells suggests a "generic" marginal zone lymphoma. EMZL are negative for CD10 and CD103, and CD5, although classically negative, can be partially expressed in a minority of cases.

Cytogenetics/FISH: Routine cytogenetic karyotyping is not very useful in EMZL lymphoma due to the low number and low proliferative rate of the neoplastic cells in the marrow in most cases. Although EMZL does have genetic abnormalities that are detectable by FISH, this is not generally required on the bone marrow; FISH studies are generally only performed on the primary diagnostic extranodal tissue sample. Trisomy 3, 12 and 18 are frequently present but may be non-specific [9,14,22] (Table 11.6).

> *Caveat*: The t(14;18)(q32;q21) of EMZL is indistinguishable from the translocation in FL at chromosomal resolution since *MALT1* and *BCL2* are located in the same chromosome band and are only 4.5 Mb apart.

Molecular diagnostics: *IG* PCR may be required to differentiate a reactive lymphoid follicle from neoplastic cells. However, it must be stressed that PCR should not be used routinely as a screening tool for any lymphoid aggregates in the marrow. It should be reserved for those cases where the lymphoid aggregates have some atypical features, such as an expanded perifollicular region by cells with a monocytoid appearance.

Residual bone marrow disease and therapeutic monitoring

Disease monitoring for EMZL does not usually require examination of the bone marrow. Restaging bone marrow studies may be undertaken if the marrow was initially involved at diagnosis; similar methods would then be performed as in the original staging bone marrow exam.

Pre-transplant bone marrow assessment

Transplantation is not a standard treatment choice for EMZL.

Nodal marginal zone lymphoma

Nodal marginal zone lymphoma (NMZL) is a small B-cell neoplasm of post-germinal center cells that has monocytoid cytological and architectural features and a non-specific phenotype (similar to EMZL lymphoma). By definition, NMZL involves nodal but not extranodal or splenic tissues. Due to this strict definition, clinical features are required to subclassify a marginal zone lymphoma; widespread marginal zone lymphoma with lymph node involvement can represent systemic involvement of EMZL or a NMZL (SMZL does not involve lymph nodes outside the splenic region). The BM features are largely non-specific as there are no distinct morphological, immunophenotypic or genetic features.

Primary diagnosis or initial staging bone marrow

Morphology: NMZL cells can be very difficult to identify on blood and bone marrow aspirate smears. Classically they are small to medium sized and have small round nuclei with moderately abundant cytoplasm. No specific architectural pattern is present on the bone marrow core biopsy but the most common is nodular non-paratrabecular lymphoid aggregates with occasional paratrabecular aggregates [19,20]. The cytology is heterogeneous with admixed large cells. These larger immunoblasts can be quite prevalent and, as in EMZL, should not be over-interpreted as transformation to a more aggressive neoplasm without additional morphological evidence. The neoplastic cells may surround reactive germinal centers.

Ancillary tests in nodal marginal zone lymphoma

> Typical immunophenotype:
>   Positive: CD19, CD20, CD79a.
>   Negative: CD10, BCL-6, cyclin-D1, CD23.
>   Variable: CD5 can be variably positive.
> Immunohistochemistry panel: CD3, CD5, CD10, CD20,
>   CD43, BCL-2, CD138, kappa, lambda.

Immunohistochemistry: The IHC features of NMZL are indistinguishable from EMZL and SMZL lymphomas. The cells express pan-B-cell antigens (CD19, CD20, CD22, CD79a) and monotypic kappa or lambda surface immunoglobulin. The majority of cases express BCL-2 and half express CD43. CD10, BCL-6, cyclin D1 and CD23 are negative. CD5 and IgD are classically negative but can be expressed independently in a small portion of cases. Annexin A1 and TRAP are negative. Assessment of kappa and lambda light chain expression by IHC or ISH may be useful to assess associated plasma cells for a monotypic population.

Flow cytometry: The main role of FC is to distinguish between MZL and reactive lymphoid infiltrates. As with EMZL, a light chain restricted CD19, CD20-positive B-cell population lacking CD5, CD10, CD25 and CD103 is suggestive but not definitive for a marginal zone lymphoma.

Cytogenetics/FISH: No specific abnormalities are associated with NMZL. Trisomy 3 may be seen but is non-specific. The EMZL-associated translocations are not present.

Molecular diagnostics: IG PCR may be useful in rare cases when the discrimination between a reactive lymphoid infiltrate and involvement by lymphoma is problematic and this has not been resolved by flow cytometry.

Residual bone marrow disease and therapeutic monitoring

If the bone marrow was involved at diagnosis, flow cytometry can be performed to monitor the presence of light chain-restricted B-cells and to detect continued presence of cells with the known antigenic profile of the lymphoma. B-cell numbers may also be measured by flow cytometry to monitor the efficacy of antibody-based immunotherapy.

Pre-transplant bone marrow assessment

Transplantation is not a standard treatment choice for NMZL.

Diffuse large B-cell lymphoma

Diffuse large B-cell lymphoma (DLBCL) is a heterogeneous group of large cell lymphomas with different diagnostic criteria and a lower rate of bone marrow involvement than small mature B-cell lymphomas [1,5]. The most common type of DLBCL contains

sheets of large centroblast-like cells with moderately abundant cytoplasm. These are derived from post-antigen stimulated cells from the germinal center or post-germinal center and they retain the antigen expression profile consistent with the level of differentiation. In most cases, the neoplastic B-cell has undergone *IG* rearrangement and somatic mutation. Chromosome translocations involving *BCL6* on 3q27 occur in 30–40% of cases and t(14;18)(q32;q21); *IGH-BCL2* in approximately 20% [1,9,14]. These translocations result in over expression of the *BCL6* and *BCL2* oncogenes by juxtaposition next to an *IGH* regulatory element. *MYC* rearrangements are present in approximately 5–10% of DLBCL; it has been suggested that these cases may be better classified as "B-cell lymphoma unclassifiable with features intermediate between diffuse large B-cell lymphoma and Burkitt lymphoma" [14]. This is a new WHO category which has been proposed for those neoplasms that do not fulfill the requirements for Burkitt lymphoma but have some morphological or genetic features of a more aggressive process; the features are detailed in Table 11.7. This category is also proposed if there are concurrent anomalies in *BCL6*, *BCL2* and *MYC*, the so-called 'double hit' lymphoma [14].

Some specific types of DLBCL which have characteristic bone marrow features are:

- *EBV-associated DLBCL*: This subtype of DLBCL should be considered if there is significant plasmablastic morphology and associated necrosis or in the setting of prior transplantation or immunodeficiency from any cause.
- *T-cell rich B-cell lymphoma (TCRBCL)*: This subtype has distinct morphology and presentation. It is often associated with a fever of unknown origin and vague lymphoreticular involvement. A bone marrow examination may provide the diagnosis when unsuspected.
- *Intravascular B-cell lymphoma* (IVBCL): This can be an elusive diagnosis due to the lack of clinically evident tissue involvement. The marrow may be the best or only site with diagnostic material.

Primary diagnosis or initial staging bone marrow

Morphology: Morphological evaluation of the marrow is the single most important assessment for a primary diagnosis or staging of DLBCL for multiple reasons:

Table 11.7. Comparison between Burkitt lymphoma, BL/BL and diffuse large B-cell lymphoma (adapted from [38]).

Standard IHC panel:	CD10, BCL-6, BCL-2, Ki-67
Cytogenetic anomalies:	t(8;14), t(2;8), t(8;22), t(14;18), t(3q27), complex karyotype
FISH panel:	*MYC* bap, *MYC* fusion, *BCL2-IGH* fusion, *BCL6* bap, *IGH* bap, *IGL* bap

	Burkitt lymphoma	**BL/BL**	**DLBCL**
CD10 IHC	+	+/−	+/−
BCL-6 IHC	+	+/−	+/−
BCL-2 IHC	−	+/−	+/−
Ki67 IHC	> 95%	< 95%	< 90%
IGH-MYC rearrangement	+	+	−
Non *IGH-MYC* rearrangement	−	+	−
MYC + BCL2 rearrangement	−	+	−
BCL2 rearrangement	−	+	+
BCL6 rearrangement	−	+	+
Simple karyotype	+	+	
Complex karyotype	−	+	

bap: breakapart.

1. If the bone marrow is involved, it is often readily detected on H&E core biopsy sections.
2. It is possible to classify if the lymphoma in the marrow is concordant with or discordant from the lymphoma classification in the diagnostic tissue site.
3. If the marrow is involved (solely or concurrently) by a small cell infiltrate in a patient with a tissue diagnosis of DLBCL, two considerations with separate prognostic significance are possible:
   i. A single neoplasm with transformation from a small mature B-cell process to a large cell process, or,
   ii. Synchronous presentation of two separate neoplasms.

The type of small B-cell neoplasm in the marrow and the expression of similar antigens in the large cells may help differentiate these two possibilities.

Morphological patterns of BM involvement by DLBCL include:

1. *"Common" DLBCL* forms large clusters or sheets of neoplastic cells which may be associated with extensive necrosis. This is also the pattern for plasmablastic lymphoma.
2. *TCRBCL* involves the BM in lightly eosinophilic lymphohistiocytic collections with fewer admixed neoplastic large cells. Based on this pattern the differential diagnosis includes classical Hodgkin lymphoma, T-cell lymphoma or granulomatous infections.
3. *Intravascular B-cell lymphoma* can be detected as a subtle infiltration of sinusoids and blood vessels in the BM by large atypical cells usually marginalized to the vessel walls or filling the lumen (Figure 11.4j).

In DLBCL the aspirate has lower sensitivity than the trephine biopsy for detecting bone marrow disease, similar to FL and MCL. When present in the aspirate the cells are identified by their large size, basophilic cytoplasm, pleomorphic nuclei and commonly one or more nucleoli.

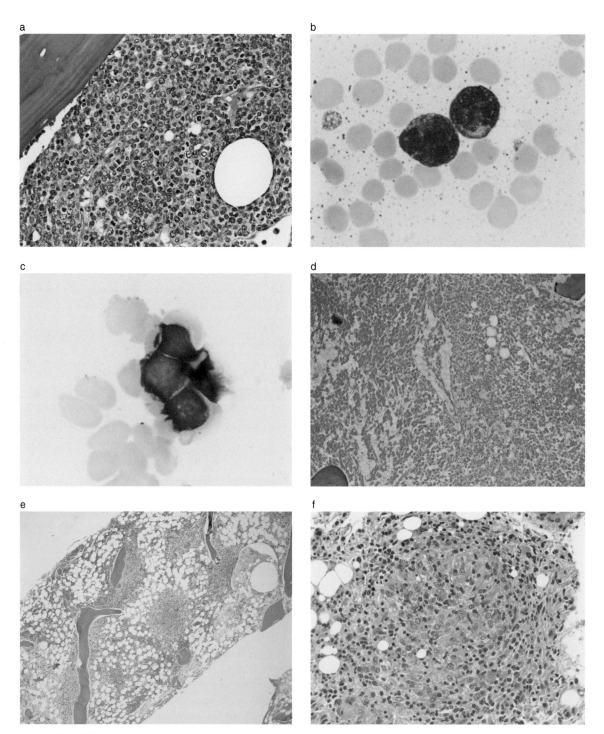

Figure 11.4. Diffuse large B-cell lymphoma in the bone marrow.
a. Sheets of DLBCL cells in the core biopsy, hematoxylin and eosin (H&E) 400×.
b. DLBCL in the aspirate are large atypical cells with coarse chromatin and irregular nuclear contours, Wright–Giemsa 1000×.
c. Touch preparations of bone marrow artificially make the cells appear blast-like.
d. Necrosis in a marrow sample, a frequent finding in DLBCL, H&E 200×.
e. The TCRBCL variant, creates lymphohistiocytic nodular aggregates, H&E 40×.
f. TCRBCL variant 200×.
g. IHC for CD20 highlights the few but large neoplastic B-cells in TCRBCL, 200×.
h. The abundant reactive T-cells, CD3 in TCRBCL 200×.
i. Intravascular B-cell lymphoma in the bone marrow. Large atypical cells are present in vessels, H&E 400×.
j. Intravascular B-cell lymphoma, CD20 100×.
k. Flow cytometric immunophenotyping of DLBCL may be negative or may show a CD10 variable B-cell population which lacks surface light chain expression (k1–3).

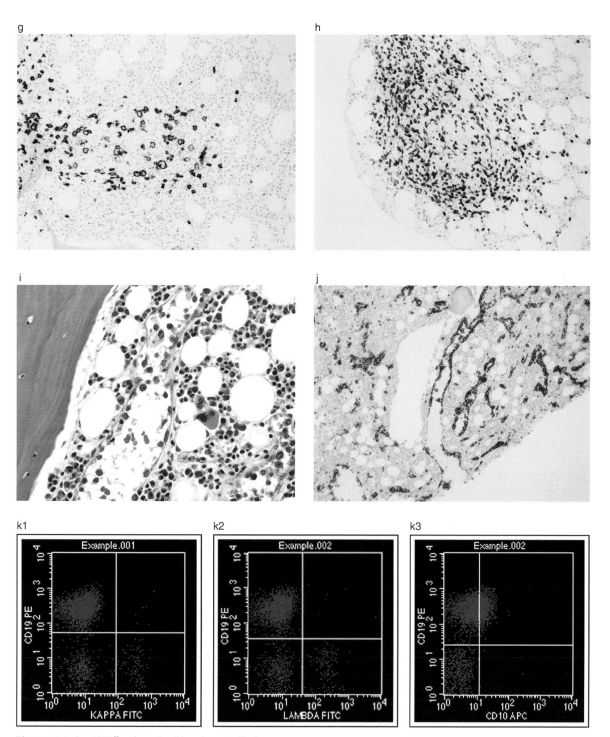

Figure 11.4. (cont.) Diffuse large B-cell lymphoma in the bone marrow.

Ancillary tests in diffuse large B-cell lymphoma

Typical immunophenotype:
    Positive: CD19, CD20, CD45 (strong).
    Variable: CD10, BCL6, BCL-2, MUM-1, EBV.
Immunohistochemistry panel: CD3, CD10, CD20,
        CD30, BCL-6, BCL-2, MUM-1, Ki67.
EBER – if necrosis, plasmablastic differentiation or
    immunodeficiency state.

Immunohistochemistry: The typical immunophenotype of DLBCL is CD19-, CD20- and CD45-positive. CD10 and BCL-6 are expressed in the germinal center subtype whereas MUM1/IRF4 is expressed in the non-germinal center/activated B-cell subtype. BCL-2 is positive in a subset of cases and is usually partial. CD5 is positive in a small collection of transformed and *de novo* cases. Staining for B-cell markers in the bone marrow biopsy is not traditionally performed to screen for marrow involvement as some see no increase in sensitivity over careful morphological assessment [23]; others however advocate that it increases sensitivity of detection by 20% [24,25]. Care must be taken to differentiate normal B-cell precursors (hematogones) from neoplastic B-cells and to select additional B-cell markers following rituximab (anti-CD20) treatment; PAX-5, CD19 or CD79a are useful in this setting. Prognostication associated with germinal center B-cell-like or activated B-cell-like subtypes is best performed on a tissue biopsy and not the BM. If B-ALL is a consideration, TdT is helpful in confirming an immature cell population. Burkitt lymphoma should be CD10-positive and BCL-2-negative with a very high percent of Ki67-positive cells; it is important to note that Ki67 alone is non-discriminatory as a high Ki67 result (>99%) can be seen in DLBCL.

In situ hybridization: It is useful to perform *in situ* hybridization (ISH) for EBER when there is a high likelihood of EBV association (plasmacytic/blastic differentiation, necrosis, immunodeficiency states – including elderly patients) as the result has therapeutic and prognostic significance. Kappa and lambda ISH may be helpful in plasmablastic lymphoma.

Flow cytometry: The DLBCL cells are large and do not fare well with the processing stressors, usually resulting in decreased sensitivity, and discordance between flow and histology. A negative flow study does not exclude DLBCL, and FCI of the marrow is generally not useful for classification of DLBCL. FCI can however be useful to detect light chain restriction of B-cells indicating the presence of a clonal B-cell population; this can increase the sensitivity of detection of bone marrow disease by 10% [24,25]. Even so, a positive result in the absence of morphology should be interpreted with caution, leading to additional confirmatory studies. Additionally, if an abnormal B-cell population is detected by flow cytometry, the phenotype is non-specific and the differential diagnosis includes FL, blastoid MCL, BL and maturing B-ALL. Additionally, DLBCL and FL commonly have negative surface Ig expression and may be difficult to differentiate from hematogones. Permeabilizing the cells to access intracellular antigen will frequently show cytoplasmic light chain restriction in a neoplastic population; hematogones will remain light chain negative. If B-ALL is a consideration, dim to negative CD45 expression and TdT positivity favor B-ALL.

Cytogenetics/FISH

Karyotyping: Karyotyping of the bone marrow is not generally useful in DLBCL. FISH is the preferred approach if there is a need to assess the marrow for chromosomal abnormalities.

FISH: It is recommended that FISH be performed on the primary diagnostic material and not the marrow; FISH may be required on the bone marrow if this is the primary site of disease, or to confirm the presence of marrow involvement using a probe to detect the abnormalities identified on the primary tissue. If BL is a morphological and immunophenotypic consideration, FISH for *MYC* 8q24 can be performed to exclude the diagnosis. FISH can also be performed on the marrow for *BCL6* and t(14;18)(q32;q21); *IGH-BCL2*; however, as stated above, it is preferable to perform these on extramedullary tissue if possible [9,25]. *BCL6* is common in DLBCLs and can be fused to several partner genes, with immunoglobulin and non-immunoglobulin partner genes reported. The t(14;18)(q32;q21); *IGH-BCL2* (approximately 20% of DLBCLs) [9] is associated with neoplasms which originate from germinal center B-cells. A positive IHC result for BCL-6 and BCL-2 protein over-expression loosely correlates with the presence of the corresponding translocation by FISH; however, cases with positive IHC staining for these oncoproteins can be present in the absence of the FISH translocation and vice versa [26].

Molecular diagnostics: *IG* PCR can be used to detect clonal *IG* gene rearrangement for bone marrow staging of DLBCL and to differentiate a neoplastic diagnosis from reactive conditions. The presence of a clonal *IG* gene rearrangement in the marrow has been reported to be associated with a poorer survival, even when there is no histological evidence of bone marrow disease. Rare DLBCL cases show co-expression of B- and T-cell antigens and the additional clonality data from PCR can support lineage assignment. For patients with chromosomal translocation involving *BCL6*, over-expression of *BCL6* mRNA can be detected using quantitative RT-PCR techniques. The *BCL2-IGH* rearrangement may be detected by PCR, as described above for follicular lymphoma.

> *Caveat*: Historically, *IG* PCR has been used to aid the discrimination between CHL and B-cell NHL as they were negative in the former and usually positive in the latter; however, newer primer sets now frequently detect clonal peaks in CHL.

Residual bone marrow disease and therapeutic monitoring

Bone marrow monitoring is similar to management for lymphoma in general with the emphasis on morphology. Flow cytometry can be used for light chain analysis. Molecular testing (for *IG* clonality or specific chromosomal aberrations) can be performed to exclude ongoing presence of a clonal B-cell population in the marrow but is not widely utilized for minimal residual disease.

Pre-transplant bone marrow assessment

In vivo and *in vitro* purging of lymphoma cells may offer improved outcomes in transplant patients.

Burkitt lymphoma

Burkitt lymphoma (BL) is a very aggressive neoplasm derived from germinal center B-cells. Morphologically it has a "starry sky" appearance and is composed of monomorphic intermediate-sized cells with deeply

basophilic vacuolated cytoplasm. It is associated with a 8q24 *MYC* rearrangement with the immunoglobulin *IGH*, *IGK* or *IGL* genes, t(8;14), t(2;8) or t(8;22), respectively. Approximately 10% of otherwise classic cases may be negative for *MYC* by FISH studies [14]. The typical immunophenotype is expression of CD19, CD10, CD20 and BCL-6 antigens, and negativity for BCL-2 and TdT. Characteristically more than 90% of BL cells are Ki67-positive. There are three BL variants:

- *Endemic BL* seen in pediatric cases in Africa and New Guinea. This is predominantly extranodal disease and usually does not involve the peripheral blood. It is sometimes present in the bone marrow.
- *Sporadic BL* with a worldwide incidence and a predilection for a younger population. It is most common in extranodal sites and can involve the bone marrow in cases with high tumor burden.
- *Immunodeficiency-associated BL* seen with HIV infection.

All three clinical variants carry a high risk for involvement of the central nervous system [14]. Rarely BL can be predominantly bone marrow-based without evidence of primary tissue-based disease. In neoplasms with high-grade morphological features or with a positive *MYC* anomaly, a challenging differential diagnosis may arise between BL and DLBCL; additional data are necessary to help accurately categorize the process. As stated previously, *MYC* rearrangements are present in approximately 5–10% of DLBCLs and these cases may be better classified as B-cell lymphoma unclassifiable, with features intermediate between diffuse large B-cell lymphoma and Burkitt lymphoma [14].

Primary diagnosis or initial staging bone marrow

Morphology: A bone marrow aspirate smear and trephine imprints are very useful to assess the morphological features of BL. The cells are of intermediate size with deeply basophilic cytoplasm containing lipid vacuoles (positive on Oil Red O cytochemical staining). The clot section/particle preparation and trephine biopsy show large collections or sheets of medium-sized cells (equal to a macrophage nucleus) with a syncytial or squared-off cytoplasmic appearance. The mitotic rate is high and often there are admixed tingible

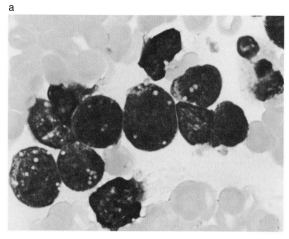
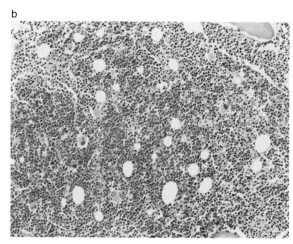

Figure 11.5. Burkitt lymphoma in the bone marrow.
a. Bone marrow aspirate smear shows intermediate-sized cells with deeply basophilic vacuolated cytoplasm.
b. Core biopsy with sheets of intermediate sized cells. The starry sky pattern is often not a feature in the marrow.

body macrophages creating a starry sky appearance; however, the classic starry sky pattern is not as striking in bone marrow as in tissue (Figure 11.5).

Ancillary tests in Burkitt lymphoma

Typical immunophenotype:
Positive: CD19, CD10, CD20, CD38, CD43, BCL-6, surface Ig, Ki67 (>90%).
Negative: BCL-2, TdT.
Immunohistochemistry panel: CD3, CD10, CD20, BCL-6, BCL-2, TdT, Ki-67.

Immunohistochemistry: Despite some morphological similarities with lymphoblasts, the phenotype is different. BL shows bright expression of CD20, CD45 and restricted light chain expression; PAX-5, CD79a, CD19, CD10, BCL-6, CD38 and CD43 are also positive and Ki-67 is > 90% positive. BCL-2 and TdT should be negative. B-ALL, by definition is TdT-positive, has dim CD45 and typically does not express CD20 or surface light chains.

Flow cytometry: FCI can efficiently phenotype BL. The neoplastic cells are bright for CD45, CD20 and CD10 and show light chain restriction; TdT is negative. This phenotype is the same as for FL and DLBCL but there are cytological differences.

Cytogenetics/FISH: In the appropriate morphological and clinical setting, a *MYC-IG* translocation by karyotype or FISH is diagnostic of BL. FISH is more useful

than karyotyping due to the rapidity and high sensitivity of the assay. A breakapart probe will detect the *MYC* 8q24 translocation but will not identify whether the partner gene is *IGH*, *IGK*, *IGL* or a non-immunoglobulin gene. Non-*IG* translocation partners are not typically seen in BL and their presence favors the classification of B-cell lymphoma unspecified category [27] (see Table 11.7). *MYC* amplifications and complex anomalies are also more indicative of a diagnosis other than BL.

Caveat: MYC-IG translocations are not restricted to BL and are seen in DLBCL, B-cell prolymphocytic leukemia (B-PLL) and some transformations of small B-cell neoplasms. Ten percent of otherwise classic cases of BL can be negative for *MYC-IG* by FISH.

Molecular diagnostics: Molecular studies for a *MYC-IG* fusion are cumbersome due to the high variability of breakpoints spanning large regions of DNA. Therefore FISH is more reliable, sensitive and specific for detecting *MYC* abnormalities. *IG* PCR for B-cell clonality is rarely required as morphology establishes malignancy.

Residual bone marrow disease and therapeutic monitoring

Bone marrow aspirate and trephine morphology, flow cytometry, FISH and molecular genetics can all be used to monitor disease following therapy. Molecular studies using combined PCR methods have been studied for minimal residual disease testing in pediatric patients [28]. CSF morphology is routinely monitored in BL. The cells are morphologically distinctive (see Figure 11.9c). Confirmatory flow, FISH or *IG* PCR studies can also be performed on the CSF but are rarely required. In addition, the small CSF volume and typical low cellularity commonly leads to insufficient cells for reliable results.

Pre-transplant bone marrow assessment

Flow cytometry for light chain-restricted CD10-positive B-cells, and *IG* PCR can be performed on follow-up pre-transplant blood and/or bone marrow samples to detect persistent disease prior to collection of cells for autologous transplantation.

Hodgkin lymphoma

Hodgkin lymphoma is divided into two main categories:

1. Classical Hodgkin lymphoma (CHL).
2. Nodular lymphocyte predominant Hodgkin lymphoma (NLPHL).

Classical Hodgkin lymphoma

Classical Hodgkin lymphoma is a neoplasm of B-cell derivation in which there are very few large neoplastic cells in a reactive inflammatory background. The neoplastic cells are CD30- and PAX-5-positive with variable rates of CD20 and CD15 expression. No specific genetic alteration has been associated with CHL. The bone marrow is involved in <10% of cases and as the pattern of infiltration is patchy it is recommended that bilateral core biopsies be performed [2]. The frequency with which the marrow is involved varies by subtype:

1. *Histological subtype* (Table 11.1): Patients with immunodeficiency-associated mixed cellularity (MC) and lymphocyte-depleted (LD) subtypes have the highest likelihood of having marrow involvement. However, as nodular sclerosis (NS) CHL is more common, in absolute numbers more marrows are involved with NS CHL.
2. *Sites of disease*: CHL with isolated cervical lymphadenopathy tends to occur in younger patients and these have much lower rates of marrow involvement than those with predominantly hidden primary sites, e.g. retroperitoneum and mediastinum.

3. The presence of B symptoms may also help predict the stage and marrow involvement.

Caveat: A primary diagnosis of classical Hodgkin lymphoma in the bone marrow should be made with caution. This is due to the paucity of lesional cells in the marrow and the similarity of architectural pattern that can be seen with other lymphoma types. A provisional diagnosis of CHL in the marrow must be correlated with diagnosis at another tissue site, if possible, due to the therapeutic differences for classical Hodgkin versus non-Hodgkin lymphomas.

Primary diagnosis or initial staging bone marrow

Morphology: At diagnosis the majority of patients with CHL do not have marrow involvement. The bone marrow is reactive with granulocytic hyperplasia, eosinophilia and a plasmacytosis; Reed Sternberg/Hodgkin cells are not present. When the marrow is involved there are distinctive focal lymphohistiocytic collections and commonly with significant reticulin fibrosis in the involved areas. The neoplastic areas in the marrow contain significant numbers of plasma cells, lymphocytes, eosinophils and histiocytes and few large atypical neoplastic cells. The neoplastic cells have large nuclei with prominent eosinophilic nucleoli; these are usually infrequent and can be difficult to identify in the marrow. These lymphohistiocytic aggregates are an important clue to the diagnosis; however they are not diagnostic as other types of lymphoma such as TCRBCL and PTCL can manifest the same pattern. Therefore immunohistochemistry is an integral part of the diagnosis (see below). CHL does not present as isolated interstitial large atypical cells within normal background hematopoiesis, as is seen in ALCL, or as isolated large immunoblasts associated with reactive appearing lymphoid aggregates. The lymphohistiocytic lesions are usually not readily aspirated, and only rarely are diagnostic Reed–Sternberg/Hodgkin cells present in the aspirate smear (see Figure 11.6).

Ancillary tests in classical Hodgkin lymphoma

Typical immunophenotype:
Positive: CD30, PAX-5, MUM1
Variable: CD15, CD20
Negative: CD45, CD79a, CD43, OCT-2, BOB.1

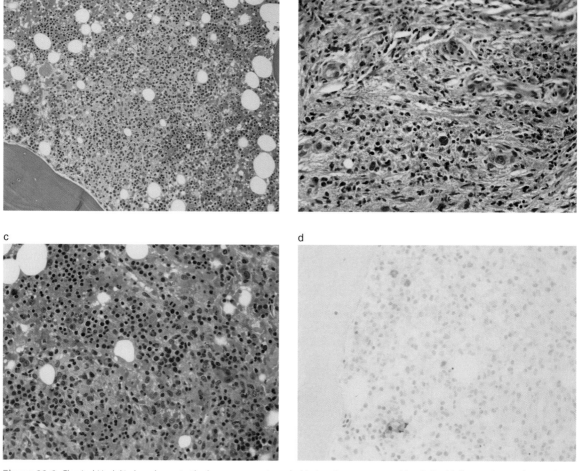

Figure 11.6. Classical Hodgkin lymphoma in the bone marrow. Lymphohistiocytic aggregates with admixed inflammation are key to the diagnosis.

a. Focal infiltrate, hematoxylin and eosin (H&E) 100×.

b. Associated with extensive fibrosis, H&E 100×.

c. Neoplastic cells can be difficult to see or can show typical Reed–Sternberg cell morphology, H&E 400×.

d. IHC for CD30 200× showing a golgi pattern. Note that only few neoplastic cells are present and that associated plasma cells are positive.

e. IHC for PAX-5. The neoplastic cells are classically slightly weaker than normal background B-cells 200×.

f. EBV-ISH 200× which may be useful in some cases. CD15 may or may not be positive, also in a golgi pattern.

g. Aspirate smear showing atypical large Hodgkin or Reed–Sternberg cells, Wright–Giemsa 1000×.

h. Aspirate smear showing atypical large Hodgkin or Reed–Sternberg cells, Wright–Giemsa 1000×.

Immunohistochemical panel (if morphology is suspicious of involvement): CD3, CD15, CD20, CD30, PAX5 and CD45. EBER, MUM-1 and additional stains as needed.

Immunohistochemistry: Immunohistochemistry is only required when the bone marrow trephine morphology is suggestive of involvement by CHL, as described above. If there are no suspicious lymphohistiocytic aggregates, IHC is not required as the Hodgkin cells do not occur in a normal hematopoietic background without disturbing the marrow architecture. The large neoplastic cells are usually strongly CD30- and MUM-1-positive. CD15 is usually positive and CD20 is positive in approximately 40% of cases and usually shows variable staining intensity within the neoplasm [14]. Both CD30 and CD15 show membranous and Golgi staining patterns. PAX-5 typically has slightly dimmer staining than

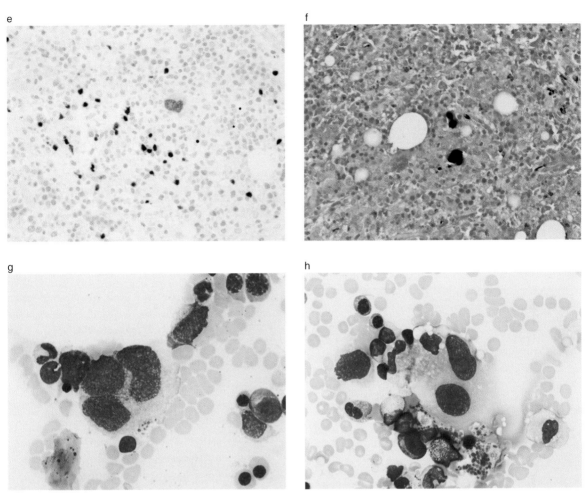

Figure 11.6. (cont.)

the normal background B-cells. CD45 and EMA are characteristically negative. T-cell antigens are usually negative but rarely can be weakly positive. When being assessed as part of a staging procedure, this phenotypic profile confirms the lymphohistiocytic aggregates are due to marrow infiltration by CHL. When the bone marrow is the primary site of disease the main differential diagnoses include TCRBCL, PTCL and reactive histiocytic aggregates. The large cell phenotype of CD20 strong, CD30 patchy or negative and CD45 positive favors TCRBCL. Variable large cell staining for CD3, CD20, CD30 and CD45 with polytypic kappa and lambda favors the heterogenous immunoblasts seen in a reactive process. *In situ* hybridization for EBER may be useful; EBV positivity varies in frequency according to subtype, with the

immuno-deficiency-associated types much more frequently positive.

Caveats: Plasma cells can be CD30-positive and granulocytes are CD15-positive.

Flow cytometry: Flow cytometry has no role in the analysis of the bone marrow in CHL.

Cytogenetics/FISH: Cytogenetics/FISH studies do not add value in CHL.

Molecular diagnostics: *IG* PCR is not typically needed and is rarely performed on the bone marrow sample for two reasons. Firstly, the bone marrow aspirate sample frequently does not contain the neoplastic cells, and, secondly although CHL is a B-cell neoplasm, *IG* PCR will only detect a clonal population when sensitive primer sets are used [29].

Nodular lymphocyte predominant Hodgkin lymphoma

Nodular lymphocyte predominant Hodgkin lymphoma (NLPHL), a neoplasm of B-cell derivation characterized by "popcorn cells," has frequent relapses, responds well to therapy and has an excellent prognosis. The scattered large malignant ("popcorn") cells have convoluted nuclei and a phenotype similar to the neoplastic cells of TCRBCL, i.e. CD20, BCL-6- and CD45-positive. There are no specific cytogenetic or molecular anomalies. NLPHL rarely involves the bone marrow (<1% of cases reported) and therefore a primary diagnosis should not be made on a marrow biopsy. If a patient with a tissue diagnosis of NLPHL has lymphomatous involvement of the marrow, the primary diagnosis should be reviewed and TCRBCL considered. Nonetheless, NLPHL that involves the marrow may have a more aggressive course.

Primary diagnosis or initial staging bone marrow

Morphology: When NLPHL involves the marrow the bone marrow trephine biopsy will have nodular aggregates of small lymphocytes with occasional large atypical cells. These are the malignant lymphocyte predominant (LP, "popcorn" or L&H) cells which are characterized by folded nuclei with multiple basophilic nucleoli. The bone marrow aspirate is rarely involved.

Ancillary tests in nodular lymphocyte predominant Hodgkin lymphoma

Typical immunophenotype:
   Positive: CD20, CD45, BCL-6, PAX-5, OCT-2, BOB.1, Ig light chain, IgD (subset of cases).
   Negative: CD15, CD30.
Immunohistochemistry panel: CD20, CD30, BCL6, CD45, OCT-2, BOB.1, IgD, PD-1 (CD279), additional B-cell markers as needed.

Immunohistochemistry: The phenotype of the neoplastic cells in NLPHL is similar to the B-cells in TCRBCL. They express pan-B-cell antigens (CD19-, CD22-, CD79a-positive), CD45, BCL-6, OCT-2 and BOB.1. CD15 and CD30 are negative. PD-1-positive T-cells may ring the neoplastic cells.

Flow cytometry: Flow cytometry does not add value in the detection of NLPHL involving the bone marrow.

Cytogenetics/FISH: These are not required in the diagnosis or assessment of NLPHL involving the bone marrow.

Molecular diagnostics: LP cells, being neoplastic B-cells, have clonally rearranged *IG* genes. However, because of the small number of neoplastic cells in involved tissue, *IG* PCR will generally be negative unless sensitive primers are used. Hence molecular studies do not add value in the diagnosis or detection of NLPHL involving the bone marrow as in NLPHL.

Residual bone marrow disease and therapeutic monitoring of CHL and NLPHL

Repeat bone marrow examination for morphological analysis should be performed as follows:

1. On completion of therapy to confirm eradication of previously detected bone marrow disease.
2. Restaging of relapse in an extramedullary site.
3. Investigation of unexplained cytopenias, e.g. due to bone marrow infiltration, secondary or therapy-related myelodysplasia or marrow aplasia.

If positive, an abbreviated IHC panel is used as complete characterization will have been performed previously.

Pre-transplant bone marrow assessment of CHL and NLPHL

Refractory or relapsed CHL is frequently considered for transplantation after salvage therapy. Pre-transplant assessment is predominantly based on clinical and imaging findings such as PET scans, B-symptoms and LDH levels. Evaluation of bone marrow prior to transplant should be similar to the initial staging bone marrow. There is no role for flow cytometric immunophenotyping, PCR, or FISH on the marrow prior to transplantation. If a treatment-related myeloid disorder is suspected, karyotyping may be helpful. Transplantation is not standard treatment for NLPHL.

Anaplastic large cell lymphoma

Anaplastic large cell lymphoma (ALCL) is a T-cell malignancy composed of large cells that have pleomorphic horseshoe-shaped nuclei and abundant cytoplasm. Three types of ALCL are described based on disease location and association with anaplastic lymphoma kinase (*ALK*) rearrangement:

1. Systemic neoplasms associated with a translocation involving the *ALK* gene (ALCL, *ALK*-positive).
2. Systemic neoplasms with no anomaly in the *ALK* gene (ALCL, *ALK*-negative).
3. Primary cutaneous ALCL which is *ALK*-negative.

These disorders share morphological features and all have strong expression of CD30 antigen. They have morphological similarities with peripheral T-cell lymphoma with which they must be distinguished due to prognostic differences [30]. Bone marrow analysis is required for staging the systemic types of ALCL. For primary cutaneous ALCL a bone marrow is not essential; it can be used to confirm limitation to the skin but this is not universally accepted as being necessary [31].

Primary diagnosis or initial staging bone marrow

Morphology: The bone marrow features of anaplastic large cell lymphoma are variable. They most commonly have sheets of atypical medium to large cells with horseshoe-shaped nuclei and perinuclear clearing ("hallmark" cells) and frequently there are admixed phagocytic macrophages (Figure 11.7). Less commonly cases have more occult scattered large cells; these can be difficult to detect on morphology alone and require IHC to highlight the neoplastic cells [32]. The rare lymphohistiocytic variant of ALCL can have pink histiocytic aggregates with admixed plasma cells and eosinophils; the differential diagnosis with this appearance is classical Hodgkin lymphoma.

Ancillary tests in anaplastic large cell lymphoma

Typical immunophenotype:
Positive: CD30 (strong), CD25, EMA.
Variable: ALK, CD3, CD2, CD4, CD5, CD45RO, CD45, TIA-1, granzyme B.
Negative: EBER.

Immunohistochemistry panel: CD3, CD20, CD30, granzyme B. CD43, PAX-5, ALK as needed.
Caveats: CD4, TIA-1, CD43, CD13 and CD33 can be difficult to interpret in the bone marrow due to monocyte/myeloid staining. Non-hematopoietic neoplasms can be CD30-positive.

Immunohistochemistry: The neoplastic cells in ALCL are always CD30-positive with the strongest staining seen in the large cells (including in the small cell variants). Although ALCL is a T-cell lymphoma, CD3 is commonly negative (75% of cases) and should not be used as a screening antibody. Other T-cell antibodies, such as CD2, CD4, CD5 and CD45RO, are variably positive. CD43 can be helpful but can be difficult to interpret in the bone marrow due to expression of the antigen by granulocytes. The cytotoxic associated antigens TIA-1, granzyme B and perforin are commonly positive. It is important to note that CD13 and CD33 can be expressed in ALK-positive ALCL [33].

Immunohistochemistry of the bone marrow should be used as follows:

1. *Staging marrow*: It is recommended that IHC for CD30 be performed routinely for bone marrow staging; this improves the sensitivity of disease detection [32]. ALK will also be helpful in a subset of cases. It is important to note that the ALK staining pattern (i.e. nuclear, cytoplasmic, membranous) varies with different ALK translocation partners (Table 11.8).
2. *Diagnostic marrow*: If the BM is the primary site of disease, more extensive immunophenotyping is required to confirm the diagnosis of ALCL. CD30, ALK and a panel of T-cell-associated antibodies should be used. T-cell associated markers and CD45 can be negative in a number of cases. Demonstration of T-cell differentiation may be possible by detection of (in descending order of frequency) CD2, CD7, CD3, CD4, CD5, or CD8 and CD45RO or CD43 may also help assign lineage. The differential diagnosis of ALCL in the marrow includes:
   i. Anaplastic large B-cell lymphoma, a B-cell malignancy with anaplastic cytology and ALK-negative.
   ii. ALK-positive B-cell lymphoma, a neoplasm of B-cell lineage with an unusual phenotype (CD138-positive; CD20- and CD30-negative) with granular cytoplasmic ALK positivity.

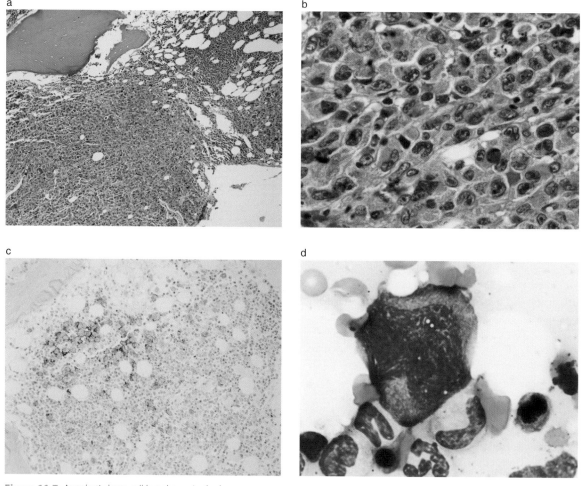

Figure 11.7. Anaplastic large cell lymphoma in the bone marrow.
a. Bone marrow core biopsy showing sheets of large anaplastic cells, hematoxylin and eosin (H&E).
b. Cytology of the classic hallmark cell in ALCL.
c. IHC for CD30 highlights the ALCL cells and increases the sensitivity for detection of marrow disease, 100×.
d. Aspirate smear showing an ALCL cell, Wright–Giemsa 1000×.

Flow cytometry: FCI does not significantly add to the diagnostic or staging assessment of ALCL cases. This is because the neoplastic cells are large and can be difficult to detect by flow cytometry. A small series showed 83% of cases were detectable by flow but there were few captured neoplastic cells; a complex sequential gating strategy had to be used to identify and characterize the cells [34]. Both CD13 and CD33 can be seen on ALCL cells by flow cytometry, most commonly in ALK-positive cases [33].

Cytogenetics/FISH: ALCL is associated with chromosomal translocations involving ALK and these can be detected by conventional karyotyping or FISH. A FISH breakapart ALK probe should be used so that the ALK translocation can be identified irrespective of the translocation partner (Table 11.8). Karyotyping and FISH are not generally required for bone marrow staging.

Molecular diagnostics: Molecular genetic methods can be performed on the bone marrow to detect t(2;5);*NPM-ALK* either for staging or monitoring purposes. Genomic breakpoints lie within *NPM* intron 4 and *ALK* intron 16, allowing detection of the rearrangement by RT-PCR or by long-range PCR of

Table 11.8. *ALK* gene translocation partners and ALK antibody IHC staining patterns in ALCL (adapted from [14]).

Anomaly	Partner gene	ALK staining pattern	Percent of cases
t(2;5)(p23;q35)	*NPM*	Nuclear, cytoplasmic	84%
t(1;2)(q25;p23)	*TPM3*	Cytoplasmic/peripheral	13%
Inv(2)(p23q35)	*ATIC*	Cytoplasmic	1%
t(2;3)(p23;q21)	*TFG*	Cytoplasmic	1%
t(2;17)(p23;q23)	*CLTC*	Cytoplasmic (granular)	<1%
t(X;2)(q11–12;p23)	*MSN*	Membrane	<1%
t(2;19)(p23;p13.1)	*TPM4*	Cytoplasmic	<1%
t(2;22)(p23;q11.2)	*MYH9*	Cytoplasmic	<1%
t(2;17)(p23;q25)	*ALO17*	Cytoplasmic	<1%

genomic DNA. Both nested RT-PCR and real-time RT-PCR assays are able to detect the fusion transcript at a sensitivity of one cell in 10^6. PCR is much less commonly used than immunohistochemistry and FISH for marrow assessment. *TCR*-PCR can be useful for diagnostic dilemmas to discriminate between ALCL and B-cell lymphoma or CHL.

Residual bone marrow disease and therapeutic monitoring

Restaging bone marrow examinations may be performed in cases with documented bone marrow disease at diagnosis or at relapse. The marrow assessment is similar to that in the original diagnostic sample or staging marrow. Although real time RT-PCR of *NPM-ALK* expression has been evaluated for minimal residual disease monitoring in pediatric ALCL cases, this is not currently used routinely [35].

Pre-transplant bone marrow assessment

If restaging is required, pre-transplant evaluation is similar to that performed in an initial staging assessment; an abbreviated IHC panel can be used. If a bone marrow is performed all cases should be assessed by IHC for CD30-positive cells as involvement of the BM can be occult. Pre-transplant flow cytometry, PCR and FISH studies do not add useful information and are not required. If a treatment-related myeloid disorder is suspected, a full karyotype may be helpful.

Angioimmunoblastic T-cell lymphoma

Angioimmunoblastic T-cell lymphoma (AITL) is an aggressive neoplasm characterized by systemic symptoms. The neoplastic cell is derived from mature follicular helper T-cells of the lymphoid follicle and expresses a T-helper cell phenotype (CD3-, CD4-, CD2-, CD5-positive) together with follicular T-cell antigens (CD10, CXCL13 and PD-1 [CD279]). Associated EBV-positive B-immunoblasts may be present and are polytypic but can expand to a monoclonal population in some cases. No specific cytogenetic anomalies are associated with AITL. Bone marrow involvement by AITL is variable (Table 11.1). The diagnosis can be subtle with the lymphomatous involvement often "masked" by reactive inflammatory cells that are secondary to systemic dysregulation [36,37]. These confounding morphological features may lead to erroneous diagnoses of chronic myeloproliferative neoplasms, myeloma and hypereosinophilic disorders. Bone marrows may contain > 30% plasma cells and suggest a diagnosis of myeloma; however, the plasma cells in AITL are polytypic [36].

Primary diagnosis or initial staging bone marrow

Morphology: The neoplastic AITL cells are commonly present in the bone marrow aspirate but are difficult to identify on morphology alone. They typically are small with eccentric, indented or cleaved nuclei and

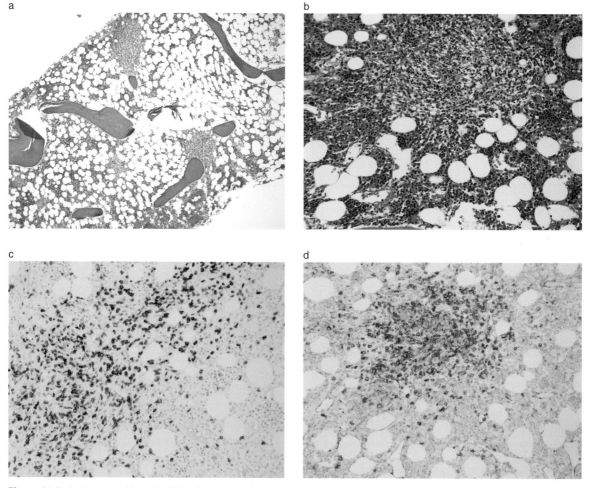

Figure 11.8. Angioimmunoblastic T-cell lymphoma in the bone marrow.
a. AITL showing a mixed infiltrative pattern with stellate nodular and paratrabecular aggregates, hematoxylin and eosin (H&E), 40×.
b. Bone marrow biopsy H&E, 200×.
c. Atypical cell contours are accentuated by IHC for CD3 200×.
d. AITL cells are CD4-positive 200×.

gray cytoplasm sometimes with fine vacuoles. Flow cytometry is required to confirm their presence. The lymphomatous cells are best seen on H&E bone marrow trephine sections. The infiltrates classically have a paratrabecular location and a stellate nodular appearance (Figure 11.8). The neoplastic T-cells are usually small-to medium-sized with minimal cytological atypia and clear cytoplasm. There is an admixed polymorphous reactive infiltrate of CD8-positive T-cells, histiocytes, immunoblasts, plasma cells and eosinophils. If the histiocytes are numerous, they can impart a granulomatous appearance. The typical expanded follicular dendritic cell meshwork associated with AITL in lymph nodes is not seen in the bone marrow.

Ancillary tests in angioimmunoblastic T-cell lymphoma

Typical immunophenotype:
Positive: CD2, CD3, CD4, CD5, CD10, CXCL13, PD-1 (CD279). Admixed CD20-positive large B-cells may be EBV-positive.
Immunohistochemistry panel: CD2, CD3, CD4, CD5, CD8, CD20, PD-1 (CD279), βF1. CXCL-13, CD10, EBER, as needed.

e

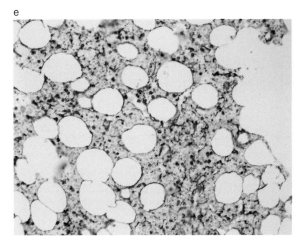

f

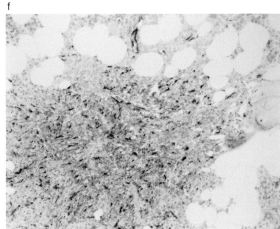

g

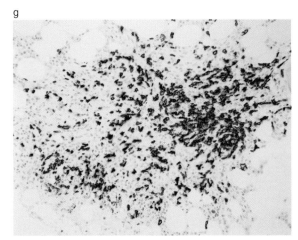

Figure 11.8. (cont.) Angioimmunoblastic T-cell lymphoma in the bone marrow showing immunohistochemical reactivity patterns.

e. IHC for CD10 200×, and (f) CXCL-13 200× is less useful due to high background and decreased expression in bone marrow.

g. CD20, 200× showing intermixed small B-cells which may lead to a false diagnosis of reactive mixed lymphoid infiltrates.

Immunohistochemistry: Immunohistochemistry for CD3 and CD20 is critical to locate and assign a lineage to the atypical cells. CD3 is helpful to highlight the atypical cytological contours of the T-cells and PD-1 to establish that the T-cells are abnormal [37]. CD10, CXCL13 and EBER, although useful diagnostically in tissue biopsies, are less useful as markers of AITL in the bone marrow; however, if the T-cells do express CD10 this suggests the diagnosis of AITL [36,37]. Confirmation of the diagnosis generally requires a tissue biopsy. In contrast to other T-cell lymphomas, AITL frequently do not show aberrant loss of T-cell antigens; an exception is βF1.

Caveat: CD10 is positive in the marrow meshwork and is expressed by granulocytes, making the interpretation of staining of lymphoid cells difficult.

Flow cytometry: FCI can be used to identify AITL in blood and bone marrow aspirates by the aberrant expression of CD10 by T-cells (CD2, CD3 positive).

Cytogenetics/FISH: AITL does not have an associated specific translocation therefore cytogenetics and FISH do not add value. Trisomy 3, 5 and an extra copy of X are recurrent anomalies.

Molecular diagnostics: *TCR*-PCR can be used to confirm the presence of clonal T-cells in the blood and/or bone marrow. The clonal bands or peaks (depending on the method used) can be compared to peaks of clonal populations detected at other sites of involvement. Identical fragment sizes in tissue from separate locations lend further evidence for a neoplastic clone.

Disease or therapeutic monitoring

Bone marrow is usually monitored by morphology, IHC for the antigens known to be expressed by the AITL cells and TCR clonality. Flow cytometry can be used on the blood and bone marrow aspirate to monitor continued presence of the abnormal CD10-positive T-cells.

Pre-transplant assessment

If marrow reassessment is required prior to transplantation the evaluation is similar to that performed in the initial staging. However, an abbreviated IHC panel can be used targeting the known antigen expression

profile. If a treatment-related myeloid disorder is suspected, a karyotype may be helpful.

General principles of cerebrospinal fluid examination

It is rare for a primary diagnosis of lymphoma to be made on a cerebrospinal fluid (CSF) sample. The CSF is most commonly examined as a staging or monitoring procedure for lymphomas that are known to have a high predilection for central nervous system (CNS) involvement. Most CSF samples are obtained during administration of prophylactic intra-thecal therapy and not necessarily in the setting of known

a

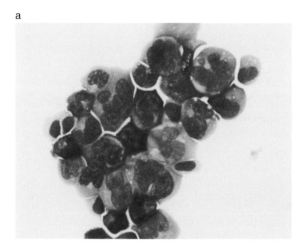

b

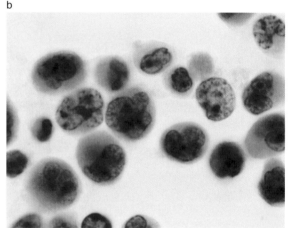

c

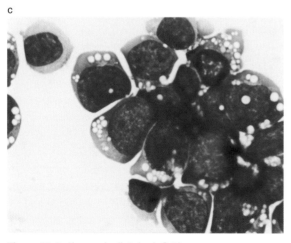

d

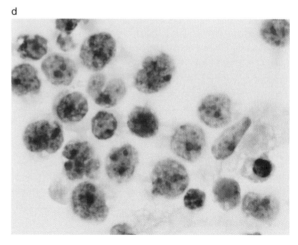

Figure 11.9. Abnormal cells in body fluids.

a, b. T-cell lymphoma in the CSF showing atypical nuclear contours and coarse chromatin, cytospin. (a) Wright–Giemsa, 800× (b) and (b) Papanicolaou stain, 1000×.

c, d. Burkitt lymphoma showing cytoplasmic vacuoles in metachromatic stains, cytospin. (c) Wright–Giemsa, 1000× (d) and coarse chromatin on Papanicolaou stain 1000×.

involvement. These fluids should be triaged quickly as the cells degrade within a day after collection.

Morphology: The cellularity of normal CSF is very low. Hypercellularity can be a clue to involvement by lymphoma but this can also be due to a reactive lymphocytosis; these must be differentiated and some helpful features are:

1. Reactive CSF lymphocytosis usually has cells of varying size with a variable amount of cytoplasm and may be accompanied by neutrophils.
2. Malignant lymphoid infiltrates are usually monomorphous with few neutrophils. These populations may be sufficiently atypical for a definitive morphological diagnosis if the process has been characterized elsewhere. Others may require additional ancillary testing for confirmation (Figure 11.9).

Lymphomas that commonly involve the CSF are:

1. *Burkitt lymphoma* which has the distinctive deeply basophilic and vacuolated cytoplasm (Figure 11.9c,d).
2. *Some T-cell lymphomas*, which usually have medium- to large-sized cells with markedly atypical nuclear contours.

Caveats: If many red blood cells are present, peripheral blood contamination may be the source of the neoplastic cells and not the CSF. Also, rarely vertebral bone marrow can be inadvertently sampled during the procedure, especially in children, with hematopoietic precursors confounding the CSF picture. Correlation with the clinical history and peripheral blood smear findings is important in these cases. Also, cytocentrifuge preparations can cause nuclear features to look slightly more immature (fine chromatin pattern) and should not be over-interpreted.

Ancillary tests in cerebrospinal fluid analysis

Immunohistochemistry: A paraffin-embedded cell block can be prepared from the CSF and used for IHC analysis. Cell blocks can be very useful in cases where morphological identification of the cells together with the antigen expression profile is imperative. There can however be higher background staining than tissue.

Flow cytometry: Flow cytometry is extremely useful if there are sufficient cells in the sample and these are viable. Flow cytometry can be used to rapidly obtain the phenotype of the neoplastic population and to determine whether a B-cell population has restricted

Table 11.9. Relative utility of ancillary techniques in the diagnosis of lymphoma involving the bone marrow.

Diagnosis	Most useful	Potentially useful	Rarely useful
FL	BM biopsy	IHC, FISH, IGH, FCI	
MCL	BM aspirate, FCI, BM biopsy, IHC		
SMZL	FCI, BM biopsy, IHC	IGH	
EMZL	FCI, BM biopsy, IHC	IGH	
NMZL	FCI, BM biopsy, IHC	IGH	
DLBCL	BM biopsy, IHC	BM aspirate, FCI, FISH	IGH
BL	BM aspirate, FCI, BM biopsy, IHC, FISH	Karyotype	IGH
CHL	BM biopsy, IHC		BM aspirate, FC, FISH, IGH
NLPHL	BM biopsy, IHC		BM aspirate, FCI, FISH, IGH
AITL	BM biopsy, IHC	BM aspirate, FCI, TCR	
ALCL	BM aspirate, BM biopsy, IHC	FCI, TCR	FISH

BM aspirate: aspirate morphology; FCI: flow cytometry; BM biopsy: bone marrow core biopsy morphology/architecture; IHC: immunocytochemistry; FISH: fluorescence *in situ* hybridization; *IGH*: PCR for immunoglobulin; TCR: PCR for T-cell receptor.

light chain expression (clonal). Normocellular fluids usually do not contain sufficient cells for a reliable analysis. Also, if the sample is degraded and cell viability is low the study is not valid as neoplastic cells may be present and not be detected.

Cytogenetics/FISH: As CSF is fresh fluid, karyotyping and FISH can be performed but is rarely indicated.

Molecular diagnostics: PCR and Southern blot are available if required for diagnosis but are not routinely used.

Conclusion

The diagnosis and staging of lymphoma in the bone marrow can be challenging. The use of morphology together with a number of ancillary techniques in an educated fashion increases the efficiency and accuracy. Unnecessary testing should be avoided due to the cost and the potential for misinterpretation and erroneous conclusions. Table 11.9 summarizes the various lymphoma entities described in this chapter and the ancillary techniques that give the highest yield of information for each diagnosis.

References

1. Zhang QY, Foucar K. Bone marrow involvement by Hodgkin and non-Hodgkin lymphomas. *Hematol Oncol Clin N Am* 2009;**23**(4):873–902.

2. Wang J, Weiss LM, Chang KL *et al.* Diagnostic utility of bilateral bone marrow examination: significance of morphologic and ancillary technique study in malignancy. *Cancer* 2002;**94**(5):1522–31.

3. Evans PA, Pott Ch, Groenen PJ *et al.* PCR-based clonality testing in B-cell malignancies by use of multiple immunoglobulin gene targets. Report of the BIOMED-2 Concerted Action BHM4-CT98–3936. *Leukemia* 2007;**21**(2):207–14.

4. Aksentijevich I, Flinn IW. Monoclonal antibody therapy with autologous peripheral blood stem cell transplantation for non-Hodgkin's lymphoma. *Cancer Control* 2002;**9**(2):99–105.

5. Arber DA, George TI. Bone marrow biopsy involvement by non-Hodgkin's lymphoma: frequency of lymphoma types, patterns, blood involvement, and discordance with other sites in 450 specimens. *Am J Surg Pathol* 2005;**29**(12):1549–57.

6. Iancu D, Hao S, Lin P *et al.* Follicular lymphoma in staging bone marrow specimens: correlation of histologic findings with the results of flow cytometry

7. Schmidt B, Kremer M, Götze K *et al.* Bone marrow involvement in follicular lymphoma: comparison of histology and flow cytometry as staging procedures. *Leuk Lymphoma* 2006;**47**(9):1857–62.

8. Gu K, Chan WC, Hawley RC. Practical detection of t(14;18)(IgH/BCL2) in follicular lymphoma. *Arch Pathol Lab Med* 2008;**132**(8):1355–61.

9. Campbell LJ. Cytogenetics of lymphomas. *Pathology* 2005;**37**(6):493–507.

10. Belaud-Rotureau MA, Parrens M, Carrere N *et al.* Interphase fluorescence in situ hybridization is more sensitive than BIOMED-2 polymerase chain reaction protocol in detecting *IGH-BCL2* rearrangement in both fixed and frozen lymph node with follicular lymphoma. *Hum Pathol* 2007;**38**(2):365–72.

11. Mandigers CM, Meijerink JP, van 't Veer MB *et al.* Dynamics of circulating t(14;18)-positive cells during first-line and subsequent lines of treatment in follicular lymphoma. *Ann Hematol* 2003;**82**(12):743–9.

12. Hirt C, Schüler F, Kiefer T, Schwenke C *et al.* Rapid and sustained clearance of circulating lymphoma cells after chemotherapy plus rituximab: clinical significance of quantitative t(14;18) PCR monitoring in advanced stage follicular lymphoma patients. *Br J Haematol* 2008;**141**(5):631–40.

13. Arcaini L, Montanari F, Alessandrino EP *et al.* Immunochemotherapy with in vivo purging and autotransplant induces long clinical and molecular remission in advanced relapsed and refractory follicular lymphoma. *Ann Oncol* 2008; **19**(7):1331–5.

14. Swerdlow SH, Campo E, Harris NL *et al.* (eds.). *WHO Classification of Tumours of Haematopoietic and Lymphoid Tissues*, 4th edn. Lyon: IARC Press; 2008.

15. Thomas PW, Avet-Loiseau H, Oscier D. A subset of t(11;14) lymphoma with mantle cell features displays mutated IgVH genes and includes patients with good prognosis, non-nodal disease. *Blood* 2003; **101**(12):4975–81.

16. de Boer CJ, Kluin-Nelemans JC, Dreef E *et al.* Involvement of the *CCND1* gene in hairy cell leukemia. *Ann Oncol* 1996;**7**(3):251–6.

17. Fu K, Weisenburger DD, Greiner TC *et al.* Lymphoma/ Leukemia Molecular Profiling Project. Cyclin D1-negative mantle cell lymphoma: a clinicopathologic study based on gene expression profiling. *Blood*. 2005;**106**(13):4315–21.

18. Brizova H, Kalinova M, Krskova L, Mrhalova M, Kodet R. Quantitative monitoring of cyclin D1 expression: a molecular marker for minimal residual

disease monitoring and a predictor of the disease outcome in patients with mantle cell lymphoma. *Int J Cancer* 2008;**123**(12):2865–70.

19. Inamdar KV, Medeiros LJ, Jorgensen JL *et al.* Bone marrow involvement by marginal zone B-cell lymphomas of different types. *Am J Clin Pathol* 2008;**129**(5):714–22.

20. Orchard J, Garand R, Davis Z *et al.* Bone marrow histology in marginal zone B-cell lymphomas: correlation with clinical parameters and flow cytometry in 120 patients. *Ann Oncol* 2009;**20**(1):129–36.

21. Dong HY, Weisberger J, Liu Z, Tugulea S. Immunophenotypic analysis of CD103+ B-lymphoproliferative disorders: hairy cell leukemia and its mimics. *Am J Clin Pathol* 2009;**131**(4):586–95.

22. Remstein ED, Dogan A, Einerson RR *et al.* The incidence and anatomic site specificity of chromosomal translocations in primary extranodal marginal zone B-cell lymphoma of mucosa-associated lymphoid tissue (MALT lymphoma) in North America. *Am J Surg Pathol* 2006;**30**(12):1546–53.

23. Baiyee D, Warnke R, Natkunam Y. Lack of utility of CD20 immunohistochemistry in staging bone marrow biopsies for diffuse large B-cell lymphoma. *Appl Immunohistochem Mol Morphol* 2009;**17**(2):93–5.

24. Duggan PR, Easton D, Luider J, Auer IA. Bone marrow staging of patients with non-Hodgkin lymphoma by flow cytometry: correlation with morphology. *Cancer* 2000;**88**(4):894–9.

25. Talaulikar D, Dahlstrom JE. Staging bone marrow in diffuse large B-cell lymphoma: the role of ancillary investigations. *Pathology* 2009;**41**(3):214–22.

26. Skinnider BF, Horsman DE, Dupuis B, Gascoyne RD. Bcl-6 and Bcl-2 protein expression in diffuse large B-cell lymphoma and follicular lymphoma: correlation with 3q27 and 18q21 chromosomal abnormalities. *Hum Pathol* 1999;**30**(7):803–8.

27. Bellan C, Stefano L, Giulia de F, Rogena EA, Lorenzo L. Burkitt lymphoma versus diffuse large B-cell lymphoma: a practical approach. *Hematol Oncol* 2009;**27**(4):182–5.

28. Busch K, Borkhardt A, Wössmann W, Reiter A, Harbott J. Combined polymerase chain reaction methods to detect c-myc/IgH rearrangement in childhood Burkitt's lymphoma for minimal residual disease analysis. *Haematologica* 2004;**89**(7):818–25.

29. Hebeda KM, Van Altena MC, Rombout P, Van Krieken JH, Groenen PJ. PCR clonality detection in Hodgkin lymphoma. *J Hematop* 2009;**2**(1):34–41.

30. Savage KJ, Harris NL, Vose JM *et al.* International Peripheral T-Cell Lymphoma Project. ALK− anaplastic large-cell lymphoma is clinically and immunophenotypically different from both ALK+ ALCL and peripheral T-cell lymphoma, not otherwise specified: report from the International Peripheral T-Cell Lymphoma Project. *Blood* 2008;**111**(12):5496–504.

31. Benner MF, Willemze R. Bone marrow examination has limited value in the staging of patients with an anaplastic large cell lymphoma first presenting in the skin. Retrospective analysis of 107 patients. *Br J Dermatol* 2008;**159**(5):1148–51.

32. Weinberg OK, Seo K, Arber DA. Prevalence of bone marrow involvement in systemic anaplastic large cell lymphoma: are immunohistochemical studies necessary? *Hum Pathol* 2008;**39**(9):1331–40.

33. Bovio IM, Allan RW. The expression of myeloid antigens CD13 and/or CD33 is a marker of ALK+ anaplastic large cell lymphomas. *Am J Clin Pathol* 2008;**130**(4):628–34.

34. Muzzafar T, Wei EX, Lin P *et al.* Flow cytometric immunophenotyping of anaplastic large cell lymphoma. *Arch Pathol Lab Med* 2009;**133**(1):49–56.

35. Kalinova M, Krskova L, Brizova H *et al.* Quantitative PCR detection of NPM/ALK fusion gene and CD30 gene expression in patients with anaplastic large cell lymphoma – residual disease monitoring and a correlation with the disease status. *Leuk Res* 2008;**32**(1):25–32.

36. Grogg KL, Morice WG, Macon WR. Spectrum of bone marrow findings in patients with angioimmunoblastic T-cell lymphoma. *Br J Haematol* 2007;**137**(5):416–22.

37. Khokhar FA, Payne WD, Talwalkar SS *et al.* Angioimmunoblastic T-cell lymphoma in bone marrow: a morphologic and immunophenotypic study. *Hum Pathol* 2010;**41**(1):79–87.

38. Bellan C, Stefano L, Giulia de F, Rogena EA, Lorenzo L. Burkitt lymphoma versus diffuse large B-cell lymphoma: a practical approach. *Hematol Oncol* 2010;**28**(2):53–6.

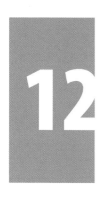

Plasma cell neoplasms

Rafael Fonseca and Riccardo Valdez

Introduction

Plasma cell neoplasms result from the clonal expansion of terminally differentiated B-cells that have the capacity to secrete a monoclonal immunoglobulin (Ig). This chapter will discuss the appropriate use of diagnostic techniques in the diagnosis and assessment of multiple myeloma, monoclonal gammopathy of undetermined significance, smoldering myeloma, plasma cell leukemia and Waldenström macroglobulinemia.

Multiple myeloma

Multiple myeloma (MM) is a plasma cell malignancy characterized by the proliferation of plasma cells (PC), mostly within the bone marrow (BM) [1]. The disease peaks in incidence in the seventh decade of life [2]. While still considered an incurable diagnosis for most patients, patients are surviving longer due to the availability of new treatments [3,4]. In a subset of patients, mostly those treated with more aggressive interventions such as combinations of novel agents and autologous stem cell transplant (SCT), the disease may be curable [5]. MM is part of a spectrum of disorders characterized by this proliferation of clonal PC which includes monoclonal gammopathy of undetermined significance (MGUS) and smoldering MM (SMM). In MGUS, patients have a minimal plasmacytosis and the monoclonal PCs cause no harm to the individual; it is usually detected incidentally. Patients with MGUS can go on for years, often decades, without ever having further expansion of the monoclonal PCs [6]. Patients with SMM have a more advanced plasmacytosis, yet have no discernible evidence of end organ damage due to this expansion. Pathologically the diagnosis of SMM is made when a patient has greater than 10% plasma cells in the BM but still has

no complications [7]. MGUS and SMM will be discussed in more detail later in this chapter.

Complications of MM arise due to tumoral effects or the effect of the protein produced by the plasma cells. The tumoral effects of the clonal PC expansion result in anemia and bone destruction [8]. The bone destruction, manifest by hypercalcemia (due to the release of matrix calcium) and loss of bone structure, is characterized by lytic bone lesions, osteoporosis or pathologic fractures. The main consequence of the protein production and its physicochemical characteristics is impairment of renal function resulting from the light chains damaging the tubules [9]. Other paraneoplastic complications such as amyloidosis or POEMS syndrome can also occur but will not be discussed further.

Diagnosis of multiple myeloma

An accurate diagnosis of the disease is critical to establish optimal management. Unlike many other hematological malignancies, decisions regarding treatment do not rest solely on the pathologic findings. In fact the pathologic analysis per se is insufficient to allow decisions regarding need for treatment [10]. The pathological analysis has to be coupled with information emanating from the clinical interview and other laboratory parameters. It is for this reason that close communication between the pathologist and the clinician is crucial. It is particularly important for the clinician not to initiate treatment alone on the BM report diagnosis being consistent with MM. At the time of diagnosis, at a minimum, a patient should have a complete blood count and chemistry (evaluating calcium and creatinine), β_2-microglobulin, serum and urine electrophoresis and immunofixation as needed, quantitative immunoglobulins and serum free light chains

Diagnostic Techniques in Hematological Malignancies, ed. Wendy N. Erber. Published by Cambridge University Press. © Cambridge University Press 2010.

Table 12.1. Laboratory evaluation of multiple myeloma at diagnosis.

Laboratory test	Specific features/comments
Blood count and film with differential count	At diagnosis Plasma cell enumeration (% plasma cells) Presence of rouleaux Ongoing regular monitoring for response to therapy
Bone marrow aspirate	Plasma cell morphology Plasma cell enumeration
Bone marrow trephine	Pattern of bone marrow infiltration Immunocytochemistry for CD138; +/− CD56, light chains Repeat to monitor response to therapy
Flow cytometry	At diagnosis to establish plasma cell phenotype For ploidy and to assess proliferation rate
Cytogenetics/FISH	To detect genetic abnormalities associated with prognosis Minimal panel: t(4;14), t(14;16), del17p
Biochemistry	β2-microglobulin SPEP, immunofixation, UPEP Serum free light chains Quantitative immunoglobulins Renal function Calcium
Radiology	Skeletal survey +/− MRI

SPEP: Serum protein electrophoresis; UPEP: Urine protein elecrophoresis

(Table 12.1). In addition all patients need to have a complete bone marrow evaluation including aspirate and biopsy and FISH analysis. Patients need to have a thorough radiological evaluation for bone lesions. In this chapter we will deal with a description of tests commonly used in the evaluation of patients with MM and what a work-up recommendation might be.

Blood count and film

The blood count in patients presenting with myeloma commonly shows mild pancytopenia with red cell macrocytosis (MCV 100–105 fl). On the blood film there is generally rouleaux formation and background staining due to the presence of a paraprotein. There may be circulating plasma cells and the number bears some correlation with prognosis. The number of circulating plasma cells is also used to discriminate between plasma cell myeloma ($<2 \times 10^9$/L) and plasma cell leukemia ($\geq 20\%$ of leukocytes or $\geq 2 \times 10^9$/L). The morphology of circulating neoplastic plasma cells varies from well-differentiated, resembling those in bone marrow, to pleomorphic with atypical features, such as small size with minimal cytoplasm (lymphoplasmacytoid), large, cleaved, indented or lobated nuclei and presence of nucleoli.

Bone marrow aspirate and trephine biopsy

Bone marrow examination, with both aspirate and trephine biopsy, is one of the most important components of the laboratory evaluation in individuals suspected of having MM or a related condition. While MM is known to be a patchy disease, as commonly evidenced by radiographic findings including MRI studies demonstrating heterogeneous bony mottling, the diagnosis can usually be established with a high quality unilateral bone core biopsy and aspirate. Bilateral procedures, as sometimes performed for lymphoma staging, are unnecessary in MM. Obtaining a core biopsy and aspirate (rather than just one or the other) improves the chances of obtaining a truly representative sampling of this patchy disease.

Bone marrow aspirate: The bone marrow aspirate in MM will show a variable plasmacytosis. As the pattern of marrow infiltration is commonly focal, a "squash" preparation is generally helpful in ascertaining the

a

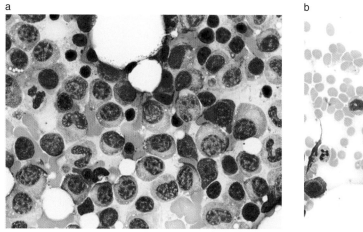

b

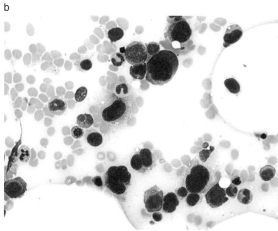

Figure 12.1. Characteristic plasma cell morphology in the bone marrow aspirate of multiple myeloma.
a. Bone marrow aspirate "squash" preparation showing a marked plasmacytosis of relatively monomorphic intermediate-sized cells.
b. Pleomorphic plasma cells including multinucleated plasma cells.

degree of marrow infiltration (Figure 12.1). However, it is standard practice to perform the plasma cell count on the aspirate smears where 30% or greater plasma cells are generally present. The plasma cell morphology can resemble normal plasma cells but morphological atypia is common with features such as:

1. *Cell size*: vary from small lymphoplasmacytoid cells with minimal cytoplasm to large plasma cells with abundant cytoplasm.
2. *Nuclear : cytoplasmic ratio*: high in lymphoplasmacytoid cells to very low.
3. *Cytoplasm*: usually basophilic and may contain vacuoles (Russell bodies or Mott cells), crystals or other azurophilic inclusions (Figure 12.2). "Flame" plasma cells which have reddish peripheral cytoplasm due to distension of the endoplasmic reticulum by immunoglobulin, most commonly IgA.
4. *Nuclei*: less condensed chromatin, bi- or multinuclearity and presence of nucleoli.
5. Anaplastic plasma cells with morphology that may be difficult to recognise as plasma cells.

Although many important pieces of hematological data are obtained during the evaluation of a bone marrow aspirate specimen, an accurate estimate of percentage of PCs in the bone marrow is the single most important aspect of the evaluation in patients with a suspected plasma cell disorder. An accurate PC percentage can be obtained in most cases through careful cytological examination and manual

differential cell count (usually based on 500 cells) of a Romanowsky stained bone marrow aspirate smear; this is generally more accurate than estimating plasma cell number on a hematoxylin and eosin (H&E) stained biopsy section.

Bone marrow trephine: The pattern of bone marrow infiltration in MM may be focal (interstitial or nodular) or diffuse (Figure 12.3). With disease progression the plasma cell infiltrate extends and diffusely replaces normal hematopoietic activity. The plasma cells tend to be relatively monomorphic, intermediate-large sized cells with eccentric nuclei and amphophilic cytoplasm with a pale-staining Golgi region on H&E staining. Giemsa staining can be useful to highlight plasma cells due to the prominent cytoplasmic basophilia. Multinuclear and giant plasma cells can be seen. The nuclear chromatin is condensed with coarse clumping ("clock face" appearance) and a nucleolus may be present. Plasma cell inclusions such as Dutcher bodies (pseudo-nuclear inclusions) and cytoplasmic inclusions, such as vacuoles or Russell bodies may be present. The trephine biopsy generally gives a better indication of the extent of disease than the aspirate.

Immunocytochemistry using CD138 antibodies, which are relatively specific for plasma cells, can be used to highlight the plasma cells, determine the extent of disease and to quantify plasma cells. Immunocytochemistry on the trephine can also be used to determine whether the PC are neoplastic. CD56 positivity is an indicator that the plasma cells are

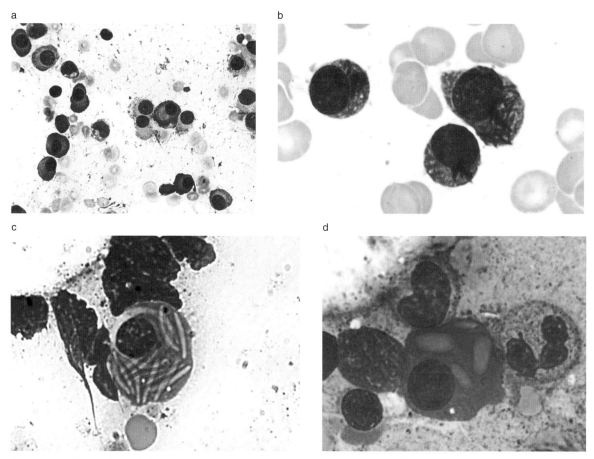

Figure 12.2. Plasma cell morphology in bone marrow aspirates showing varied morphological features. These features generally bear little clinical significance but may represent pitfalls for accurate diagnosis.
a. Flame plasma cell showing the eosinophilic (red) coloration at the edges of the basophilic cytoplasm. This feature has been associated with IgA-type plasma cells.
b. Plasma cells with Auer rod-like inclusions.
c. Plasma cell with multiple crystalline inclusions.
d. Plasma cell with large crystalline inclusions.

neoplastic, as is kappa or lambda (cytoplasmic) light chain restriction. There may be an increase in reticulin, particularly with extensive disease.

Correlation of aspirate and trephine: The two specimen types must be correlated for the most accurate results. In cases where an inadequate or hemodilute aspirate was obtained, the bone core biopsy becomes more central to determining the extent of plasmacytosis. It should be noted that there is sometimes discordance between the percentage of PCs in the aspirate smears and that in the core biopsy section. This can be for a variety of reasons, including focal disease, hemodilute aspirate smears, inaspirable marrow due to extensive disease or increased reticulin, suboptimal

core biopsy but good aspirate (Figure 12.4). A hemodilute marrow aspirate is a common explanation for an artificially low PC percentage. The impact of hemodilution increases as higher volume bone marrow aspirates are obtained to complete necessary ancillary studies including flow cytometry, cytogenetic and fluorescence *in situ* hybridization testing. For the purposes of clinical prognostication, it is therefore recommended that the higher number of PC from the two specimen types always be used.

Some caveats are worth noting when considering a BM biopsy in an individual suspected of having MM or a related disorder. Patients who present with multiple plasmacytomas may not have evidence of a clonal PC population in a random site bone marrow

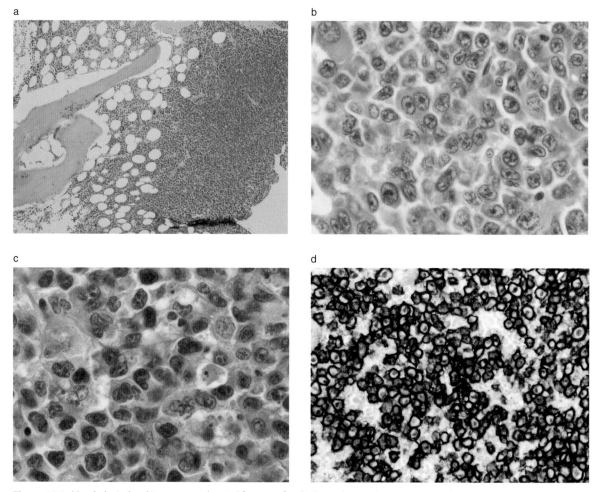

Figure 12.3. Morphological and immunocytochemical features of multiple myeloma in bone marrow trephines.
a. Example of nodular pattern of marrow involvement in myeloma.
b. Characteristic appearance of neoplastic plasma cells at high magnification.
c. Anaplastic myeloma cells. The morphology can be non-specific without immunocytochemical analysis.
d. CD138 (immunoperoxidase staining) positivity of the plasma cells in myeloma.

biopsy and aspirate when evaluated by outline morphological methods alone. Adjunct testing such as immunocytochemistry or fluorescence *in situ* hybridization may be required to assess for the presence of a low level PC clone in such cases. A number of pathological and immunophenotypic characteristics of PCs have been associated with variable outcomes in MM (e.g. plasmablastic morphology [11]), but none are in wide clinical use due to low levels of reproducibility and the current availability of better prognostic tools (see below).

Morphological subtypes of MM: Although the morphology of most cases of myeloma is characteristic and easy to diagnose, there are some specific morphological subtypes, detectable on both aspirate and trephine biopsy, which have atypical cytological features; these have been reported to be associated with prognosis and include:

1. *Lymphoplasmacytic morphology*: This is seen in approximately 15% of MM cases and comprises small well-differentiated plasma cells. This is associated with t(11;14)(q13;q32) and expression of CD20 antigen and cyclin D1 (see below).
2. *Plasmablastic myeloma*: Approximately 10% of cases have immature plasma cell morphology, i.e. variable cell size, with a higher nuclear :

a

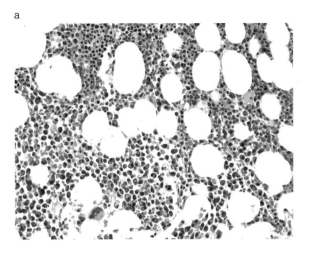

b

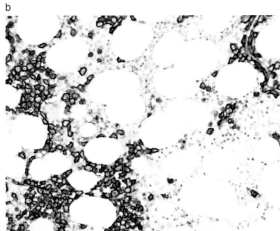

c

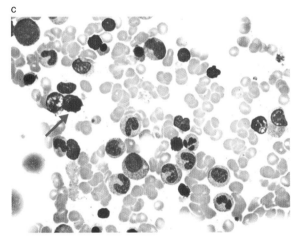

Figure 12.4. Discordance between the number of plasma cells in the bone marrow trephine biopsy and aspirate smears due to the patchy nature of marrow infiltration.
a. Bone marrow trephine biopsy showing patchy plasma cell infiltrates admixed with normal background bone marrow elements.
b. Bone marrow trephine biopsy stained with CD138 highlighting the patchy interstitial plasmacytosis.
c. A representative field of the corresponding bone marrow aspirate smear showing myeloid cells and only a single plasma cell (arrow).

cytoplasmic ratio, fine chromatin and nucleolus (Figure 12.5).

3. *Anaplastic myeloma*: The plasma cells are poorly differentiated with marked morphological atypia. The plasma cells can mimic other hematological malignancies (including lymphoma and acute leukemia) and require immunophenotyping to make the diagnosis. These tend to be highly aggressive.

Flow cytometry and proliferation assays

The phenotype of normal and neoplastic plasma cells differ and therefore flow cytometry can be used in the diagnosis of MM. It is now common practice for a portion of the BM aspirate to be analyzed by flow cytometric analysis [12–14] (Table 12.2 and Figures 12.6 and 12.7). Applications of flow cytometry include to:

1. Detect and enumerate plasma cells, using CD38 and CD138 as plasma cell-associated antibodies.
2. Distinguish normal from neoplastic plasma cells based on phenotype, i.e. CD19 antigen is expressed by normal plasma cells but absent from neoplastic cells. CD56 is positive in 90% of MM and negative on normal plasma cells.
3. Identify specific types of MM, e.g. CD20-positive disease associated with t(11;14).
4. Detect cytoplasmic kappa or lambda light chain restriction, thereby inferring clonality.
5. Detect markers associated with prognosis, e.g. expression of CD27 antigen associated with good prognosis, CD28 with poor prognosis, or lack of CD56 and poor prognosis.
6. Determine the proliferation rate based on Ki67 (MIB-1) expression or plasma cell labeling index,

Table 12.2. Phenotype of normal and neoplastic plasma cells.

Antigen	Normal plasma cells	Neoplastic plasma cells
CD19	Positive	Negative
CD20	Negative	Positive with t(11;14)
CD27	Negative	Positive in 50% cases
CD28	Negative	Positive in 30–50% cases
CD38	Positive	Positive
CD45	Majority negative	Negative
CD56	Negative	Positive in 90% cases
CD138	Positive	Positive

a

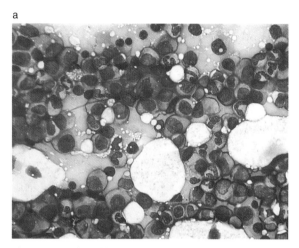

b

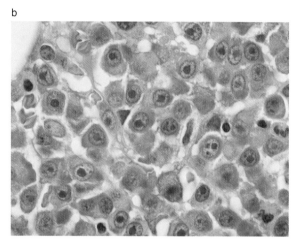

Figure 12.5. Plasmablastic multiple myeloma.
a. Bone marrow aspirate showing immature nuclear chromatin of the neoplastic plasma cells.
b. Bone marrow trephine showing prominent nucleoli in the plasma cells.

i.e. the percent PC in S-phase of the cell cycle using bromodeoxyuridine incorporation.
7. Calculate the plasma cell DNA index (Figure 12.8).
8. Detect disease-associated antigens which can be used for monitoring residual disease.
9. Detect antigens which may be targets for antibody-based therapy, e.g. CD138, CD27 or CD28.

Routine flow cytometric immunophenotyping, however, generally only plays only a minor role in the diagnosis of MM. Clonality assessment (and quantitation) of PCs is most often accomplished directly through the use of antibodies and immunocytochemistry or probes and *in situ* hybridization on fixed bone marrow biopsy material, or, indirectly through serum protein electrophoresis and immunofixation testing of serum and/or urine. One of the reasons flow cytometry is not more widely used in routine diagnosis is because of the tendency for PCs to be fragile and lost during the processing steps involved in preparing the aspirate for analysis by the flow cytometer. This can result in reporting a falsely low number of clonal plasma cells or failure to identify a PC clone due to low numbers, both of which may cause confusion. Newer and more standardized sample preparation methods are being developed to overcome this technical issue. This will be necessary as

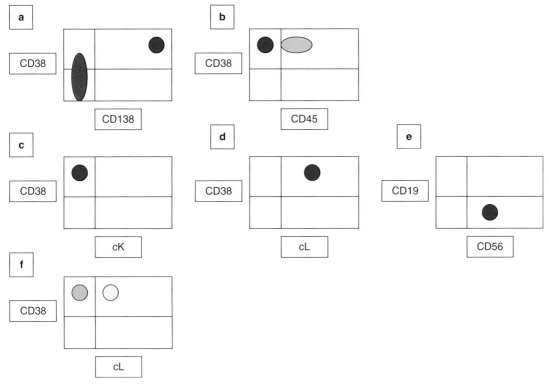

Figure 12.6. Schematic depiction of phenotypic markers and sample gating strategies used to assess plasma cells by flow cytometry.
a. Plasma cells are identified by bright co-expression of CD38 and CD138 (dark blue circle). Note that the normal subset of lymphocytes are also CD38-positive but CD138-negative.
b. Gating on CD38-positive cells shows the plasma cell population to be CD45-negative or dim.
c. The CD38-positive plasma cells are negative for cytoplasmic kappa.
d. The CD38-positive plasma cells show cytoplasmic lambda light chain restriction.
e. Analysis of the dual CD38/CD138-positive plasma cells shows them to express CD56 and lack CD19 expression, the phenotype of neoplastic plasma cells.
f. Gating on cells with bright CD38 and dim CD45 expression demonstrates an additional population of clonal plasma cells in that quadrant.

accurate phenotypic characterization and quantitation of neoplastic PCs becomes a more important part of the management of MM patients, particularly in regard to minimal residual disease (MRD) testing. This is most relevant for patients undergoing stem cell transplantation [15], evaluation of those suspected to be in stringent CR, and monitoring patients in clinical trials. While FCI is not currently an essential test in the routine diagnostic evaluation of patients with clear-cut MM, it does have an important role in the evaluation of patients with IgM or IgA paraproteinemias, which may be associated with B-cell non-Hodgkin lymphomas with or without plasma cell differentiation (e.g. lymphoplasmacytic lymphoma and marginal zone lymphoma).

Proliferation assays, such as the plasma cell labeling index test, can provide useful diagnostic and prognostic information in patients with MM and related disorders; however, these tests are not routinely performed in most clinical laboratories. The development of flow cytometry-based proliferation assays and/or the identification of surrogate markers of proliferation may make this type of analysis more commonplace in the future.

Genetic assays

Genetic factors are the preferred method to establish prognostic categories in myeloma [16]. Testing for genetic aberrations, especially by FISH, has therefore become an integral part of the initial evaluation of the disease.

Karyotype

The presence of abnormal metaphases by karyotype analysis has been identified as a powerful prognostic feature in MM. It is now well accepted that the presence of any cytogenetic abnormalities is associated with an

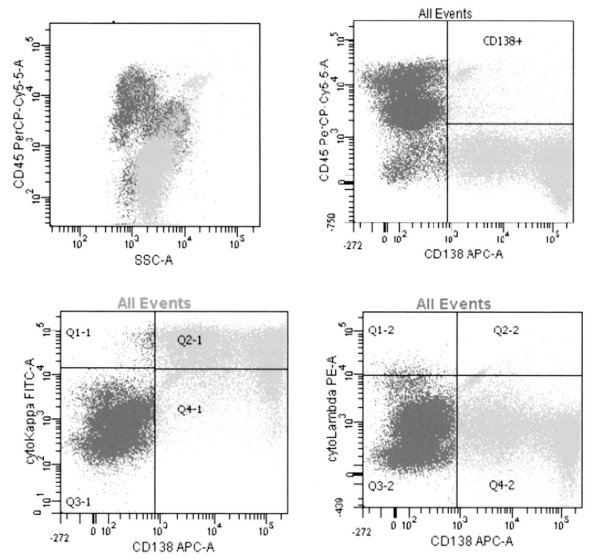

Figure 12.7. Flow cytometry histograms showing CD138, CD45 and cytoplasmic kappa and lambda gating strategies for assessing plasma cells. The plasma cells (light blue) are CD45-negative, CD138-positive with kappa light chain restriction.

inferior outcome in MM [17]. Dewald and colleagues first reported the impact of abnormal cytogenetics and outcome in MM, and noted that the percent of abnormal metaphases correlated with outcome [17]. Later Tricot and colleagues identified the presence of any abnormalities and chromosome 13 aberrations as major determinants of outcome [18]. In subsequent studies of large cohorts of patients the presence of abnormalities, especially structural, and hypodiploidy emerged as important prognostic determinants in MM [19].

While these chromosomal abnormalities carry this prognostic significance the use of karyotyping is fraught with several limitations. Karyotyping in MM usually yields normal results, as the metaphases being analyzed originate from the myeloid elements of the BM, and not the myeloma cells which have a much lower proliferation rate [17,20]. Metaphase FISH and multicolor karyotyping are not much more informative than standard cytogenetic analysis due to this problem that the majority of metaphases originate from the myeloid elements and not the PC. It has been shown that the ability to obtain abnormal metaphases correlates closely with both the extent of BM involvement by PCs and with their proliferation [21]. Many consider

Table 12.3. Fluorescence *in situ* hybridization (FISH)-detectable genetic abnormalities in multiple myeloma.

Genetic abnormality	Genes involved	Frequency	Prognosis
1. Primary genetic events			
t(4;14)(p16;q32)	*FGFR3–IgH*	15%	Unfavorable
t(14;16)(q32;q23)	*IgH–cMAF*	5%	Unfavorable
Hyperdiploidy	Numerical abnormalities		Favorable
t(11;14)(q13;q32)	*CCND1–IgH*	15%	Neutral
2. Secondary genetic events			
13q deletions and monosomy		50%	
17p13 deletions	p53	10% (at diagnosis)	Unfavorable
Chromosome 1 abnormalities	1q gains 1p losses	Common	Unfavorable
12p deletions	CD27 gene	10%	Unfavorable

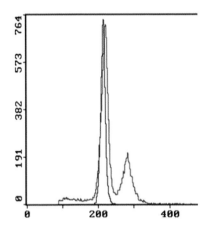

Figure 12.8. Flow cytometry histogram showing the DNA content of normal cells (blue line) and those from a myeloma patient (red line). The myeloma sample has one large peak of normal (diploid) cells and a second peak of hyperdiploid myeloma cells (DNA index of 1.4).

the presence of any cytogenetic abnormality a surrogate of these two MM features. In addition the "chromosome anatomy" of certain abnormalities, such as t(4;14) (p16;q32), make them invisible on metaphase spreads, even when metaphase abnormalities are detected [22]. Recommendations of which genetic test to perform remains controversial, with some advocating continued use of metaphase spreads as prognostic tools and some recommending the use of interphase cytogenetics and novel genomic technologies. Whilst this debate

continues, it should be clear to the treating physician that the presence of any abnormality is indicative of a more aggressive MM.

Fluorescence *in situ* hybridization

With the advent of interphase molecular cytogenetic techniques the aforementioned limitations of metaphase cytogenetics were overcome [23]. FISH panels have now been developed and can be used to establish disease subtype categorization (Table 12.3). It is important to note that FISH testing in MM needs to be coupled with a method to accurately identify the PC (Figure 12.9). FISH may be coupled with immunofluorescence detection of PCs using FICTION (e.g. cIg-FISH), morphology and other stains (e.g. Giemsa) or cell sorting (e.g. with CD138 bead selection). These approaches are essential to ensure that only the genetics of the PCs is assessed [23,24]. In the absence of one of these methods to confidently identify the PC the test lacks sensitivity and its diagnostic reliability is lost.

Minimal FISH panel: A minimal panel for FISH testing in MM should include, at the very least, probes to detect del(17p13), t(4;14)(p16;q32) and t(14;16) (q32;q23) [25]. The presence of any one of these factors is now widely used as an indicator of high risk or poor prognosis MM. Testing for the translocations needs to be done only once as the subtype of MM does not change over time [25]. Testing for del(17p13) could be

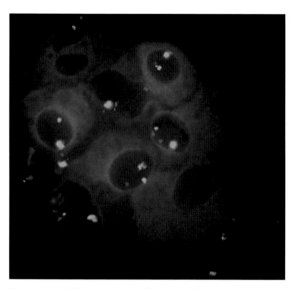

Figure 12.9. FISH using probes for p53 (red; R) and centromere 17 (green; G) combined with immunofluorescence for CD138 (Alexa Fluor 35) highlighting the plasma cells (blue). Abnormal plasma cells can be seen with a 1R2G pattern, indicating deletion of p53. The normal cells show a 2R2G signal pattern.

considered as a test that can be repeated. While no formal clinical validations have been done it is clear that deletions of 17p13 can arise during follow-up and identify patients with more aggressive disease.

Extended FISH panel: An extended FISH panel can be used to detect genetic defects that have modest effects on outcome. This would encompass other markers of genetic categories such as deletion of chromosome 13 (−13), t(11;14)(q13;q32), hyperdiploidy and others. These markers can sometimes serve useful diagnostic purposes [25]. For instance patients with MM and t(11;14)(q13;q32) can have lymphoplasmacytic morphology, express CD20 and upregulated cyclin D1, occasionally creating a possibility of a diagnosis of lymphoproliferative disorder, other than MM (Figure 12.10) [26]. In these cases the presence of t(11;14)(q13;q32) together with a monoclonal protein makes the diagnosis of MM certain. Similarly the presence of t(11;14)(q13;q32) in patients with an IgM monoclonal protein virtually excludes the diagnosis of Waldenström macroglobulinemia and establishes IgM MM [27,28].

Detection of abnormalities of chromosome 13 by FISH (monosomy or interstitial deletion) often creates confusion for the treating physician and deserves explanation. While detection of −13 by FISH has

been associated with a diminished prognosis, its effects are not strong enough for these patients to be categorized as high-risk MM [29]. It is therefore important to recognize that the presence of −13 alone cannot be used to guide treatment decisions in MM.

A number of new genomic markers have been identified in myeloma using array-based comparative genomic hybridization (aCGH) [30–32]. Notable amongst these are amplifications of chromosomes 1 (1q) or 5q and 12p deletions. Using these markers a French group has been able to identify subsets of patients with dissimilar outcomes. While these markers were identified via aCGH they are eminently applicable to interphase-based strategies that could potentially be used with other known prognostic markers to identify groups of patients with prognostic relevance. Further testing and validation of such markers is underway.

Genomic technologies

The advent of RNA-based microarrays allows a detailed assessment of the transcriptional profile of MM cells [16]. Several lessons have already been learned from such efforts. The first is that MM is composed of well-defined subgroups of the disease that usually share a founder genetic lesion (e.g. an *IgH* translocation subtype) that results in a uniform transcriptional profile [33]. Accordingly seven to eight subgroups of the disease have been identified. Second is that GEP allows for the best prognostication of MM [16,33]. Investigators have developed a high-risk profile based on GEP signature data that identifies 15% of patients who have the most aggressive variants of the disease, and for whom new treatment modalities are needed. GEP has also allowed further insights into the biology of the disease such as with the discovery of bone lesions associated with dysregulated DKK1. GEP is also being used to identify predictors of therapeutic benefit (e.g. response rate, duration of response).

Gene expression profiling is not currently available as a routine clinical laboratory test for a variety of reasons, including practical limitations (e.g. the need for a purification step to separate MM cells from background bone marrow elements prior to RNA extraction and the necessity for a large number of cells for testing) and regulatory issues. GEP testing is being performed in research laboratories, and further technological advances perfected in that arena (such as

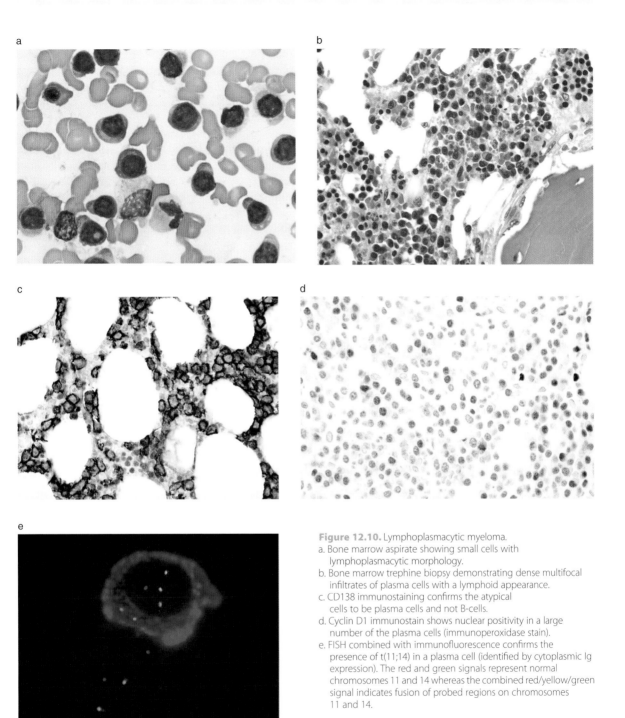

Figure 12.10. Lymphoplasmacytic myeloma.
a. Bone marrow aspirate showing small cells with lymphoplasmacytic morphology.
b. Bone marrow trephine biopsy demonstrating dense multifocal infiltrates of plasma cells with a lymphoid appearance.
c. CD138 immunostaining confirms the atypical cells to be plasma cells and not B-cells.
d. Cyclin D1 immunostain shows nuclear positivity in a large number of the plasma cells (immunoperoxidase stain).
e. FISH combined with immunofluorescence confirms the presence of t(11;14) in a plasma cell (identified by cytoplasmic Ig expression). The red and green signals represent normal chromosomes 11 and 14 whereas the combined red/yellow/green signal indicates fusion of probed regions on chromosomes 11 and 14.

the ability to perform the GEP with fewer cells). This will help pave the way for GEP to be fully developed and validated for use in accredited clinical laboratories for MM and other cancer types in the near future.

Protein analysis

The integration of proteomic markers into the clinical assessment of multiple myeloma presents opportunities and challenges [34]. The monoclonal proteins associated with MM and related conditions are the ideal proteomic marker in that they are disease-, patient- and clone-specific. Indeed the protein variation introduced by the process of somatic hypermutation makes the specificity of monoclonal proteins unsurpassable as ideal protein biomarkers. Furthermore these proteins can be measured with tests that have enough amplitude that make them reliably quantitative, and thus of clinical use. As such the identification and quantification of monoclonal proteins has been the mainstay for diagnosis and monitoring of the disease for the past 40 years [35].

Serum protein electrophoresis and immunofixation

Serum protein electrophoresis (SPEP) is essential for the diagnosis and monitoring of MM and other plasma cell and monoclonal protein disorders (Figure 12.11). It is a test that is widely available and reliably allows the identification of monoclonal proteins that exceed a serum concentration of approximately 30 g/L. Following electrophoresis, a non-specific protein dye is used for protein labeling and visualization of bands. Monoclonal protein bands can then be identified and quantified in the gamma and less frequently the beta regions of the SPEP gel. SPEP can serve as a useful initial screening procedure when MM is suspected. It is important to highlight that the SPEP results alone do

not have enough negative predictive value to exclude underlying MM or associated conditions. In some instances the concentration of the monoclonal proteins is so low that it can only be detected by more sensitive methods such as immunofixation, serum free light chain assay or urine protein electrophoresis. The specificity of SPEP is, however, high and detection of a monoclonal protein band should prompt a comprehensive evaluation by a clinical hematologist.

SPEP results are reliable enough that measurement of monoclonal bands by this method is routinely used in clinical practice [35]. The monoclonal band is commonly referred to as the M-spike (for "monoclonal" or "myeloma" spike). The spikes are quantified by measuring the area under the curve and calculated via integration. Quantitation is easiest and most reliable when the monoclonal protein migrates to the gamma globulin region. This is more common with IgG monoclonal proteins than with IgA or IgM monoclonal proteins which often migrate to the beta region. Beta region spikes are sometimes difficult to see on SPEP gels, and increases in beta region proteins may warrant evaluation by immunofixation even if a distinct band (restriction) is not seen. Subsequent measurements of beta region spikes may be best accomplished by quantitative immunoglobulin analysis.

While SPEP will show evidence of a band of restricted mobility ("BORM") in one of the protein regions, immunofixation is required to confirm that it is a true monoclonal protein band and to further characterize the heavy and light chain components. In the immunofixation test, monoclonal antibodies specific to the major Ig heavy chains (G, A, M) and the two Ig light chains (kappa and lambda) are used. Immunofixation can therefore characterize a monoclonal protein. It is also more sensitive than SPEP and is therefore capable of detecting smaller amounts of monoclonal protein. A negative immunofixation test following therapy is therefore used accordingly as a marker of deep therapeutic response.

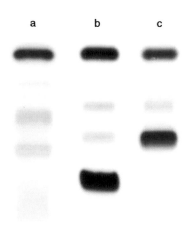

Figure 12.11. Serum protein electrophoresis gels showing:
a. Normal serum protein pattern.
b. Large monoclonal protein band (spike) in the gamma region. Note the lightness of the remainder of the gamma region due to suppression of background immunoglobulins.
c. Large monoclonal protein band in the beta region. While distinct in this example, many beta region spikes are difficult to distinguish from background beta proteins, and therefore, quantitative immunoglobulin measurement may be a more accurate way to monitor such a paraprotein over time.

Quantitative immunoglobulins

Quantitative serum immunoglobulin determination should be performed routinely during the evaluation of individuals with MM and related disorders. Quantitation is performed by nephelometry, an automated test performed that uses the principle of light scatter. While nephelometry can provide accurate levels of serum immunoglobulins, it cannot be used to determine if increased immunoglobulin levels are monoclonal or polyclonal. Thus the test is only useful when used in conjunction with SPEP and immunofixation and when the monoclonal protein concentrations exceed the upper limit of normal. It is important to remember that the values obtained by nephelometry and SPEP should not be considered interchangeable when monitoring disease. As mentioned above, quantitative immunoglobulin determination can be particularly useful for monitoring patients with IgA or IgM monoclonal proteins that migrate into the beta region of an SPEP; nephelometry is likely to provide a more consistent result compared with SPEP in such instances. Quantitative immunoglobulin analysis is also useful for assessing the degree of background immunoglobulin suppression in an individual with sizable monoclonal proteins.

Urine protein electrophoresis

Determination of monoclonal proteins in the urine can serve as an adjunct in the evaluation of patients with MM and associated disorders. Urine electrophoresis can be performed and a 24-hour excretion of monoclonal protein calculated. The test is complicated by the need to have a 24-hour urine collection by patients. The future of this test is being challenged by the recent availability of the serum free light chain assay for the diagnosis and monitoring of MM. In addition to serving as a tool for quantification of monoclonal proteins, urine protein electrophoresis can also measure albuminuria. This is of help in cases of light chain-associated amyloidosis-associated nephrotic syndrome and to monitor for drug toxicity.

Serum free light chain assays

The serum free light chain assay (Freelite™) has revolutionized the capacity to detect and monitor MM protein [36,37]. The test measures epitopes not exposed when the light chain is bound to heavy chains and thus measures the free fraction of light chain immunoglobulins. The smaller size of the free light chain (also known as Bence Jones protein) makes this free light chain small enough to be filtered at the glomeruli and create hazards for renal health. Determination of the concentration of the free light chain serves as an adjunct in establishing risk for renal damage in MM patients. Its sensitivity has also made a diagnosis of true "non secretory MM" extremely rare.

Clearance of free light chains is mediated via the kidney and elevation of their concentration is seen in patients with renal disease. Monitoring the ratio between kappa and lambda free light chains serves as a useful adjunct to determine whether the observed elevation is clonal or not; however, in most cases, this is not difficult given the extreme variation (elevation) of the associated monoclonal free light chain. Monitoring the ratio thus becomes less relevant, and close attention to the actual concentration of the monoclonal free light chain is sufficient. New tests that measure the bound heavy and light chains are being developed to be used instead of some of the aforementioned tests.

Staging of multiple myeloma

Staging of MM has evolved over the years with most classifications being mostly indicative of tumor burden. For many years the disease has been classified using the Durie–Salmon classification, which was primarily aimed at determining tumor burden [38]. This classification uses the combination of host and tumor features such as the hemoglobin, serum calcium concentration, concentration of the monoclonal proteins and presence of radiological abnormalities (Table 12.4). The classification was the hallmark for comparison of patients enrolled in clinical trials but was limited in its prognostic abilities, and difficult to remember. To improve this the International Myeloma Working group developed the International Staging System (ISS) (Table 12.4) [39]. The ISS was developed as a meta-analysis of over 10 000 patients treated with various modalities and is solely based on the combination of the β_2-microglobulin and albumin levels [39]. It has been extensively used since its publication and represents a practical way of estimating prognosis. It is worth mentioning that despite the simplicity of the ISS classification it has been estimated that up to one-third of MM patients do not have β_2-microglobulin measured at the time of diagnosis. It is important to note that as for other bone marrow-based hematological malignancies, the anatomic location is not relevant and hence does not form part of routine staging; the only exception to this may be solitary plasmacytomas. However, with sophisticated testing it is increasingly clear that true isolated plasmacytomas are rare, with most cases representing a localized growth of otherwise disseminated clonal cells.

Risk stratification

Multiple approaches for risk stratification of MM have been proposed, including the aforementioned ISS classification [39]. Over the years most risk-stratified approaches have incorporated genetic and genomic

Table 12.4. Multiple myeloma staging systems.

Stage	Durie–Salmon staging [38]	International Staging System [39]

I	All of the following:
	Hemoglobin >10 g/dL
	Serum calcium normal (<12 mg/dL)
	On roentgenogram, normal bone structure or solitary bone plasmacytoma only
	Low M-component production rates
	  IgG <5 g/dL
	  IgA <3 g/dL
	  Urine light chain M-component on electrophoresis <4 g/24 h
		β_2-microglobulin <3.5 mg/L, and albumin ≥3.5 g/dL

II	Overall data as minimally abnormal as shown for Stage I, and no single value as abnormal as defined for stage III	All others
III	One or more of the following: Hemoglobin <8.5 g/dL Serum calcium >12 mg/dL Advanced lytic bone lesions High M-component production rates IgG >7 g/dL IgA >5 g/dL Urine light chain M-component on electrophoresis >12 g/24 h Subclassification A = relatively normal renal function (serum creatinine value <2.0 mg/dL) B = abnormal renal function (serum creatinine ≥2.0 mg/dL)	β_2-microglobulin ≥5.5 mg/dL

markers to identify groups of patients with dissimilar outcomes [40]. Initially this included the incorporation of karyotypic abnormalities including any genetic abnormality, deletion of chromosome 13 and hypodiploidy. More recently risk stratification has incorporated FISH for t(4;14)(p16;q32), t(14;16)(q32;q23) and deletions of chromosome 17 [40]. Globally these three genetic markers have been proposed as good identifiers of outcome and utilized in ongoing clinical trials [41]. Several groups have now highlighted the importance of identifying these genetic subtypes associated with prognosis for the long-term management planning of patients. Whether these established genetic aberrations remain prognostic with the incorporation of novel therapies remains to be determined, and it seems that bortezomib may overcome the prognostic significance of some of these markers [41,42].

While these genetic features provide an approximation to predicted outcome a large proportion of the clinical variability remains unaccounted for. Gene expression profiling approaches and integrating array-based comparative genomic hybridization have

been shown to further improve prognostic prediction [16,43]. In time a simplified approach that is based on integration of this information will allow a practical scheme of determining prognosis for patients.

Response criteria in myeloma

Traditional response criteria in MM reflected the limited treatments available. These were best represented by criteria such as those developed by cooperative groups such as SWOG and ECOG [44]. More recently the European Bone Marrow Transplant registry developed criteria that encompassed deeper responses attained with stem cell transplantation [45]. Subsequently the International Myeloma Working Group developed response criteria and these are listed in Table 12.5 [10]. These criteria define complete response (CR), stringent CR (sCR), very good partial response (VGPR), partial response (PR), stable disease (SD) and progressive disease (PD). The definitions of these will evolve over time, reflecting increased understanding of the disease.

Table 12.5. International Myeloma Working Group response criteria in multiple myeloma (adapted from [10]).

Response category	Response criteria
Stringent CR	CR as defined below plus: Normal FLC ratio and Absence of clonal cells in bone marrow by immunocytochemistry or immunofluorescence
CR	Negative immunofixation on the serum and urine and disappearance of any soft tissue plasmacytomas and <5% plasma cells in bone marrow
VGPR	Serum and urine M-protein detectable by immunofixation but not on electrophoresis or 90% or greater reduction in serum M-protein plus urine M-protein level <100 mg per 24 h
PR	≥50% reduction of serum M-protein and reduction in 24-h urinary M-protein by ≥90% or to <200 mg per 24 h. If the serum and urine M-protein are unmeasurable, a ≥50% decrease in the difference between involved and uninvolved FLC levels is required in place of the M-protein criteria. If serum and urine M-protein are unmeasurable, and serum free light assay is also unmeasurable, ≥50% reduction in plasma cells is required in place of M-protein, provided baseline bone marrow plasma cell percentage was ≥30% In addition to the above listed criteria, if present at baseline, a ≥50% reduction in the size of soft tissue plasmacytomas is also required
Stable disease	Not meeting criteria for CR, VGPR, PR or progressive disease

CR = Complete response; PR = Partial response; VGPR = Very good partial response; FLC = Free light chain.

Disease monitoring

There is no standardized set of tests that must be performed for the ongoing monitoring of MM during therapy. Monoclonal protein levels, Ig quantitation and serum free light chains should be performed at regular intervals to assess therapeutic response. Repeating bone marrow examinations is only needed if uncertainty arises about disease response status and at the time of relapse. In most centers a repeat bone marrow examination is performed at day 100 post autologous stem cell transplant to assess the extent of response. In responding patients, including those who have completed stem cell transplant, monitoring is usually done every 2–3 months with laboratory tests alone.

Monoclonal gammopathy of undetermined significance and smoldering multiple myeloma

Diagnostic features

Monoclonal gammopathy of undetermined significance: Monoclonal gammopathy of undetermined

significance (MGUS) is defined by the presence of a monoclonal protein (<30 g/L), a clonal bone marrow plasmacytosis (<10%) and no end-organ damage. The blood count is normal but there may be rouleaux as a result of the monoclonal protein. The plasma cells in the marrow may be cytologically normal or show atypical features as seen in MM. In the bone marrow trephine the plasma cells may be present in small clusters or interstitial foci and these can be highlighted with CD138 immunocytochemistry (Figure 12.12). The monoclonal protein is most commonly IgG and there is a normal concentration of the other immunoglobulins. The phenotype of the neoplastic plasma cells in MGUS resembles that of MM (CD19-negative, CD56-positive, cytoplasmic kappa or lambda restricted expression). However, in contrast to MM, there are usually residual normal polyclonal plasma cells (CD19-positive, CD56-negative) in the marrow. The same cytogenetic abnormalities as seen in MM can be detected in MGUS.

Smoldering multiple myeloma: Smoldering multiple myeloma (SMM) meets the diagnostic criteria of MM

a

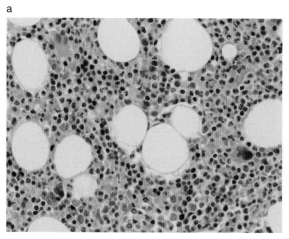

b

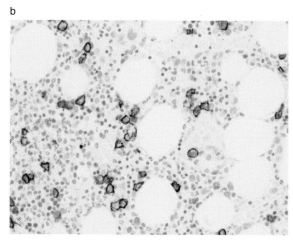

Figure 12.12. Monoclonal gammopathy of undetermined significance.
a. There is a low level plasmacytosis in the bone marrow trephine (approximately 10% of cells). These can be difficult to detect on hematoxylin and eosin staining.
b. CD138 immunoperoxidase staining highlights the bone marrow plasmacytosis. The plasma cells are present in small clusters and as single cells.

but is asymptomatic and there is no organ-related damage. The number of plasma cells is generally 10–20%, higher than MGUS.

Traditionally obtaining a BM sample to evaluate a patient with MGUS or SMM had been considered dispensable. It has now become apparent that bone marrow examination is required to distinguish between MGUS and SMM as this cannot be done with other laboratory tests [7]. The distinction between MGUS and SMM is important due to the much higher risk of progression to MM from SMM [7]. It is therefore recommended that any patient with a life expectancy of 5 years or more should have a BM sample obtained for analysis. The finding of SMM should prompt further evaluation for sentinel signs of possible progression to MM. It is recommended that patients with SMM be evaluated more frequently than those with MGUS. Since progression to MM can occur via renal failure or catastrophic bone fractures careful monitoring is recommended.

Diagnostic differences between MGUS/SMM and MM

The pathological features of MGUS/SMM and MM are the same. The only distinguishing feature is the percent bone marrow plasmacytosis [7]. The other laboratory features are less valuable distinguishing between MGUS/SMM and MM, as follows:

1. *Plasma cell proliferation rates*: these are higher in MM than in MGUS/SMM but this test is not used routinely in clinical practice [46].
2. *Flow cytometry*: incapable of separating between the entities as the neoplastic plasma cell phenotype (CD19-negative; CD56-positive; cytoplasmic light chain restriction) is seen in both MGUS/SMM and MM.
3. *Genetics*: the same genetic features are observed in both MM and MGUS/SMM and therefore cannot be used to differentiate between these entities [47,48]. Accordingly initiation of therapy should not be based solely on detection of these genetic aberrations. The only aberrations which are seen in MM and not in MGUS, are chromosome 17 deletions. Since deletions of 17p are a strong predictor of poor survival, MGUS/SMM patients with this genetic abnormality should be monitored for possible evolution to active MM.

Risk of progression of MGUS/SMM to MM

The risk of progression from MGUS to MM is much lower than for SMM. The risk for progression for MGUS is estimated at 1% per year and is fixed, and overall 25% at 25 years. For SMM the risk is 10% per year for the first 5 years, 3% per year for the next 5 years and then drops to 1% per year as in MGUS [7] giving an overall risk of progression of nearly 70% at

10 years. The risk of progression from MGUS to MM is largely determined by biology, with features such as:

1. Lower risk for IgG proteins than others.
2. Tumor burden, e.g. elevated free light chains or higher concentration of serum monoclonal proteins [49].
3. Number of clonal plasma cells (versus polyclonal plasma cells) can be used to estimate risk of progression for SMM [50].

Plasma cell leukemia

Plasma cell leukemia (PCL) is the most aggressive plasma cell neoplasm. It is manifest by the presence of circulating plasma cells making up ≥20% of total leukocytes in the peripheral blood or an absolute peripheral plasmacytosis of ≥2 ×10⁹/L (Figure 12.13) [51]. The circulating plasma cells can show a wide range of cytological features such as mature-appearing and bland or plasmablastic. The latter may be mistaken for myeloblasts, especially in heavily treated patients where the differential diagnosis includes therapy-related myelodysplastic syndrome or acute myeloid leukemia. It should be noted that plasma cells cannot be specifically identified by automated hematology analyzers, and that identification and quantitation of circulating plasma cells must be done through morphological review of the peripheral blood smear. There are two types of plasma cell leukemia:

1. Primary (pPCL) arises *de novo* with no preceding history of MM. Rouleaux is less common and the plasma cell morphology can be more heterogeneous.
2. Secondary (sPCL) arises in the context of pre-existing MM [51,52]. sPCL is the most extreme manifestation of extramedullary MM. Patients tend to also have extensive involvement of the bone marrow and can have deposits at other sites such as the liver or spleen when thoroughly evaluated.

At the genetic level most pPCL is composed of MM cells with *IgH* translocations, particularly with t(11;14)(q13;q32) [52,53]. sPCL can have any of the genetic aberrations observed in MM including hyperdiploidy [52]. A large fraction of patients exhibit abnormalities of the genes of the p53 pathway (deletion/mutation) [52]. In agreement with previously noted associations of these genetic features with the monoclonal protein type, there is a predilection for IgG lambda or lambda-alone disease [53]. The immunophenotype of the neoplastic plasma cells tends to lack aberrant expression of the cell surface marker CD56 seen in MM [52,54].

Waldenström macroglobulinemia

Waldenström macroglobulinemia (WM), also known as lymphoplasmacytic lymphoma (LPL), is a late B-cell neoplasm that shares features with MM [55]. The neoplastic cells produce a monoclonal protein which is usually of the IgM type [55]. This is a fundamental difference from MM and occurs because the monoclonal cells have expanded before heavy chain switching ("pre-switch"); therefore, the malignancy while related to MM is ontologically different. Accordingly the biology of the disease is different from MM and more akin to other late B-cell neoplasms like chronic lymphocytic leukemia/small lymphocytic lymphoma.

Diagnostic features

The clinical and pathological findings of WM are varied and there is no specific or pathognomonic feature [56]. Hyperviscosity and organomegaly are common and the concentration of the IgM paraprotein can be high.

Morphology of blood and bone marrow

The blood count and film show anemia and rouleaux and there may be a lymphocytosis (Figure 12.14). The circulating lymphocytes are predominantly small and mature and some show plasmacytoid features (eccentric

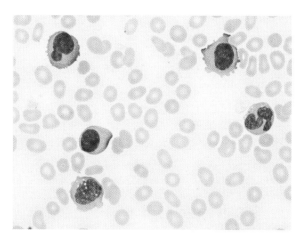

Figure 12.13. Blood film of a case of primary plasma cell leukemia.

nuclei, basophilic cytoplasm and Golgi zone). The bone marrow is infiltrated by lymphocytes, lymphoplasmacytoid cells and plasma cells; there is commonly a reactive mast cell infiltrate with normal morphology. In the bone marrow trephine the infiltrate may be interstitial or nodular. Dutcher bodies may be present.

Most cases of WM therefore have the morphology of lymphoplasmacytic lymphoma (LPL), although some can have the morphology of extranodal marginal zone lymphoma. While these two B-cell lymphomas are distinct entities, they share some common morphological features including the presence of a heterogeneous population of small lymphocytes, plasmacytoid lymphocytes, and plasma cells, which

are sometimes clonal (particularly in LPL) [57]. Lymphoplasmacytic lymphoma is the most common pathological designation for WM involving primarily the bone marrow [56].

Immunophenotype

The phenotype of WM is that of a mature B-cell lymphoma that typically expresses the B-cell antigens CD19, CD20, CD79a with surface immunoglobulin (IgM, without IgD) and light chain restriction. The cells may be CD38 positive but typically do not express CD5 (helping to distinguish them from CLL/SLL and mantle cell lymphoma) or CD10 antigens (helping to distinguish them from germinal center cell lymphomas

a
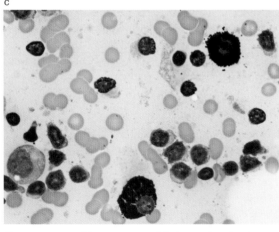

b
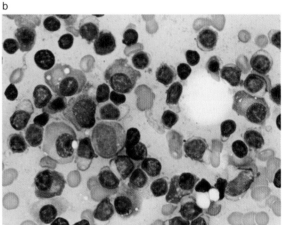

c

d
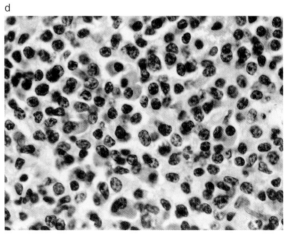

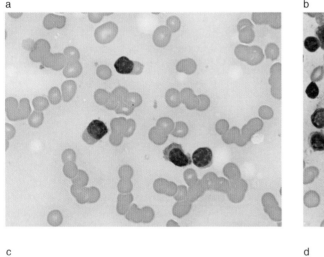

Figure 12.14. Waldenström macroglobulinemia (lymphoplasmacytic lymphoma).
a. Blood film showing rouleaux, background protein staining and lymphoplasmacytoid cells.
b. Bone marrow aspirate showing the infiltrate comprised predominantly of lymphocytes, with admixed lymphoplasmacytic cells and plasma cells.
c. Mast cells with normal morphology are commonly increased in the bone marrow.
d. Bone marrow trephine biopsy showing the lymphocytes, lymphoplasmacytic cells and plasma cells.

such as follicular lymphoma) [56]. CD11c, CD25 and CD103 are also negative. Expression of plasmacytic markers (CD38 and CD138) is common in the plasma cell component of WM lymphomas.

A subset of MM patients has bone marrow morphology that mimics WM/LPL (small lymphoplasmacytoid cells), and this may potentially lead to an erroneous diagnosis of B-cell lymphoma. So-called LPL-like MM can be distinguished from LPL in most cases through the use of flow cytometry, cyclin D1 immunohistochemistry, and FISH for t(11;14). The distinction can be made as follows:

1. *True LPL*: dominant CD20-positive B-cell clone by flow cytometry, cyclin D1-negative and t(11;14)-negative (see Figure 12.10).
2. *MM with LPL-like features*: major clonal plasma cell population that is CD138-positive, cyclin D1-positive. t(11;14) is detectable by interphase FICTION (immunoFISH) performed on cytoplasmic immunoglobulin-selected plasma cells. The small plasmacytoid cells may be CD20-positive.

Genetics

The genetic nature of WM is different from that of MM in that none of the typical MM genetic aberrations such as *IgH* translocations or hyperdiploidy are observed [28,58,59]. In some rare instances secondary MM associated changes can also be detected in WM; these include abnormalities of chromosome 13 or deletion of 17p13 [28,58,59]. The most common genetic aberration in WM is loss of the long arm of chromosome 6 [28,58,59]. While this is a lesion which is also detected in many other B-cell neoplasms the frequency is higher in WM, approaching 50%. Recent discoveries have shown that genes implicated in constitutive genetic activation of the NF-kB pathway are also common in WM [60]. There is no evidence to suggest clinical utility of these markers, but it appears that cases with 6q deletions represent more advanced disease [61].

References

1. Harousseau JL, Shaughnessy J Jr, Richardson P. Multiple myeloma. *Hematology* 2004;**1**:237–56.
2. Rajkumar SV, Kyle RA. Multiple myeloma: diagnosis and treatment. *Mayo Clin Proc* 2005;**80**(10):1371–82.
3. Kastritis E, Zervas K, Symeonidis A *et al.* Improved survival of patients with multiple myeloma after the introduction of novel agents and the applicability of the International Staging System (ISS): an analysis of the Greek Myeloma Study Group (GMSG). *Leukemia* 2009;**23**(6):1152–7.
4. Kumar SK, Rajkumar SV, Dispenzieri A *et al.* Improved survival in multiple myeloma and the impact of novel therapies. *Blood* 2008;**111**(5):2516–20.
5. Barlogie B, Tricot G, Anaissie E *et al.* Thalidomide and hematopoietic-cell transplantation for multiple myeloma. *New Engl J Med* 2006;**354**(10):1021–30.
6. Kyle RA, Therneau TM, Rajkumar SV *et al.* A long-term study of prognosis in monoclonal gammopathy of undetermined significance. *New Engl J Med* 2002;**346**(8):564–9.
7. Kyle RA, Remstein ED, Therneau TM *et al.* Clinical course and prognosis of smoldering (asymptomatic) multiple myeloma. *New Engl J Med* 2007;**356**(25):2582–90.
8. Kyle RA, Rajkumar SV. Multiple myeloma. *New Engl J Med* 2004;**351**(18):1860–73.
9. San Miguel JF, Lahuerta JJ, Garcia-Sanz R *et al.* Are myeloma patients with renal failure candidates for autologous stem cell transplantation? *Hematol J* 2000;**1**(1):28–36.
10. Durie BG, Harousseau JL, Miguel JS *et al.* International uniform response criteria for multiple myeloma. *Leukemia* 2006;**20**(9):1467–73.
11. Greipp PR, Bennett JM, Gaillard JP *et al.* Poor survival in plasmablastic myeloma in Eastern Cooperative Oncology Group study E9487: cell kinetic, ploidy, biological marker, and clinical correlations (Meeting abstract). *Proc Annu Meet Am Soc Clin Oncol* 1995;**14**.
12. San Miguel JF, Almeida J, Mateo G *et al.* Immunophenotypic evaluation of the plasma cell compartment in multiple myeloma: a tool for comparing the efficacy of different treatment strategies and predicting outcome. *Blood* 2002;**99**(5):1853–6.
13. Paiva B, Vidriales MB, Perez JJ *et al.* Multiparameter flow cytometry quantification of bone marrow plasma cells at diagnosis provides more prognostic information than morphological assessment in myeloma patients. *Haematologica* 2009;**94**(11):1599–602.
14. Paiva B, Vidriales MB, Mateo G *et al.* The persistence of immunophenotypically normal residual bone marrow plasma cells at diagnosis identifies a good prognostic subgroup of symptomatic multiple myeloma patients. *Blood* 2009;**114**(20):4369–72.
15. Diez-Campelo M, Perez-Simon JA, Perez J *et al.* Minimal residual disease monitoring after allogeneic

transplantation may help to individualize post-transplant therapeutic strategies in acute myeloid malignancies. *Am J Hematol* 2009; **84**(3):149–52.

16. Shaughnessy JD Jr, Zhan F, Burington BE *et al.* A validated gene expression model of high-risk multiple myeloma is defined by deregulated expression of genes mapping to chromosome 1. *Blood* 2007; **109**(6):2276–84.

17. Dewald GW, Kyle RA, Hicks GA, Greipp PR. The clinical significance of cytogenetic studies in 100 patients with multiple myeloma, plasma cell leukemia, or amyloidosis. *Blood* 1985;**66**(2):380–90.

18. Tricot G, Barlogie B, Jagannath S *et al.* Poor prognosis in multiple myeloma is associated only with partial or complete deletions of chromosome 13 or abnormalities involving 11q and not with other karyotype abnormalities. *Blood* 1995;**86**(11):4250–6.

19. Smadja NV, Bastard C, Brigaudeau C, Leroux D, Fruchart C. Hypodiploidy is a major prognostic factor in multiple myeloma. *Blood* 2001; **98**(7):2229–38.

20. Sawyer JR, Waldron JA, Jagannath S, Barlogie B. Cytogenetic findings in 200 patients with multiple myeloma. *Cancer Genet Cytogenet* 1995;**82**(1):41–9.

21. Rajkumar SV, Fonseca R, Dewald GW *et al.* Cytogenetic abnormalities correlate with the plasma cell labeling index and extent of bone marrow involvement in myeloma. *Cancer Genet Cytogenet* 1999;**113**(1):73–7.

22. Chesi M, Nardini E, Brents LA *et al.* Frequent translocation t(4;14)(p16.3;q32.3) in multiple myeloma is associated with increased expression and activating mutations of fibroblast growth factor receptor 3. *Nature Genetics* 1997;**16**(3):260–4.

23. Ahmann GJ, Jalal SM, Juneau AL *et al.* A novel three-color, clone-specific fluorescence in situ hybridization procedure for monoclonal gammopathies. *Cancer Genet Cytogenet* 1998;**101**(1):7–11.

24. Avet-Loiseau H, Andree-Ashley LE, Moore D 2nd *et al.* Molecular cytogenetic abnormalities in multiple myeloma and plasma cell leukemia measured using comparative genomic hybridization. *Genes Chromosomes Cancer* 1997;**19**(2):124–33.

25. Fonseca R, Bergsagel PL, Drach J *et al.* International Myeloma Working Group molecular classification of multiple myeloma: spotlight review. *Leukemia* 2009; **23**(12):2210–21.

26. Garand R, Avet-Loiseau H, Accard F *et al.* t(11;14) and t(4;14) translocations correlated with mature lymphoplasmacytoid and immature morphology, respectively, in multiple myeloma. *Leukemia* 2003;**17**:2032–5.

27. Avet-Loiseau H, Garand R, Lode L, Harousseau J-L, Bataille R. Translocation t(11;14)(q13;q32) is the hallmark of IgM, IgE, and nonsecretory multiple myeloma variants. *Blood* 2003;**101**(4):1570–1.

28. Schop RF, Kuehl WM, Van Wier SA *et al.* Waldenström macroglobulinemia neoplastic cells lack immunoglobulin heavy chain locus translocations but have frequent 6q deletions. *Blood* 2002; **100**(8):2996–3001.

29. Fonseca R, Blood E, Rue M *et al.* Clinical and biologic implications of recurrent genomic aberrations in myeloma. *Blood* 2003;**101**(11):4569–75.

30. Keats JJ, Fonseca R, Chesi M *et al.* Promiscuous mutations activate the noncanonical NF-kappaB pathway in multiple myeloma. *Cancer Cell* 2007; **12**(2):131–44.

31. Annunziata CM, Davis RE, Demchenko Y *et al.* Frequent engagement of the classical and alternative NF-kappaB pathways by diverse genetic abnormalities in multiple myeloma. *Cancer Cell* 2007;**12**(2):115–30.

32. Carrasco DR, Tonon G, Huang Y *et al.* High-resolution genomic profiles define distinct clinico-pathogenetic subgroups of multiple myeloma patients. *Cancer Cell* 2006;**9**(4):313–25.

33. Zhan F, Huang Y, Colla S *et al.* The molecular classification of multiple myeloma. *Blood* 2006; **108**(6):2020–8.

34. Katzmann JA, Clark R, Sanders E, Landers JP, Kyle RA. Prospective study of serum protein capillary zone electrophoresis and immunotyping of monoclonal proteins by immunosubtraction. *Am J Clin Pathol* 1998;**110**(4):503–9.

35. Katzmann JA, Clark R, Wiegert E *et al.* Identification of monoclonal proteins in serum: a quantitative comparison of acetate, agarose gel, and capillary electrophoresis. *Electrophoresis* 1997;**18** (10):1775–80.

36. Bradwell AR, Carr-Smith HD, Mead GP, Harvey TC, Drayson MT. Serum test for assessment of patients with Bence Jones myeloma. *Lancet* 2003; **361**(9356):489–91.

37. Abraham RS, Clark RJ, Bryant SC *et al.* Correlation of serum immunoglobulin free light chain quantification with urinary Bence Jones protein in light chain myeloma. *Clin Chem* 2002;**48**(4):655–7.

38. Durie BG, Salmon SE. A clinical staging system for multiple myeloma. Correlation of measured myeloma cell mass with presenting clinical features, response to treatment, and survival. *Cancer* 1975; **36**(3):842–54.

39. Greipp PR, San Miguel J, Durie BG *et al*. International staging system for multiple myeloma. *J Clin Oncol* 2005;**23**(15):3412–20.

40. Stewart AK, Bergsagel PL, Greipp PR *et al*. A practical guide to defining high-risk myeloma for clinical trials, patient counseling and choice of therapy. *Leukemia* 2007;**21**(3):529–34.

41. San Miguel JF, Schlag R, Khuageva NK *et al*. Bortezomib plus melphalan and prednisone for initial treatment of multiple myeloma. *New Engl J Med* 2008;**359**(9):906–17.

42. Jagannath S, Richardson PG, Sonneveld P *et al*. Bortezomib appears to overcome the poor prognosis conferred by chromosome 13 deletion in phase 2 and 3 trials. *Leukemia* 2007;**21**(1):151–7.

43. Chng WJ, Braggio E, Mulligan G *et al*. The centrosome index is a powerful prognostic marker in myeloma and identifies a cohort of patients that might benefit from aurora kinase inhibition. *Blood* 2008;**111**(3):1603–9.

44. Durie BG. Is magnitude of initial response predictive for survival in multiple myeloma? *Ann Oncol* 1991;**2**(3):166.

45. Blade J, Samson D, Reece D *et al*. Criteria for evaluating disease response and progression in patients with multiple myeloma treated by high-dose therapy and haemopoietic stem cell transplantation. Myeloma Subcommittee of the EBMT. European Group for Blood and Marrow Transplant. *Br J Haematol* 1998;**102**(5):1115–23.

46. Greipp PR, Kyle RA. Clinical, morphological, and cell kinetic differences among multiple myeloma, monoclonal gammopathy of undetermined significance, and smoldering multiple myeloma. *Blood* 1983;**62**(1):166–71.

47. Avet-Loiseau H, Facon T, Daviet A *et al*. 14q32 translocations and monosomy 13 observed in monoclonal gammopathy of undetermined significance delineate a multistep process for the oncogenesis of multiple myeloma. Intergroupe Francophone du Myelome. *Cancer Res* 1999; **59**(18):4546–50.

48. Fonseca R, Bailey RJ, Ahmann GJ *et al*. Genomic abnormalities in monoclonal gammopathy of undetermined significance. *Blood* 2002; **100**(4):1417–24.

49. Kyle RA, Therneau TM, Rajkumar SV *et al*. Long-term follow-up of 241 patients with monoclonal gammopathy of undetermined significance: the original Mayo Clinic series 25 years later.[see comment]. *Mayo Clinic Proceedings* 2004; **79**(7):859–66.

50. Perez-Persona E, Mateo G, Garcia-Sanz R *et al*. Risk of progression in smouldering myeloma and monoclonal gammopathies of unknown significance: comparative analysis of the evolution of monoclonal component and multiparameter flow cytometry of bone marrow plasma cells. *Br J Haematol* 2009;**148**(1):110–4.

51. Noel P, Kyle RA. Plasma cell leukemia: an evaluation of response to therapy. *Am J Med* 1987;**83**(6):1062–8.

52. Tiedemann RE, Gonzalez-Paz N, Kyle RA *et al*. Genetic aberrations and survival in plasma cell leukemia. *Leukemia* 2008;**22**(5):1044–52.

53. Avet-Loiseau H, Daviet A, Brigaudeau C *et al*. Cytogenetic, interphase, and multicolor fluorescence in situ hybridization analyses in primary plasma cell leukemia: a study of 40 patients at diagnosis, on behalf of the Intergroupe Francophone du Myelome and the Groupe Francais de Cytogenetique Hematologique. *Blood* 2001;**97**(3):822–5.

54. Garcia-Sanz R, Orfao A, Gonzalez M *et al*. Primary plasma cell leukemia: clinical, immunophenotypic, DNA ploidy, and cytogenetic characteristics. *Blood* 1999;**93**(3):1032–7.

55. Fonseca R, Hayman S. Waldenström macroglobulinaemia. *Br J Haematol* 2007;**138**(6):700–20.

56. Owen RG, Johnson SA, Morgan GJ. Waldenström's macroglobulinemia: laboratory diagnosis and treatment. *Hematol Oncol* 2000;**18**(2):41–9.

57. Treon SP, Dimopoulos M, Kyle RA. Defining Waldenström's macroglobulinemia. *Semin Oncol* 2003;**30**(2):107–9.

58. Schop RF, Jalal SM, Van Wier SA *et al*. Deletions of 17p13.1 and 13q14 are uncommon in Waldenström macroglobulinemia clonal cells and mostly seen at the time of disease progression. *Cancer Genet Cytogenet* 2002;**132**(1):55–60.

59. Schop RF, Van Wier SA, Xu R *et al*. 6q deletion discriminates Waldenström macroglobulinemia from IgM monoclonal gammopathy of undetermined significance. *Cancer Genet Cytogenet* 2006; **169**(2):150–3.

60. Braggio E, Keats JJ, Leleu X *et al*. Identification of copy number abnormalities and inactivating mutations in two negative regulators of nuclear factor-kappaB signaling pathways in Waldenström's macroglobulinemia. *Cancer Res* 2009;**69**(8):3579–88.

61. Ocio EM, Schop RF, Gonzalez B *et al*. 6q deletion in Waldenström macroglobulinemia is associated with features of adverse prognosis. *Br J Haematol* 2007; **136**(1):80–6.

Chronic myeloid leukemia

Emma J. Gudgin and Brian Huntly

Introduction

Chronic myeloid leukemia (CML) (named "chronic myelogenous leukemia, *BCR-ABL1* positive" in the WHO Classification) is a clonal myeloproliferative disease of hematopoietic stem cells. It is caused by a characteristic cytogenetic abnormality, the Philadephia chromosome (Ph), which results from a reciprocal translocation between the long arms of chromosomes 9 and 22 (Figure 13.1) [1]. This translocation results in the transfer of the Abelson (*ABL1*) proto-oncogene on chromosome 9 to an area of chromosome 22 termed the breakpoint cluster region (*BCR*), containing the *BCR* gene, thereby generating the *BCR-ABL1* fusion oncogene [2]. This produces an abnormal tyrosine kinase protein that causes the disordered myelopoiesis found in CML [3]. Work over the past 30 years on the pathogenesis of CML has led to a rationally designed therapy and the development of targeted tyrosine kinase inhibitors such as imatinib mesylate [4–8]. This agent, which first came into clinical use in 1998, has revolutionized the treatment of CML. Imatinib works as a competitive inhibitor of binding at the ABL1 kinase domain ATP pocket, binds to the inactive conformation of BCR-ABL1 and causes subsequent cell death.

The incidence of CML is 1–1.5 cases/100 000 per year, and accounts for approximately 15% of all leukemias [9]. The median age of diagnosis is 45–55 years [10], although CML can occur at any age, and there is a slightly higher incidence in men [11]. Although the molecular pathogenesis is well defined, the cause of the chromosomal translocation is not known. There is a slight increased risk with radiation exposure but no other risk factors have been identified [12].

Chronic myeloid leukemia is divided into three phases. The initial phase is the relatively indolent chronic phase (CP), which if untreated has a median duration of 3–5 years. This is followed by the aggressive advanced phases of the disease, divided into accelerated phase (AP) and blast phase; the latter is an acute leukemia, and is further characterized by a block in differentiation. The vast majority of patients present in chronic phase, many as an incidental finding on a full blood count. Common presenting features include fatigue, weight loss, night sweats, mild anemia and symptoms relating to splenomegaly resulting from extramedullary hematopoiesis. A minority of patients are diagnosed with advanced phases of the disease without any history of antecedent CP. Symptoms here usually relate to more severe anemia, thrombocytopenia and splenomegaly. It is likely that imatinib has changed the natural history of the disease and appears to have the majority of its effect by prolonging CP, however, how long this will be on average remains to be seen.

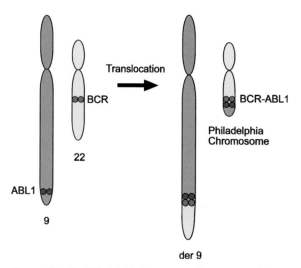

Figure 13.1. The Philadelphia chromosome. The majority of the *ABL1* gene (red) on chromosome 9 (blue) is translocated into the *BCR* locus (green) on chromosome 22 (yellow), to form the *BCR-ABL1* fusion oncogene (see Figure 13.4 for molecular resolution).

Diagnostic Techniques in Hematological Malignancies, ed. Wendy N. Erber. Published by Cambridge University Press.
© Cambridge University Press 2010.

Diagnosis of chronic myeloid leukemia

Chronic myeloid leukemia, chronic phase

Blood and bone marrow morphology: The majority of patients with CML are diagnosed in chronic phase (CP). The diagnosis is initially made on the characteristic blood count and film appearances (Table 13.1 and Figure 13.2a, b). The major blood film abnormalities are a neutrophil leukocytosis with granulocytic progenitors at all stages of differentiation being present. There is a bimodal peak of myelocytes and mature neutrophils. There is a basophilia but the basophils can sometimes be difficult to identify as they are commonly hypogranular. A mild eosinophilia, frequently showing basophilic as well as eosinophilic granules ("baso-eosinophils") and monocytosis are common; there is no dysplasia. Blast cells are usually present but account for less than 5% of leukocytes in chronic phase. The red cells are normochromic and normocytic. The platelet count may be normal or there may be thrombocytosis; thrombocytopenia is uncommon.

The bone marrow is markedly hypercellular due to granulocytic hyperplasia but with normal differentiation. Eosinophils and basophils are prominent and erythropoiesis appears relatively reduced. The megakaryocytes are distinctive in CML: they are smaller than normal and the nuclei are hypolobated (mono- or bi-lobed nuclei are a feature). Sea-blue histiocytes, indicating long-standing granulocytic hyperplasia, and pseudo-Gaucher cells may be present. Bone marrow trephine features include granulocytic hyperplasia, a thickened paratrabecular cuff of immature granulocytic progenitors and megakaryocytic hyperplasia with the distinctive "dwarf" morphology (Figure 13.2c, d). Small clusters of interstitial immature cells may be present even in chronic phase. It is however not essential

Table 13.1. Blood, bone marrow aspirate and trephine biopsy features of chronic myeloid leukemia in chronic phase.

	Quantitative features	Qualitative features
Leukocyte count	Leukocytosis up to 1000 × 10^9/L, median 100 × 10^9/L Blasts usually < 2% Basophilia Eosinophilia (common) Monocytosis (mild)	All stages of granulocytic development present in the blood Mature neutrophils and myelocytes predominate (bimodal peak) Eosinophils with basophilic granules
Hemoglobin	Low or normal Rarely increased	
Platelets	Normal or raised (upto 1000 × 10^9/L)	
BM aspirate and trephine	Greatly increased cellularity	
BM granulopoiesis	Marked granulocytic hyperplasia Blasts usually <5%	Thick paratrabecular cuff of immature granulocytes Small interstitial islands of blast cells may be present
BM megakaryocytes	Megakaryocytes may be reduced, normal or increased	Small, hypolobated "dwarf" or "micro" megakaryocytes may be prominent Increased megakaryocytes may be associated with moderate to severe fibrosis
BM erythropoiesis	Relatively reduced	Normoblastic
Other BM features	Sea-blue histiocytes (occasional) Pseudo-Gaucher cells (rare)	

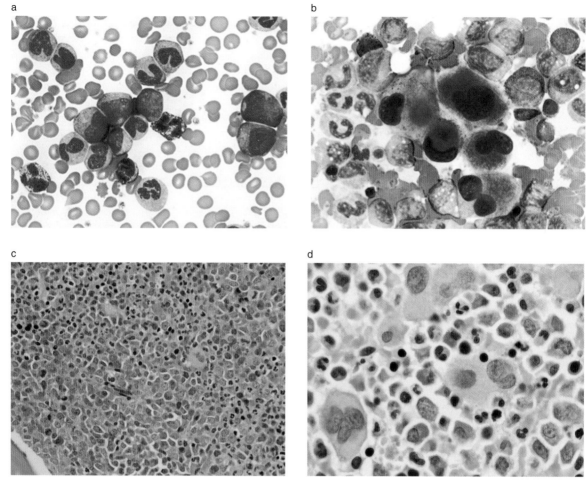

Figure 13.2. Morphology of chronic myeloid leukemia.
a. Peripheral blood smear of chronic phase CML, hematoxylin and eosin (H&E), 100×.
b. Bone marrow aspirate showing small hypolobular megakaryocytes, H&E, 100×.
c. Bone marrow trephine biopsy showing granulocytic hyperplasia. There is a thickened paratrabecular cuff of early myeloid precursors.
d. High power view of the bone marrow trephine showing megakaryocytic hyperplasia with "dwarf" (small) forms and hypolobated nuclei.

to perform a bone marrow trephine at diagnosis of CML although it can give a useful baseline of disease status.

Immunophenotyping: Immunophenotyping does not have a routine role in the diagnosis of CML. However, phenotypic assessment of blast cells may be useful where these constitute more than 5% of nucleated cells. Immunocytochemistry can be used to determine the phenotype of nodular aggregates of interstitial blast cells in bone marrow trephine biopsies.

Cytogenetics: Confirmation of the diagnosis of CML is obtained by identification of the Philadelphia (Ph) chromosome. This can be performed by karyotypic analysis of metaphase cells from bone marrow, as shown in Figure 13.3a (using Giemsa or G-banding), or detection of the *BCR-ABL1* fusion by fluorescence *in situ* hybridization (FISH) on interphase cells (Figure 13.3b) from peripheral blood or bone marrow. Ideally, both karyotyping and FISH should be performed at diagnosis. Full karyotypic analysis is necessary to look for further chromosomal abnormalities that may be present at

a

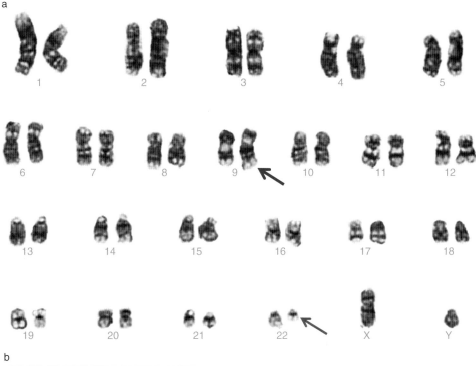

b

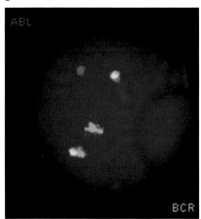

Figure 13.3. a. Karyotype showing the Philadelphia chromosome t(9;22) derivative chromosome 22 (red arrow), and the derivative chromosome 9 (blue arrow).
b. Dual color FISH of chronic phase CML, showing one normal *ABL1* signal on chromosome 9 (single red signal), one normal *BCR* signal on chromosome 22 (single green signal) and two fusion signals (red, green and yellow fused signals) one from *ABL1-BCR* on chromosome 9 and the other from *BCR-ABL1* on chromosome 22.

diagnosis; more commonly these occur in, and help to define, advanced stage disease. In less than 5% of cases the Ph chromosome is not detectable by Giemsa banding; however, in the majority of these the *BCR-ABL1* fusion is detectable by FISH (Figure 13.4). Cases that lack a classical Ph chromosome may still rearrange a *BCR-ABL1* oncogene, either through insertion of 5' *BCR* into the *ABL1* locus on chromosome 9, or 3' *ABL1* into the *BCR* locus on chromosome 22. There may also be a variant translocation involving other chromosomes in addition to 9 and 22. In the former case the change in size of chromosomes 9 and 22 is minimal and the karyotype appears normal. In the latter the most obvious karyotypic change may not involve chromosomes 9 and/or 22. FISH with probes for the *ABL1* and *BCR* loci is therefore very helpful in this situation. FISH is also important for detecting abnormal chromosomal deletions, e.g. deletion of the reciprocal translocation *ABL1-BCR*

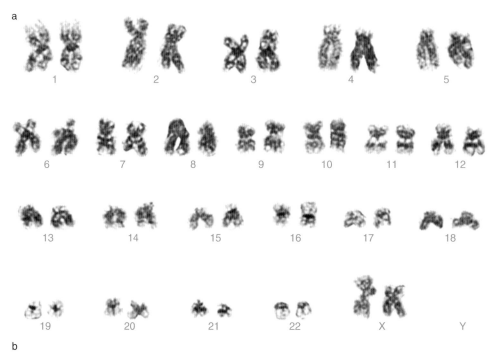

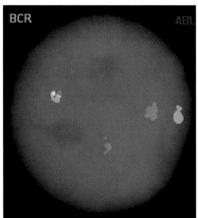

Figure 13.4. "Masked" Philadelphia translocation.
a. Apparently normal karyotype.
b. FISH showing abnormal chromosome 22 (green, yellow and red conjoined signals).

on chromosome 9q, which may be present at diagnosis.

Molecular genetics: *BCR-ABL1* transcripts can also be detected by polymerase chain reaction (PCR) techniques (see Chapter 5 for details). Both qualitative reverse transcriptase-PCR and quantitative real-time PCR (qRT-PCR) can be used at diagnosis. qRT-PCR is preferable as it gives a baseline against which comparisons can be made when used for molecular monitoring of therapy. However, the sensitivity of detection of *BCR-ABL1* can vary significantly between samples. This may be due to:

1. Differences in the amount of sample mRNA extracted.
2. Integrity of the RNA.
3. Efficiency with which the RNA is reverse transcribed into cDNA.

Therefore, to allow reproducibility between samples at different time points, a ratio is calculated: the level of *BCR-ABL1* cDNA in the sample is related to the level of cDNA of another constitutively expressed "housekeeping" gene, which ideally is expressed at the same or similar level in leukemic and normal cells. This allows for differences in the amount and quality of the mRNA to be accounted for. There is ongoing debate about the most appropriate control gene that should be used. *ABL1* is used in most laboratories, although others such as *BCR* and $\beta_2$microglobulin have been proposed [13].

The breakpoints within the *BCR* gene occur in three main regions (Figure 13.4). The commonest is the major breakpoint cluster region, or M-BCR, within a 5.8 kb area spanning *BCR* exons e12–e16 (previously referred to as exons b1–b5); due to alternative splicing either e13 or e14 fusion mRNA may be produced. Translocations involving the M-BCR, minor breakpoint cluster region (m-BCR) and the μ-BCR give rise to BCR-ABL1 mRNA transcripts of different lengths (Figure 13.5). The ABL1 portion is fairly constant, although breakpoints in *ABL1* can occur anywhere over a large (greater than 300 kb) area at its 5' end. Wherever the breakpoint in *ABL1*, the mRNA transcribed is virtually always BCR joined to *ABL1* exon a2, although rare exceptions do exist. Most patients with CML, and approximately one third of patients with Ph-positive acute lymphoblastic leukemia (ALL), have breakpoints in the M-BCR. This results in the generation of e13a2 or e14a2 transcripts which are translated to a 210 kDa chimeric protein, P210. In the majority of patients with Ph-positive ALL, the e1a2 transcript

is formed, which produces a 190 kDa fusion protein P190. Due to alternative splicing, a small amount of P190 may be found in over 90% of CML patients [14]. P190 is also the main abnormal fusion protein produced in a small number of CML patients, who have increased monocytes, which may resemble chronic myelomonocytic leukemia; this suggests that the site of the breakpoint can influence the phenotype of the disease [15,16]. In keeping with this, the rare P230 fusion protein is particularly associated with increased neutrophils, resembling chronic neutrophilic leukemia [17].

In a small number of patients with the clinical features of CML, no Ph chromosome or *BCR-ABL1* rearrangement or transcripts can be detected. These patients are referred to as Ph-negative, *BCR-ABL1*-negative or "Atypical CML, *BCR-ABL1*-negative" and are now considered to be a separate disease entity, due to obvious differences in biology. They usually do not fit the standard morphological pattern, typically showing less basophilia, a less pronounced excess of myelocytes and neutrophils and a degree of dysplasia. A minority may have other kinase fusion proteins, which may be imatinib sensitive, such as FIP1L1-PDGRFα or β. In such patients, full karyotyping and molecular investigation for potential imatinib-sensitive alternative kinase fusions should

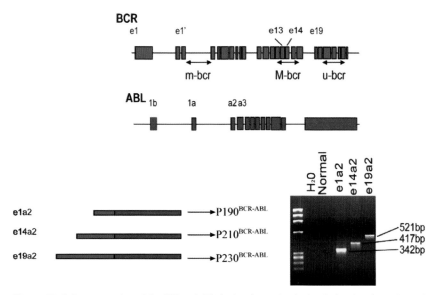

Figure 13.5. Representation of the *BCR* and *ABL1* loci at the molecular level, showing the major, minor and μ breakpoint sites. Exons are represented as filled boxes, and introns as lines. The insert shows the three main fusion mRNA transcribed: e1a2, e14a2 or e13a2 and e19a2 are translated to P190, P210 and P230 respectively. The different mRNA lengths are visualized by running on a 1% agarose gel containing ethidium bromide.

be performed. Atypical CML, *BCR-ABL1* negative is discussed further in Chapter 15.

Accelerated and blast phase

Patients known to have CML may develop clinical features suggesting advancing disease in addition to splenomegaly, such as bone pain, weight loss and night sweats. The World Health Organization defines accelerated phase (AP) disease as the presence of one or more of the following [9]:

1. Myeloblasts making up 10–19% of nucleated cells in the blood or bone marrow.
2. Basophils comprising ≥20% of the peripheral blood leukocyte count.
3. Cytogenetic evidence of clonal evolution.
4. Platelets persistently ≤100 × 10^9/L or ≥ 1000 × 10^9/L despite appropriate CML therapy.
5. Increasing splenomegaly and increasing leukocyte count despite appropriate CML therapy.

In addition to the WHO, there are several other classification systems for the definition of the different phases of CML. The European Leukaemia Network expert panel criteria [18], which are also widely used, does not classify cytogenetic evidence of clonal evolution as defining AP in the absence of other features of disease progression. Other features that are suggestive, but not diagnostic of disease that is progressing to AP include the development of marked dysgranulopoiesis or bone marrow fibrosis.

A peripheral blood blast count of ≥ 20%, defines blast phase (BP), or blast crisis, and clinically is considered an acute leukemia. Other diagnostic features of blast phase are the presence of large interstitial nodular aggregates of blast cells in the bone marrow trephine biopsy and an extramedullary blast cell proliferation. In approximately 75% of cases the blast cells are of myeloid lineage, and may include blasts of the basophil, eosinophil and megakaryocyte lineages. In the remaining 25% the blast cells are lymphoid in origin, most commonly of B-cell lineage. Expression of aberrant lineage markers is not uncommon, but true bilineage transformation is rare.

Prognosis and risk stratification

Several prognostic factors can be identified at diagnosis, the most important of which is the phase of disease. In CP, other clinical and laboratory information obtained prior to treatment may be used to generate a prognostic score, as devised by Sokal [19] or Hasford [20] (Table 13.2). These utilize patient age, spleen size and blood count parameters to stratify patients into risk groups with both scoring systems dividing patients into low-, intermediate- or high-risk disease. Although devised for patients treated with interferon-α and hydroxycarbamide, both scoring systems can be used to predict the cytogenetic response to standard dose imatinib [21,22]. The Sokal score has been reported to also predict major molecular responses and overall survival (OS) in imatinib-treated patients [23]. Other factors such as a high initial *BCR-ABL1* expression level, and baseline cytogenetic changes such as additional copies of the Ph chromosome may be associated with an adverse prognosis [23]. The European Leukaemia Network [18] have described "warning features":

1. At diagnosis:
   a. High-risk Sokal or Hasford score (Table 13.2)
   b. Additional cytogenetic abnormalities (ACA) in Ph-positive cells
2. At 12 months: less than major molecular response
3. At any time:
   a. Any sustained rise in transcript level
   b. Other cytogenetic abnormalities (OCA) in Ph-positive cells

These merit more stringent response monitoring, however it should be noted that these characteristics have not been formally demonstrated to alter prognosis in patients treated up-front with tyrosine kinase inhibitors.

Following the initiation of treatment, the level and timing of hematological, cytogenetic and molecular responses to therapy also strongly predict response (Tables 13.3 and 13.4); early cytogenetic response is the most important of these parameters in response prediction [24–26]. Minimal residual disease is most accurately measured by *BCR-ABL1* transcript levels. Undetectable *BCR-ABL1* transcripts are associated with better progression-free survival, whereas a documented and sustained rise in transcript level is associated with loss of response to therapy.

Table 13.2. Sokal and Hasford prognostic scoring systems (Online calculator available at http://www.icsg.unibo.it/rrcalc.asp).

	Sokal score	Hasford score
Age	0.0116 (age – 43.4 years)	0.6666 if age ≥ 50 years
Spleen size (cm below costal margin)	0.0345 (spleen size – 7.51)	0.042 × spleen size
Platelet count × 10^9/L	0.188 [(platelets/700)^2 – 0.563]	1.0956 if platelets ≥ 1500 10^9/L
PB blasts, %	0.0887 (blasts – 2.1)	0.0584 × myeloblasts
PB basophils, %		0.20399 when basophils > 3%
PB eosinophils, %		0.0413 × eosinophils
Relative risk	Score = Exponential of total of above scores	Score = total of above scores × 100
Low risk	<0.8	≤780
Intermediate risk	0.8–1.2	781–1480
High risk	>1.2	>1480

Table 13.3. European Group for Blood and Marrow Transplantation (EBMT) allogeneic transplantation risk score [39].

	Prognostic factors	Score
Donor	HLA identical sibling	0
	Other	1
Stage	First chronic phase	0
	Accelerated phase	1
	Blast crisis	2
Age	< 20	0
	20–40	1
	> 40	2
Sex match	Male recipient/ female donor	1
	Any other combination	1
Time from diagnosis to transplantation	< 12 months	0
	> 12 months	1

Table 13.4. European Group for Blood and Marrow Transplantation (EBMT) data for outcome of allogeneic hematopoietic stem cell transplantation for CML at 2 years in patients transplanted between 2000–2003: survival, transplant-related mortality and relapse.

EBMT risk score	2-year survival	Transplant-related mortality	Relapse incidence
0–1	80%	17%	16%
2–4	60%	32%	22%
>4	38%	41%	31%

1. Hematological remission rate: 98%.
2. Major cytogenetic remission rate: 92%.
3. Complete cytogenetic remission rate: 87%.
4. Progression-free survival (PFS): 84% [24].

As the majority of interferon-α patients crossed over into the imatinib treatment group, overall survival differences were difficult to demonstrate in this trial, but retrospective analyses show a clear overall survival benefit [27,28]. Similar results to the IRIS trial were obtained from two other single institution studies [29,30]. The results from these trials may however represent the best results achievable as the patients in these studies may not have been representative of the CML population as a whole. A population-based study showed a significantly worse level of response for all criteria [31], more in keeping with individual center

Treatment

Patients presenting with CML in chronic phase are initially treated with imatinib. This has become the standard of care since the landmark International Randomized Study of Interferon and STI571 (IRIS) trial [6] which randomized over 1000 early CP CML patients between imatinib (previously known as STI571) and interferon-α. After 5 years of follow-up, the imatinib group showed the following responses, as defined in Table 13.5:

Table 13.5. European Leukaemia Network (ELN) definitions of hematological, cytogenetic and molecular responses.

Complete hematological response	Cytogenetic response (CgR)		Molecular response (MolR)
WCC < 10 × 10⁹/L	% of Ph+ cells:		Complete (CMolR):
Platelet count < 450 × 10⁹/L	Complete (CCgR):	0%	No detectable *BCR-ABL* transcripts
No immature granulocytes in PB	Partial (PCgR):	1–35%	
Basophils < 5% of blood leukocytes	Minor (MCgR):	36–65%	Major (MMolR):
No palpable splenomegaly	Minimum (minCgR):	66–95%	*BCR-ABL*: control gene ratio < 0.1
	None:	> 95%	

practice. The current "gold standard" for CML patients presenting in CP is to treat with imatinib 400 mg/day. However, even is being challenged in prospective clinical trials assessing higher doses of imatinib [32,33] and newer second generation kinase inhibitors in comparison to imatinib [34,35].

Although imatinib treatment has already surpassed initial expectations, the long-term outcome of this therapy is not yet fully known, and treatment failures and resistance do occur. Overall in both IRIS and another recent study, approximately one-third of patients had discontinued imatinib treatment due to drug intolerance or, more commonly, treatment failure or the development of resistance after an initial response [36]. Such resistance is multi-factorial, with the most important factors likely to be:

1. Development of *BCR-ABL1* kinase domain mutations which interfere with imatinib binding or the conformation of *BCR-ABL1*.
2. Clonal evolution leading to *BCR-ABL1* over-expression and activation of alternative oncogenic pathways.
3. Multidrug resistance gene expression resulting in reduced intracellular concentrations of imatinib may also play a role [37].

Disease monitoring

Laboratory monitoring of hematological, cytogenetic and molecular responses is essential in guiding therapeutic decisions in CP CML (Figure 13.6). The type and frequency of disease monitoring (discussed in the next section) reflect therapeutic response with more frequent monitoring recommended for patients with "warning" features. Other treatment options are considered in cases of excessive toxicity, or failure or suboptimal response as described in Figure 13.7.

The most appropriate therapy for patients failing imatinib is not yet fully clear, with several available options. The optimal therapy will depend on patient age and allogeneic stem cell donor availability. Second generation kinase inhibitors and other targeted therapies are in clinical use or in development. These agents can overcome the majority of kinase domain mutations; dose escalation of imatinib may also be beneficial in this situation. Allogeneic stem cell transplantation (SCT) provides long-term, disease-free survival in approximately 50% of eligible patients treated in CP [38], but at the risk of major toxicity and mortality (Tables 13.3 and 13.4). The European Group for Blood and Marrow Transplantation (EBMT) is a large registry which collates survival data from a large number of patients undergoing stem cell transplantation procedures. Data registry has demonstrated that survival post stem cell transplant depends on five main factors, as listed in Table 13.3 [39]. An EBMT allogeneic transplantation risk scoring system was devised based on these data; a score of 7 carries the highest risk of death, and 0 the lowest. This is illustrated in Table 13.4, which shows the EBMT outcome data for CML patients at 2 years following allogeneic transplantation based on the EBMT score. The use of reduced intensity conditioning regimes to decrease treatment-related toxicity may improve outcomes and allow transplantation in older patients with higher EBMT scores [40]; however, currently its scope remains experimental. Classical cytotoxic drugs such as hydroxycarbamide may also be used, but would only control the WCC, and other experimental agents may be considered [41].

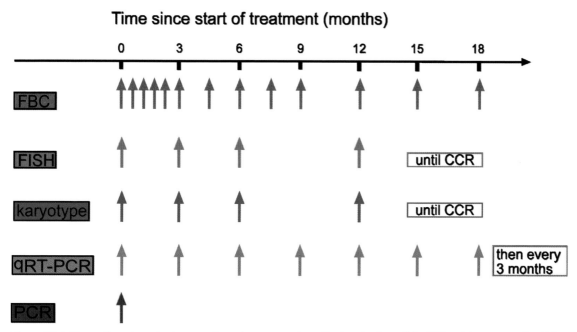

Figure 13.6. Diagnostic and monitoring tests for patients presenting with chronic phase CML. FISH and karyotyping should be performed on BM and qRT-PCR on peripheral blood. At any time, if qRT-PCR shows an increase in the level of *BCR-ABL1* transcripts, this should be repeated immediately. An obviously rising transcript level is an indication for a bone marrow aspirate, FISH and full karyotype, to assess phase of disease, cytogenetic relapse and to look for ACA. In addition tyrosine kinase mutation screening should also be performed at this time.

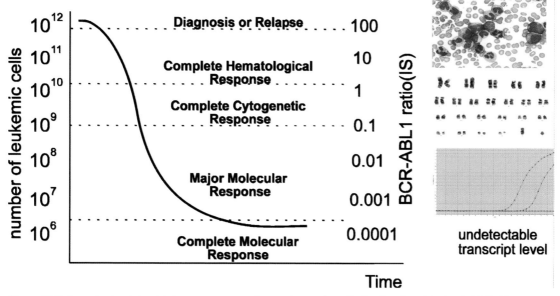

Figure 13.7. Approximate relationship between response, the putative number of leukemic cells and the level of *BCR-ABL1* transcripts. Possible monitoring methods are depicted on the right of the figure.

Monitoring of chronic phase CML

It has long been established that there is a correlation between a reduction in disease "bulk" and progression-free survival (PFS) and OS in CML. However, previous non-transplant treatments have been largely ineffective in producing deep and sustained cytogenetic and molecular responses. The advent of tyrosine kinase inhibitor therapy has resulted in excellent cytogenetic and molecular responses being achieved routinely. This has resulted in new approaches to quantify disease response. Patients treated with imatinib show a marked variation in the speed of response, and the level to which the leukemic cells are reduced (Figure 13.7). Closely monitoring response to treatment is therefore important because the depth to which the leukemia burden is reduced correlates with a reduced incidence of progression to advanced phase disease [42]. Also patients who respond poorly, or who lose a previous response may be rapidly identified and alternative therapeutic strategies considered. The European Leukaemia Network [18] has defined response criteria, as outlined in Table 13.5. The definitions of "failure" and "suboptimal" responses to therapy are illustrated in Figure 13.8.

1. If only a sub-optimal response is achieved the patient should be offered other treatments whenever available.
2. In failure of imatinib therapy the long-term treatment outcome from continuing imatinib is not likely to be ideal. Other treatments should be considered.

Hematological monitoring: In a newly diagnosed CP CML patient, hematological response to imatinib should be assessed by performing a blood count as follows:

1. Fortnightly until complete hematological response (CHR) is achieved and confirmed, and,
2. Every 3 months, unless otherwise required.

The value of regular monitoring of bone marrow aspirate and trephine biopsy appearances is debatable. A bone marrow morphological scoring system has been devised for disease monitoring which strongly correlates with complete cytogenetic response [43]. Persistent high-level morphological abnormalities early on herald a high likelihood of treatment failure.

Cytogenetic monitoring: Cytogenetic response should be assessed as follows:

1. At 3 and 6 months [18];
2. Then every 6 months until complete cytogenetic remission (CCgR) is achieved and confirmed;
3. Then at least every 12 months.

The best method of measuring cytogenetic response is debated. Both karyotyping and FISH can be used but the two techniques are not necessarily directly comparable (Table 13.6). Karyotyping typically only examines 20 cells and therefore the sensitivity of the test is relatively low, and the confidence interval for the results high. Metaphases from bone marrow are required, which may grow less well in culture than

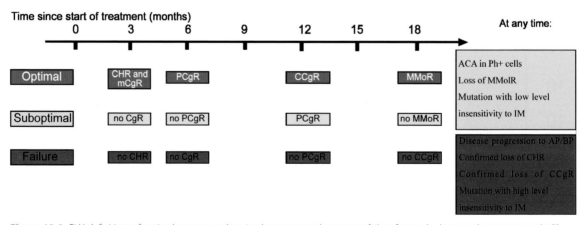

Figure 13.8. ELN definitions of optimal response, suboptimal response and treatment failure for newly diagnosed patients in early CP CML treated with 400 mg imatinib daily.

Table 13.6. Comparison of karyotyping, fluorescence *in situ* hybridization (FISH) and molecular monitoring of *BCR-ABL1* [62].

	Karyotyping	FISH	qRT-PCR
Sensitivity	5–10%	0.1–1%	0.001–0.01%
Accuracy	± 15%	± 2–5%	± 2–5 fold
Blood or marrow	BM metaphases	PB or BM	PB or BM
False positivity	Rare	Yes: 2–5%	Yes: ≤ 0.1%
False negativity	Yes	Yes	Yes
Detection of ACA	Yes	No	No
Detection of OCA	Yes	No	No

ACA = additional chromosomal abnormalities; OCA = other cytogenetic abnormalities; PB = peripheral blood; BM = bone marrow.

normal cells after exposure to imatinib. Karyotyping, however, does have the advantage of detecting additional cytogenetic abnormalities in Ph-positive cells and other cytogenetic abnormalities in Ph-negative cells. FISH, on the other hand, has the advantage of evaluating many more cells (typically 100–200) which improves the sensitivity of detection to between 1 in 100 to 1 in 1000 cells. The false positive rate is relatively high at 2–5% [37], although this can be reduced when three or four probes are used. This is particularly important when evaluating for complete cytogenetic response. Another advantage of FISH is that peripheral blood may be used, rather than bone marrow, as interphase cells are assessed. It should also be noted that Ph-positive cells may clear faster from blood than the bone marrow. The response criteria developed by the European Leukaemia Network were based on conventional bone marrow cytogenetics and from many clinical trials. Therefore bone marrow karyotyping rather than FISH is suggested for the majority of patients. One exception to this is when the genetic abnormalities at diagnosis are only detectable on FISH. In practice genetic monitoring by karyotyping may not be feasible for routine monitoring as it is time consuming and labor intensive. It may therefore be appropriate to reserve karyotyping for patients with warning features or those showing a suboptimal response.

The development of additional cytogenetic abnormalities in a proportion of Ph-positive cells demonstrates "clonal evolution." Examples of non-random ACAs are:

1. An extra Ph chromosome.
2. Trisomy 8.
3. Isochromosome 17.
4. Trisomies of chromosomes 19 and 20.
5. 20q abnormalities.

Additional cytogenetic abnormalities are more common in advanced phase (accelerated or blast phase) disease, and are associated with a higher hematological relapse rate, lower complete cytogenetic remission rate and shorter overall survival at 2 years [44]. In CP they are therefore a warning sign of impending treatment failure, and suggest the need for closer monitoring and consideration of other therapeutic strategies or a dose increase of imatinib.

Other cytogenetic abnormalities occur in Ph-negative cells in approximately 5% of patients who have achieved CCgR with imatinib [45–47]. OCA include:

1. Trisomy 8.
2. Trisomy 8 with other abnormalities.
3. Deletion of chromosome 7.

The development of OCAs may be related to the evolution of a myelodysplastic clone. Over a median follow-up of 51 months, the prognosis for patients with OCA in the absence of myelodysplasia was the same as those without OCA [48]. However, patients with known OCA require more frequent monitoring of cytogenetics, *BCR-ABL1* transcripts [18] and blood and bone marrow morphology, as the long-term clinical significance is not yet known. For this reason prospective monitoring for the development of OCA remains controversial.

BCR-ABL1 transcript monitoring: Molecular response is determined by measuring the *BCR-ABL1* transcript ratio compared to a control gene by qRT-PCR. For this RNA extracted from peripheral blood buffy coat cells or BM can be used; in practice blood cells are almost always used. The results are given either as:

1. The ratio of *BCR-ABL1* to control gene transcript numbers on a log10 scale × 100%, or,
2. "Log reduction" from a standardized baseline derived from results obtained in a series of untreated patients [49].

In the IRIS trial molecular responses were defined as a log reduction in the number of *BCR-ABL1* transcripts, with a 3 log reduction being shown to be associated with increased progression-free survival (PFS).

To minimize variability in qRT-PCR results serial measurements should be performed on the same tissue (usually blood rather than marrow), by the same high-quality laboratory, and using reliable collection and transport procedures. To achieve inter-laboratory standardization, an International Scale (IS) for molecular monitoring has been proposed. The International Scale will require validation of two known reference samples of plasmids, lyophilized cells or cell extracts. Each laboratory would then have a conversion factor for its own results, to enable true comparisons in international and national databases [50].

Molecular responses by *BCR-ABL1* to control gene ratio should be assessed every 3 months. If the level of *BCR-ABL1* transcripts appears to be rising, the test should be repeated immediately without waiting another 3 months. If treatment fails, or there is a suboptimal therapeutic response, as defined by the European Leukaemia Network response criteria (Figure 13.6), the following analyses should be performed:

1. Mutation analysis to look for kinase domain mutations; this should be performed using the same cDNA that was used for the qRT-PCR analysis.
2. Bone marrow aspirate morphology.
3. Cytogenetics (karyotype) to determine phase of disease, cytogenetic status and to look for ACA.

The additional information gained from these tests will subsequently contribute to informed therapeutic decisions.

Mutation detection: Resistance to imatinib is often caused by selection of mutations in the *BCR-ABL1* kinase domain, altering residues that are directly or indirectly critical for imatinib binding [51–54]. The most common method of detecting point mutations of the kinase domain in clinical practice is by allele-specific oligonucleotide PCR (ASO-PCR). In this technique DNA is amplified with both normal and mutation-specific forward oligonucleotide primers (ASO) and a common reverse primer. The allele-specific primers are designed such that they are complementary to one of the several possible mutations; only the perfectly matched oligonucleotide is therefore able to act as a primer for amplification. To date over 90 different mutations in the kinase domain have been described and the clinical significance of many is unknown. Since each mutation requires a specific primer, screening is generally only performed for the most common mutations [55,56]. Alternative methods of mutation detection are by direct sequencing of the DNA kinase domain, or by denaturing high performance liquid chromatography; these technologies are not usually available outside large research facilities and hence are not suitable in clinical practice.

The frequency of mutations in imatinib-resistant patients varies between 42% [57] and 90% [52]. This wide range is because of the different methods used to detect mutants, the clinical definition of resistance, and the phase of disease, with more mutations seen in advanced phase CML. Although mutations are more common in patients with advanced disease and chronic phase patients with increasing *BCR-ABL1* transcript levels [53,58], mutant clones may remain at very low levels or disappear entirely. Mutations may therefore not necessarily be associated with an increased chance of relapse or disease progression [59,60]. Different mutations have different biochemical and clinical properties, and therefore require different clinical strategies to treat them. For example,

1. Some mutations do not confer any resistance to imatinib and so are clinically irrelevant.
2. Some can be overcome by increased doses of imatinib.
3. Some mutations, such as the T315I mutation, are resistant to imatinib and second-generation TK inhibitors.

It is for this reason that the significance of a mutation must be interpreted in the clinical context of the specific patient. However, T315I mutations are uniformly problematic and allogeneic transplantation or experimental therapies should be considered in these patients.

Disease monitoring of accelerated and blast phase CML

There are fewer data available on treatment outcomes and monitoring of patients who present with advanced phase CML. Patients presenting with accelerated phase disease, who therefore have not been previously treated with imatinib, may be given 600–800 mg/day imatinib, as long as no imatinib-resistant mutation is present. Hematological, cytogenetic and molecular monitoring should be performed more frequently than described above for CP disease. The aim of therapy in these patients is to generate a second (or later) chronic phase, then consideration for consolidation with allogeneic transplantation if appropriate. If the disease presents, or has progressed to blast phase, then the treatment and monitoring is similar to that for acute leukemia (see Chapters 7 and 8). However the expected duration of response following disease control with imatinib and cytotoxic chemotherapy is likely to be relatively short, and therefore allogeneic transplantation should be considered.

Conclusion

Chronic myeloid leukemia is probably the most comprehensively studied and best understood malignancy today. It is a model of scientific knowledge directing rational drug design and dramatically altering the lives of many patients living with this malignancy. The hematology laboratory plays a key role in this process: making the diagnosis, determining prognosis, predicting changes in the disease natural history and monitoring response to therapy.

Acknowledgments

The authors wish to thank Bridget Manasse, Anthony Bench and Wendy Erber for providing the cytogenetic and morphology images.

References

1. Nowell PC, Hungerford DA. A minute chromosome in human chronic granulocytic leukemia. *Science* 1960;**132**:1497–501.

2. Heisterkamp N, Groffen J, Stephenson JR et al. Chromosomal localization of human cellular homologues of two viral oncogenes. *Nature* 1982;**299** (5885):747–9.

3. Daley GQ, Van Etten RA, Baltimore D. Induction of chronic myelogenous leukemia in mice by the P210bcr/abl gene of the Philadelphia chromosome. *Science* 1990;**247**(4944):824–30.

4. Goldman JM, Melo JV. Chronic myeloid leukemia – advances in biology and new approaches to treatment. *New Engl J Med* 2003;**349**(15):1451–64.

5. Druker BJ, Tamura S, Buchdunger E et al. Effects of a selective inhibitor of the Abl tyrosine kinase on the growth of *Bcr-Abl* positive cells. *Nat Med* 1996;**2** (5):561–6.

6. O'Brien SG, Guilhot F, Larson RA et al. Imatinib compared with interferon and low-dose cytarabine for newly diagnosed chronic-phase chronic myeloid leukemia. *New Engl J Med* 2003;**348**(11):994–1004.

7. Sawyers CL, Hochhaus A, Feldman E et al. Imatinib induces hematologic and cytogenetic responses in patients with chronic myelogenous leukemia in myeloid blast crisis: results of a phase II study. *Blood* 2002;**99**(10):3530–9.

8. Druker BJ, Talpaz M, Resta DJ et al. Efficacy and safety of a specific inhibitor of the BCR-ABL tyrosine kinase in chronic myeloid leukemia. *New Engl J Med* 2001;**344**(14):1031–7.

9. Vardiman JW, Melo JV, Baccarani M, Thiele J. Chronic myelogenous leukaemia, *BCR-ABL1* positive. In Jaffe ES, Harris, NL, Stein H, Vardiman JW (eds.), *Tumours of Haematopoietic and Lymphoid Tissues*. Lyon: IARC Press; 2008:32–7.

10. Faderl S, Talpaz M, Estrov Z, Kantarjian HM. Chronic myelogenous leukemia: biology and therapy. *Ann Intern Med* 1999;**131**(3):207–19.

11. Berger U, Maywald O, Pfirrmann M et al. Gender aspects in chronic myeloid leukemia: long-term results from randomized studies. *Leukemia* 2005;**19** (6):984–9.

12. Corso A, Lazzarino M, Morra E et al. Chronic myelogenous leukemia and exposure to ionizing radiation – a retrospective study of 443 patients. *Ann Hematol* 1995;**70**(2):79–82.

13. Beillard E, Pallisgaard N, van der Velden VH et al. Evaluation of candidate control genes for diagnosis and residual disease detection in leukemic patients using 'real-time' quantitative reverse-transcriptase polymerase chain reaction (RQ-PCR) – a Europe against cancer program. *Leukemia* 2003;**17** (12):2474–86.

14. Saglio G, Pane F, Gottardi E et al. Consistent amounts of acute leukemia-associated P190 BCR/ABL transcripts are expressed by chronic myelogenous leukemia patients at diagnosis. *Blood* 1996;**87** (3):1075–80.

15. Melo JV. The diversity of BCR-ABL fusion proteins and their relationship to leukemia phenotype. *Blood* 1996;**88**(7):2375–84.

16. Melo JV, Myint H, Galton DA, Goldman JM. P190 *BCR-ABL* chronic myeloid leukaemia: the missing link with chronic myelomonocytic leukaemia? *Leukemia* 1994;**8**(1):208–11.

17. Pane F, Frigeri F, Sindona M *et al.* Neutrophilic-chronic myeloid leukemia: a distinct disease with a specific molecular marker (BCR/ABL with C3/A2 junction). *Blood* 1996;**88**(7):2410–14.

18. Baccarini M, Cortes J, Pane F *et al.* Chronic myeloid leukaemia: an update of concepts and management recommendations of European LeukemiaNet. *J Clin Oncol* 2009;**27**(35):6041–51.

19. Sokal JE, Cox EB, Baccarani M *et al.* Prognostic discrimination in "good-risk" chronic granulocytic leukemia. *Blood* 1984;**63**(4):789–99.

20. Hasford J, Pfirrmann M, Hehlmann R *et al.* A new prognostic score for survival of patients with chronic myeloid leukemia treated with interferon alfa. Writing Committee for the Collaborative CML Prognostic Factors Project Group. *J Natl Cancer Inst* 1998;**90**(11):850–8.

21. Rosti G, Trabacchi E, Bassi S *et al.* Risk and early cytogenetic response to imatinib and interferon in chronic myeloid leukemia. *Haematologica* 2003;**88**(3):256–9.

22. Hasford J, Pfirrmann M, Hehlmann R *et al.* Prognosis and prognostic factors for patients with chronic myeloid leukemia: nontransplant therapy. *Semin Hematol* 2003;**40**(1):4–12.

23. Bonifazi F, de Vivo A, Rosti G *et al.* Chronic myeloid leukemia and interferon-alpha: a study of complete cytogenetic responders. *Blood* 2001;**98**(10):3074–81.

24. Druker BJ, Guilhot F, O'Brien SG *et al.* Five-year follow-up of patients receiving imatinib for chronic myeloid leukemia. *New Engl J Med* 2006;**355**(23):2408–17.

25. Branford S, Rudzki Z, Harper A *et al.* Imatinib produces significantly superior molecular responses compared to interferon alfa plus cytarabine in patients with newly diagnosed chronic myeloid leukemia in chronic phase. *Leukemia* 2003;**17**(12):2401–9.

26. Kantarjian H, O'Brien S, Shan J *et al.* Cytogenetic and molecular responses and outcome in chronic myelogenous leukemia: need for new response definitions? *Cancer* 2008;**112**(4):837–45.

27. Roy L, Guilhot J, Krahnke T *et al.* Survival advantage from imatinib compared with the combination interferon-alpha plus cytarabine in chronic-phase chronic myelogenous leukemia: historical comparison between two phase 3 trials. *Blood* 2006;**108**(5):1478–84.

28. Kantarjian HM, O'Brien S, Cortes J *et al.* Imatinib mesylate therapy improves survival in patients with newly diagnosed Philadelphia chromosome-positive chronic myelogenous leukemia in the chronic phase: comparison with historic data. *Cancer* 2003;**98**(12):2636–42.

29. Kantarjian HM, Talpaz M, O'Brien S *et al.* Survival benefit with imatinib mesylate versus interferon-alpha-based regimens in newly diagnosed chronic-phase chronic myelogenous leukemia. *Blood* 2006;**108**(6):1835–40.

30. de Lavallade H, Milojkovic D, Khorashad JS *et al.* Outcome, prognostic factors and long-term follow-up in 207 chronic phase CML patients receiving front-line imatinib 400 mg at a single institution. *ASH Annual Meeting Abstr* 2007;**110**(11):1045.

31. Lucas CM, Wang L, Austin GM *et al.* A population study of imatinib in chronic myeloid leukaemia demonstrates lower efficacy than in clinical trials. *Leukemia* 2008;**22**(10):1963–6.

32. Kantarjian H, Talpaz M, O'Brien S *et al.* High-dose imatinib mesylate therapy in newly diagnosed Philadelphia chromosome-positive chronic phase chronic myeloid leukemia. *Blood* 2004;**103**(8):2873–8.

33. Cortes J, Baccarani M, Guilhot F *et al.* A phase iii, randomized, open-label study of 400 mg versus 800 mg of imatinib mesylate (im) in patients (pts) with newly diagnosed, previously untreated chronic myeloid leukemia in chronic phase (CML-CP) using molecular endpoints: 1-year results of TOPS (Tyrosine Kinase Inhibitor Optimization and Selectivity) study. *ASH Annual Meeting Abstr* 2008;**112**(11):335.

34. Cortes J, O'Brien S, Jones D *et al.* Efficacy of nilotinib (formerly AMN107) in patients (pts) with newly diagnosed, previously untreated Philadelphia chromosome (Ph)-positive chronic myelogenous leukemia in early chronic phase (CML-CP). *ASH Annual Meeting Abstr* 2008;**112**(11):446.

35. Cortes J, O'Brien S, Borthakur G *et al.* Efficacy of dasatinib in patients (pts) with previously untreated chronic myelogenous leukemia (CML) in early chronic phase (CML-CP). *ASH Annual Meeting Abstr* 2008;**112**(11):182.

36. de Lavallade H, Apperley JF, Khorashad JS *et al.* Imatinib for newly diagnosed patients with chronic myeloid leukemia: incidence of sustained responses in an intention-to-treat analysis. *J Clin Oncol* 2008;**26**(20):3358–63.

37. Apperley JF. Part I: mechanisms of resistance to imatinib in chronic myeloid leukaemia. *Lancet Oncol* 2007;**8**(11):1018–29.

38. Silver RT, Woolf SH, Hehlmann R *et al.* An evidence-based analysis of the effect of busulfan, hydroxyurea, interferon, and allogeneic bone marrow transplantation in treating the chronic phase of chronic

myeloid leukemia: developed for the American Society of Hematology. *Blood* 1999;**94**(5):1517–36.

39. Gratwohl A, Hermans J, Goldman JM *et al.* Risk assessment for patients with chronic myeloid leukaemia before allogeneic blood or marrow transplantation. Chronic Leukemia Working Party of the European Group for Blood and Marrow Transplantation. *Lancet* 1998;**352**(9134):1087–92.

40. Crawley C, Szydlo R, Lalancette M *et al.* Outcomes of reduced-intensity transplantation for chronic myeloid leukemia: an analysis of prognostic factors from the Chronic Leukemia Working Party of the EBMT. *Blood* 2005;**106**(9):2969–76.

41. Goldman JM. How I treat chronic myeloid leukemia in the imatinib era. *Blood* 2007;**110**(8):2828–37.

42. Hughes TP, Kaeda J, Branford S *et al.* Frequency of major molecular responses to imatinib or interferon alfa plus cytarabine in newly diagnosed chronic myeloid leukemia. *New Engl J Med* 2003;**349**(15):1423–32.

43. Lugli A, Ebnoether M, Cogliatti SB *et al.* Proposal of a morphologic bone marrow response score for imatinib mesylate treatment in chronic myelogenous leukemia. *Hum Pathol* 2005;**36**(1):91–100.

44. Cortes JE, Talpaz M, Giles F *et al.* Prognostic significance of cytogenetic clonal evolution in patients with chronic myelogenous leukemia on imatinib mesylate therapy. *Blood* 2003;**101**(10):3794–800.

45. Bumm T, Muller C, Al-Ali HK *et al.* Emergence of clonal cytogenetic abnormalities in Ph- cells in some CML patients in cytogenetic remission to imatinib but restoration of polyclonal hematopoiesis in the majority. *Blood* 2003;**101**(5):1941–9.

46. O'Dwyer ME, Gatter KM, Loriaux M *et al.* Demonstration of Philadelphia chromosome negative abnormal clones in patients with chronic myelogenous leukemia during major cytogenetic responses induced by imatinib mesylate. *Leukemia* 2003;**17**(3):481–7.

47. Bacher U, Hochhaus A, Berger U *et al.* Clonal aberrations in Philadelphia chromosome negative hematopoiesis in patients with chronic myeloid leukemia treated with imatinib or interferon alpha. *Leukemia* 2005;**19**(3):460–3.

48. Deininger MW, Cortes J, Paquette R *et al.* The prognosis for patients with chronic myeloid leukemia who have clonal cytogenetic abnormalities in Philadelphia chromosome-negative cells. *Cancer* 2007;**110**(7):1509–19.

49. Hughes T, Deininger M, Hochhaus A *et al.* Monitoring CML patients responding to treatment with tyrosine kinase inhibitors: review and recommendations for harmonizing current methodology for detecting BCR-ABL transcripts and kinase domain mutations and for expressing results. *Blood* 2006;**108**(1):28–37.

50. Cross NC, Hughes TP, Hochhaus A, Goldman JM. International standardisation of quantitative real-time RT-PCR for BCR-ABL. *Leuk Res* 2008;**32**(3):505–6.

51. Gorre ME, Mohammed M, Ellwood K *et al.* Clinical resistance to STI-571 cancer therapy caused by BCR-ABL gene mutation or amplification. *Science* 2001;**293**(5531):876–80.

52. Shah NP, Nicoll JM, Nagar B *et al.* Multiple BCR-ABL kinase domain mutations confer polyclonal resistance to the tyrosine kinase inhibitor imatinib (STI571) in chronic phase and blast crisis chronic myeloid leukemia. *Cancer Cell* 2002;**2**(2):117–25.

53. Branford S, Rudzki Z, Walsh S *et al.* High frequency of point mutations clustered within the adenosine triphosphate-binding region of BCR/ABL in patients with chronic myeloid leukemia or Ph-positive acute lymphoblastic leukemia who develop imatinib (STI571) resistance. *Blood* 2002;**99**(9):3472–5.

54. von Bubnoff N, Schneller F, Peschel C, Duyster J. BCR-ABL gene mutations in relation to clinical resistance of Philadelphia-chromosome-positive leukaemia to STI571: a prospective study. *Lancet* 2002;**359**(9305):487–91.

55. O'Hare T, Eide CA, Deininger MW. BCR-ABL kinase domain mutations, drug resistance, and the road to a cure for chronic myeloid leukemia. *Blood* 2007;**110**(7):2242–9.

56. Pavlovsky C, Kantarjian H, Cortes JE. First-line therapy for chronic myeloid leukemia: past, present, and future. *Am J Hematol* 2009;**84**(5):287–93.

57. Hochhaus A, Hughes T. Clinical resistance to imatinib: mechanisms and implications. *Hematol Oncol Clin North Am* 2004;**18**(3):641–56, ix.

58. Press RD, Willis SG, Laudadio J, Mauro MJ, Deininger MW. Determining the rise in BCR-ABL RNA that optimally predicts a kinase domain mutation in patients with chronic myeloid leukemia on imatinib. *Blood* 2009;**114**(13):2598–605.

59. Sherbenou DW, Wong MJ, Humayun A *et al.* In chronic myeloid leukemia (CML) patients with complete cytogenetic response to imatinib, BCR-ABL kinase domain mutations are relatively rare and not consistently associated with subsequent relapse. *ASH Annual Meeting Abstr* 2005;**106**(11):434.

60. Jabbour E, Kantarjian H, Jones D *et al.* Frequency and clinical significance of BCR-ABL mutations in patients with chronic myeloid leukemia treated with imatinib mesylate. *Leukemia* 2006;**20**(10):1767–73.

61. Gratwohl A, Brand R, Apperley J *et al*. Allogeneic hematopoietic stem cell transplantation for chronic myeloid leukemia in Europe 2006: transplant activity, long-term data and current results. An analysis by the Chronic Leukemia Working Party of the European Group for Blood and Marrow Transplantation (EBMT). *Haematologica* 2006;**91**(4):513–21.

62. Kantarjian H, Schiffer C, Jones D, Cortes J. Monitoring the response and course of chronic myeloid leukemia in the modern era of BCR-ABL tyrosine kinase inhibitors: practical advice on the use and interpretation of monitoring methods. *Blood* 2008;**111**(4):1774–80.

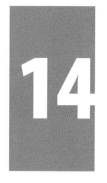

Myeloproliferative neoplasms

Philip A. Beer and Anthony R. Green

Introduction

The myeloproliferative neoplasms (MPNs) are a group of clonal stem cell disorders with similarities at the phenotypic and molecular level. Clinically these disorders are characterized by over-production of one or more mature myeloid elements and a variable tendency to develop acute myeloid leukemia (AML). Polycythemia vera (PV), essential thrombocythemia (ET) and primary myelofibrosis (PMF) overlap clinically and share a tendency to undergo phenotypic shift, such that patients with ET may develop PV, and ET or PV may undergo myelofibrotic transformation. A degree of phenotypic overlap is also seen in patients with chronic eosinophilic leukemia (CEL) and systemic mastocytosis (SM). At the molecular level, the myeloproliferative neoplasms are characterized by dysregulated tyrosine kinase signaling due to localized mutations (affecting *JAK2*, *MPL* or *KIT*) or chromosomal rearrangements (affecting *ABL1*, *PDGFRA/B* or *FGFR1*). Chronic myeloid leukemia (CML) has been discussed separately in Chapter 13.

Polycythemia vera

Epidemiology and pathogenesis

Polycythemia vera is characterized by over-production of erythrocytes, a variable increase in granulocytes and/or platelets and a risk of thrombotic and hemorrhagic complications. The annual incidence is around 1–2.5 per 100 000 population, with a peak between 50 and 70 years of age, and a slight male predominance [1]. Polycythemia vera may be diagnosed by chance, following a thrombotic event or during investigation for symptoms such as pruritus, gout, headaches or visual disturbance. Thrombotic complications are the main cause of morbidity and mortality. A minority of patients develop progressive disease

such as transformation to myelofibrosis, myelodysplasia or AML. Acquired mutations in *JAK2* are present in the vast majority of PV patients, comprising *JAK2* V617F in 97% and mutations in *JAK2* exon 12 in the majority of the remainder. Whereas mutations in *JAK2* exon 12 appear specific to patients presenting with erythrocytosis, the *JAK2* V617F mutation is also present in around 50% of patients with ET or PMF [2,3].

Investigation and diagnosis

Recent advances in understanding of the molecular basis of PV have led to a dramatic change in how this condition is diagnosed.

JAK2 mutation analysis: A raised hemoglobin in association with a pathogenetic mutation in *JAK2* is sufficient to confirm a diagnosis of PV according to the British Committee for Standards in Haematology (BCSH) criteria. Testing for the *JAK2* V617F mutation is therefore recommended as the initial investigation in all patients with a raised hemoglobin. The method used should be sensitive enough to detect a mutant allele burden of around 1%, as in some patients, the neoplastic clone represents a minority of blood cells. Suitable techniques include allele-specific PCR or real-time PCR, and the test can be performed on peripheral blood DNA or cDNA. Screening for *JAK2* exon 12 mutations is recommended in all cases where a *JAK2* V617F mutation is not detected. Screening for *JAK2* exon 12 mutations is complicated by the existence of over 20 different disease-associated alleles and the occurrence of a low mutant allele burden in some patients. Screening methods should therefore be able to detect all allelic variants within the exon 12 region with an adequate degree of sensitivity, and include pyrosequencing and high-resolution melt curve analysis [4]. The identification of activating mutations in *JAK2* has raised the possibility of targeted

Diagnostic Techniques in Hematological Malignancies, ed. Wendy N. Erber. Published by Cambridge University Press.
© Cambridge University Press 2010.

Table 14.1. World Health Organization (WHO) and British Committee for Standards in Haematology (BCSH) criteria for the diagnosis of polycythemia vera.

WHO 2008 [20]	BCSH 2007 [21]
Polycythemia vera Requires A1 + A2 + any B or A1 + two B	**JAK2-positive polycythemia vera** Requires A1 + A2
A1 Hb >18.5 g/dL (♂) or >16.5 g/dL (♀) or Hb or Hct > 99th percentile or red cell mass > 125% predicted or Hb >17 g/dL (♂) or >15 g/dL (♀) associated with 2 g/dL increase from baseline not attributed to correction of iron deficiency	**A1** High Hct (> 0.52 in men, > 0.48 in women) or raised red cell mass (> 125% predicted)
A2 Mutation in *JAK2*	**A2** Mutation in *JAK2*
	***JAK2*-negative polycythemia vera** Requires A1–A3 + either another A or two B
	A1 Raised red cell mass (> 125% predicted) or hematocrit > 0.60 in men, > 0.56 in women **A2** Absence of mutation in *JAK2* **A3** No cause of secondary erythrocytosis **A4** Palpable splenomegaly **A5** Acquired genetic abnormality (excluding *BCR-ABL1*) in the hematopoietic cells
B1 Bone marrow biopsy showing pan-myelosis **B2** Low serum erythropoietin **B3** Endogenous erythroid colony growth *in vitro*	**B1** Thrombocytosis (> 450 × 10⁹/L) **B2** Neutrophil leukocytosis (> 10 × 10⁹/L in non-smokers; > 12.5 × 10⁹/L in smokers) **B3** Radiological evidence of splenomegaly **B4** Endogenous erythroid colonies *or* low serum erythropoietin

therapy for PV. To date, clinical trials of JAK2 inhibitors have mainly enrolled patients with primary or post-ET/PV myelofibrosis (see PMF section for further details), although limited data suggest some efficacy in PV patients who are refractory to other treatment modalities.

World Health Organization (WHO) criteria for the diagnosis of *JAK2*-positive PV differ slightly from those of the BCSH in that they require one or more of the following additional supporting features:

1. Typical bone marrow histology.
2. Low serum erythropoietin (Epo).
3. Growth of erythroid colonies *in vitro* in the absence of Epo (endogenous erythroid colonies, EEC) (Table 14.1).

Blood film and bone marrow examination: Patients with a persistently raised hematocrit (> 0.52 in males, > 0.48 in females) should generally be referred for further investigation. Examination of the blood film may reveal features of iron deficiency or the presence of large platelets. At diagnosis the bone marrow aspirate in PV generally shows hyperplasia of the erythroid, granulocyte and megakaryocyte lineages (pan-myelosis) with pleomorphic megakaryocyte

morphology (Figure 14.1a). Stainable iron is usually absent. Bone marrow trephine histology shows increased cellularity with trilineage hyperplasia, pleomorphic megakaryocyte morphology and loose megakaryocyte clusters (Figure 14.1b). Immunocytochemistry may be useful to delineate the presence of pan-myelosis, with staining for myeloperoxidase and glycophorin (CD235) highlighting granulocytic and erythroid lineages respectively. Staining with a megakaryocyte-associated antibodies (e.g. CD41, CD61 or Factor VIIIRAg) will highlight megakaryocytic hyperplasia and pleomorphism, and may identify small megakaryocytes that may not be evident on hematoxylin and eosin staining. It should be noted, however, that there are no specific morphological features for PV and these overlap with other MPNs and reactive conditions. In patients with a *JAK2* exon 12 mutation, erythroid hyperplasia is evident but the granulocyte and megakaryocyte lineages are often normal (Figure 14.2a, b). In PV patients positive for either V617F or exon 12 mutations, reticulin may be normal or slightly increased, although occasional patients harbor significant reticulin fibrosis in the absence of other features of myelofibrotic transformation. Cytogenetic

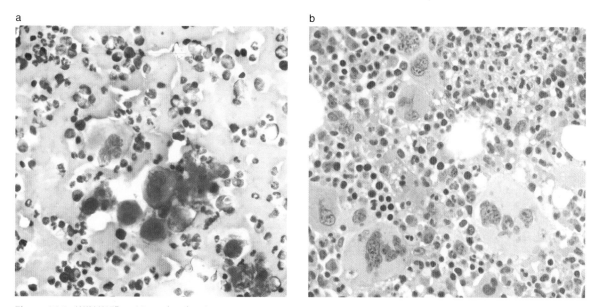

Figure 14.1. *JAK2* V617F-positive polycythemia vera.
a. Bone marrow aspirate showing a cluster of pleomorphic megakaryocytes.
b. Bone marrow trephine section showing pan-myelosis with clusters of pleomorphic megakaryocytes.

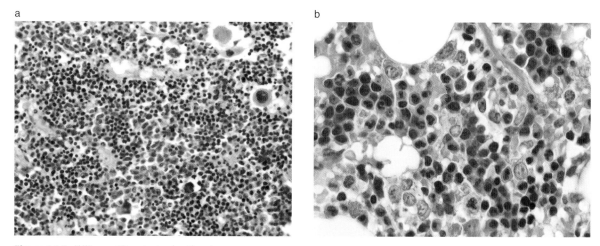

Figure 14.2. *JAK2* exon 12 mutant polycythemia vera.
a and b. Bone marrow trephine biopsy sections from PV with the *JAK2* exon 12 N542-E543del mutation showing erythroid hyperplasia.

analysis is not indicated in the initial assessment, but is useful in the investigation of *JAK2*-negative erythrocytosis and at disease progression (see below).

Erythropoietin and progenitor assays: The majority of PV patients have serum erythropoietin (Epo) levels below the normal range at initial diagnosis, although levels may normalize swiftly following venesection or cytoreductive therapy. A low serum Epo concentration is not specific for PV, and may be seen with inherited erythropoietin receptor mutations, ET or idiopathic erythrocytosis. Growth of EEC *in vitro* can be observed in the majority of PV patients at initial diagnosis but may be masked by cytoreductive therapy. EEC formation may also be seen in patients with ET or PMF, and in those with inherited Epo receptor mutations. The limited availability and lack of standardization reduces the overall diagnostic utility of the EEC assay.

Given that detection of a *JAK2* mutation confirms a clonal blood disorder, the requirement in the

WHO diagnostic criteria for an additional supportive feature is presumably aimed at distinguishing PV from other *JAK2*-positive MPNs (primarily ET and PMF). However, none of these additional features are specific for PV, as noted above. As such, the presence of a *JAK2* mutation in a patient with a high hemoglobin is considered sufficient to make a diagnosis of PV, as per BCSH guidelines (Table 14.1).

JAK2-negative erythrocytosis: It is currently unclear if *JAK2*-negative PV exists as a genuine entity, and as such the clinical features of this condition are unknown. The WHO and BCSH criteria differ in several important respects in their approach to the diagnosis of *JAK2*-negative PV. First, WHO criteria do not require measurement of red cell mass (or the presence of a hematocrit indicative of a raised red cell mass: > 0.60 in men, > 0.56 in women). Second,

investigation for causes of secondary erythrocytosis is not mandated by WHO criteria. The WHO diagnosis of *JAK2*-negative PV therefore rests on the presence of a raised hemoglobin along with two supporting features to distinguish clonal from secondary erythrocytosis. However, the supporting features, comprising bone marrow pan-myelosis, low serum Epo or EEC formation (Table 14.1), lack specificity for clonal hematopoiesis (see above) and these criteria risk labeling inherited or reactive erythrocytosis as a clonal blood disorder. Confirmation of a raised red cell mass by radionuclide studies is therefore recommended for all patients with a raised hemoglobin in the absence of a *JAK2* mutation. Such studies will distinguish a true erythrocytosis, associated with an increased red cell mass, from apparent polycythemia, where the hemoglobin concentration is increased due to a contracted plasma volume in the presence of a normal red

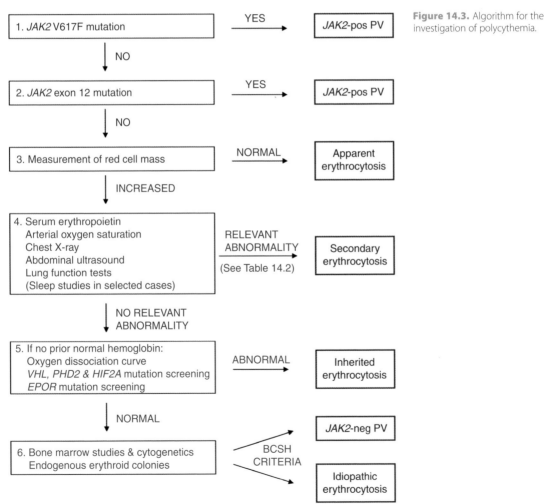

Figure 14.3. Algorithm for the investigation of polycythemia.

Table 14.2. Causes of erythrocytosis.

Polycythemia vera

Idiopathic erythrocytosis

Inherited erythrocytosis
  High oxygen-affinity hemoglobin
  2,3-bisphosphoglycerate mutase deficiency
  Erythropoietin receptor mutation
  Oxygen sensing pathway mutation (*VHL*, *PHD2* or *HIF2A*)

Hypoxia-associated
  Generalized hypoxia: lung disease, cardiac disease, high altitude habitat
  Localized renal hypoxia: renal artery stenosis, intrinsic renal disease
  Intermittent hypoxia: obstructive sleep apnea

Ectopic erythropoietin secretion
  Benign tumors: uterine leiomyoma
  Malignant tumors: hepatocellular carcinoma, cerebellar hemangioblastoma

Drug-associated
  Exogenous erythropoietin
  Androgen preparations

cell mass. A true erythrocytosis is established by a red cell mass > 125% of predicted, and mandates an exhaustive search for secondary causes in patients lacking a *JAK2* mutation (Figure 14.3). In this context, a high serum Epo is highly suggestive of a secondary erythrocytosis, whereas a normal serum Epo is unhelpful. As noted above, reduced serum Epo levels may be seen in PV, inherited Epo receptor mutations or idiopathic erythrocytosis. Other causes of a secondary erythrocytosis are listed in Table 14.2.

In patients with a true erythrocytosis lacking a mutation in *JAK2*, a diagnosis of *JAK2*-negative PV should be considered as per BCSH criteria (Table 14.1). Although bone marrow cytogenetic examination is not routinely required in the diagnosis of *JAK2*-positive PV, such studies are useful in suspected *JAK2*-negative PV, as an acquired cytogenetic abnormality confirms the presence of clonal hematopoiesis. A reasonable approach is the initial use of fluorescence *in situ* hybridization (FISH) studies to look for common MPN-associated abnormalities such as del(20q), del(13q), add(8) and add(9), and proceeding to full karyotypic analysis if FISH studies are uninformative. Patients with a true erythrocytosis who do not fulfill diagnostic criteria for PV and have no identifiable secondary cause are currently classified as idiopathic erythrocytosis.

Risk stratification and therapeutic monitoring

An increased leukocyte count or high *JAK2* mutant allele burden at diagnosis have been associated with an increased risk of subsequent thrombosis, although the utility of these observations in guiding therapy is not yet clear. Current guidelines recommend anti-platelet therapy for all patients with PV, along with regular venesection for those with an isolated erythrocytosis, or cytoreductive agents for those with thrombocytosis, progressive splenomegaly or constitutional symptoms [5].

Consensus guidelines on the monitoring of response to therapy are available. These take into consideration therapeutic efficacy at the clinical/hematological, bone marrow histological and molecular levels [6]. A clinical/hematological response involves resolution of physical symptoms and normalization of the blood count, and is the aim of treatment in the majority of cases. Successful therapy may also result in normalization of bone marrow cellularity. At present, however, the implications of a histological response have not been fully evaluated, and reassessment of bone marrow histology is not usually performed routinely. Interferon-α therapy has been associated with a fall in the peripheral blood mutant allele burden; however the significance of this reduction is currently unclear, and quantitation of mutant *JAK2* (e.g. by pyrosequencing or real-time PCR) is not currently recommended outside the setting of a clinical trial.

Disease progression

Myelofibrotic transformation complicates around 10% of patients with PV, and may be suspected by the presence of increasing splenomegaly, reduced requirements for cytoreductive therapy or the development of anemia. Myelofibrotic transformation of PV is phenotypically indistinguishable from PMF and the diagnostic process and criteria are similar (Table 14.3; see PMF section for a full discussion).

Evolution to AML complicates around 5% of patients with PV (Figure 14.4a, b). The diagnostic process generally starts with examination of the blood film, the presence of > 20% blasts in the blood being diagnostic of leukemic transformation. Examination of the bone marrow is indicated in patients where the peripheral blood blast count is < 20% (where transformation to myelofibrosis or myelodysplasia should also be considered) or

Table 14.3. Criteria for the diagnosis of myelofibrotic transformation of essential thrombocythemia or polycythemia vera.

Requires A1 + A2 and any two B criteria

A1 Previous diagnosis of ET or PV

A2 Reticulin ≥ 3 (on a 0–4 scale)

B1 New palpable splenomegaly or increase in spleen size of ≥ 5 cm

B2 Unexplained anemia with 2 g/dL decrease from baseline hemoglobin

B3 Leukoerythroblastic blood film

B4 Tear-drop red cells

B5 Constitutional symptoms [a]

B6 Histological evidence of extramedullary hematopoiesis

[a] Drenching night sweats, weight loss >10% over 6 months or diffuse bone pain.

a   b

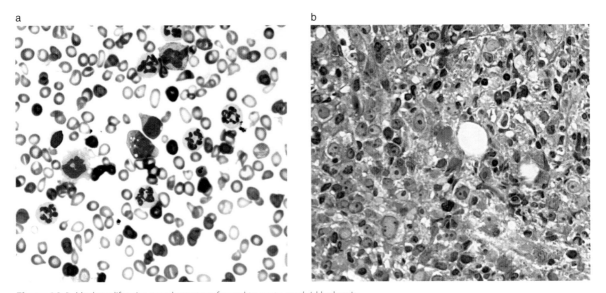

Figure 14.4. Myeloproliferative neoplasms transformed to acute myeloid leukemia.
a. Blood film showing acute myeloid leukemia following myelofibrotic transformation of PV.
b. Bone marrow trephine biopsy showing leukemic transformation of PV.

where high-dose chemotherapy is being considered. As with *de novo* AML, the presence of > 20% of blast cells in the bone marrow is diagnostic of leukemic transformation. Flow cytometric analysis of peripheral blood or bone marrow may be useful to confirm both the presence of excess immature cells and to determine their lineage (see AML chapter for recommendations on antibody panels). Bone marrow karyotypic analysis is also commonly performed, although it should be noted that the strong prognostic significance of different karyotypic abnormalities seen in *de novo* AML may not be applicable to post-MPN AML, where the overall prognosis is generally poor. Of note, patients with a *JAK2*-mutant MPN may develop AML that is negative for the *JAK2* mutation, although the prognostic significance of this observation is currently unknown.

Essential thrombocythemia

Epidemiology and pathogenesis

Essential thrombocythemia (ET) is characterized by an isolated thrombocytosis and a risk of thrombotic and hemorrhagic complications. The annual incidence of ET is in the order of 1–2.5 per 100 000 population and appears slightly more common in females [1]. Patients may present at any age, although ET is largely a disorder of later life with a peak incidence between the ages of 50 and 70 years. Presentation in childhood is rare but well recognized. Essential thrombocythemia is often diagnosed following the incidental finding of a high platelet count, although a proportion of patients present with thrombotic or hemorrhage complications. A minority of patients develop progressive disease such as transformation to myelofibrosis, myelodysplasia or AML. The *JAK2* V617F mutation is found in approximately 50% of patients [2,3]. Mutations in exon 10 of *MPL*, the thrombopoietin receptor, are found in around 4% of patients with ET and a similar proportion with PMF (but not in PV) with five different *MPL* alleles (*MPL* S505N and *MPL* W515L/K/A/R) reported to date. Of note, *MPL* S505N may also be observed as an inherited allele in kindreds with familial thrombocytosis [7,8]. Rarely, ET patients harbor more than one mutation, for example both *JAK2* V617F and *MPL* W515L [9].

Investigation and diagnosis

Essential thrombocythemia has traditionally been a diagnosis of exclusion, requiring the absence of reactive conditions and other myeloproliferative and myelodysplastic syndromes that may present with thrombocytosis (Table 14.4). The identification of mutations in *JAK2* and *MPL* now allows for the positive identification of

this disorder in over a half of all cases. Diagnostic criteria for ET are presented in Table 14.5. The BCSH criteria are similar to WHO 2008 but differ in three important respects [10]. First, in the presence of a pathogenetic mutation the BCSH criteria do not necessarily require bone marrow studies, as although mutations in *JAK2* or *MPL* are not specific for ET, PV can be excluded by normal iron studies and PMF by the absence of associated clinical and laboratory features (see below). Second, BCSH criteria do not use bone marrow histology to subdivide ET into "true-ET" and "prefibrotic myelofibrosis" as the existence of the latter

Table 14.4. Causes of thrombocytosis.

Myeloid malignancy
  Essential thrombocythemia
  Polycythemia vera
  Primary myelofibrosis
  Chronic myeloid leukemia
  Refractory anemia with ring sideroblasts associated with marked thrombocytosis
  Myelodysplastic syndrome associated with isolated del (5q)

Reactive (secondary) thrombocytosis
  Blood loss or iron deficiency
  Infection or inflammation
  Disseminated malignancy
  Drug effect (vincristine, epinephrine, all-trans-retinoic acid)
  Splenectomy or congenital absence of spleen
  Hemolytic anemia

Familial thrombocytosis
  Mutations in *TPO*, *MPL* or unknown genes

Spurious thrombocytosis
  Cryoglobulinemia
  Cytoplasmic fragmentation in acute leukemia
  Red cell fragmentation

Table 14.5. World Health Organization (WHO) and British Committee for Standards in Haematology (BCSH) criteria for the diagnosis of essential thrombocythemia.

WHO 2008 [20]	BCSH 2010 [10]
Requires A1–A4	Requires A1–A3 or A1 + A3–A5
A1 Sustained platelet count >450 × 10^9/L	**A1** Sustained platelet count >450 × 10^9/L
A2 Bone marrow showing increased numbers of enlarged, mature megakaryocytes	**A2** Presence of an acquired pathogenetic mutation (e.g. in *JAK2* or *MPL*)
A3 Not meeting WHO criteria for PV, PMF, CML, MDS or other myeloid neoplasm	**A3** No other myeloid malignancy, especially PV, PMF, CML or MDS
A4 Acquired mutation or clonal marker *or* no reactive cause for thrombocytosis	**A4** No reactive cause for thrombocytosis and normal iron stores
	A5 Bone marrow aspirate and trephine biopsy showing increased megakaryocytes displaying a spectrum of morphology with predominant large megakaryocytes with hyperlobated nuclei and abundant cytoplasm. Reticulin is generally not increased (grades 0–2/4 or grade 0/3)

proposed entity remains controversial and the underlying histological criteria are difficult to apply reproducibly, even by experienced hematopathologists [11]. Third, the BCSH classification includes patients with bone marrow reticulin of greater than grade 2 (on a 0–4 scale) who lack other features of PMF or myelofibrotic transformation; such patients are not classified under the current WHO criteria.

JAK2 and MPL mutation analyses: The combination of an isolated thrombocytosis with a pathogenetic mutation, in the absence of iron deficiency (which may mask PV) or features of PMF (see below), is generally sufficient to make a diagnosis of ET. Testing for the *JAK2* V617F mutation is recommended as the initial investigation in all patients with thrombocytosis (see PV section for choice of assay). Screening for *MPL* exon 10 mutations is recommended in *JAK2*-negative cases. Strategies for detection may include testing only for the most common mutation (*MPL* W515L), for example by allele-specific or real-time PCR. An alternative and more

comprehensive approach is to use a technology such as pyrosequencing or high-resolution melt curve analysis to detect all mutations within exon 10. The identification of activating mutations in the cytokine receptor signaling pathway (*JAK2* and *MPL*) has raised the possibility of targeted therapy. To date, clinical trials of JAK2 inhibitors have mainly enrolled patients with primary or post-ET/PV myelofibrosis (see PMF section for further details), although limited data suggest some efficacy in ET patients who are refractory to other treatment modalities. Occasional patients with CML present with an isolated thrombocytosis in the absence of leukocytosis. Given the major therapeutic implications, testing for *BCR-ABL1* should be considered in all patients who lack mutations in *JAK2* and *MPL*.

In patients with suspected ET who lack *JAK2* and *MPL* mutations, exclusion of reactive causes is particularly important (Table 14.4). In this context a careful history, assessment of inflammatory markers (e.g. C-reactive protein and/or erythrocyte sedimentation rate) and bone marrow histology are all recommended in order to confirm the diagnosis (Figure 14.5).

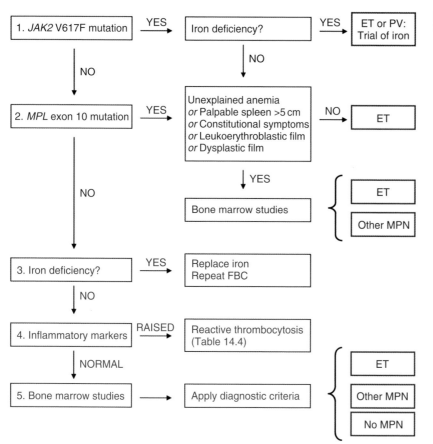

Figure 14.5. Algorithm for the investigation of thrombocytosis.

Serum biochemistry, cytokines and progenitor assays: Assessment of body iron stores is required in all patients with thrombocytosis, to exclude iron-deficient PV in those with a *JAK2* mutation, and to look for iron deficiency as a cause of reactive thrombocytosis in those lacking a pathogenetic mutation. Measurement of serum ferritin is suitable for first-line testing. Measurement of biochemical markers of systemic inflammation, such as C-reactive protein and erythrocyte sedimentation rate, are also recommended in all patients. These tests are important in assessing the reliability of serum ferritin, as iron studies are altered in the presence of acute and chronic inflammation. Systemic inflammatory disorders are also an important cause of reactive thrombocytosis in patients lacking a pathogenetic mutation (Table 14.4).

Serum thrombopoietin levels are normal or slightly elevated in ET and have no diagnostic utility. Serum Epo levels are low in a proportion of patients with ET, especially those with a *JAK2* V617F mutation. Growth of cytokine-independent erythroid and/or megakaryocyte colonies is observed in approximately 50% of ET patients, although limited availability and lack of standardization reduces the diagnostic utility of these assays.

Blood film and bone marrow examination: Examination of the blood film is recommended in all patients with thrombocytosis, primarily to exclude features of other myeloid disorders associated with thrombocytosis (Table 14.4). The blood film in ET is often normal apart from the thrombocytosis. Morphological platelet abnormalities, such as platelet anisocytosis, the presence of large platelets, and hypogranularity, may be seen in a proportion of patients. However, the blood film alone is rarely diagnostic. The presence of anemia, tear-drop erythrocytes or circulating progenitor cells (or the presence of significant palpable splenomegaly) raise the possibility of PMF and mandate bone marrow aspirate and trephine biopsy. The presence of dysplastic features also necessitates bone marrow studies to exclude a myelodysplastic disorder, such as that associated with a deletion of chromosome 5q.

Bone marrow aspirate and trephine biopsy are recommended in all cases of suspected ET lacking a mutation in *JAK2* and *MPL*, both to identify typical features of ET and to exclude other myeloid malignancies that may present with an isolated thrombocytosis. Although bone marrow studies may not be essential to confirm a diagnosis of *JAK2*- or *MPL*-positive ET, assessment of reticulin fibrosis carries prognostic significance (see below).

At diagnosis the bone marrow aspirate often shows large and giant (present in small numbers) megakaryocytes with hyperlobated nuclei (Figure 14.6a); hematopoiesis is generally otherwise normal. Iron staining may be helpful in excluding iron deficiency or the presence of ring sideroblasts. Bone marrow trephine histology typically shows an increase in megakaryocyte frequency with megakaryocyte clustering, some large and giant megakaryocytes and nuclear hyperlobation, usually in the absence of significant reticulin fibrosis (Figure 14.6b). Cellularity is generally normal or slightly increased, but occasional cases may show a hypocellular marrow, for example those with mutations in *MPL* [7,12].

Cytogenetics: As with PV, chromosomal analysis, by G-banding or FISH, is helpful in those lacking mutations in *JAK2* and *MPL*, primarily to exclude lesions associated with other myeloid disorders such as t(9;22) (CML) or deletions of chromosome 5q ('5q-minus syndrome'). Other karyotypic abnormalities, mainly comprising deletions of chromosomes 20q or 13q or additional copies of chromosomes 8 or 9, are found in 5% of ET patients and establish the existence of clonal hematopoiesis. A reasonable approach is the initial use of FISH studies to look for common abnormalities, proceeding to full karyotypic analysis if these studies are uninformative.

Variants of essential thrombocythemia: The WHO classification recognizes refractory anemia with ring sideroblasts associated with marked thrombocytosis (RARS-T) as a provisional entity as a myelodysplastic/myeloproliferative disorder. RARS-T is similar to ET both clinically and pathogenetically, displaying thrombotic complications, large megakaryocytes with hyperlobated nuclei and a similar prevalence of mutations in *JAK2* and *MPL*. It may be that RARS-T represents a morphological variant of ET. Alternatively RARS-T may represent a morphological manifestation of oligoclonal disease [9], with a *JAK2* or *MPL* mutant ET clone coexisting with an MDS clone. Given the risk of thrombotic complications, RARS-T is probably best managed as a variant of ET.

The *JAK2* V617F mutation has been reported in patients presenting with mesenteric vein thrombosis and a normal blood count, particularly young/middle-

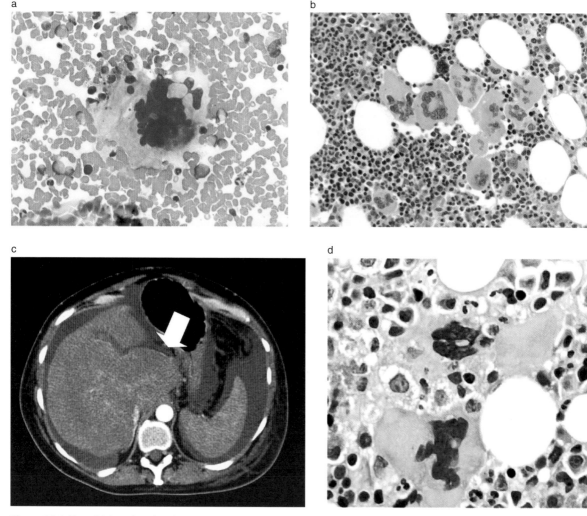

Figure 14.6. Essential thrombocythemia.

a. Bone marrow aspirate in *JAK2* V617F-positive ET showing a giant megakaryocyte with a low nuclear : cytoplasmic ratio and hyperlobated nucleus.

b. Bone marrow trephine biopsy showing increased cellularity and clusters of large, hyperlobated megakaryocytes.

c. Contrast enhanced abdominal CT scan showing features of established hepatic vein thrombosis in a 53-year-old female, including hypertrophy of the caudate lobe (arrow) with atrophy of the remaining liver and surrounding ascites; the spleen is of normal size.

d. Bone marrow trephine biopsy from the same patient showing normal cellularity and increased megakaryocytes with occasional hyperlobated forms. Although the patient was *JAK2* V617F-positive, other investigations, including blood count, red cell mass and cytogenetic analysis, were normal.

aged females. In some cases, a diagnosis of PV is masked by an increase in plasma volume, often due to the presence of splenomegaly secondary to portal hypertension. In other cases the red cell mass is normal, suggesting the presence of a pre-clinical MPN. In such cases, bone marrow histology may suggest an underlying MPN, and long-term follow-up is recommended as many patients will subsequently develop a clinically overt MPN, most commonly ET (Figure 14.6c, d).

Risk stratification and therapeutic monitoring

Cytoreductive therapy in ET is aimed primarily at reducing the frequency of thrombotic complications. Patients are currently stratified according to known risk factors, the best established of which are age over 60 years or history of prior thrombosis. An increased leukocyte count at diagnosis has been reported as an independent predictor of thrombosis in both ET and

PV. Patients with *JAK2* V617F-positive ET also exhibit higher rates of venous and arterial thrombosis compared with those without the mutation. The presence of an *MPL* mutation predicted for higher rates of arterial thrombosis compared to *JAK2/MPL*-negative patients in the Italian but not the PT-1 cohort [7,12]. Increased bone marrow reticulin fibrosis at diagnosis has been identified as an independent predictor of both thrombotic and hemorrhagic complications [13]. The predictive utility of the platelet count remains unclear, and an association between the degree of thrombocytosis and risk of thrombosis or hemorrhage is not well established.

As with PV, response to therapy may be considered on clinical/hematological, bone marrow histological and molecular levels [6]. In patients requiring cytoreductive therapy, treatment is generally adjusted to maintain the platelet count within normal limits. Routine reassessment of bone marrow response is not generally indicated in patients with stable disease. Anagrelide therapy has been associated with increasing bone marrow fibrosis and a risk of myelofibrotic transformation compared to hydroxycarbamide [14]. As the increase in fibrosis is reversible in some cases on cessation of anagrelide [13], regular assessment of bone marrow histology, e.g. every 2–3 years, is recommended for those receiving this drug.

Disease progression

Rates of myelofibrotic and AML transformation are similar to those seen in PV, and are diagnosed according to the same criteria (see PV section for a full discussion).

Primary myelofibrosis

Epidemiology and pathogenesis

Primary myelofibrosis (PMF) is characterized by megakaryocyte proliferation and bone marrow fibrosis with consequent extramedullary hematopoiesis and bone marrow failure. PMF is less common than PV or ET, with an annual incidence of approximately 0.1–0.5 per 100 000 population, peaking between the ages of 50 and 70 years [1]. Presentation in childhood is extremely rare. Complications such as leukemic transformation (seen in around 30% of cases) and bone marrow failure result in a median overall survival of 3–5 years. The mutation spectrum in PMF is similar to ET, with the *JAK2* V617F mutation present in around 50% of patients and *MPL* mutations present in a further 5–8%.

Investigation and diagnosis

Diagnostic criteria for PMF are presented in Table 14.6. In both WHO and BCSH criteria, a diagnosis of PMF requires typical bone marrow appearances along with additional supportive clinical and/or laboratory features. The predictive utility of the different supportive features has not been formally tested, although in patients with significant bone marrow fibrosis the two sets of criteria show a high degree of concordance. The main difference between the two is the inclusion of patients without significant bone marrow fibrosis in the WHO 2008 classification. This inclusion is based on the notion that the early stages of PMF, termed "pre-fibrotic" or "cellular phase" myelofibrosis, may be recognized by their typical histological appearances. However the reproducibility of this classification has been called into question [11], and its clinical utility remains unproven. Of note, patients without significant bone marrow fibrosis were generally excluded from studies of survival in PMF [15,16], and it is therefore not known if prognostic indices in common usage are applicable to patients with pre-fibrotic or cellular phase myelofibrosis (see below).

Splenomegaly: Palpable splenomegaly is present in most cases of PMF, and the degree of enlargement varies markedly between patients. Although long-standing bone marrow fibrosis due to any etiology may be associated with a degree of splenic enlargement, massive splenomegaly is suggestive of PMF or myelofibrotic transformation of another MPN.

Blood film and bone marrow examination: The blood count in PMF is highly variable: hemoglobin levels may be normal or decreased, and leukocyte and platelet counts may be normal, decreased or increased. Blood film examination usually shows circulating erythroid and myeloid progenitors (leukoerythroblastic film), tear-drop erythrocytes and large poorly stained hypogranular platelets (Figure 14.7a). It should be noted that circulating progenitor cells and tear-drop erythrocytes are features of bone marrow fibrosis *per se* (primary or secondary) and are not specific for PMF.

Bone marrow studies are central to the diagnosis of PMF, to confirm the presence of bone marrow fibrosis and to rule out other malignant or reactive conditions (Table 14.7). Aspiration of particulate bone marrow is often unsuccessful due to the presence of fibrosis. Where an adequate aspirate is obtained the particles may be

Table 14.6. Criteria for the diagnosis of primary myelofibrosis.

WHO 2008 [20]	Modified from Campbell and Green [2]
Requires A1–A3 and any two B criteria	A1 + A2 and any two B criteria
A1 Megakaryocyte atypia and fibrosis *or* megakaryocyte atypia, increased granulocytic and decreased erythroid cellularity without fibrosis	**A1** Reticulin ≥ 3 (on a 0–4 scale)
A2 Not meeting WHO criteria for PV, CML, MDS or other myeloid neoplasm	**A2** Pathogenetic mutation (e.g. in *JAK2* or *MPL*) *or* absence of *BCR-ABL1*
A3 Acquired mutation or clonal marker *or* no reactive cause for fibrosis	
B1 Leukoerythroblastic blood film	**B1** Palpable splenomegaly
B2 Increase in serum LDH[a]	**B2** Unexplained anemia
B3 Anemia	**B3** Tear-drop red cells
B4 Palpable splenomegaly	**B4** Leukoerythroblastic blood film
	B5 Constitutional symptoms[b]
	B6 Histological evidence of extramedullary hematopoiesis

[a] Lactate dehydrogenase.
[b] Weight loss > 10% over 6 months, drenching sweats or diffuse bone pain.

markedly hypercellular but with hypo- or acellular trails. Other typical aspirate appearances include granulocytic hyperplasia, reduced erythroid activity and megakaryocytic hyperplasia with dysplastic morphology.

Examination of bone marrow histology and staining for the presence of reticulin fibers is essential in all cases; demonstration of grade 3 or 4 reticulin fibrosis (on a 0–4 scale) is required to make a diagnosis of PMF. Bone marrow trephine histology shows a range of morphological appearances. In the early stages of disease, the bone marrow is hypercellular with granulocytic hyperplasia and abundant, dysplastic megakaryocytes often residing in tight clusters which may be paratrabecular. Megakaryocytes may have an angulated shape and a high nuclear : cytoplasmic ratio with hypolobated nuclei (Figure 14.7b). Over time the bone marrow cavity is gradually replaced by collagen fibrosis (as demonstrated by the reticulin stain), such that in advanced disease few hematopoietic elements can be identified (Figure 14.7c). There may be sinusoidal expansion and intrasinusoidal hematopoietic cells (Figure 14.7d). New bone formation (termed osteomyelosclerosis) may be observed, particularly in the later stages of the disease.

Other malignant or reactive conditions associated with bone marrow fibrosis are listed in Table 14.7. Bone marrow fibrosis secondary to malignant infiltration may be localized (secondary carcinoma, systemic mastocytosis) or generalized (hairy cell leukemia, acute leukemia, CML). In the majority of cases, the diagnosis will be apparent from bone marrow histology and confirmed by appropriate immunostaining of the infiltrate, although exclusion of CML requires testing for the *BCR-ABL1* fusion. Hyperparathyroidism or severe vitamin D deficiency may result in diffuse bone marrow fibrosis and anemia, although other features of PMF are generally absent; bone marrow fibrosis resolves with correction of the metabolic abnormality. Autoimmune bone marrow fibrosis is a rare disorder which may be indistinguishable from PMF. Most but not all patients have a pre-existing autoimmune disease, usually systemic lupus erythematosis or systemic sclerosis. Other clues to an autoimmune etiology include the absence of palpable splenomegaly, lymphoid aggregates in the bone marrow or auto-antibodies in the blood; complete resolution of bone marrow fibrosis with steroids or other immunosuppressive therapy is the norm. Gray platelet syndrome is an extremely rare autosomal dominant disorder where leakage of platelet alpha-granules, containing growth factors such as PDGF and TGF-β, is associated with large gray-colored circulating platelets, a variable bleeding tendency and the development of bone marrow fibrosis in a proportion of patients.

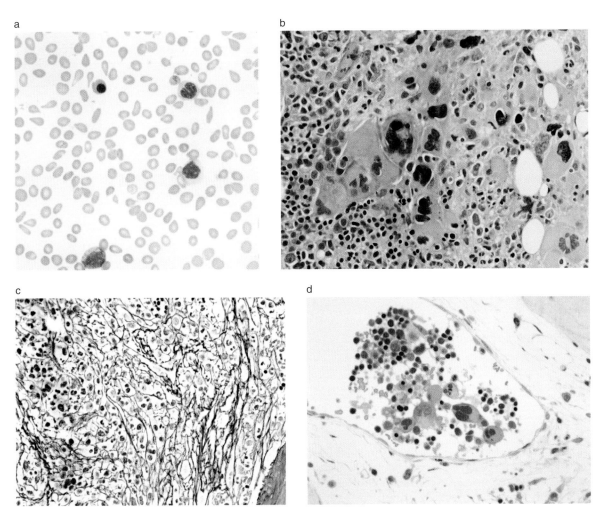

Figure 14.7. Primary myelofibrosis.
a. Blood film appearances in PMF, showing tear-drop erythrocytes and circulating myeloid and erythroid progenitors.
b. Bone marrow trephine biopsy showing hypercellularity, dysorganized hematopoiesis and tight clusters of dysplastic megakaryocytes.
c. Bone marrow trephine biopsy (Gomori silver stain) showing a coarse network of reticulin fibers (grade 4).
d. Bone marrow trephine biopsy showing hematopoietic cells within an expanded sinusoid.

A proportion of patients diagnosed with chronic phase ET or PV harbor increased levels of bone marrow reticulin in the absence of other features of PMF or myelofibrotic transformation. The presence of reticulin fibrosis in patients with ET or PV should be clearly distinguished from the clinical syndromes of PMF and myelofibrotic transformation, both of which require the presence of additional clinical and/or laboratory features such as splenomegaly, anemia, circulating progenitors or tear-drop erythrocytes (Tables 14.3 and 14.6).

Immunocytochemistry: Immunocytochemical staining may be useful in PMF to delineate the different myeloid lineages within a disordered bone marrow. Staining for myeloperoxidase and glycophorin (CD235) will highlight the granulocytic and erythroid lineages respectively. Staining with a megakaryocyte antibodies (e.g. CD41, CD61 or Factor VIIIRAg) will highlight megakaryocyte hyperplasia and pleomorphism, and often identifies small or dysplastic megakaryocytes that may not be evident on hematoxylin and eosin staining. CD34 immunostaining is useful to enumerate the proportion of immature cells within the bone marrow in order to exclude progression to acute leukemia. Abnormal megakaryocytes can be CD34-positive in PMF.

Cytogenetics: Chromosomal analysis, by G-banding of FISH, can usually be performed on peripheral blood

Table 14.7 Causes of bone marrow fibrosis.

Myeloid malignancy
  Primary myelofibrosis
  Myelofibrotic transformation of essential thrombocythemia or polycythemia vera
  Accelerated phase of chronic myeloid leukemia
  Myelodysplasia with fibrosis
  Acute panmyelosis with fibrosis (a subtype of acute myeloid leukemia)
  Systemic mastocytosis

Other malignancy
  Hairy cell leukemia
  Secondary carcinoma

Bone disease
  Hyperparathyroidism
  Vitamin D deficiency (rickets and osteomalacia)

Autoimmune disease (e.g. systemic lupus erythematosus, systemic sclerosis)

Previous radiotherapy

Gray platelet syndrome

Granulomatous disease (e.g. tuberculosis, sarcoid)

Table 14.8. Prognostic factors in primary myelofibrosis.

IWGMRT Score[a] (2009) [15]	Other indicators of poor prognosis
Age > 65 years	WBC count < 4 × 10^9/L
Constitutional symptoms[b]	Absolute monocytosis
	Increased circulating CD34+ cells
Hemoglobin < 10 g/dL	Cytogenetic abnormalities (other than
WBC count > 25 × 10^9/L	del(20q) or del(13q))
	JAK2 V617F mutation (not all studies)
Peripheral blood blast count > 1%	Prior splenectomy

Number of risk factors (median survival):
0 risk factors: low risk (135 months)
1 risk factor: intermediate-1 (95 months)
2 risk factors: intermediate-2 (48 months)
≥ 3 risk factors: high risk (27 months)

[a] International Working Group for Myelofibrosis Research and Treatment.
[b] Weight loss > 10%, unexplained fever or excessive sweats for > 1 month.

where bone marrow cannot be aspirated. Karyotypic abnormalities are present in up to 50% of PMF patients and may be of prognostic significance (see below). CML may occasionally present with bone marrow fibrosis and should be excluded in all cases of suspected PMF that are negative for mutations in *JAK2* and *MPL*, either by chromosomal analysis or molecular testing for the *BCR-ABL1* fusion.

JAK2 and MPL mutation analysis: The *JAK2* V617F mutation is present in approximately 50% of PMF patients, and testing is recommended in all suspected cases. Mutations in *MPL* exon 10 are present in a further 5–8% of cases, and testing is useful in *JAK2* V617F-negative disease. *JAK2* exon 12 mutations have not yet been reported in patients with PMF, however, myelofibrotic transformation of *JAK2* exon 12-positive PV has been described.

Risk stratification and therapeutic monitoring

The prognosis in PMF is highly variable, although patients can be stratified by various clinical and laboratory features (Table 14.8). Presence of a *JAK2* V617F mutation predicts for decreased transfusion

requirement and higher white cell and platelet counts compared with those with *JAK2* wild-type disease. *JAK2* V617F-positive PMF has been associated with a worse overall survival, although this remains controversial. Mutations in *MPL* exon 10 predict for increased transfusion requirements compared with both *JAK2* V617F-positive and *JAK2/MPL* mutation-negative patients without a clear impact on survival. Levels of circulating CD34+ progenitor cells provide prognostic information in PMF, and may be enumerated as a proportion of CD45+ leukocytes by flow cytometry.

Since the identification of the *JAK2* V617F mutation, several small molecule inhibitors of JAK2 have been tested in animal models and early clinical trials. As JAK2 is the sole tyrosine kinase responsible for signaling via the erythropoietin and thrombopoietin receptors, JAK2 inhibition results in a predictable, dose-dependent anemia and thrombocytopenia. As such, JAK2 inhibitors have a narrow therapeutic window which limits their clinical utility. JAK2 inhibitor therapy commonly results in a reduction in spleen size in PMF, with occasional patients achieving independence from red cell transfusion. A proportion of patients also report improvement in constitutional symptoms, an effect that may be related to inhibition of JAK1 signaling and a consequent reduction in cytokine secretion.

Response to therapy may be considered at the clinical, hematological and bone marrow histological levels [17]. For the majority of patients, however, therapy is aimed at alleviating symptoms, with efficacy judged by quality of life, full blood count and palpation of the spleen. Further assessment of response may be indicated in the setting of a clinical trial, and may include radiological assessment of spleen size, examination of bone marrow histology or measurement of mutant allele burden.

Disease progression and assessment for bone marrow transplantation

Evolution to AML complicates around 30% of patients with PMF, and is diagnosed in the presence of > 20% blast cells in the peripheral blood or bone marrow. The choice of further investigations will depend on the general condition of the patient and whether intensive therapy is being considered (see PV section for a full discussion). A proportion of patients develop progressive disease without transformation to acute leukemia, often characterized by an increasing leukocyte count, falling hemoglobin and progressive extramedullary hematopoiesis.

Allogeneic bone marrow transplantation (BMT) is currently the only curative treatment for PMF, but availability is limited by the toxicity of this treatment modality and the older age of most patients. Bone marrow transplantation is generally reserved for those with poor prognosis disease, and pre-transplant work-up should include a full assessment of prognostic factors (Table 14.8). In patients with *JAK2*- or *MPL*-positive PMF, quantitation of mutant allele burden serves as a simple marker of disease control following BMT; suitable techniques include real-time PCR or pyrosequencing.

Chronic eosinophilic leukemia

Epidemiology and pathogenesis

Chronic eosinophilic leukemia (CEL) is a rare disorder characterized by peripheral blood eosinophilia, a male predominance and variable end-organ damage secondary to eosinophil degranulation. The main challenge for the diagnostician is the separation of clonal eosinophilia from the myriad reactive causes of a raised eosinophil count (Table 14.9).

Table 14.9. Causes of peripheral blood eosinophilia.

Infection, especially parasitic

Allergic and hypersensitivity disorders (including pulmonary hypersensitivity)

Vasculitis and autoimmune disorders (e.g. Churg–Strauss syndrome, rheumatoid arthritis)

Myeloid malignancy
  Chronic eosinophilic leukemia
  Myelodysplastic/myeloproliferative disorders
  Chronic myeloid leukemia
  Systemic mastocytosis
  Acute myeloid leukemia

Lymphoid malignancy
  T-cell lymphoma or occult T-cell clone
  B-lymphoblastic leukemia/lymphoma with t(5;14)(q31;q32); *IL3-IGH*
  Hodgkin lymphoma

Disseminated carcinoma

Idiopathic: hypereosinophilic syndrome

Chronic eosinophilic leukemia is characterized at the molecular level by rearrangements involving the receptor tyrosine kinases PDGFRA, PDGFRB or FGFR1 [18]. Rearrangement of *PDGFRA* is seen in 20–50% of patients with persistent eosinophilia and no secondary cause, and is due to a small intrachromosomal deletion which fuses *FIP1L1* to *PDGFRA*. *PDGFRB* rearrangements, due to chromosomal translocation, are rare and heterogeneous, with over 20 different fusion partners reported. *FGFR1*-rearranged disease is extremely rare and involves at least 12 different translocation partners.

Rearrangements of *PDGFRA* are associated with proliferation of eosinophil and occasionally mast cell lineages. *PDGFRB*-rearranged disease often involves other myeloid lineages, and the disease may be classified as atypical chronic myeloid leukemia with eosinophilia or chronic myelomonocytic leukemia with eosinophilia. *FGFR1*-rearranged disease is associated with a wide range of phenotypes, including CEL, AML and lymphoblastic lymphoma, which often arise sequentially within an individual patient.

Investigation and diagnosis

Diagnosis of CEL requires distinction from other myeloid malignancies and reactive conditions (Table 14.9). The process of investigation will depend in part on the

Table 14.10. Approach to the investigation of eosinophilia.

Patient history

Foreign travel	Animal contact
Medication (including non-prescription)	Systems review
Rashes	

Clinical examination

Respiratory	Gastrointestinal
Cardiac	Nervous system
Lymphatic	

Stage one investigations

Blood count and blood film	Autoantibodies:
Inflammatory markers	Nuclear, extractable nuclear antigen and DNA antibodies
Immunoglobulins including IgE	Anti-neutrophil cytoplasmic antibodies
Chest X-ray	Rheumatoid factor

Foreign travel or émigré

Hot stool: ova, cysts and parasites × 3
Strongyloides serology
Serology relevant to specific area of travel

Stage two investigations: bone marrow studies

Bone marrow morphology	Cytogenetic analysis by G-banding
FISH and/or molecular studies:	T-cell studies:
PDGFRA rearrangement	T-cell receptor rearrangement
BCR-ABL1	T-cell immunophenotype
KIT D816V	

Further investigations: end-organ damage

Lung function tests
ECG
Echocardiogram
Cardiac MRI

Table 14.11. World Health Organization classification of patients with peripheral blood eosinophilia ($> 1.5 \times 10^9$/L) [20].

Diagnostic entity	Criteria
PDGFRA-rearranged myeloid neoplasm with eosinophilia	Detection of *FIP1L1-PDGFRA* in blood or bone marrow by molecular or cytogenetic technique
PDGFRB-rearranged myeloid neoplasm with eosinophilia	Detection of *PDGFRB*-rearrangement
FGFR1-rearranged myeloid neoplasm with eosinophilia	Detection of *FGFR1*-rearrangement
Chronic eosinophilic leukemia	1. No reactive eosinophilia (see Table 14.9) 2. No other myeloid or lymphoid malignancy 3. No T-cell population with clonal TCR or aberrant phenotype 4. *Either* clonal bone marrow abnormality or increased blasts in peripheral blood (2–19%) or bone marrow (6–19%)
Hypereosinophilic syndrome	Meets above criteria 1–3 but not criteria 4

TCR = T-cell receptor.

diagnostic of CEL according to WHO criteria (Table 14.11). In the absence of one of these molecular lesions, a diagnosis of CEL requires exclusion of other MPNs that may be associated with eosinophilia (especially CML) and causes of reactive eosinophilia, including the presence of an occult T-cell clone. Even if these disorders are excluded, CEL can only be diagnosed in the presence of either a clonal cytogenetic abnormality (other than *BCR-ABL1*) or an increase in blast cells in blood or bone marrow. Patients with persistent eosinophilia without a secondary cause who do not meet criteria for CEL are currently classified as hypereosinophilic syndrome (HES) (Table 14.11) and this entity is therefore likely to be heterogeneous. Hypereosinophilic syndrome patients should therefore be reassessed regularly for the presence of new clinical or laboratory findings that may illuminate the underlying diagnosis.

Blood film and bone marrow examination: The blood count in CEL shows an elevated eosinophil count usually with normal hemoglobin and platelet levels,

clinical history and physical examination and may not involve a hematologist at the outset (Table 14.10). Patients with CEL may be diagnosed by chance or with symptomatic complications of eosinophil degranulation affecting the skin (urticaria, rashes), heart (endomyocardial fibrosis and thrombosis), nervous system (various manifestations: peripheral or central, focal or generalized) or lung (pulmonary fibrosis, infiltrates or pleural effusion). Of note, the presence of end-organ damage is not specific for CEL and may occur as a consequence of any cause of persistent eosinophilia, be it clonal or reactive.

The presence of eosinophilia in association with rearrangement of *PDGFRA*, *PDGFRB* or *FGFR1* is

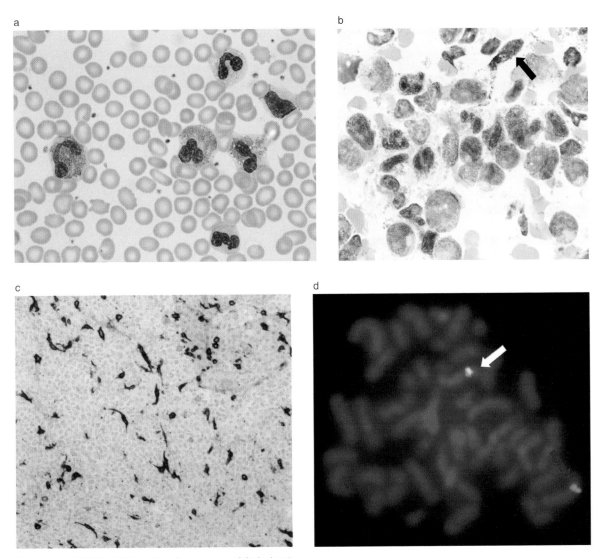

Figure 14.8. *PDGFRA-FIP1L1*-positive chronic eosinophilic leukemia.
a. Blood film showing partially degranulated eosinophils.
b. Bone marrow aspirate showing increased eosinophil precursors and occasional mast cells (arrow).
c. Bone marrow trephine biopsy stained with CD117 highlighting a diffuse infiltrate of mast cells, some with spindle-shaped morphology.
d. Metaphase FISH showing a normal chromosome 4q signal (white arrow) and loss of the red probe on the other chromosome 4q (red arrow) due to an interstitial deletion resulting in a *PDGFRA-FIP1L1* fusion. Courtesy of Bridget Manasse, Addenbrooke's Hospital, Cambridge, UK.

although anemia and thrombocytopenia may be present in late-stage disease or where there is significant splenic enlargement. Levels of neutrophils and/or monocytes may also be increased, particularly in association with rearrangement of *PDGFRB*. On blood film examination, eosinophils may show abnormal morphology including hypersegmented nuclei (three or more segments), ring nuclei or partial loss of cytoplasmic granules (Figure 14.8a), although none of these features reliably distinguish CEL from reactive causes

of eosinophilia. Dysplasia in non-eosinophil lineages and/or the presence of circulating primitive cells are suggestive of a clonal blood disorder.

Bone marrow studies are recommended in cases of persistent eosinophilia where other causes have been excluded (Table 14.9). The bone marrow aspirate in CEL shows an increase in eosinophils at all stages of maturation, with eosinophil myelocytes often showing prominent basophilic granulation (Figure 14.8b). An increase in neutrophil and/or monocyte lineages with or without dysplasia may also be seen, especially in association with rearrangement of *PDGFRB*. The trephine biopsy appearances are similar to the aspirate, with a variable increase in overall cellularity. An increase in mast cells may also be evident, especially in *PDGFRA*-rearranged disease, generally as a scattered infiltrate of morphologically normal cells (Figure 14.8c). In some cases focal mast cell infiltrates may be seen, for example surrounding blood vessels, and rare cases of *FIP1L1-PDGFRA*-associated disease may meet morphological criteria for systemic mastocytosis. Similar to the peripheral blood film, bone marrow eosinophil morphology alone is generally unable to distinguish clonal from reactive conditions, although the presence of dysplasia in non-eosinophil lineages or an increased blast count favors a clonal proliferation.

Cytogenetics: Chromosomal analysis is recommended in all cases of suspected CEL. G-banding analysis will detect rearrangements of *PDGFRB* and *FGFR1*, although the *FIP1L1-PDGFRA* fusion is inapparent due to the small size of the intrachromosomal deletion and requires FISH (Figure 14.8d) or molecular detection (RT-PCR for the fusion transcript, which can also be performed on peripheral blood). FISH probes are also available for the detection of *PDGFRB*-rearrangements. CML, which may occasionally present with a predominant eosinophil proliferation, can be excluded by G-banding, FISH studies or molecular analysis for the *BCR-ABL1* fusion. Acquired karyotypic abnormalities such as trisomy 8 or isochromosome 17q may be seen in CEL and establish the presence of clonal hematopoiesis.

T-cell receptor gene rearrangement: Occult clonal T-cell proliferations are a recognized cause of eosinophilia, often in association with skin rashes and a raised serum IgE but without palpable lymphadenopathy. Molecular analysis of bone marrow for clonal rearrangement of the T-cell receptor is therefore recommended in cases lacking rearrangements of *PDGFRA/B* or *FGFR1*. T-cell immunophenotyping should also be considered, particularly when a lymphocytosis is detected in the aspirate sample.

Risk stratification and therapeutic monitoring

Therapy for CEL is aimed primarily at protecting patients from the long-term complications of a raised eosinophil count, particularly end-organ damage to the heart and lungs. Baseline investigation of the heart (cardiac MRI or echocardiogram) and lungs (lung function testing with or without CT imaging) may be indicated in the presence of relevant symptoms or clinical signs. There may also be a role for repeating cardiac and respiratory investigations at regular intervals (e.g. every 1–3 years) although this will be guided by response to therapy of the individual patient.

PDGFRA and PDGFRB are both inhibited by the tyrosine kinase inhibitor imatinib. Imatinib therapy in disorders carrying rearrangements of *PDGFRA/B* generally results in a prompt and sustained normalization of the eosinophil count. Monitoring of therapeutic response by bone marrow FISH studies should be considered for all imatinib-treated patients, for example every 6 months until complete cytogenetic remission is achieved. Molecular quantitation of the *FIP1L1-PDGFRA* fusion is also possible using bone marrow or peripheral blood, and may be used to monitor response to therapy once complete cytogenetic remission has been achieved. Disease relapse on imatinib has been reported in patients with *PDGFRA*-rearranged CEL, due to acquisition of mutations in *FIP1L1-PDGFRA* resulting in decreased imatinib sensitivity.

Disease progression

PDGFRA- and PDGFRB-rearranged CEL both carry a good prognosis, with AML transformation reported only rarely, and imatinib therapy providing protection from eosinophil-associated end-organ damage. FGFR1 is not inhibited by imatinib or other currently available tyrosine kinase inhibitors. Moreover this condition is associated with a dismal prognosis, with progression to AML or development of lymphoblastic lymphoma almost invariable within a year of diagnosis. Early allogeneic bone marrow transplantation is the only useful treatment modality currently available, although small molecular inhibitors of FGFR1 are under development.

Systemic mastocytosis

Epidemiology and pathogenesis

Systemic mastocytosis (SM) is characterized by focal proliferations of neoplastic mast cells in bone marrow, skin and various other organs. The annual incidence of this rare condition is less than 1 per 1 000 000 population. Clinical manifestations are heterogeneous

Table 14.12. Causes of bone marrow mastocytosis.

Myeloid malignancy
   Systemic mastocytosis
   Mast cell leukemia
   Chronic eosinophilic leukemia

Lymphoproliferative disorders

Chronic infection or inflammation

Aplastic anemia/paroxysmal nocturnal hemoglobinuria

Familial mastocytosis

and include skin rashes, mediator-related symptoms (hypotension/syncope, diarrhoea, flushing and anaphylaxis) and end-organ damage (bone marrow failure, bone destruction, liver failure, splenomegaly with hypersplenism and gastrointestinal malabsorption). Organ failure is the main source of morbidity and mortality, although a minority of patients develop AML. Acquired mutations in *KIT* are present in the vast majority of SM patients, comprising *KIT* D816V in 90%, other variants at D816 in 5–10%, and changes at I817 and D820 in occasional patients.

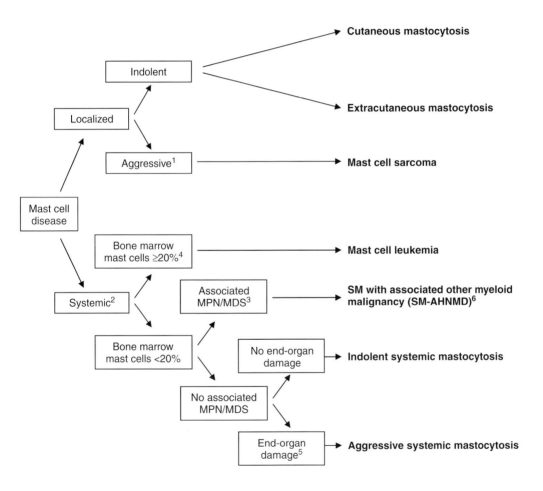

[1]Evidence of tissue destruction
[2]Meeting WHO criteria for systemic mastocytosis (Table 14.13)
[3]Meeting WHO criteria for systemic mastocytosis and a separate myeloproliferative or myelodysplastic neoplasm
[4]Or peripheral blood mast cells ≥10%
[5]Evidence of impaired bone marrow or liver function, osteolytic lesions, pathological fractures, splenomegaly with hypersplenism or malabsorption
[6]SM-AHNMD: Systemic mastocytosis with associated clonal, hematological non-mast-cell lineage disease

Figure 14.9. Algorithm for the diagnosis of neoplastic mast cell disorders.

Investigation and diagnosis

Demonstration of tissue infiltration by abnormal mast cells is key to the diagnosis of SM. The nature of the tissue examined will depend on the presenting features and may include skin, liver or bone marrow. In the bone marrow, low-level mast cell infiltrates, generally with normal morphology, can occasionally be seen in some reactive and lymphoproliferative disorders (Table 14.12). In SM typical appearances in tissue and bone marrow biopsies comprise multifocal, dense infiltrates of mast cells with abnormal spindle-shaped morphology. The subclassification of mast cell disease depends on the extent of the disease (local versus generalized), the presence or absence of a non-mast-cell hematopoietic proliferation and the presence of end-organ damage (indolent versus aggressive disease) (Figure 14.9 and Table 14.13). In patients presenting with skin disease (most commonly urticaria pigmentosa) in the absence of systemic symptoms or features of end-organ damage, further investigation may not be required. In this situation, measurement of serum tryptase may be useful as consistently raised levels generally indicate the involvement of other organs (see below).

Blood film and bone marrow examination: The blood film in SM may be normal or show features of an accompanying myeloproliferative or myelodysplastic/myeloproliferative neoplasm (see below). The presence of ≥ 10% mast cells in the blood indicates a diagnosis of mast cell leukemia, a rare disorder that may occur *de novo* or as a complication of SM. Bone marrow studies are recommended in all cases where an abnormal mast cell infiltrate has been identified on tissue biopsy, in order to correctly stage the extent of the disease. In cases where the bone marrow is infiltrated, abnormal mast cells showing angular nuclei and hypogranular cytoplasm may be present in small numbers in the bone marrow aspirate, although they often remain trapped within bone marrow particles (Figure 14.10a).

Bone marrow trephine histology is one of the major diagnostic criteria for systemic mastocytosis (Table 14.13). In systemic mastocytosis there are multifocal dense clusters of spindle-shaped cells with surrounding collagen fibrosis and a cuff or central

Table 14.13. World Health Organization criteria for the diagnosis of systemic mastocytosis [20].

A1 + any B criterion *or* any three B criteria

A1	Multifocal, dense mast cell infiltrates (≥ 15 mast cells) in bone marrow and/or extracutaneous organs
B1	Greater than 25% of mast cells show atypical morphology (spindle-shaped or immature)
B2	Acquired mutation at *KIT* D816 in blood, bone marrow or extracutaneous organ
B3	Mast cells express CD2 and/or CD25
B4	Serum tryptase > 20 ng/mL (only in absence of an associated clonal myeloid disorder)

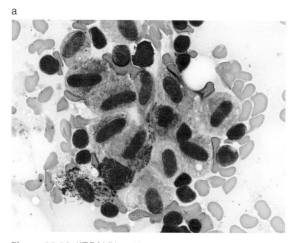

a

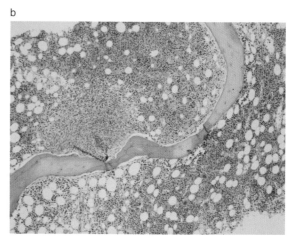

b

Figure 14.10. *KIT* D816V-positive systemic mastocytosis.
a. Mast cells in a bone marrow aspirate showing hypogranular mast cells and spindle-shaped morphology.
b. Bone marrow trephine biopsy showing mast cells embedded in collagen fibrosis adjacent to normal hematopoiesis.

core of mature lymphocytes (Figure 14.10b). This differs from reactive conditions where the mast cells are morphologically normal and appear as scattered isolated forms. Mast cells can be highlighted by staining with Giemsa or toluidine blue stains (although malignant mast cells may stain poorly in decalcified tissues due to degranulation), or immunostaining for mast cell tryptase or the KIT receptor CD117. Immunostaining for CD2 and CD25 is also recommended, as aberrant expression of one or both of these antigens is typical of neoplastic mast cells. Between the mast cell clusters, the bone marrow may appear normal or hypercellular. Eosinophils are often increased, either within the mast cell infiltrates or throughout the marrow cavity. Bone destruction and/or new bone formation may also be present.

In approximately 30% of cases, the bone marrow mast cell infiltrate is associated with features of a coexisting myeloproliferative or myelodysplastic/ myeloproliferative neoplasm, referred to in the WHO classification as 'systemic mastocytosis with associated clonal, hematological non-mast-cell lineage disease' (SM-AHNMD). The accompanying myeloid proliferation, most commonly resembling chronic myelomonocytic leukemia (CMML) or atypical chronic myeloid leukemia (aCML, Figure 14.11), is classified

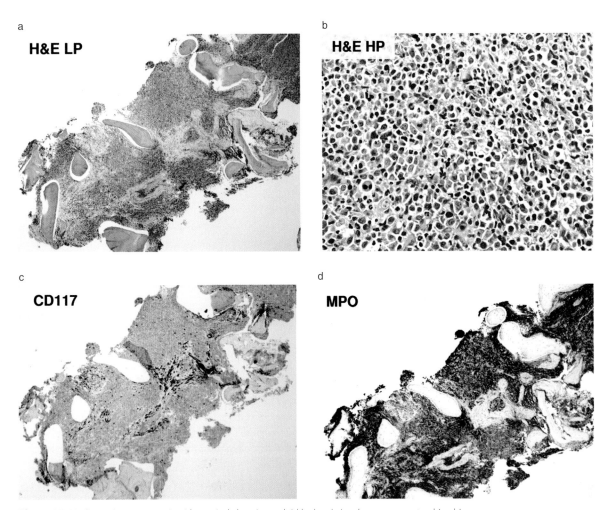

Figure 14.11. Systemic mastocytosis with atypical chronic myeloid leukemia in a bone marrow trephine biopsy.
a. Hematoxylin and eosin (H&E) stain showing diffuse hypercellularity with patchy areas of enhanced eosinophilia.
b. Higher power view (H&E stain) showing granulocytic hyperplasia in the diffusely hypercellular areas; these are the chronic myeloid leukemia.
c. The eosinophilic areas in the H&E are mast cells, as highlighted by strong CD117 positivity.
d. The surrounding granulocytic hyperplasia is highlighted by myeloperoxidase (MPO) staining.

independently of the mast cell disease according to standard criteria.

A generalized increase in bone marrow mast cells may also be seen in patients with *FIP1L1-PDGFRA*-positive CEL (see above). In most cases, the mast cells are scattered throughout the bone marrow (Figure 14.8c), although in occasional cases they may form clusters or show spindle-shaped morphology, such that a diagnosis of systemic mastocytosis is suspected. Testing for the *FIP1L1-PDGFRA* fusion, either by cytogenetic or molecular techniques, is therefore recommended in cases of suspected SM that are negative for mutations in *KIT*.

Cytogenetics: Clonal cytogenetic abnormalities are occasionally detected, usually in patients with SM-AHNMD, and include +8, −7/7q, −5/5q and other non-specific myeloid-associated aberrations. Cytogenetic analysis can therefore be restricted to cases with an associated myeloid proliferation. For the sake of efficiency, a reasonable approach would be to use a panel of FISH probes to detect common myeloid-associated abnormalities (e.g. 5q, 7q, chromosome 8 and 20q).

KIT mutation analysis: Testing for *KIT* mutations can be performed on bone marrow or other tissues where an abnormal mast cell infiltrate has been detected. The method used should be of suitable sensitivity as the burden of clonal disease in bone marrow is often low; for this reason testing of peripheral blood is not advisable due to the risk of false negative results. Testing for

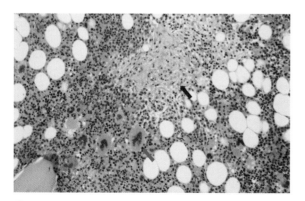

Figure 14.12. Systemic mastocytosis with essential thrombocythemia, showing a coexisting mast cell infiltrate (red arrow) and large, hyperlobated megakaryocytes (blue arrow). In this patient, *KIT* D816V and *JAK2* V617F mutations were present in distinct clonal expansions [9]. Courtesy of Dr. Jonathan Cullis, Salisbury District Hospital, UK.

the common *KIT* D816V mutation is recommended in all cases, and a search for other *KIT* mutations may be considered in negative cases. A proportion of patients with an accompanying myeloid disorder, particularly those with CMML, harbor both a *JAK2* V617F and *KIT* D816V mutation. Of note, in a case of SM with associated ET, mutations in *JAK2* and *KIT* were present in separate clonal proliferations (Figure 14.12) [9]. It is likely, therefore, that SM-AHNMD represents morphologically apparent oligoclonal disease, as has been suggested for RARS-T (see ET section).

Acquired mutations affecting a different region of *KIT* (codons 550–584) are associated with gastrointestinal stromal tumors (GIST). Of interest, inherited mutations in this region (e.g. del559–560) give rise to a rare autosomal dominant syndrome characterized by coexisting GIST and mast cell disease, although occasionally patients present with mast cell disease in isolation. A family history of gastrointestinal tumors or mast cell disease should therefore be sought in young patients presenting with *KIT* D816V-negative SM.

Although native KIT is inhibited by the tyrosine kinase inhibitor imatinib, mutations at D816 render the receptor resistant to this agent. Second-generation tyrosine kinase inhibitors such as dasatinib show activity against mutant KIT *in vitro*; however, results from clinical trials have been disappointing. Newer molecules with improved activity are under development. Where SM is diagnosed in the absence of a *KIT* mutation, a trial of imatinib may be considered if therapy is required. Inherited *KIT* mutations retain sensitivity to imatinib, and a trial of imatinib may be considered for those with familial mastocytosis should therapy become necessary.

Serum tryptase: Measurement of serum tryptase is recommended in all cases of suspected SM. It should be noted that allergic reactions are associated with an increase in serum tryptase that may take several days to return to normal. Serum tryptase level may be normal when the disease is restricted to the skin but is generally increased if other organs are involved.

End-organ damage: Screening for end-organ damage should be guided by patient symptoms and physical examination, and may included a skeletal survey, dual energy X-ray absorptiometry (DEXA) scan or radiological assessment of liver and spleen.

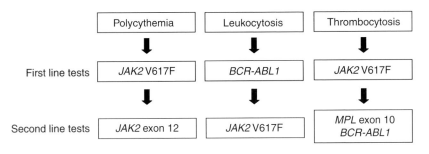

Figure 14.13. Algorithm for the molecular investigation of a suspected myeloproliferative neoplasm.

Risk stratification and therapeutic monitoring

The prognosis in SM is highly variable. Patients with indolent SM (SM without evidence of end-organ damage) appear to have a normal life expectancy. The absence of skin disease correlates with widespread organ infiltration and is associated with reduced survival. Other indicators of poor prognosis include anemia, thrombocytopenia, hypoalbuminemia, weight loss, eosinophilia or >5% mast cells in the bone marrow aspirate. The prognosis of any accompanying non-mast-cell lineage myeloid disease (SM-AHNMD) should also be considered as this may impart a poor prognosis to a patient with otherwise indolent mast cell disease.

Therapy is aimed at alleviating the symptoms of mediator release and inhibiting the mast cell proliferation in patients with evidence of end-organ damage. Response to treatment is generally assessed by patient symptoms and evidence of end-organ damage [19]. Routine reassessment of bone marrow histology is not routinely indicated outside the setting of a clinical trial. Serum tryptase levels correlate with disease burden and serial assessment may provide a useful proxy for therapeutic efficacy.

An integrated approach to the diagnosis of myeloproliferative neoplasms

The recent past has witnessed considerable advances in our understanding of the molecular basis of MPNs. These insights have led to the development of new diagnostic tests and an improved understanding of the relationship between the different disease entities. These advances are perhaps most evident in the diagnostic process, where the emphasis is shifting away from histological criteria and towards a molecular approach to disease classification. Testing for molecular lesions is now recommended as first line in the investigation of most MPNs, and in many cases it is possible to make a precise diagnosis from a simple blood test. Using this approach, molecular diagnostic tests are applied sequentially, depending on the nature of the blood count abnormality (Figure 14.13). Testing for mutations can be performed on DNA or complementary DNA (cDNA) depending on the specific assay used, with screening for fusion genes such as *BCR-ABL1* or *PDGFRA-FIP1L1* requiring cDNA. Adequate amounts of both DNA and cDNA can easily be obtained from a 5–10 mL sample of anticoagulated peripheral blood. Such samples are usually stable for 24–48 hours, facilitating referral to a central diagnostic laboratory.

There are several advantages to using molecular diagnostics as first-line tests in the investigation of a suspected MPN. First, molecular investigations are generally quick and simple to perform, and turnaround times can be kept short. Second, molecular testing is relatively cheap, and a positive test may obviate the need for more expensive investigations such as cytogenetic studies. Third, the algorithm allows for reflex testing if the first-line study is negative, further speeding up the diagnostic process. Finally, newly characterized pathogenetic lesions can easily be incorporated into the investigation algorithm. Overall, this approach is likely to save on physician time, patient visits to the out-patient department and the overall cost of the diagnostic process.

References

1. McNally RJ, Rowland D, Roman E, Cartwright RA. Age and sex distributions of hematological malignancies in the U.K. *Hematol Oncol* 1997;**15**(4):173–89.

2. Campbell PJ, Green AR. The myeloproliferative disorders. *New Engl J Med* 2006;**355**(23):2452–66.

3. Levine RL, Pardanani A, Tefferi A, Gilliland DG. Role of *JAK2* in the pathogenesis and therapy of myeloproliferative disorders. *Nat Rev Cancer* 2007;7(9):673–83.

4. Jones AV, Cross NC, White HE, Green AR, Scott LM. Rapid identification of *JAK2* exon 12 mutations using high resolution melting analysis. *Haematologica* 2008;93(10):1560–4.

5. McMullin MF, Bareford D, Campbell P *et al*. Guidelines for the diagnosis, investigation and management of polycythaemia/erythrocytosis. *Br J Haematol* 2005;130(2):174–95.

6. Barosi G, Birgegard G, Finazzi G *et al*. Response criteria for essential thrombocythemia and polycythemia vera: result of a European LeukemiaNet consensus conference. *Blood* 2009;113(20):4829–33.

7. Beer PA, Campbell PJ, Scott LM *et al*. MPL mutations in myeloproliferative disorders: analysis of the PT-1 cohort. *Blood* 2008;112(1):141–9.

8. Ding J, Komatsu H, Wakita A *et al*. Familial essential thrombocythemia associated with a dominant-positive activating mutation of the *c-MPL* gene, which encodes for the receptor for thrombopoietin. *Blood* 2004;103(11):4198–200.

9. Beer PA, Jones AV, Bench AJ *et al*. Clonal diversity in the myeloproliferative neoplasms: independent origins of genetically distinct clones. *Br J Haematol* 2009;144(6):904–8.

10. Harrison CN, Bareford D, Butt N *et al*. Guideline for investigation and management of adults and children presenting with a thrombocytosis. *Br J Haematol* 2010;149(3):352–75.

11. Wilkins BS, Erber WN, Bareford D *et al*. Bone marrow pathology in essential thrombocythemia: interobserver reliability and utility for identifying disease subtypes. *Blood* 2008;111(1):60–70.

12. Vannucchi AM, Antonioli E, Guglielmelli P *et al*. Characteristics and clinical correlates of *MPL* 515W>

L/K mutation in essential thrombocythemia. *Blood* 2008;112(3):844–7.

13. Campbell PJ, Bareford D, Erber WN *et al*. Reticulin accumulation in essential thrombocythemia: prognostic significance and relationship to therapy. *J Clin Oncol* 2009;27(18):2991–9.

14. Harrison CN, Campbell PJ, Buck G *et al*. Hydroxyurea compared with anagrelide in high-risk essential thrombocythemia. *New Engl J Med* 2005;353(1):33–45.

15. Cervantes F, Dupriez B, Pereira A *et al*. New prognostic scoring system for primary myelofibrosis based on a study of the International Working Group for Myelofibrosis Research and Treatment. *Blood* 2009;113(13):2895–901.

16. Dupriez B, Morel P, Demory JL *et al*. Prognostic factors in agnogenic myeloid metaplasia: a report on 195 cases with a new scoring system. *Blood* 1996;88(3):1013–18.

17. Tefferi A, Barosi G, Mesa RA *et al*. International Working Group (IWG) consensus criteria for treatment response in myelofibrosis with myeloid metaplasia, for the IWG for Myelofibrosis Research and Treatment (IWG-MRT). *Blood* 2006;108(5):1497–503.

18. Atlas of Genetics and Cytogenetics in Oncology and Haematology {database on the Internet}. Available from: http://AtlasGeneticsOncology.org

19. Valent P, Akin C, Sperr WR *et al*. Aggressive systemic mastocytosis and related mast cell disorders: current treatment options and proposed response criteria. *Leuk Res* 2003;27(7):635–41.

20. Swerdlow SH, Campo E, Harris NL *et al*. (eds.). *WHO Classification of Tumours of Haematopoietic and Lymphoid Tissues*, 4th edn. Lyon: IARC Press; 2008.

21. McMullin MF, Reilly JT, Campbell P *et al*. on behalf of the National Cancer Research Institute, Myeloproliferative Disorder Subgroup and Kate Ryan on behalf of the British Committee for Standards in Haematology. Amendment to the guideline for diagnosis and investigation of polycythaemia/erythrocytosis. *Br J Haematol* 2007;138(6):821–2.

15 Myelodysplastic syndromes and myelodysplastic/myeloproliferative neoplasms

Raphael Itzykson, Hervé Roudot and Pierre Fenaux

Myelodysplastic syndromes and myelodysplastic/myeloproliferative neoplasms

Myelodysplastic syndromes (MDS) are a group of clonal disorders of the hematopoietic stem cell (HSC) characterized by ineffective hematopoiesis. This leads to peripheral blood cytopenias, and an excess of marrow blast cells. In some cases this can progress to acute myeloid leukemia (AML). Myelodysplastic syndromes are thought to result from the accumulation of genetic or epigenetic lesions (such as promoter hypermethylation) initially in a very immature progenitor cell. This leads to a proliferative advantage of the MDS clone over normal immature progenitors. MDS lineage-committed progenitors display both abnormal terminal differentiation and an increased susceptibility to apoptosis. These two features explain the clinical consequences of blast cell accumulation and peripheral blood cytopenias [1].

The diagnosis of MDS is generally suggested by the presence of peripheral blood (PB) cytopenias. However, the diagnosis requires the integration of the blood manifestations with the clinical history and physical examination. Although the etiology of MDS is generally unknown, antecedent cytotoxic therapy or radiation exposure and congenital bone marrow failure syndromes can predispose to MDS. Physical examination is in general normal in MDS, while splenomegaly can be found in myelodysplastic/myeloproliferative neoplasms (MDS/MPN). Careful morphological review of bone marrow for dysplasia is central to the diagnosis of MDS and MDS/MPN, and cytogenetic analysis for prognosis. Molecular

genetics and flow cytometry assays are under evaluation, and, in future, may provide information for further refinement of the prognosis. The specific features of each of these diagnostic modalities will be discussed.

The classification of MDS has undergone significant changes over the past 30 years. Prior to the introduction of the first international classification in 1982 by the French American British (FAB) group, a number of descriptive terms were used to describe MDS [2]. The FAB classification provided an internationally accepted nomenclature. This was revised by a WHO expert committee in 2001, and again in 2008, to include novel features which refined MDS prognosis, e.g. multi-lineage dysplasia [3,4]. The WHO classification lowered the bone marrow blast cell threshold for AML from 30% to 20%, and introduced the term MDS/MPN to encompass a heterogeneous set of entities previously included in MDS (including chronic myelomonocytic leukemia – CMML). MDS/MPN share MDS features, such as marrow dysplasia and peripheral cytopenias, but also have proliferative characteristics of hyperleukocytosis, organomegaly, and underlying genetic lesions in cell proliferation pathways, notably in the Ras pathway.

Prognostic evaluation of MDS largely relies on an International Prognostic Scoring System (IPSS). This was established on the basis of an international cohort of patients (IMRAW cohort) that was managed symptomatically. The IPSS utilizes the number of cytopenias, the percentage of blast cells in the marrow, and cytogenetics. From this the IPSS separates patients into four risk categories (low, intermediate-1,

Diagnostic Techniques in Hematological Malignancies, ed. Wendy N. Erber. Published by Cambridge University Press.
© Cambridge University Press 2010.

Table 15.1. International Prognostic Scoring System (IPSS) [5].

Score	0	0.5	1	1.5
Cytopenias	0–1	2–3		
% bone marrow blasts	<5%	5–10%		11–19%
Karyotype	Favorable	Intermediate	Unfavorable	

IPSS group	Low	Intermediate-1	Intermediate-2	Unfavorable
Score	0	0.5–1	1.5–2	2.5+
Proportion of patients	33	38	22	7
Overall survival (median, years)	5.7	3.5	1.2	0.4
Time to AML (median, years)	5.7	2.7	0.95	0.3

intermediate-2, and high) (Table 15.1) [5]. The IPSS has since been validated in patient cohorts receiving active treatments, including intensive chemotherapy and allogeneic stem cell transplantation. IPSS categories are often grouped into "lower-risk" MDS (IPSS low and intermediate-1), and "higher-risk" MDS (IPSS intermediate-2 and high). Lower-risk MDS are patients with prolonged survival and where the main objective is to manage chronic cytopenias, notably anemia; for this group of patients aggressive treatments, especially allogeneic stem cell transplantation (ASCT) should be deferred. In higher-risk MDS, treatments aimed at altering the disease history and prolonging survival, such as ASCT and the hypomethylating agent azacytidine, are required [6]. Alternative prognostic classifications have been proposed to better capture the heterogeneity of "lower-risk" MDS [7]. One of these uses a score based on the WHO classification (WHO-based prognostic scoring system, WPSS). In this approach red blood cell (RBC) transfusion requirements and bone marrow multi-lineage dysplasia are substituted for the number of cytopenias utilized by the IPSS, and, the relative contribution of cytogenetics compared with blast percentage is also modified [8].

Diagnostic criteria for MDS and MDS/MPN

Three criteria must be met for the diagnosis of MDS:

1. Persistent (>6 months) and significant *cytopenia*(s) i.e. Hb <10 g/dL, absolute neutrophil count (ANC) <1.8 × 10^9/L and platelets <100 × 10^9/L.

2. Significant bone marrow *dysplasia*, or *blast excess* or a typical cytogenetic abnormality.
3. Exclusion of differential diagnoses [9].

The term "idiopathic cytopenias of undetermined signification" (ICUS) has been coined for cases when the cytopenias or dysplasias do not reach the diagnostic thresholds required to diagnose MDS and differential diagnoses have been excluded. The natural history of ICUS remains unclear, but as it may evolve into MDS, blood and bone marrow monitoring is indicated. Some criteria have been proposed to identify those ICUS cases that are *bona fide* MDS, but none has been prospectively validated [10].

Benign secondary dysplasias must be distinguished from primary MDS. Common causes include:

1. *Vitamin deficiency*, such as megaloblastic anemias due to folate deficiency or hydroxycobalamin deficiency.
2. *Copper deficiency*.
3. *Toxic exposure* including to heavy metals, such as chronic arsenic exposure, or excessive zinc supplementation.
4. *Drugs*: anti-folate drugs, mycophenolate mofetil and growth factors such as G-CSF.
5. *Viral infections* such as HIV-associated myelodysplasia [11].

Some cases of MDS display erythroid hypoplasia, requiring other causes of erythroblastopenia to be excluded (e.g. parvovirus B19 infection, congenital dyserythropoietic anemia). Lymphoproliferative disorders such as hairy cell leukemia, or large granular lymphocytic leukemia can also present as isolated cytopenias; these can be excluded on morphology and flow cytometry. Hyperleukocytosis of MDS/MPN, with or without mild monocytosis, must be distinguished from secondary causes as seen in inflammation, infection (e.g. tuberculosis) or carcinoma.

Peripheral blood and bone marrow morphology in MDS and MDS/MPN

Peripheral blood

Red cells: Dysplastic features in the peripheral blood are often the first indicator of MDS (Table 15.2). The majority of MDS patients (80–90%) present with normocytic or macrocytic, non-regenerative anemia (without polychromasia) and which is frequently isolated. Very rarely MDS can present with a hypochromic microcytic anemia resulting from acquired hemoglobin H disease which is caused by somatic mutations in the ATRX gene ("α-thalassemia MDS" [12]). Intramedullary apoptosis from ineffective erythropoiesis can cause increased lactate dehydrogenase and hyper-bilirubinemia. Rarely, hemolysis can occur in MDS from acquired pyruvate kinase deficiency or from a Paroxysmal Nocturnal Hemolysis (PNH) clone. Erythroid dysplasia can cause elevated

hemoglobin F and loss of ABO antigens; the latter can lead to blood grouping difficulties and discrepancies between forward and reverse groups.

Leukocytes and platelets: Isolated thrombocytopenia and neutropenia are less common in MDS than isolated anemia. Thrombocytopenia (25% cases) can be accompanied by decreased platelet function; when platelet numbers and bleeding symptoms are discordant, platelet aggregation tests may be indicated. Immune thrombocytopenia may occur in MDS, and this can be assessed by isotopic platelet labeling. Thrombocytosis is associated with particular genetic lesions, including deletion 5q, 3q26 anomaly and *JAK2* mutations. Neutropenia (~50% cases) in MDS is commonly accompanied by impaired neutrophil function, such as chemotaxis, phagocytosis and reduced bactericidal power. Circulating blast cells are frequent in MDS cases with excess marrow blast cells. However, even in lower-risk MDS, small numbers of blasts (1–2%) can be seen in the blood and these are prognostically meaningful [13]. These above-mentioned peripheral blood numerical and morphological abnormalities may suggest MDS but are insufficient on their own to make a diagnosis. A bone marrow examination is required to make the diagnosis of MDS.

Myelodysplastic/myeloproliferative neoplasms should be considered when there is coexistence of hyperleukocytosis with cytopenias and dysplastic morphological features. Monocytosis of $>1 \times 10^9$/L (and representing >10% WBC) with neutrophilia and <10% neutrophil precursors is suggestive of CMML or its juvenile form (JMML), while presence of >10% immature myeloid progenitors is found in atypical chronic myeloid leukemia (aCML). Blast cells may also be seen in the circulation in CMML, JMML and aCML but these make up less than 20% of leukocytes.

Bone marrow aspirate cytology

Cytological examination of aspirated bone marrow is essential to make a diagnosis of MDS. The bone marrow trephine (BMT) biopsy is useful to assess overall marrow cellularity and to evaluate the presence of fibrosis. Optimal diagnosis requires well-prepared bone marrow smears stained with May–Grünwald Giemsa (MGG) and Perls' stains, and morphological expertise. Increasing the number of analyzed cells improves the reproducibility of dysplasia assessment and reduces the confidence interval of blast percentage [14]. Consensus thresholds are:

Table 15.2. Dysplastic features of peripheral blood and bone marrow according to World Health Organization diagnostic criteria [90].

Dyserythropoiesis	Dysgranulopoiesis
Nucleus	Small or unusually large size
Budding	Nuclear hypolobation (pseudo-Pelger–Huët)
Internuclear bridging	Irregular hypersegmentation
Karryorhexis	Hypogranularity, agranularity
Multinuclearity	Pseudo-Chediak–Higashi granules
Hyperlobulation	Auer rods
Megaloblastosis	
Cytoplasm	**Dysmegakaryopoiesis**
Ring sideroblasts	Micro-megakaryocytes
Vacuolization	Hypolobated nucleus
Periodic acid Schiff positivity	Multi-nucleation

Table 15.3. World Health Organization classification of myelodysplastic syndromes (MDS) [90].

Feature	RCUD	RARS	RCMD	RAEB-1	RAEB-2	MDS-U	del(5q) syndrome
Cytopenias	1 (rarely 2)	Anemia	1+	1+	1+	1+	1+
Peripheral blood blast cells	<1%	0	<1%	<5%	5–19%	<1%	<1%
Bone marrow dysplasia	1	Erythroid only	2+	1+	1+	<10% lineage	typical
Ring sideroblasts	<15%	>15%	< or >15%	< or >15%	< or >15%	<15%	<15%
Bone marrow blast cells	<5%	<5%	<5%	5–9%	10–19%	<5%	<5%
Cytogenetics	Often normal	Often normal	Any	Any	Any	Typical of MDS	Isolated del5q

RCUD = Refractory cytopenia with uni-lineage dysplasia.
RARS = Refractory anemia with ring sideroblasts.
RCMD = Refractory cytopenia with multi-lineage dysplasia.
RAEB = Refractory anemia with excess blasts.

1. Blood: 200 leukocytes and 500 if circulating blast cells are present (this may require a buffy coat preparation).
2. Bone marrow (MGG stain): 500 nucleated cells, including at least 100 non-erythroid cells and 30 megakaryocytes.
3. Perls' Prussian Blue stain: 100 erythroid cells.

The various aspects of bone marrow examination (detailed below) can be integrated to diagnose and classify MDS and MDS/MPN according to WHO criteria (MDS: Table 15.3; MDS/MPN: Table 15.4).

Dysplasia: Presence of dysplasia is the first key criterion for the diagnosis of MDS and MDS/MPN and for determining prognosis. Dysplastic changes are often, but not always, correlated to the blood cytopenias. A given lineage is considered dysplastic if two or more dysplastic features are found on ≥ 10% cells. Typical bone marrow dysplastic features are summarized in Table 15.2. Multi-lineage dysplasia is defined as the coexistence of dysplasias in two or more lineages. Multi-lineage dysplasia cases frequently have excess blasts. However, multi-lineage dysplasia defines a subgroup of MDS patients without blast excess who have a worse prognosis [8].

Ring sideroblasts: Ring sideroblasts are defined as sideroblasts with ≥ 5 siderotic granules surrounding

at least one third of the nuclear circumference [15]. They are not specific for MDS as they can also be seen in a variety of conditions including alcohol consumption, copper deficiency or zinc excess and X-linked recessive inherited sideroblastic anemia. Ring sideroblasts are considered significant when they represent >15% of erythroid cells; this is a common finding in MDS with excess blasts. In the absence of excess blasts, ring sideroblasts define an entity with a favorable prognosis, termed "refractory anemia with ring sideroblasts" (RARS). Perls' staining can also reveal increased macrophage storage iron in MDS, mainly resulting from ineffective erythropoiesis or chronic red blood cell transfusions.

Other features: Auer rods have historically been recognized as a poor prognostic marker in MDS and remain so in the current WHO classification. Some morphological features are strongly suggestive of a specific underlying cytogenetic or genetic aberration. For example, characteristic dysgranulopoiesis combining pseudo-Pelger-Huët anomaly and small vacuolated neutrophils is associated with 17p deletions and p53 tumor suppressor gene mutations [16]. The "5q– syndrome", recognized by the WHO classification as a distinct entity, also has a distinct morphology (see below). Finally, the very rare cases presenting as MDS/MPN with marrow eosinophilia often have rearrangements of the PDGFβ receptor, and are

Table 15.4. World Health Organization criteria for myelodysplastic/myeloproliferative neoplasms (MDS/MPN) [90].

Diagnostic feature	CMML-1	CMML-2	aCML	JMML	MDS/MPN-U	RARS-T
Peripheral blood monocytes	$>1 \times 10^9$/L		<10%	$>1 \times 10^9$/L		
Left shift and myelocytes	<10%		>10%	[a]		
Leukocytes ($\times 10^9$/L)	Any		>13	$>10^a$	$>13^a$	
Platelets ($\times 10^9$/L)					$>450 \times 10^9$/L^a	$>450 \times 10^9$/L
Peripheral blood blasts	<5%	5–19%	<20%	<20%		
Ring sideroblasts >15%	No		No	No		Yes
Bone marrow blasts	<10%	10–19%	<20%	<20%		
Dysplasia	One or +^{a}		Dysgranulopoiesis		Yes^a	
t(9;22) or *BCR-ABL1* fusion	No		No	No	No	No
PDGFRA/B rearrangement	No		No		No	No
Cytogenetics				-7^a		
Gene mutation				PTPN11 RAS NF1		*JAK2* V617F
GM-CSF progenitor hypersensitivity				Yes^a		

^{a} Minor diagnostic criteria.
CMML = Chronic myelomonocytic leukemia.
aCML = Atypical chronic myeloid leukemia, *BCR-ABL1* negative.
JMML = Juvenile myelomonocytic leukemia.
MDS/MPN-U = Myelodysplastic/Myeloproliferative neoplasm, unclassifiable.
RARS-T = Refractory anemia with ring sideroblasts associated with marked thrombocytosis.

considered as specific entities because of their sensitivity to the tyrosine kinase inhibitor imatinib [17].

Granulo-monocytic proliferation: In MDS/MPN there is bone marrow hypercellularity with striking granulocytic proliferation which parallels the blood hyperleukocytosis. It should be noted that in the bone marrow, the monocytic proliferation of CMML/JMML can be difficult to identify on morphology alone. The identification of the monocytic progenitors in the marrow may require the use of esterase cytochemical staining or immunocytochemistry utilizing markers of the monocytic lineage. In CMML/JMML, dysplasia is mainly present in the granulocytic lineage but can affect other lineages, resulting in macrocytic or normocytic anemia or thrombocytopenia. In atypical CML the morphology and presentation can mimic that of typical CML, except for the invariable presence of dysgranulopoiesis.

Blast cell count: Precise enumeration of bone marrow blast cells is the second central criterion for diagnostic and prognostic classification of MDS. Blasts are defined by a high nuclear : cytoplasmic ratio and diffuse chromatin pattern, and can be "agranular" (B1) or "granular" (B2) (see also Table 15.4) [15]. A third class of blasts (B3), defined by the presence of numerous (>20) azurophilic granules, should be included in the blast percentage; these can be distinguished from promyelocytes by the lack of a Golgi structure [18]. In the setting of erythroid hyperplasia (i.e. when erythroid lineage cells make up >50% of nucleated cells), the denominator for the blast cell percentage is the total of non-erythroid cells. Peripheral blood and bone marrow blast counts in CMML/JMML should include promonocytes (but not promyelocytes) [19], and these are of prognostic significance in CMML.

Bone marrow trephine histology

Histological examination of the BMT biopsy is commonly performed in the initial diagnostic work-up of suspected MDS. However some restrict the BMT to situations where bone marrow aspiration has failed (e.g. "blood tap") or low-cellularity smears. The BMT features to be discussed are cellularity, fibrosis and abnormally localized immature myeloid precursors as well as the role of immunocytochemistry.

Hypocellularity: The BMT allows objective evaluation of bone marrow cellularity, which physiologically declines with age. Application of a standardized age correction to cellularity reduces the incidence of "hypoplastic" MDS from 29% to 7% [20,21]. Hypoplastic MDS must be distinguished from aplastic anemia and this can be difficult [14]. In this context, the presence of circulating blast cells and megakaryocytic or granulocytic dysplasia favor hypoplastic MDS. However, mild erythroid dysplasia can be seen in both MDS and aplastic anemia. Other features that support a diagnosis of MDS are:

1. Abnormal sideroblasts, i.e. increased number with abnormal patterns of siderotic granules or ring sideroblasts.
2. The presence of two or more blast cell clusters (defined below).
3. Cytogenetic aberrations, especially of chromosomes 5 or 7 (which often requires assessment by fluorescence *in situ* hybridization (FISH). This may need to be performed on peripheral blood cells, as karyotype culture of bone marrow often fails). However, these typical MDS anomalies can also arise after immunosuppressive treatment in aplastic anemia, and loss of chromosome Y or trisomy 8 can sometimes be the consequence of aging or immune aggression in both diseases [22].

In cases where it is difficult to confidently distinguish between hypoplastic MDS and aplastic anemia, CD34 and PCNA immunostaining of the BMT [23], or flow cytometry (if sufficient numbers of cells are available) may help. However, small PNH clones can be encountered in both diseases. In fact, as immune aggression has been proposed to participate in the pathophysiology of a subgroup of MDS [22], it is likely that there is a diagnostic "gray zone" between aplastic anemia and MDS.

The independent prognostic value of hypoplasia in MDS is debated [24,25]. Recognition of hypoplastic MDS, though not formalized in the WHO classification, can influence therapeutic decisions, as some investigators have reported responses to immunosuppression. Conversely, hypoplasia may induce severe hematological toxicity with other MDS drugs, such as azacytidine.

Bone marrow fibrosis: Fibrosis can be semi-quantitatively assessed by staining for reticulin fibres, for instance with Gomori's silver stain. A four-grade system has been proposed, ranking fibrosis from grade 0 to III (absent, mild, moderate or severe) [21]. Fibrosis is considered significant if grade II or III. Fibrotic MDS (MDS-F) must be distinguished from:

1. Acute panmyelosis with myelofibrosis (APMF), an entity with an abrupt onset with cytopenias, bone pain and fever.
2. Acute megakaryoblastic leukemia, which is rare in adults, and can be identified by positive cytochemistry with acid phosphatase and α-naphthyl acetate esterase, detection of platelet peroxidase by electron microscopy, or megakaryocyte immunostaining [26].
3. Primary myelofibrosis (PMF). Compared to PMF, MDS-F has low circulating CD34+ cell counts, infrequent *JAK2* V617F mutations and lower bone marrow cellularity [27].

Fibrosis is common in therapy-related MDS, where it is seen with multi-lineage dysplasia and adverse cytogenetics (although fibrosis is a cause of karyotype failure). The fibrosis itself may be an independent adverse prognostic factor for both survival and leukemic transformation [27]. Fibrosis leads to difficulties in counting blasts, but as its prognostic effect is also apparent in patients with blast excess, fibrosis appears to be an additional prognostic tool, rather than a separate MDS entity.

Abnormally localized immature myeloid progenitors: Abnormal hematopoietic progenitor cell localization in the bone marrow has been described in MDS, and possibly reflects defective hematopoiesis. Clusters (3–5 cells) or aggregates (>5 cells) of blast cells away from the endosteum or vascular niches, in the central portion (interstitium) of the bone marrow, have been called abnormally localized immature myeloid progenitors (ALIP) [28]; ALIP have been proposed as both diagnostic and prognostic markers, but suffer from a poor inter-observer reproducibility [27].

Immunocytochemistry: Immunocytochemistry with a CD34 antibody can be used to identify immature hematopoietic progenitors and megakaryocytes, and to assess the blast cell percentage. However, it must be noted that in some cases of MDS the blast cells are CD34-negative; CD117 has been proposed as a surrogate marker in these cases. Some authors suggest that CD34-positive cell clusters may better reflect prognosis than the overall percentage of CD34-positive cells [27]. It is important to remember that CD34 also stains endothelial cells, and therefore additional markers of vessels are required to distinguish angiogenesis from progenitors. Assessing angiogenesis may prove of interest in future, as microvessel density is increased in MDS [29], and distinct angiogenesis patterns have been identified in CMML [30].

Cytogenetics and molecular genetics in MDS and MDS/MPN

Conventional cytogenetics

Giemsa-banding karyotyping: Conventional cytogenetics by G-banding karyotyping is abnormal in approximately half of MDS patients [31]. The proportion of abnormal karyotypes has slightly increased over the years with refinements in culture conditions and standardization of the number of metaphases studied. Abnormal karyotypes, especially those of unfavorable prognosis, are more frequent in MDS cases with excess blast cells. The cytogenetic aberrations seen are highly heterogeneous. The most frequent types of abnormalities, by decreasing order, are:

1. Total or partial chromosome losses (most frequent).
2. Total or partial chromosome gains.
3. Unbalanced translocations.
4. Balanced translocations (rare).

Normal karyotypes, which have a favorable prognosis in MDS, are seen in 75% of patients with refractory anemia and less commonly in refractory anemia with excess blasts (RAEB) (25–50%). Karyotyping has a number of applications in the analysis of MDS:

1. A typical MDS chromosomal abnormality may assist in a morphologically challenging diagnosis.
2. Providing prognostic information.
3. Influencing therapeutic decision making [32], e.g. karyotype is a predictor of response to erythropoietin in lower-risk MDS [33].

Some chromosomal alterations occur frequently and overall represent 40% of all abnormal karyotypes. These are (Table 15.5):

1. Partial or total deletion of chromosome 5 (−5/5q−).
2. Partial or total deletion of chromosome 7 (−7/7q−).
3. Trisomy 8 (+8).
4. Partial deletion of chromosome 20 (20q−).
5. Loss of the Y chromosome (−Y).

These common chromosomal abnormalities, although not specific of MDS (as they also occur in AML or MPN), have defined prognostic value in the standard IPSS cytogenetic risk classification [5]. Trisomy 8 and −Y can also occur in constitutional mosaicism; a constitutional karyotype on blood with

Table 15.5. Cytogenetic abnormalities in myelodysplastic syndromes (MDS), their frequency and prognosis.

	Frequency	Prognosis	Reference
Trisomy 8	10%	Intermediate	[5,31,35]
del(7q)/−7	10%	Unfavorable	[5,35]
del(5q)	15%	Favorable	[5]
del(20q)	5%	Favorable	[5,31,35]
del(12p)	1%	Favorable	[31,35]
−Y	5%	Favorable	[5,31,35]
i(17q) or t(17p)	2%	Intermediate/Unfavorable	[35]
inv[3] or t(3;3)	2%	Intermediate	[35]
Complex	15%	Unfavorable	[5,31,35]

phytohemagglutinin as the mitogen should therefore be performed in these cases to ensure the correct interpretation of a cytogenetic response after intensive therapy or ASCT. Alterations in chromosome 5 and 7 and other uncommon abnormalities in AML are considered as "myelodysplasia-related changes" in the current WHO classification [4], as they may reflect an underlying undiagnosed myelodysplasia. The remaining 60% of abnormal karyotypes show rare chromosomal alterations (<2% each) and these have been arbitrarily assigned a neutral prognostic value in the IPSS. The prognostic associations of these have recently been studied in large cohorts [31,34] allowing assignment of well-defined prognosis to ~95% of MDS patients (Table 15.5).

Uncovering the cytogenetic heterogeneity of MDS has refined diagnostic entities and given new prognostic information. This has paved the way for the molecular dissection of MDS and the identification of specific therapeutic interventions. Some drugs, for example, have been shown to have differential activity in MDS according to karyotype, the exemplar being lenalidomide in del(5q) patients. Since balanced translocations are uncommon in MDS, relatively few genes potentially involved in the pathogenesis of MDS have been discovered with cytogenetics. Molecular genetic techniques have, however, led to the identification of minimal regions of chromosome interstitial deletion, where a shortlist of candidate genes can be studied functionally [35].

FISH: FISH has been a useful technique for gaining a better understanding of the pathophysiology of MDS in the following ways:

1. Demonstrating that recurrent genetic abnormalities are present in immature hematopoietic cells.
2. Providing insight into the target cell involved in transformation of the MDS to acute leukemia [36].
3. Confirming the selective intramedullary apoptosis of MDS committed progenitors [37].

In routine clinical practice, interphase FISH can help identify the most frequent abnormalities when insufficient mitoses are obtained for karyotyping. Centromeric probes can detect monosomies and trisomies of chromosomes 5, 7 and 8. Probes can also uncover recurrent interstitial deletions in 5q, 7q, 20q and 17p. A negative FISH result is not informative as it does not exclude an underlying genetic defect.

The prognostic significance of the 10–15% cryptic deletions that can be identified by FISH in patients with otherwise normal karyotypes has not been prospectively studied. Multi-color FISH can help better define complex karyotypes, without known prognostic impact. FISH can be used for monitoring the cytogenetic response following therapy, most notably in the setting of lenalidomide for 5q– syndrome [38].

Clonal evolution: Modification or changes to the karyotype (clonal evolution) is a relatively rare event in MDS (10–20% of cases). When clonal evolution does occur it is often associated with disease progression.

Common chromosomal alterations in MDS

del(5q) and the "5q– syndrome": Interstitial deletion of the long arm of chromosome 5, or del(5q), is the most frequent cytogenetic aberration in MDS, occurring in 15% of patients. The "5q– syndrome," first described by Van den Berghe *et al.* in 1974 [39], is characterized by an isolated del(5q) on conventional cytogenetics and absence of peripheral blood or bone marrow blast excess, and is now a recognized entity in the WHO classification ("MDS with isolated del(5q)"; Table 15.3).

The distinct morphological features of the "5q– syndrome" include:

1. Thrombocytosis (one third of patients).
2. Macrocytic anemia.
3. Megakaryocytes with hypolobated nuclei.
4. Erythropoiesis is commonly hypoplastic with minimal dyserythropoiesis.
5. Minimal dysgranulopoiesis.

The "5q– syndrome" has a favorable prognosis in the IPSS, with a prolonged overall survival (median survival 12 years) and a low risk (<10%) of progression to AML. The prognosis is in fact dominated by the consequences of chronic red blood cell transfusions. Patients with "5q– syndrome" have a dramatic response to the immuno-modulatory agent lenalidomide, with two-thirds reaching long-term transfusion independence [38]. Lenalidomide seems to exert its action through a clonal suppression effect, the molecular mechanisms of which are under study [40].

The interstitial deletion of 5q is of variable size, but invariably affects bands q31–q33. A common deletion region in 5q33 spanning over 1.5 Mb and encompassing 42 genes has been delineated [41]. The lack of a recurrent point mutation or a cryptic deletion on the normal 5q allele is in favor of a haplo-insufficiency model whereby loss of a single copy of one or, more probably, several genes causes the 5q– syndrome. Several candidate genes have been implicated including *SPARC*, *CTNNA1*, *EGR1* and *RPS14* [32].

Patients with blast excess or with additional cytogenetic aberrations can also have del(5q). The prognosis of these patients is much poorer than for isolated "5q– syndrome" [31], even with lenalidomide therapy [38,42]. Some authors have proposed that a distinct common deleted region, located in 5q31, is involved in these cases of MDS [43].

del(20q): MDS with del(20q) commonly presents with thrombocytopenia and has a favorable prognosis in the IPSS. It is commonly accompanied by loss of chromosome Y, which can also be found in healthy elderly subjects [44]. Del(20q) is not specific for MDS as it also occurs in MPN.

Trisomy 8: Trisomy 8 is seen in 10% of MDS and sometimes results from germinal mosaicism. It is often subclonal and fluctuates independently of blast cell counts [45]. This suggests it is a secondary lesion in MDS.

Monosomy 7/del(7q): Chromosome 7 anomalies (10% of MDS) include del(7q), monosomy 7 and more rarely t(1;7). These are second in frequency to del(5q) and almost invariably have a poor prognosis in terms of both survival and transformation risk. Different minimal regions of deletion have been described in 7q35–36, possibly with distinct prognostic values. Monosomy 7 can transform aplastic anemia or constitutional bone marrow failure syndromes (Fanconi anemia and Down syndrome), or arise after radiation or toxic exposure. It is also the most frequent alteration in childhood MDS where it is often accompanied by a degree of myeloproliferation. There is *in vitro* evidence that 7q is a genetically unstable region and that G-CSF treatment may select a del(7q) clone. Patients with –7/del(7q) have impaired neutrophil function and therefore may present with severe infections despite having only moderate neutropenia. These patients respond poorly to intensive chemotherapy but interesting results have been described with hypomethylating agents [6].

Complex karyotypes: Complex karyotypes (15% of MDS) are conventionally defined as the coexistence

of ≥ 3 genetic anomalies in a single clone and are thought to result from alterations in DNA repair or checkpoint signaling. Complex karyotypes are, by essence, heterogeneous. The prognosis worsens with each additional aberration, rather than by the chromosomes involved (most frequently 5, 7 and 17). In AML, the presence of monosomies has been shown to better predict prognosis than karyotypic complexity [46], however this analysis has not been undertaken in MDS where monosomies are in fact more frequent. Complex karyotypes are highly chemo-resistant, but interesting results with hypomethylating agents have been observed but require confirmation.

Other poor prognostic genetic abnormalities: There are other genetic abnormalities associated with poor prognosis which are not included in the IPSS. These include the 3q26 alterations, inv(3)(q21;q26) and t(3;3)(q21;q26), which rearrange the *MDS1/EVI1* locus with complex oncogenic roles [47], and may present with thrombocytosis. Alterations of 17p, resulting from unbalanced translocations or isochromosome 17, affect the p53 locus and also are in the high-risk cytogenetic category; they are generally part of complex karyotypes.

Cytogenetics and fusion transcripts of MDS/MPN

In MDS/MPN the karyotype is most often normal. When abnormalities are detected these are generally non-specific lesions, such as monosomy 7, in JMML and CMML, or del(20q) or del(12p) in CMML. It is important that t(9;22) and *BCR-ABL1* transcripts (by RT-PCR) are absent to exclude a diagnosis of typical CML (see Chapter 13). Similarly, significant marrow eosinophilia in cases of CMML is associated with the very rare t(5;12) translocation fusing the *ETV6* and *PDGFB* genes. These cases must be reconsidered as hypereosinophilic MPN, or CMML with eosinophilia and a *PDGFRA* or *PDGFRB* rearrangement by PCR.

Molecular genetics and genomics

Gene mutations: Mutations in oncogenes or tumor suppressor genes can be identified in up to 60% of MDS cases. The implicated genes that are currently known are not specific for MDS, and can be mutated in *de novo* AML or in MPN; they therefore cannot be used as diagnostic criteria. This differs from many of the MDS/MPN entities where gene mutations are important in the diagnosis (Table 15.4). In contrast to AML, a molecular genetic prognostic classifier has not emerged in MDS.

As in AML, the mutations in MDS can be broadly categorized on the basis of the cellular pathways involved. "Class I" mutations affect cytokine signaling pathways, and "class II mutations" transcription factors that drive hematopoiesis. Class I mutations are thought to confer a proliferative advantage to the MDS clone, while Class II mutations are causal for dysplasia. Of the Class I genes, mutations of the cytokine receptors *FLT3* (5% cases), *FMS* (M-CSF receptor; <5% cases) and *KIT* (<1%) are all rare in MDS. Mutations in *KIT* can be regarded as identifying atypical mastocytosis, cases that will respond to tyrosine kinase inhibitors [48]. The emergence of active tyrosine kinase inhibitors against *FLT3* may, in future, encourage systematic genotyping in MDS. The *JAK2* mutations of MPN can also be found in some MDS. Approximately 50% of patients with RARS with marked thrombocytosis (RARS-T), a provisional MDS/MPN syndrome, have *JAK2* mutations [49].

Members of the Ras pathway are Class I genes which govern cell proliferation, differentiation, motility and apoptosis in response to cytokines and are frequently altered in MDS/MPN. *NRAS* mutations are found in low frequency in MDS, mainly in cases transformed to AML, but in 40–50% of CMML. This is even more striking in JMML, as virtually all cases harbor one mutually exclusive mutation in Ras pathway genes *PTPN11* (35%), *NRAS* (20%), *KRAS* (20%) or *NF1* (20%). Mutations of the remaining allele of *NF1* and *PTPN11* are present in JMML cases secondary to congenital neurofibromatosis type 1 and Noonan syndrome, respectively. Systematic profiling of *RAS* mutational status in MDS is currently of limited use, largely because pharmacological targeting by farnesyl-transferase inhibitors has low efficacy [50].

Since dysplasia in terminal stages of differentiation is a hallmark of MDS, it could be inferred that Class II genes affecting hematopoiesis would be specific to MDS. So far, specific type II mutations have not been described. Mutations in *AML1/RUNX1*, a gene also involved in immature AML, occur in 15–40% of MDS and CMML cases, most often in advanced cases. These mutations appear to cooperate with high-risk cytogenetics and *RAS* mutations, especially in therapy-related MDS. The polycomb gene *ASXL1* is also a potential regulator of hematopoiesis and is mutated in 10% of MDS and 40% of CMML cases [51]. Though dysregulation of apoptosis seems cardinal in MDS, no molecular lesion involving apoptosis genes has been identified in MDS. The one exception is mutations in the pleiotropic tumor suppressor gene p53, mainly in 17p– cases.

Gene over-expression: Molecular biology can also detect abnormal gene transcript levels by quantitative PCR assays. Over-expression of the *EVI1* gene is found in one-third of MDS patients, particularly those with excess blast cells; this over-expression can be present even without obvious 3q26 rearrangements on conventional cytogenetic analysis. It has been proposed that arsenic trioxide, an active agent in MDS [52], may target the EVI1 protein for degradation. As in AML, the WT1 transcription factor is over-expressed in virtually all cases of MDS with blast excess, and approximately one-third of lower-risk MDS. The leukemogenic potential of this lesion is still unclear, but WT1 over-expression can provide a useful tool for minimal residual disease (MRD) monitoring in the context of intensive therapy, as in AML [53].

Clonality assays: Clonality assays based on gene imprinting (HUMARA assays) were the first molecular tools to confirm the clonal nature of MDS with a normal karyotype. These assays can still be used as diagnostic co-criterion [9], but novel genomic tools are now available that can both confirm clonality and provide valuable prognostic information. Clonal T-cell expansions have also been described in up to 50% of MDS patients [54]. These clones can be autoreactive, for instance in the context of trisomy 8 [55], and their identification could pinpoint patients likely to benefit from IST [56].

High-throughput genomics: Microarray gene expression profiling (GEP), as described in Chapter 5, has been applied to sorted CD34-positive cells in MDS to elucidate the molecular pathways involved in common chromosomal anomalies [57]. Preliminary attempts to establish the diagnosis of MDS on the basis of the GEP of total marrow mononuclear cells has shown disappointing results, with only 50% of cases being classified as MDS; the GEP profiles of the remainder were spread between AML and normal marrow categories. A subset of MDS cases without excess blasts presents with an AML GEP, and these have been shown to have inferior outcome [58]. Gene expression profiling can predict the response of del(5q) patients to lenalidomide therapy [59]. Thus, prospective study of GEP in MDS may be valuable in the future. However the requirement to sort cell populations prior to microarray poses a major technical limitation.

Two novel high-throughput techniques allow pan-genomic assessment of chromosomal region gains or losses. Comparative genomic hybridization (CGH) arrays allow high-resolution detection of copy number changes, and can detect subclonal alterations that are missed by conventional cytogenetics. Comparative genomic hybridization arrays require germline DNA, for example from sorted T-cells that are usually not part of the MDS clone, or from skin biopsies, with which to compare the MDS population [60]. Single nucleotide polymorphism (SNP) arrays are another potent technique that detect copy number alterations as well as copy neutral regions of loss of heterozygosity (uniparental disomy, UPD). With the use of powerful algorithms, SNP arrays can process even highly contaminated samples (up to 70% contaminant cells), but still require control DNA to eliminate germline UPDs. Neither of these techniques will completely replace conventional cytogenetics because they are unable to detect balanced chromosomal translocations.

The above-mentioned techniques have detected cryptic deletions or amplifications which have prognostic impact [61,62]. In particular, ~60% of patients with normal karyotype MDS have cryptic alterations that have a negative affect on prognosis. Uniparental disomy can be constitutional and have no prognostic value, but may pinpoint novel tumor suppressor genes. Examples include mutations in the *c-CBL* gene in MDS/MPN [63] and the *TET2* gene, which is mutated in ~25% of MDS and up to 50% of CMML. *TET2* mutations are the most frequent genetic lesion so far detected in MDS and MDS/MPN and have recently been assigned an independent favorable prognosis in MDS [64].

Epigenetic alterations: Aberrant gene promoter hypermethylation is another established mechanism for tumor suppressor loss of function in MDS. For example, hypermethylation of the tumor suppressor gene *CDKN2B*, which alleviates the negative regulation of G1/S cell cycle transition by its gene product p15/INK4B, has been found in 30–50% of MDS, most commonly in advanced cases [65]. The favorable clinical results with hypomethylating agents in MDS, including improved overall survival with aza-cytidine therapy in higher-risk MDS [6], have prompted analysis of other epigenetic alterations in MDS. Robust and quantitative measurement of

candidate gene promoter methylation can be performed routinely with bisulfite-modified DNA pyro-sequencing, or qualitatively by methylation-specific PCR (MSP). Genes belonging to various cellular pathways have been found to be aberrantly methylated in MDS, although at lower frequencies than *CDKN2B*. Even if hemizygous, these lesions can lead to functional nullisomy if the remaining allele is targeted by a chromosomal deletion. The *FZD9* gene involved in the Wnt pathway is located in the frequently deleted 7q region and may satisfy this model [66]. Preliminary results from pan-genomic methylation methods indicate that methylation profiles in MDS are heterogeneous but distinct from normal marrow and AML, are dynamic with progression, and are globally and stably reversed by hypomethylating agents [66,67].

Immunophenotyping

Flow cytometry immunophenotyping (FCI) has been proposed as an objective surrogate technique to morphology that can be used in the diagnosis of MDS (see Chapter 3). Though it can be considered as a co-criterion in MDS [9], a consensus on FC techniques and indications in MDS is yet to emerge [68]. The technical issues concern the choice of antibody panel and the standardization of abnormalities using appropriate internal and external controls to achieve inter-laboratory reproducibility. Single color FCI first detected dysplasia as aberrant fluorescence intensity of surface antigens and showed good correlation with morphology [69]. Multicolor FC can integrate various markers to analyze lineage infidelity (e.g. aberrant expression of lymphoid markers on myeloid cells), or maturational asynchrony (e.g. persistence of CD34 expression on mature cells). Using this approach, more than one dysplastic feature must be observed to conclude that there is significant dysplasia. Despite the technical limitations, FCI is reported to be able to identify antigenic abnormalities even when morphological dysplasia is not evident [70]. Most FC studies have focused on the myeloid lineage, because a large number of antigens can be analyzed. Flow cytometry can also detect erythroid dysplasia and abnormal sideroblasts [24], but the commercially available antibody panel is restricted. Megakaryocytic markers are poorly specific due to platelet aggregation on the surface of non-megakaryocytic cells. Immature "blast" cells can be identified by side scatter and CD45 gating, and

CD34 and/or CD117 labeling. Blasts counted on gated non-erythroid cells by FC show good correlation with morphology [71], but cut-off values for clinical decision are yet to be determined.

Diagnostic applications of FCI: Flow cytometry has been proposed as a method that can be used to distinguish MDS from ICUS and aplastic anemia in hypoplastic cases [9]. A diagnostic scoring system has also been proposed based on CD34-positive cells in lower-risk MDS [71]. In MDS/MPN no specific immunophenotype has been described but FCI can help to distinguish CMML from MDS and MPN [72]. The most common phenotypic abnormalities in CMML are aberrant antigen expression profiles of the monocytoid cells, such as reduced expression of CD13, CD14, CD36 or CD64, or aberrant expression of CD2 or CD56.

Prognostic applications of FCI: A flow cytometry scoring system (FCSS) has been developed based on aberrations of the myelomonocytic lineage, blast count and the degree of impairment of myelopoiesis (reflected by the ratio of myeloid to lymphoid cells) [73]. This score has prognostic value that is independent of the IPSS in the context of ASCT [73,74]. Other scores have been established for lower-risk MDS [70]. Specific FCI patterns can also be used as markers for monitoring of MRD or response to growth factors [75].

Other applications of FCI in MDS: Flow cytometry can detect small PNH clones (<3%) in up to 17% of refractory anemias (RA) but not in other MDS categories [76]. PNH+ RA defines a group with less frequent cytogenetic aberrations, lower risk of progression, and identifies patients who could respond to immunosuppressive therapy [76]. The multi-drug resistance (MDR) phenotype can also be determined by FCI assays, such as rhodamine efflux, prior to intensive chemotherapy [77]. Flow cytometry can also be used to assess the function of the immune system in MDS, such as perturbations of T-cell subpopulations [78] and under-representation of B-cells [79]; so far these investigations have not had any prognostic or therapeutic implication. Flow cytometry can also be used to monitor alterations in intra-cellular signal transduction pathways, which can serve as prognostic markers; examples include activation of the Akt or JAK/STAT pathways [80].

Other biological techniques

Biochemical markers: Some biochemical markers are useful in determining the prognosis of MDS. Serum erythropoietin level is a strong predictor of response to erythropoietin and analogs in lower-risk MDS. Despite limited specificity, ferritin can be used to assess iron overload, and monitor iron chelation therapy. Serum lactate dehydrogenase (LDH) is also a prognostic factor in MDS, particularly in the IPSS low-risk subgroup [81].

Progenitor cell culture: In MDS there is impaired growth of immature progenitors (CFU-GEMM), erythroid progenitors (BFU-E, CFU-E) and granulomonocytic progenitors (CFU-GM). The abnormal growth patterns seen, including a decreased number of colonies or small cell clusters instead of colonies, can be used as co-criteria for the diagnosis of MDS [9]. In contrast, spontaneous colony growth (i.e. without cytokines such as EPO, GM-CSF, TPO), and hypersensitivity to GM-CSF can occur in CMML and JMML and help make these diagnoses. Progenitor cell culture can also be combined with FC as a diagnostic tool; detection of hyper-phosphorylation of STAT5 in response to GM-CSF, for example, has been proposed as a diagnostic hallmark of JMML [82].

Diagnostic classification of MDS and MDS/MPN

The WHO diagnostic categories for MDS and MDS/MPN are summarized in Table 15.3 and Table 15.4. Childhood MDS is rare and must be distinguished from JMML and myeloid proliferations of Down syndrome. The distinctive features of MDS in childhood are monosomy 7, the most common cytogenetic abnormality and which has the same adverse prognostic impact as in adults but has no salient presenting feature, and the recurrence of hypoplastic MDS. Conversely, ringed sideroblasts, del(5q) and myelofibrosis are exceedingly rare in children. MDS in children without blast excess are grouped under the term "refractory cytopenia of childhood" (RCC), characterized by persistent cytopenias, dysplasia and <5% blast cells in the bone marrow. Care must be taken to differentiate childhood MDS from congenital bone marrow failure syndromes and other congenital conditions with a hematological phenotype, including metabolic and mitochondrial disorders.

Paroxysmal nocturnal hemoglobinuria

Pathogenesis

Paroxysmal nocturnal hemoglobinuria (PNH) is a rare acquired disorder of hematopoietic stem cells. The disease is characterized by hemolytic anemia, marrow failure and episodes of venous thrombosis. Paroxysmal nocturnal hemoglobinuria is caused by a somatic mutation in the X-linked phosphatidylinositol glycan class A gene (PIG-A), resulting in a deficiency in glycosyl phosphatidylinositol-anchored proteins (GPI-AP). The lack of a GPI-AP complement regulatory protein (CD59) on the erythrocyte surface leads to hemolysis, whilst the pathophysiology of thrombosis remains poorly understood. Paroxysmal nocturnal hemoglobinuria has two major clinical presentations:

1. "Classic PNH" is predominantly hemolytic without overt marrow failure.
2. "Aplastic anemia PNH syndrome" (AA-PNH) is characterized by marrow failure [83].

The complement inhibitor eculizumab is able to alleviate hemolysis, and possibly reduce the thrombotic risk [84].

Detection of PNH clones

Flow cytometry techniques have supplanted the Ham (acidified serum) test to diagnose PNH because of their greater sensitivity and reproducibility [85]. Standard FC for the detection of a PNH clone requires two antibodies to GPI-anchored molecules, such as CD55 and CD59, which can be assessed simultaneously on both granulocytes and erythrocytes. Use of two, rather than one marker increases specificity, and excludes rare cases where there is a congenital deficiency of a GPI-anchored protein [86]. Since PNH is a stem cell disorder, all hematopoietic lineages are involved and GPI-AP-deficient clones are found among all hematopoietic lineages. Granulocytes are the cell of choice for determining the size of the PNH clone, since they are longer-lived than erythrocytes (especially when there is hemolysis), and deficient CD55 and CD59 on the surface of erythrocytes can be partially masked by recent transfusion. The size of the granulocytic clone has been correlated to thrombotic risk (see below) [87].

Different patterns of expression of CD55 and CD59 can be observed within a PNH clone by FC (see Case 5, below).

1. Type I cells have normal expression of GPI-linked proteins.
2. Type II cells have partial GPI-deficiency and are only lysed with complement activation, such as during infection.
3. Type III cells have total GPI deficiency and it is only these cells that undergo spontaneous hemolysis.

This classification merits clinical validation, and as of today, does not impact on clinical decision-making in PNH.

Alternative FCI tools for the detection of PNH clones have been proposed, such as the FLAER (fluorescently labeled aerolysin) assay. This assay, which relies on detection of a bacterial peptide which binds GPI-anchored proteins, can only be applied to granulocytes, and currently lacks standardization.

Paroxysmal nocturnal hemoglobinuria (PNH) clones associated with bone marrow failure syndromes

The refinement and increased sensitivity of FCI techniques have allowed exquisitely small PNH clones (down to 0.002% [76]) to be detected in a number of conditions, including in healthy subjects. These clones are almost always <10% and do not cause hemolysis, thus never requiring eculizumab. In the setting of aplastic anemia, the presence of a PNH clone has been associated with improved responses to immunosuppressive therapy and better prognosis [88]. It is unclear whether this is also the case for MDS [89].

Other biological techniques in PNH

It is recommended that a bone marrow examination be performed when a PNH clone is detected by FCI. A bone marrow aspirate and trephine biopsy with concomitant karyotype are indicated when the PNH clone is present in association with multiple cytopenias. Patients with isolated anemia should also have a bone marrow performed as the presence of erythroid hypoplasia and/or dysplasia may be the sole evidence of underlying aplastic anemia or MDS. Other causes of anemia may also be present in PNH patients, including renal impairment or iron deficiency as a result of chronic intravascular hemolysis; investigations such as endogenous EPO and ferritin measurement may be required. Apart from the size of the PNH clone of >50%, there is no predictive factor for thrombosis in classic PNH and there are no recommendations for systematic hemostasis and thrombophilia testing. Theoretically, the etiology of PNH can be confirmed by screening for a *PIGA* mutation; however, this is technically challenging as mutations are widespread and the result has no bearing on clinical outcome.

Monitoring of PNH clones

In classic PNH, the size of the PNH clone must be measured at diagnosis and monitored as the clone can still be expanding. During eculizumab therapy the size of the red cell clone increases to reach the size of the granulocytic clone but at variable rates; LDH levels best reflect ongoing hemolysis during therapy. PNH clone dynamics or other routine biological tests do not seem to predict response to eculizumab. In the context of aplastic anemia or MDS, PNH clones can also be monitored as they may expand during natural evolution, or after IST.

Clinical examples of MDS and MDS/MPN

The following section gives clinical examples of MDS and MDS/MPN cases to illustrate the diagnostic features described above. The blood counts of all cases are shown in Table 15.6 and the morphological abnormalities, genetic and phenotypic features described and illustrated in Figures 15.1–15.5.

Case 1: Therapy-related MDS, RAEB-2

An 86-year-old woman with a past history of breast cancer, for which she received radiotherapy, presents with fatigue and pallor. A blood count was performed (Table 15.6) and showed pancytopenia. Pseudo-Pelger–Huët neutrophils with hypogranulation, and red cell anisocytosis and poikilocytosis were seen on the blood film (Figure 15.1a). Bone marrow aspirate morphology showed significant dysmegakaryopoiesis (fragmented nuclei), dyserythropoiesis (erythroblasts with budding nuclei and cytoplasmic granules, laminated cytoplasm and internuclear bridges) and dysgranulopoiesis (hypogranulated granulocytic progenitors), with 16% blasts, mostly agranular (Figures 15.1b–f). The karyotype was 47,XX,+8 [20]. Based on these data the WHO diagnosis was therapy-related MDS, RAEB-2, and the IPSS score 2.5 (i.e. three cytopenias, 10–19% bone marrow blasts, intermediate-risk cytogenetics). As the IPSS risk is high she received azacytidine therapy.

Case 2: MDS associated with isolated del(5q)

A 60-year-old woman with Behçet disease controlled by low-dose steroids was referred to a hematologist for investigation of persistent thrombocytosis. Blood count (Table 15.6) showed mild anemia and a platelet count of 1275×10^9/L. There were no signs of inflammation, the serum ferritin value was normal and the patient had no splenomegaly. She received hydroxycarbamide followed by anagrelide therapy. She became progressively anemic and red cell

Table 15.6. Blood count results for Cases 1–5.

		Case 1	Case 2	Case 3	Case 4	Case 5
Leukocytes ($\times 10^9$/L)	Total	3.6	4.2	56.8	9.3	2.9
	Neutrophils	1.08	2.98	17.8	7.31	1.0
	Eosinophils	–	0.04	0.6	0.32	0.09
	Basophils	–	0.04	0.8	0.06	0.03
	Monocytes	0.61	0.13	7.1	0.41	0.12
	Lymphocytes	1.65	1.01	25.5	1.25	1.17
	Blast cells (%)	–	–	2%	–	–
	Erythroblasts	0.61	–	0.6	–	–
Red cells	Hb (g/dL)	6.6	9.5	7.7	7.5	8.8
	MCV (fL)	102	99		87	
	Reticulocytes ($\times 10^9$/L)			65	27	
Platelet count ($\times 10^9$/L)		22	1275	75	545	16

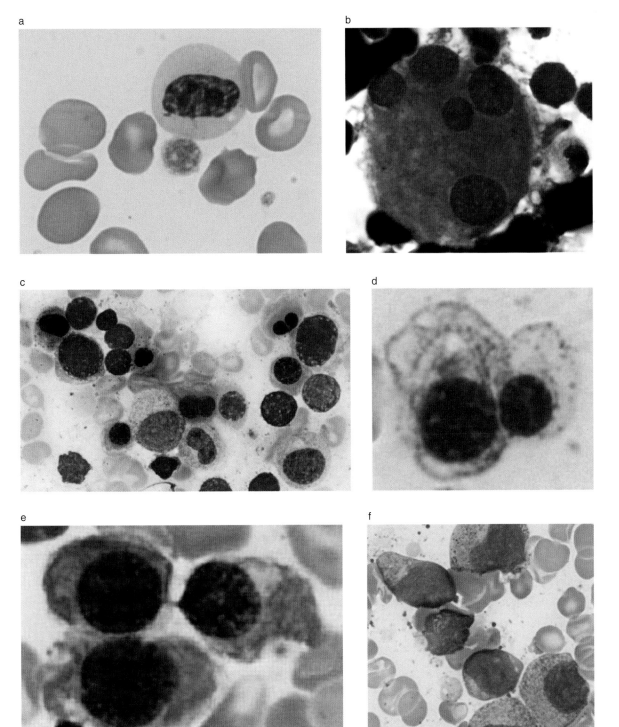

Figure 15.1. Case 1 – Therapy-related MDS, RAEB-2.
a. Pseudo-Pelger–Huët neutrophils with hypogranulation, together with red cell anisocytosis and poikilocytosis (PB smear, MGG, 100×).
b. Abnormal megakaryocyte with disrupted nuclear lobules (BM smear, MGG, 100×).
c. Erythroblasts with budding nuclei and cytoplasmic stippling (BM smear, MGG, 50×).
d. Erythroblasts with laminated granular cytoplasm (BM smear, MGG, 100×).
e. Erythroblasts with inter-nuclear bridging (BM smear, MGG, 50×).
f. Abnormal hypogranulated promyelocytes and myelocytes and agranular blasts (BM smear, MGG, 100×).
Figures 15.1a–f courtesy of Hervé Roudot, Hematology Laboratory, Hopital Avicenne, Bobigny, France.

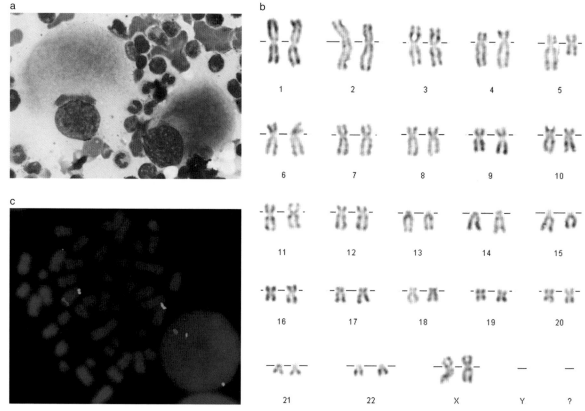

Figure 15.2. Case 2 – MDS associated with isolated del(5q).
a. Monolobated megakaryocytes (BM smear, MGG 100×). Courtesy of Hervé Roudot, Hematology Laboratory, Hospital Avicenne, Bobigny, France.
b. R-banding karyotype: 46,XX,del(5)(q31q33). Courtesy of Virginie Eclache, Hematology Laboratory, Hopital Avicenne, Bobigny, France.
c. FISH with LSI EGR1D5S721 (5q31 probe, orange), D5S23 (5p15 probe, green) dual color probe (Abbott) showing a metaphase with
    5q31deletion. Courtesy of Virginie Eclache, Hematology Laboratory, Hopital Avicenne, Bobigny, France.

transfusion-dependent (2 units packed red cells every 2 weeks). A bone marrow aspirate performed 1 month after cessation of hydroxycarbamide showed moderate dyserythropoiesis with numerous monolobated mega-karyocytes (Figure 15.2a) without excess blasts. The karyotype was 46,XX,del(5)(q31q33) [20] (Figure 15.2b), confirmed by FISH (Figure 15.2c). Lenalidomide was commenced which resulted in a sustained erythroid and cytogenetic response for 3 years.

Case 3: Juvenile myelomonocytic leukemia

A 9-month-old girl with no prior medical or relevant family history presented with subacute onset of pallor, fever, abdominal pain and rectal bleeding. On physical examination there was palpable hepato-splenomegaly, cervical lymphadenopathy and cutaneous xanthomata. A blood count showed a marked neutrophilia, lymphocytosis and monocytosis and small numbers of blast cells, mild anemia without reticulocytosis and mild thrombocytopenia (Table 15.6). The peripheral blood smear showed dysplastic monocytes (Figure 15.3a) and tear-drop poikilocytes (Figure 15.3b). Blood, urine and stool cultures were negative and biochemical analyses showed CRP 4.4 mg/L, LDH 882 U/L; HIV, CMV, EBV, toxoplasmosis and hepatitis B and C serologies were negative. HbF level was elevated at 25% (normal <1%). Bone marrow smears were hypercellular with granulocytic hyperplasia (Figure 15.3c). The karyotype was normal 46,XX [20]. Molecular screening for *KRAS* and *NRAS* mutations was negative; a mutation in exon 3 of *PTPN11* was found in bone marrow cells (Figure 15.3d). *In vitro* progenitor cell culture in methylcellulose showed spontaneous colony growth of CFU-GEMM, CFU-GM and CFU-M (Figure 15.3e). Juvenile myelomonocytic leukemia

a

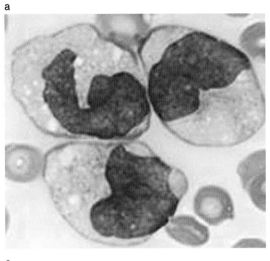

b

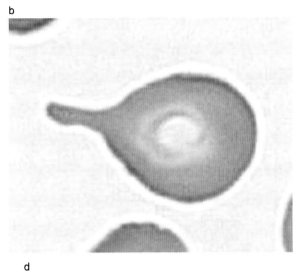

c

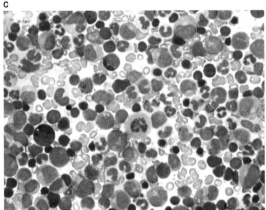

d

**PTPN11
D61V
mutation**

↓

TCAGAACACTGGTGtTTACTATGACC

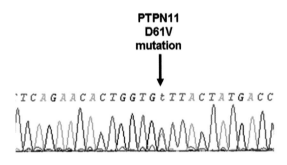

e

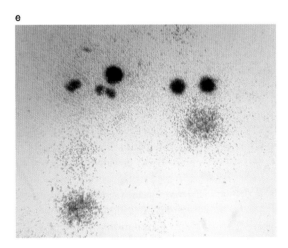

Figure 15.3. Case 3 – Juvenile myelomonocytic leukemia.
a. Dysplastic monocytes (PB smear, MGG 1000×).
b. Tear-drop poikilocyte (PB smear, MGG 1000×).
c. Granulocytic hyperplasia (BM smear, MGG 400×).
d. Electrophoretogram of *PTPN11* exon 3 sequence showing
c.182A>T substitution resulting in a mutated SHP2 D61V protein.
e. *In vitro* methylcellulose spontaneous colony growth of marrow
   progenitors showing CFU-GEMM, CFU-GM, and CFU-M (30×).
   Courtesy of B. Perez, Hematology Laboratory, Hopital Saint Louis,
   Paris, France.
Figures 15.3a–c are courtesy of O. Fenneteau, Hematology
Laboratory, Hopital Robert Debre, Paris, France and Figure 15.3d
is courtesy of H. Cavé, Hematology Laboratory, Hopital Robert Debre,
Paris, France.

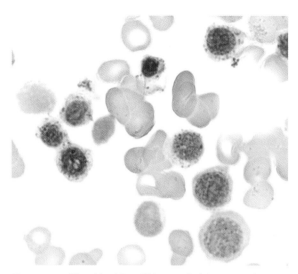

Figure 15.4. Ring sideroblasts (BM smear, Perls' stain 100×). Courtesy of Hervé Roudot, Hematology Laboratory, Hopital Avicenne, Bobigny, France.

was diagnosed and she received 6-mercaptopurine and transfusion support, and proceeded to cord blood transplantation.

Case 4: Refractory anemia with ring sideroblasts associated with marked thrombocytosis

A 68-year-old woman was referred with fatigue. A blood count showed normocytic anemia and a mild thrombocytosis (Table 15.6) and the film poikilocytosis and anisochromia. Bone marrow aspiration showed mild erythroid hyperplasia with megakaryocytic hyperplasia with pleomorphism. The Perls' stain showed 22% ring sideroblasts (Figure 15.4). The karyotype was 46,XX,del(7)(q21;q31) [17], 46,XX [3]. A hemizygous *JAK2* V617F mutation was detected on PCR. The patient failed to respond to recombinant erythropoietin and azacytidine was commenced.

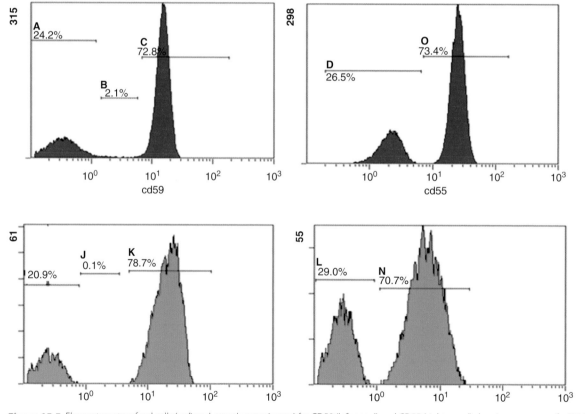

Figure 15.5. Flow cytometry of red cells (red) and granulocytes (green) for CD59 (left panel) and CD55 (right panel) showing presence of a PNH clone. Courtesy of Christophe Roumier, Hematology Laboratory, CHR Lille, France.

Case 5: Hypoplastic MDS with a PNH clone

A 46-year-old man presented with a history of prostatitis. The blood count showed marked pancytopenia and there were no specific blood film abnormalities (Table 15.6). The bone marrow (smears and trephine biopsy) was hypocellular (<20% cellularity) without significant dysplasia. The bone marrow biopsy showed heterogeneous distribution of hematopoietic cells including aplastic inter-trabecular marrow spaces. There was dyserythropoiesis and no blast excess. The karyotype was 45,X,-Y [5], 46,XY [17]. The HLA-DR15 haplotype was present, which could predict a favorable response to immunosuppressive treatment [89]. There was no T-cell or PNH clone at this time and a diagnosis of hypoplastic MDS was made. Following anti-thymocyte globulin and cyclosporine therapy the patient had significant trilineage hematological improvement (Hb >11 g/dL; platelets > 50 × 10^9/L; neutrophils >1 × 10^9/L). Following a 3-year remission a minor PNH clone was detected but without hematological consequence (Figure 15.5).

Acknowledgments

The authors would like to thank Dr. Peffault de Latour, Dr. Virginie Eclache and Dr. Benoite Perez for critical review of the manuscript.

References

1. Corey SJ, Minden MD, Barber DL *et al.* Myelodysplastic syndromes: the complexity of stem-cell diseases. *Nat Rev Cancer* 2007;**7**(2):118–29.

2. Bennett JM, Catovsky D, Daniel MT *et al.* Proposals for the classification of the myelodysplastic syndromes. *Br J Haematol* 1982;**51**(2):189–99.

3. Vardiman JW, Harris NL, Brunning RD. The World Health Organization (WHO) classification of the myeloid neoplasms. *Blood* 2002;**100**(7):2292–302.

4. Vardiman JW, Thiele J, Arber DA *et al.* The 2008 revision of the World Health Organization (WHO) classification of myeloid neoplasms and acute leukemia: rationale and important changes. *Blood* 2009;**114**(5):937–51.

5. Greenberg P, Cox C, LeBeau MM *et al.* International scoring system for evaluating prognosis in myelodysplastic syndromes. *Blood* 1997;**89**(6):2079–88.

6. Fenaux P, Mufti GJ, Hellström-Lindberg E *et al.* Efficacy of azacitidine compared with that of conventional care regimens in the treatment of higher-risk myelodysplastic syndromes: a randomised, open-label, phase III study. *Lancet Oncol* 2009;**10**:223–32.

7. Garcia-Manero G, Shan J, Faderl S *et al.* A prognostic score for patients with lower risk myelodysplastic syndrome. *Leukemia* 2008;**22**:538–43.

8. Malcovati L, Porta MG, Pascutto C *et al.* Prognostic factors and life expectancy in myelodysplastic syndromes classified according to WHO criteria: a basis for clinical decision making. *J Clin Oncol* 2005;**23**(30):7594–603.

9. Valent P, Horny HP, Bennett JM *et al.* Definitions and standards in the diagnosis and treatment of the myelodysplastic syndromes: Consensus statements and report from a working conference. *Leuk Res* 2007;**31**(6):727–36.

10. Wimazal F, Fonatsch C, Thalhammer R *et al.* Idiopathic cytopenia of undetermined significance (ICUS) versus low risk MDS: the diagnostic interface. *Leuk Res* 2007;**31**(11):1461–8.

11. Kaloutsi V, Kohlmeyer U, Maschek H *et al.* Comparison of bone marrow and hematologic findings in patients with human immunodeficiency virus infection and those with myelodysplastic syndromes and infectious diseases. *Am J Clin Pathol* 1994;**101**(2):123–9.

12. Steensma DP, Higgs DR, Fisher CA, Gibbons RJ. Acquired somatic *ATRX* mutations in myelodysplastic syndrome associated with alpha thalassemia (ATMDS) convey a more severe hematologic phenotype than germline *ATRX* mutations. *Blood* 2004;**103**(6):2019–26.

13. Knipp S, Strupp C, Gattermann N *et al.* Presence of peripheral blasts in refractory anemia and refractory cytopenia with multilineage dysplasia predicts an unfavourable outcome. *Leuk Res* 2008;**32**(1):33–7.

14. Bennett JM, Orazi A. Diagnostic criteria to distinguish hypocellular acute myeloid leukemia from hypocellular myelodysplastic syndromes and aplastic anemia: recommendations for a standardized approach. *Haematologica* 2009;**94**(2):264–8.

15. Mufti GJ, Bennett JM, Goasguen J *et al.* Diagnosis and classification of myelodysplastic syndrome: International Working Group on Morphology of myelodysplastic syndrome (IWGM-MDS) consensus proposals for the definition and enumeration of myeloblasts and ring sideroblasts. *Haematologica* 2008;**93**(11):1712–17.

16. Lai JL, Preudhomme C, Zandecki M *et al.* Myelodysplastic syndromes and acute myeloid leukemia with 17p deletion. An entity characterized by specific dysgranulopoiesis and a high incidence of P53 mutations. *Leukemia* 1995;**9**(3):370–81.

17. Apperley JF, Gardembas M, Melo JV *et al*. Response to imatinib mesylate in patients with chronic myeloproliferative diseases with rearrangements of the platelet-derived growth factor receptor beta. *New Engl J Med* 2002;**347**(7):481–7.

18. Goasguen JE, Bennett JM, Cox C *et al*. Prognostic implication and characterization of the blast cell population in the myelodysplastic syndrome. *Leuk Res* 1991;**15**(12):1159–65.

19. Goasguen JE, Bennett JM, Bain BJ *et al*. Morphological evaluation of monocytes and their precursors. *Haematologica* 2009;**94**(7):994–7.

20. Tuzuner N, Cox C, Rowe JM, Bennett JM. Bone marrow cellularity in myeloid stem cell disorders: impact of age correction. *Leuk Res* 1994;**18**(8):559–64.

21. Thiele J, Kvasnicka HM, Facchetti F *et al*. European consensus on grading bone marrow fibrosis and assessment of cellularity. *Haematologica* 2005;**90**(8):1128–32.

22. Tiu R, Gondek L, O'Keefe C, Maciejewski JP. Clonality of the stem cell compartment during evolution of myelodysplastic syndromes and other bone marrow failure syndromes. *Leukemia* 2007;**21**(8):1648–57.

23. Orazi A, Albitar M, Heerema NA, Haskins S, Neiman RS. Hypoplastic myelodysplastic syndromes can be distinguished from acquired aplastic anemia by CD34 and PCNA immunostaining of bone marrow biopsy specimens. *Am J Clin Pathol* 1997;**107**(3):268–74.

24. Della Porta MG, Malcovati L, Invernizzi R *et al*. Flow cytometry evaluation of erythroid dysplasia in patients with myelodysplastic syndrome. *Leukemia* 2006;**20**(4):549–55.

25. Yue G, Hao S, Fadare O *et al*. Hypocellularity in myelodysplastic syndrome is an independent factor which predicts a favorable outcome. *Leuk Res* 2008;**32**(4):553–8.

26. Arber DA. Realistic pathologic classification of acute myeloid leukemias. *Am J Clin Pathol* 2001;**115**(4):552–60.

27. Della Porta MG, Malcovati L, Boveri E *et al*. Clinical relevance of bone marrow fibrosis and CD34-positive cell clusters in primary myelodysplastic syndromes. *J Clin Oncol* 2009;**27**(5):754–62.

28. Tricot G, De Wolf-Peeters C, Vlietinck R, Verwilghen RL. Bone marrow histology in myelodysplastic syndromes. II. Prognostic value of abnormal localization of immature precursors in MDS. *Br J Haematol* 1984;**58**(2):217–25.

29. Korkolopoulou P, Apostolidou E, Pavlopoulos PM *et al*. Prognostic evaluation of the microvascular network in myelodysplastic syndromes. *Leukemia* 2001;**15**(9):1369–76.

30. Bellamy WT, Richter L, Sirjani D *et al*. Vascular endothelial cell growth factor is an autocrine promoter of abnormal localized immature myeloid precursors and leukemia progenitor formation in myelodysplastic syndromes. *Blood* 2001;**97**(5):1427–34.

31. Haase D, Germing U, Schanz J *et al*. New insights into the prognostic impact of the karyotype in MDS and correlation with subtypes: evidence from a core dataset of 2124 patients. *Blood* 2007;**110**(13):4385–95.

32. Itzykson R, Fenaux P. Optimal sequencing of treatments for patients with myelodysplastic syndromes. *Curr Opin in Hematol* 2009;**16**(2):77–83.

33. Park S, Grabar S, Kelaidi C *et al*. Predictive factors of response and survival in myelodysplastic syndrome treated with erythropoietin and G-CSF: the GFM experience. *Blood* 2008;**111**(2):574–82.

34. Sole F, Luno E, Sanzo C *et al*. Identification of novel cytogenetic markers with prognostic significance in a series of 968 patients with primary myelodysplastic syndromes. *Haematologica* 2005;**90**(9):1168–78.

35. Ebert BL, Pretz J, Bosco J *et al*. Identification of RPS14 as a 5q- syndrome gene by RNA interference screen. *Nature* 2008;**451**(7176):335–9.

36. Nilsson L, Eden P, Olsson E *et al*. The molecular signature of MDS stem cells supports a stem-cell origin of 5q myelodysplastic syndromes. *Blood* 2007;**110**(8):3005–14.

37. Li X, Bryant CE, Deeg HJ. Simultaneous demonstration of clonal chromosome abnormalities and apoptosis in individual marrow cells in myelodysplastic syndrome. *Int J Hematol* 2004;**80**(2):140–5.

38. List A, Dewald G, Bennett J *et al*. Lenalidomide in the myelodysplastic syndrome with chromosome 5q deletion. *New Engl J Med* 2006;**355**(14):1456–65.

39. Van den Berghe H, Cassiman JJ, David G *et al*. Distinct haematological disorder with deletion of long arm of no. 5 chromosome. *Nature* 1974;**251**(5474):437–8.

40. Wei S, Chen X, Rocha K *et al*. A critical role for phosphatase haplodeficiency in the selective suppression of deletion 5q MDS by lenalidomide. *Proc Natl Acad Sci USA* 2009;**106**(31):12974–9.

41. Boultwood J, Fidler C, Strickson AJ *et al*. Narrowing and genomic annotation of the commonly deleted region of the 5q− syndrome. *Blood* 2002;**99**(12):4638–41.

42. Ades L, Boehrer S, Prebet T *et al*. Efficacy and safety of lenalidomide in intermediate-2-or high risk myelodysplastic syndromes (MDS) with 5q deletion:

Results of a phase II study. *Blood* 2009;**113**(17):3947–52.

43. Horrigan SK, Arbieva ZH, Xie HY *et al.* Delineation of a minimal interval and identification of 9 candidates for a tumor suppressor gene in malignant myeloid disorders on 5q31. *Blood* 2000;**95**(7):2372–7.

44. Wiktor A, Rybicki BA, Piao ZS *et al.* Clinical significance of Y chromosome loss in hematologic disease. *Genes Chromosomes Cancer* 2000;**27**(1):11–16.

45. Iwabuchi A, Ohyashiki K, Ohyashiki JH *et al.* Trisomy of chromosome 8 in myelodysplastic syndrome. Significance of the fluctuating trisomy 8 population. *Cancer Genet Cytogenet* 1992;**62**(1):70–4.

46. Breems DA, Van Putten WL, De Greef GE *et al.* Monosomal karyotype in acute myeloid leukemia: a better indicator of poor prognosis than a complex karyotype. *J Clin Oncol* 2008;**26**(29):4791–7.

47. Nucifora G, Laricchia-Robbio L, Senyuk V. EVI1 and hematopoietic disorders: history and perspectives. *Gene* 2006;**368**:1–11.

48. Valent P, Sperr WR, Samorapoompichit P *et al.* Myelomastocytic overlap syndromes: biology, criteria, and relationship to mastocytosis. *Leuk Res* 2001;**25**(7):595–602.

49. Hellström-Lindberg E, Cazzola M. The role of *JAK2* mutations in RARS and other MDS. *Hematology Am Soc Hematol Educ Program* 2008;**2008**:52–9.

50. Fenaux P, Raza A, Mufti GJ *et al.* A multicenter phase 2 study of the farnesyltransferase inhibitor tipifarnib in intermediate- to high-risk myelodysplastic syndrome. *Blood* 2007;**109**(10):4158–63.

51. Gelsi-Boyer V, Trouplin V, Adelaide J *et al.* Mutations of polycomb-associated gene *ASXL1* in myelodysplastic syndromes and chronic myelomonocytic leukaemia. *Br J Haematol* 2009;**145**(6):788–800.

52. Vey N, Bosly A, Guerci A *et al.* Arsenic trioxide in patients with myelodysplastic syndromes: a phase II multicenter study. *J Clin Oncol* 2006;**24**(16):2465–71.

53. Cilloni D, Saglio G. WT1 as a universal marker for minimal residual disease detection and quantification in myeloid leukemias and in myelodysplastic syndrome. *Acta Haematol* 2004;**112**(1–2):79–84.

54. Epling-Burnette PK, Painter JS, Rollison DE *et al.* Prevalence and clinical association of clonal T-cell expansions in myelodysplastic syndrome. *Leukemia* 2007;**21**(4):659–67.

55. Sloand EM, Mainwaring L, Fuhrer M *et al.* Preferential suppression of trisomy 8 compared with normal hematopoietic cell growth by autologous lymphocytes in patients with trisomy 8 myelodysplastic syndrome. *Blood* 2005;**106**(3):841–51.

56. Kochenderfer JN, Kobayashi S, Wieder ED, Su C, Molldrem JJ. Loss of T-lymphocyte clonal dominance in patients with myelodysplastic syndrome responsive to immunosuppression. *Blood* 2002;**100**(10):3639–45.

57. Chen G, Zeng W, Miyazato A *et al.* Distinctive gene expression profiles of CD34 cells from patients with myelodysplastic syndrome characterized by specific chromosomal abnormalities. *Blood* 2004;**104**(13):4210–18.

58. Mills KI, Kohlmann A, Williams PM *et al.* Microarray-based classifiers and prognosis models identify subgroups with distinct clinical outcomes and high risk of AML transformation of myelodysplastic syndrome. *Blood* 2009;**114**(5):1063–72.

59. Ebert BL, Galili N, Tamayo P *et al.* An erythroid differentiation signature predicts response to lenalidomide in myelodysplastic syndrome. *PLoS Med* 2008;**5**(2):e35.

60. van Lom K, Hagemeijer A, Smit E *et al.* Cytogenetic clonality analysis in myelodysplastic syndrome: monosomy 7 can be demonstrated in the myeloid and in the lymphoid lineage. *Leukemia* 1995;**9**(11):1818–21.

61. Gondek LP, Tiu R, O'Keefe CL *et al.* Chromosomal lesions and uniparental disomy detected by SNP arrays in MDS, MDS/MPD, and MDS-derived AML. *Blood* 2008;**111**(3):1534–42.

62. Mohamedali A, Gaken J, Twine NA *et al.* Prevalence and prognostic significance of allelic imbalance by single-nucleotide polymorphism analysis in low-risk myelodysplastic syndromes. *Blood* 2007;**110**(9):3365–73.

63. Sanada M, Suzuki T, Shih LY *et al.* Gain-of-function of mutated *C-CBL* tumour suppressor in myeloid neoplasms. *Nature* 2009;**460**:904–8.

64. Kosmider O, Gelsi-Boyer V, Cheok M *et al.* TET2 mutation is an independent favorable prognostic factor in myelodysplastic syndromes (MDS). *Blood* 2009;**114**(15):3285–91.

65. Quesnel B, Guillerm G, Vereecque R *et al.* Methylation of the p15(INK4b) gene in myelodysplastic syndromes is frequent and acquired during disease progression. *Blood* 1998;**91**(8):2985–90.

66. Jiang Y, Dunbar A, Gondek LP *et al.* Aberrant DNA methylation is a dominant mechanism in MDS progression to AML. *Blood* 2009;**113**(6):1315–25.

67. Figueroa ME, Skrabanek L, Li Y *et al.* MDS and secondary AML display unique patterns and

abundance of aberrant DNA methylation. *Blood* 2009;**114**(16):3448–58.

68. van de Loosdrecht AA, Alhan C, Bene MC *et al.* Standardization of flow cytometry in myelodysplastic syndromes: report from the first European LeukemiaNet working conference on flow cytometry in myelodysplastic syndromes. *Haematologica* 2009;**94**(8):1124–34.

69. Maynadie M, Picard F, Husson B *et al.* Immunophenotypic clustering of myelodysplastic syndromes. *Blood* 2002;**100**(7):2349–56.

70. van de Loosdrecht AA, Westers TM, Westra AH *et al.* Identification of distinct prognostic subgroups in low- and intermediate-1-risk myelodysplastic syndromes by flow cytometry. *Blood* 2008;**111**(3):1067–77.

71. Ogata K, Kishikawa Y, Satoh C *et al.* Diagnostic application of flow cytometric characteristics of CD34+ cells in low-grade myelodysplastic syndromes. *Blood* 2006;**108**(3):1037–44.

72. Subira D, Font P, Villalon L *et al.* Immunophenotype in chronic myelomonocytic leukemia: is it closer to myelodysplastic syndromes or to myeloproliferative disorders? *Transl Res* 2008;**151**(5):240–5.

73. Wells DA, Benesch M, Loken MR *et al.* Myeloid and monocytic dyspoiesis as determined by flow cytometric scoring in myelodysplastic syndrome correlates with the IPSS and with outcome after hematopoietic stem cell transplantation. *Blood* 2003;**102**(1):394–403.

74. Scott BL, Wells DA, Loken MR *et al.* Validation of a flow cytometric scoring system as a prognostic indicator for posttransplantation outcome in patients with myelodysplastic syndrome. *Blood* 2008;**112**(7):2681–6.

75. Westers TM, Alhan C, Cali C, Ossenkoppele GJ, van de Loosdrecht AA. Quantitative dynamics of flow cytometric aberrancies during treatment with erythropoietin/G-CSF are predictive for responses in LOW/INT-I risk myelodysplastic syndromes. *Blood* 2008;**112**:5867 [Abstr].

76. Wang H, Chuhjo T, Yasue S, Omine M, Nakao S. Clinical significance of a minor population of paroxysmal nocturnal hemoglobinuria-type cells in bone marrow failure syndrome. *Blood* 2002;**100**(12):3897–902.

77. Poulain S, Lepelley P, Preudhomme C *et al.* Expression of the multidrug resistance-associated protein in myelodysplastic syndromes. *Br J Haematol* 2000;**110**(3):591–8.

78. Kordasti SY, Ingram W, Hayden J *et al.* CD4 +CD25high Foxp3+ regulatory T cells in myelodysplastic syndrome (MDS). *Blood* 2007;**110**(3):847–50.

79. Sternberg A, Killick S, Littlewood T *et al.* Evidence for reduced B-cell progenitors in early (low-risk) myelodysplastic syndrome. *Blood* 2005;**106** (9):2982–91.

80. Nyakern M, Tazzari PL, Finelli C *et al.* Frequent elevation of Akt kinase phosphorylation in blood marrow and peripheral blood mononuclear cells from high-risk myelodysplastic syndrome patients. *Leukemia* 2006;**20**(2):230–8.

81. Germing U, Hildebrandt B, Pfeilstocker M *et al.* Refinement of the International Prognostic Scoring System (IPSS) by including LDH as an additional prognostic variable to improve risk assessment in patients with primary myelodysplastic syndromes (MDS). *Leukemia* 2005;**19**(12):2223–31.

82. Kotecha N, Flores NJ, Irish JM *et al.* Single-cell profiling identifies aberrant STAT5 activation in myeloid malignancies with specific clinical and biologic correlates. *Cancer Cell* 2008;**14**(4):335–43.

83. Parker C, Omine M, Richards S *et al.* Diagnosis and management of paroxysmal nocturnal hemoglobinuria. *Blood* 2005;**106**(12):3699–709.

84. Hillmen P, Muus P, Duhrsen U *et al.* Effect of the complement inhibitor eculizumab on thromboembolism in patients with paroxysmal nocturnal hemoglobinuria. *Blood* 2007;**110**(12):4123–8.

85. Hall SE, Rosse WF. The use of monoclonal antibodies and flow cytometry in the diagnosis of paroxysmal nocturnal hemoglobinuria. *Blood* 1996;**87** (12):5332–40.

86. Yamashina M, Ueda E, Kinoshita T *et al.* Inherited complete deficiency of 20-kilodalton homologous restriction factor (CD59) as a cause of paroxysmal nocturnal hemoglobinuria. *New Engl J Med* 1990;**323**(17):1184–9.

87. Hall C, Richards S, Hillmen P. Primary prophylaxis with warfarin prevents thrombosis in paroxysmal nocturnal hemoglobinuria (PNH). *Blood* 2003;**102**(10):3587–91.

88. Sugimori C, Chuhjo T, Feng X *et al.* Minor population of CD55-CD59- blood cells predicts response to immunosuppressive therapy and prognosis in patients with aplastic anemia. *Blood* 2006;**107**(4):1308–14.

89. Sloand EM, Wu CO, Greenberg P, Young N, Barrett J. Factors affecting response and survival in patients with myelodysplasia treated with immunosuppressive therapy. *J Clin Oncol* 2008;**26**(15):2505–11.

90. Swerdlow SH, Campo E, Harris NL *et al.* (eds.). *WHO Classification of Tumours of Haematopoietic and Lymphoid Tissues*, 4th edn. Lyon: IARC Press; 2008.

Index